first edition
large animal
internal medicine

The National Veterinary Medical Series for Independent Study

first edition
large animal
internal medicine

Timothy H. Ogilvie, D.V. M., MSc

Diplomate, American College of Veterinary Internal Medicine
Professor and Chair, Department of Health Management
Atlantic Veterinary College
University of Prince Edward Island
Charlottetown, Prince Edward Island

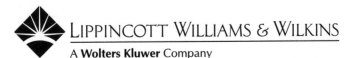

LIPPINCOTT WILLIAMS & WILKINS
A **Wolters Kluwer** Company
Philadelphia • Baltimore • New York • London
Buenos Aires • Hong Kong • Sydney • Tokyo

Editor: Elizabeth A. Nieginski
Manager, Development Editing: Julie Scardiglia
Managing Editor: Darrin Kiessling
Marketing Manager: Christine Kushner
Development Editor: Melanie Cann
Production Coordinator: Danielle Hagan
Typesetter: Maryland Composition Co., Inc.
Printer/Binder: Port City Press, Inc.

351 West Camden Street
Baltimore, Maryland 21201-2436 USA

530 Walnut Street
Philadelphia, Pennsylvania 19106-3621 USA

Accurate indications, adverse reactions and dosage schedules for drugs are provided in this book, but it is possible that they may change. The reader is urged to review the package information data of the manufacturers of the medications mentioned.

Printed in the United States of America

First Edition,
Library of Congress Cataloging-in-Publication Data
Ogilvie, Timothy H.
      Large animal internal medicine / Timothy H. Ogilvie.—1st ed.
          p.   cm.—(The National veterinary medical series for
   independent study)
      Includes index.
      ISBN 0-683-18033-9
      1. Veterinary internal medicine—Outlines, syllabi, etc.
   2. Veterinary internal medicine—Examination, questions, etc.
   I. Title. II. Series.
   SF745.045 1998
   636.089'6—dc21   97-33109
                                                           CIP

The publishers have made every effort to trace the copyright holders for borrowed material. If they have inadvertently overlooked any, they will be pleased to make the necessary arrangements at the first opportunity.

To purchase additional copies of this book, call our customer service department at **(800) 638-3030** or fax orders to **(301) 824-7390**. For other book services, including chapter reprints and large quantity sales, ask for the Special Sales Department. International customers should call **(301) 714-2324**.

Visit Lippincott Williams & Wilkins on the Internet: http://www.lww.com. Lippincott Williams & Wilkins customer service representatives are available from 8:30 am to 6:00 pm, EST.

                                                      00 01 02
                                                   2 3 4 5 6 7 8 9 10

Dedication

To my wife, Lola, and sons, Thomas and Adam

Contents

Contributors

Christopher Cebra, V.M.D., MA, MS
Diplomate, American College of Veterinary
  Internal Medicine
Assistant Professor, Large Animal Medicine
Atlantic Veterinary College
University of Prince Edward Island
Charlottetown, Prince Edward Island

Margaret Cebra, V.M.D., MS
Diplomate, American College of Veterinary
  Internal Medicine
Assistant Professor, Ambulatory Services
Atlantic Veterinary College
University of Prince Edward Island
Charlottetown, Prince Edward Island

Jeanne Lofstedt, BVSc, MS
Diplomate, American College of Veterinary
  Internal Medicine
Professor of Health Management
Associate Dean of Academic Affairs
Atlantic Veterinary College
University of Prince Edward Island
Charlottetown, Prince Edward Island

John Pringle, D.V.M., DVSc
Diplomate, American College of Veterinary
  Internal Medicine
Guest Researcher, Faculty of Veterinary
  Medicine
Swedish University of Agricultural Sciences
Uppsala, Sweden

Preface

This text is the result of the combined efforts of members of the Large Animal Medicine Service of the Department of Health Management at the Atlantic Veterinary College. We believe that students of veterinary medicine, those completing their veterinary training and preparing for licensing examinations, and those who wish to upgrade their knowledge base in large animal clinical veterinary medicine will find this book useful.

To assist readers in exam preparation and to provide a means of assessing one's knowledge of the presented material, the authors have provided study questions at the end of each chapter. In addition, a comprehensive examination containing questions similar to those found on the national board examination is included at the end of the book. Every question is followed by a complete, detailed explanation. We hope this method of review tests the general knowledge of the reader, helps serve as a stimulus to self-directed study, and serves as a useful tool for preparing for college tests, national board examinations, and clinical veterinary practice.

We have aimed to provide an overview of the diseases of clinical and economic importance in the major species of domesticated animals in North America. To maintain the book at a reasonable size, we have elected to exclude coverage of exotic species and specialized disciplines. We invite the reader to consult the many other high-quality texts that are available to find information pertaining to these more specialized topics.

Acknowledgments

I would like to acknowledge the individuals who made both the writing and publication of this text possible. They are: the contributing authors from the Large Animal Medicine Service of the Department of Health Management at the College; our veterinary students, who serve as the catalyst for keeping us current in veterinary medical education; Melanie Cann, Alethea Elkins, and the hard-working staff at Williams & Wilkins who kept us on-time and on-target with our chapters; and Mary Beth MacDonald here at the Atlantic Veterinary College, who kept us organized and our text formatted.

Chapter 1

Diseases of the Oral Cavity and Esophagus

Timothy H. Ogilvie

I. **STOMATITIS** is inflammation of the oral cavity. Conditions include **glossitis** (inflammation of the lingual mucosa), **palatitis** or **lampas** (inflammation of the palate), and **gingivitis** (inflammation of the mucosa and gums).

A. **Patient profile and history.** The patient profile is variable. Domestic animals of any breed, sex, or age may be affected by a painful mouth for a variety of reasons. The history is also highly variable and is often nonspecific for any particular condition.

B. **Clinical findings.** Inflammatory lesions of the mouth are clinically characterized by partial or complete loss of appetite, painful or slow mastication, and prehension difficulties. Sialism or ptyalism, fetid breath (if necrotic tissue is present), and local lymphadenopathy (if there has been bacterial invasion of tissue) may also be present.

C. **Etiology and pathophysiology.** Stomatitis may be caused by physical, chemical, or infectious agents.

  1. **Physical agents.** Foreign objects (e.g., corn cobs, sticks, rocks) may become lodged in the lingual groove of cattle or in the upper dental arcade of horses. Injury may also be inflicted by equipment used to administer oral medications (e.g., balling guns, dosing syringes) or by dental instruments (e.g., floats, files).

  2. **Chemical agents.** Irritant substances (e.g., mercuric preparations used as counterirritants) may be inadvertently licked or eaten by an animal.

  3. **Infectious agents.** Stomatitis may be caused by **bacteria, fungi,** or **viruses** (Table 1-1).

D. **Diagnostic plan.** A complete physical examination and history is often necessary to determine the location of the problem and define its cause. It must be determined whether the clinical signs are caused by local lesions, or whether they are manifestations of systemic disease.

E. **Laboratory tests** are usually not performed for conditions that seem to be localized to the mouth.

  1. **Hematologic work-up.** A hematologic work-up is valuable if systemic involvement is suspected.

  2. **Bacterial culture** may be helpful. For example, crushing and gram-staining the sulfur granules from the exudate of an actinobacillosis lesion will reveal *Actinobacillus lignieresii.*

F. **Differential diagnoses** include:

  1. **Neurologic diseases** (e.g., rabies, equine leukoencephalomalacia), which may cause excessive salivation

  2. **Sialadenitis**

  3. **Toxicities** (e.g., organophosphate toxicity)

  4. **Actinomycosis (lumpy jaw),** an osteomyelitis of the mandible or maxilla (see Chapter 42)

G. **Therapeutic plan**

  1. **Physical injury.** In general, lesions of the mouth and tongue that have been produced

TABLE 1-1. Infectious Causes of Stomatitis

Causative Agent	Clinical Disease
Fusobacterium necrophorum (B)	Oral necrobacillosis (necrotic stomatitis)
Actinobacillus lignieresii (B)	Actinobacillosis (wooden tongue)
Candida albicans (F)	Stomatitis, glossitis
Aphthovirus (V)	Foot and mouth disease
Enterovirus (V)	Swine vesicular disease
Vesicular stomatitis virus (V)	Vesicular stomatitis
Bovine viral diarrhea virus (V)	Bovine viral diarrhea, mucosal disease
Bovine malignant catarrh virus (V)	Bovine malignant catarrh
Rinderpest virus (V)	Rinderpest
Bovine papular stomatitis virus (V)	Bovine papular stomatitis
Contagious ecthyma virus (V)	Contagious ecthyma
Vesicular exanthema virus (V)	Vesicular exanthema of swine
Bluetongue virus (V)	Bluetongue
Epizootic hemorrhagic disease virus (V)	Epizootic hemorrhagic disease (deer)

B = bacteria; F = fungus; V = virus.

by physical agents heal rapidly without interventive therapy. Supportive care may be offered in the form of free-choice water and a soft, palatable diet for a few days.

2. **Chemical injury.** The oral cavity should be flushed with water immediately, and the animal should be observed closely to determine if any ingestion has occurred. Free-choice water and a soft, palatable ration should be offered. If anorexia (as a result of the oral cavity lesions) occurs, intravenous fluid therapy and an indwelling naso-gastric tube may be necessary to meet fluid and nutritional demands until healing occurs. With young or small patients, total parenteral nutrition may be a viable and economic option.

3. **Infection.** Specific therapies are outlined in I I.

H. **Prevention.** Many cases of stomatitis can be prevented by providing the client with information regarding management, feeding care, and hygiene.

I. **Specific conditions**
1. **Necrotic stomatitis (oral necrobacillosis)**
   a. **Patient profile and history.** Necrotic stomatitis occurs in young, milk-fed calves. The condition is often linked to unsanitary management and unhygienic feeding utensils.
   b. **Clinical findings.** Necrotic stomatitis is characterized by fever, depression, anorexia, ptyalism, and painful swallowing. In classic oral necrobacillosis, the lesions involve the buccal mucosa, giving the animal a puffy-cheeked appearance. A characteristic foul smell is associated with the exudate in the mouth.
   c. **Therapeutic plan.** Oral necrobacillosis usually responds well to penicillin G procaine (10–20,000 IU/kg intramuscularly, twice daily). Treatment may be required for 7–10 days.
2. **Actinobacillosis (wooden tongue)** is usually a sporadic condition. In cattle, the tongue, and less commonly, the pharyngeal lymph nodes, are involved, whereas in sheep, the soft tissues of the mouth, face, and neck are affected.
   a. **Clinical findings.** Onset is acute and characterized by ptyalism, excessive tongue movement, and an inability to eat.
      (1) In cattle, the tongue is swollen, hard, and painful on manipulation. The tongue may be enlarged early in the course of the disease, but later it becomes shrunken and firm.
      (2) Nodules and ulcers may be present. Suppuration occurs and pus is discharged from the affected areas.

(3) Starvation may eventually occur because of pain or the inability to prehend and masticate food.
- **b. Etiology and pathophysiology.** *Actinobacillus lignieresii*, a gram-negative rod, is a normal inhabitant of the mouth of many ruminants. The organism is thought to gain entrance to the soft tissues of the oral cavity through abrasions and penetrating wounds of the mouth and tongue, leading to the development of a granulomatous abscessation.
- **c. Differential diagnoses** for this condition include penetrating foreign bodies, bacterial phlegmon, abscesses, and tuberculosis involving the lymph nodes of the head and neck.
- **d. Therapeutic plan.** It is important to treat the condition quickly, control discharges, and isolate affected animals. The standard treatment is iodides in combination with antibiotics.
  - **(1)** Potassium iodide is administered orally (6–10 g/day for 1–10 days). Sodium chloride is administered intravenously (1 g/12 kg as a 10% solution). Treatment with sodium chloride may be repeated once.
  - **(2)** Signs of iodism (e.g., lacrimation, anorexia, coughing, flaky skin) will often develop with a course of potassium iodide therapy, necessitating adjustment of the dose.

3. Mycotic stomatitis is similar to the human disease, thrush.
- **a. Patient profile and history.** Stomatitis caused by fungi or yeasts is most commonly seen in hand-reared young (lambs, piglets) or as a sequela to long-term oral antibiotic therapy. The condition is often associated with unhygienic feeding utensils.
- **b. Clinical findings.** The lesions appear as white spots or as a velvety white membrane covering the mucosa. The white plaques progress to shallow ulcers.
- **c. Therapeutic plan.** Animals may be treated with mild oral antiseptic solutions (e.g., 2% copper sulfate). If overuse of oral antibiotics is the cause of the stomatitis, the antibiotic should be discontinued and the rationale for its initial use investigated.

4. Vesicular stomatitis
- **a. Patient profile and history.** Vesicular stomatitis occurs in cattle, horses, swine, and, occasionally, humans. The disease is most common in adult cattle.
- **b. Clinical findings.** Vesicular stomatitis is usually sporadic in occurrence, but up to 60% of a herd may develop clinical signs. The disease often develops in the summer or fall and may be cyclical in occurrence, with many years elapsing between outbreaks.
  - **(1) Cattle** exhibit fever, excessive salivation, and anorexia resulting in weight loss. By the time the disease is recognized, vesicles may have been replaced by erosions and ulcers on the lips, gums, dental pad, and tongue. Teat lesions, which cause mastitis and a drop in milk production, are also found; coronary band lesions and lameness are less common. Recovery generally occurs within 2–21 days; the lesions resolve after 1–2 months.
  - **(2) Horses** exhibit a transient pyrexia with vesicles on the lips and tongue. Hyperemia and ulceration of the coronary band area is common. Lesions may also involve the nasal turbinates and nasopharynx, causing epistaxis.
  - **(3) Swine.** Vesicles and ulcers are found on the snout, oral mucosa, and feet.
  - **(4) Humans.** Fever and influenza-like symptoms have been described.
- **c. Etiology and pathogenesis**
  - **(1) Etiology.** Vesicular stomatitis is caused by **vesicular stomatitis virus (VSV), a rhabdovirus.** The New Jersey and Indiana strains are the main serotypes.
  - **(2) Pathogenesis.** The pathogenesis of vesicular stomatitis is not fully understood, but it is hypothesized that VSV is a plant virus that undergoes modification once it is ingested by insects that feed on the plants.
    - **(a) Transmission.** Insects may spread the modified virus to other plants or directly to animals. Animals may also become infected through consumption of infected plants, by direct transmission, through human transmission, or via fomites (e.g., milking machines).

TABLE 1-2. Viral Vesicular Disease Infection Profile

Disease	Cattle	Sheep and Goats	Pigs	Horses	Humans
Vesicular stomatitis	+ + +	+	+ + +	+ + +	+
Foot and mouth disease	+ + +	+ + +	+ + +	−	+
Vesicular exanthema	−	−	+ + +	+	+
Swine vesicular disease	−	−	+ + +	−	+

− = does not occur in the species in a controlled exposure; + = sometimes occurs in the species in a controlled exposure; + + = often occurs in the species in a controlled exposure; + + + = frequently occurs in the species in a controlled exposure.

> **(i)** The seasonal disappearance of the disease in temperate regions may correspond to a decrease in the insect population or elimination of fresh forages from the diet.
> **(ii)** The disease is enzootic in areas of warm temperature, high rainfall, and heavy insect populations (e.g., the tropics or subtropics).
>
> **(b) Portal of entry.** It is thought that mucous membrane abrasions are necessary for virus penetration.

d. Diagnostic plan. Because the ulcers in this condition and the disease pattern closely resemble those of foot and mouth disease (see I I 5; Table 1-2), federal authorities must be notified and a herd quarantine must be imposed until the diagnosis is confirmed. Virus isolation, although difficult, is attempted from fresh vesicular fluids and from epithelial biopsies. Serum complement fixation and fluorescent antibody tests are used to evaluate serum.

e. Therapeutic plan. Vesicular stomatitis will usually die out within the herd, but affected animals should be isolated from herdmates. Free-choice water and good quality feed should be provided, and soothing, lanolin-based teat dips should be used on cows with teat lesions.

f. Prevention. Insect control should be employed to prevent the spread of the disease. Affected animals should be handled, fed, and milked last.

5. Foot and mouth disease

a. Patient profile and history. Cattle and swine of any age and breed are most susceptible. Foot and mouth disease primarily affects wild and domestic cloven-hooved animals in Africa, Europe, Asia, and South America. Outbreaks have occurred in previously disease-free areas (e.g., North America) as a result of movement of animals or meat products, but the outbreaks have always been successfully controlled.

b. Clinical findings

(1) Cattle. In cattle, this is a multisystemic disease characterized by fever and depression followed by stomatitis, lameness, and mastitis. Secondary bacterial infection of the lesions occurs as the thin-walled vesicles rapidly progress to ulcers.

(a) Oral lesions. Vesicles and bullae appear on the tongue, buccal mucosa, dental pad, and gingiva, causing excessive salivation and painful mastication.

(b) Foot lesions. Vesicles appear on the feet, between the claws, and on the coronary band, producing lameness.

(c) Teat lesions. Vesicular lesions develop on the teats, resulting in pain and an unwillingness of the animal to be milked.

(2) Swine, sheep, and **goats.** In these animals, the presentation is similar to that in cattle, but the clinical signs are usually milder.

c. Etiology and pathogenesis. Foot and mouth disease is caused by a picornavirus of the genus *Aphthovirus.* The virus is resistant and may persist on fomites or in meat products; it is also readily transmitted by carrier animals (e.g., swine, sheep, goats). In the latter case, the mode of transmission is via inhalation or ingestion.

d. Diagnostic plan. Federal authorities must be notified. Virus identification is accomplished using antibody detection tests (e.g., complement fixation, virus neutralization) or antigen identification assays [e.g., enzyme-linked immunosorbent assay (ELISA)]. In foot and mouth virus-free areas, a quarantine, test, and slaughter policy is usually evoked in response to identification of the disease.

e. **Prevention.** Mutations occur constantly, making a consistent vaccination program impractical. Because economic losses (as a result of production inefficiencies and trade restrictions) can be substantial, type-specific vaccines for the region are often employed in endemic areas.

6. **Swine vesicular disease**
   a. **Patient profile and history.** This disease only affects pigs and is foreign to North America. It is significant because of its clinical similarity to foot and mouth disease.
   b. **Clinical findings.** The vesicles found with this disease are most prominent around the coronary band and between the claws of the feet and less prominent in the mouth. Unlike the vesicles of foot and mouth disease, the vesicles of swine vesicular disease are thick-walled; therefore, they are not easily ruptured and may persist for 1–2 days. A transient fever accompanied by anorexia is often seen. Animals may be mildly to moderately lame.
   c. **Etiology and pathogenesis.** Swine vesicular disease is caused by an enterovirus. Because the virus can survive and persist on fomites and in meat products, control through disinfection and hygiene is difficult. Infection occurs via oral abrasions and the morbidity rate is 100%.
   d. **Diagnostic plan.** Federal authorities should be notified because of the similarity of swine vesicular disease to foot and mouth disease.
   e. **Therapeutic plan.** Treatment is not warranted for this mild disease and is rarely attempted.

7. **Vesicular exanthema**
   a. **Patient profile and history.** Only feral and domestic swine are affected, although experimental transmission has been successful in horses. The disease is limited to the Southwestern United States.
   b. **Clinical findings** include a high fever, depression, anorexia, and vesicular lesions in the mouth, on the snout, teats, udder coronary band, and heels, and between the claws. The vesicles rupture to ulcers within 24–48 hours, resulting in lameness and secondary infection. Abortion may also occur. Infection may be subclinical.
   c. **Etiology and pathogenesis.** The disease is caused by a calicivirus harbored by sea lions. The virus is thought to be periodically transmitted to the feral pig population in coastal areas (e.g., California) and then on to domestic pigs. Sources of infection are live pigs and pork products.
   d. **Diagnostic plan.** Federal authorities should be notified to rule out other vesicular diseases.
   e. **Therapeutic plan.** Treatment is rarely attempted.

8. **Bluetongue**
   a. **Patient profile and history.** Bluetongue is most common and virulent in Africa but causes disease in ruminants throughout the world. Bluetongue occurs in many locations in the United States and in parts of western Canada. It affects sheep and, occasionally, cattle.
   b. **Clinical findings**
      (1) **Sheep**
         (a) **Epidemic (acute) disease.** Fever and a bloody or mucopurulent nasal discharge are common. Swelling and edema of the mouth, lips, and tongue develop, resulting in dyspnea, dysphagia, and cyanosis of the oral membranes, followed by the development of necrotic oral ulcers. Coronitis and laminitis may lead to lameness and recumbency. Diarrhea, conjunctivitis, lacrimation, and pneumonia may also be seen. *In utero* infection may result in abortions or the birth of immune-tolerant lambs with or without signs of musculoskeletal or neurologic disorders (e.g., arthrogryposis, hydranencephaly).

 (b) **Endemic disease.** In endemic areas, sheep may have an increased incidence of abortions and a decreased level of performance.
 (2) **Cattle** usually have inapparent infections but may show some or all of the
same signs as sheep.
 c. **Etiology and pathogenesis**
 (1) **Etiology.** Bluetongue is caused by an **orbivirus, bluetongue virus (BTV).**
There are many serotypes of BTV and strains within serotypes. One closely
related virus, epizootic hemorrhagic disease virus (EHDV), causes a peracute
and fatal hemorrhagic disease in white-tailed deer and pronghorn antelope
that is very similar to bluetongue.
 (2) **Transmission.** BTV is transmitted by **biting flies** (*Culicoides* species). Cattle
and wild African ruminants are reservoirs. The virus is also found in **semen,**
leading to congenital infection.
 d. **Diagnostic plan.** Clinical diagnosis can be difficult because of the variety of clinical signs and presentations. Outbreaks should be reported to federal authorities.
Virus identification can be accomplished through:
 (1) Serologic tests (e.g., complement fixation, indirect immunofluorescence,
agar gel immunodiffusion, serum neutralization)
 (2) ELISA
 (3) Animal inoculation (e.g., sheep, chick embryo, or rodent)
 (4) Polymerase chain reaction (PCR) assays
 (5) Enzyme-linked oligonucleotide-sorbent assay (ELOSA)
 e. **Therapeutic plan.** Treatment is nonspecific and often unrewarding for the
acutely affected animal. Nursing care is recommended for the mild form of the
disease. Congenital infections are not treated.
 f. **Prevention.** Because the morbidity rate is 50%–75% and the mortality rate is
20%–50%, production losses can be of major significance; therefore, prevention
of the disease is important. A vaccine is available in the United States.

 9. **Contagious ecthyma (contagious pustular dermatitis, orf)**
 a. **Patient profile.** Contagious ecthyma is a common disease of sheep and goats.
Young animals are most commonly affected, but lesions can occur on or around
the udders of older animals that lack immunity, presumably following inoculation by nursing lambs.
 b. **Clinical findings**
 (1) Crusty, proliferative lesions are most commonly found on the mouth, muzzle, and nostrils. The lesions begin as papules that rapidly progress to vesicles, pustules, and, finally, scabs covering a granulated, inflamed base. The
lesions are sore and may fissure, crumble, and bleed.
 (2) Animals recover from the condition in approximately 3 weeks, but not before suffering ill-thrift due to decreased feed consumption and a reluctance
to nurse. The severity of the disease varies, depending on the location of the
lesions (e.g., lesions may extend into the alimentary or respiratory tract).
Generally, morbidity is high but mortality is low, unless secondary infections occur or there is extensive spread of the lesions.
 c. **Etiology and pathogenesis.** Contagious ecthyma is a highly infectious disease
caused by a parapoxvirus and spread by direct contact. It can be zoonotic; caretakers may develop scabs on their hands.
 d. **Diagnostic plan.** The diagnosis is based on the finding of typical clinical signs in
the appropriate age-range population.
 e. **Differential diagnoses** include sheep pox, goat pox, bluetongue, and ulcerative
dermatosis.
 f. **Therapeutic plan.** Contagious ecthyma is usually a self-limiting disease, but nursing care, supportive feeding, or antibiotics (to resolve secondary bacterial infections) may be needed by some patients.
 g. **Prevention**
 (1) Affected animals should be isolated from the herd or flock if possible.
 (2) Measures to limit transmission (e.g., using separate feeding utensils) should
be employed.

(3) Vaccination programs are common in large sheep-rearing areas. Commercial vaccines are available or autogenous vaccines can be prepared.

10. **Bovine papular stomatitis (BPS)**
    a. **Patient profile.** BPS is a common disease in calves or young cattle. It has a worldwide distribution.
    b. **Clinical findings**
       (1) The early sign of a transient fever usually goes unnoticed.
       (2) The initial lesions are papules that rapidly coalesce and progress to round lesions with a necrotic, grey, depressed center and a raised, reddened periphery. Lesions are found on the muzzle, the hard palate, or inside the nostrils, but not on the tongue.
          (a) The lesions may be found incidentally while examining the mouths of young cattle, or they may be associated with a period of weight loss and diarrhea ("rat-tail" syndrome, which affects feeder cattle).
          (b) The lesions may persist for weeks.
    c. **Etiology.** BPS is caused by **parapoxvirus.**
    d. **Diagnostic plan.** The diagnosis is based on the characteristic lesions and the usual lack of any other clinical findings in young cattle. It is important that this benign disease not be confused with other, more serious, diseases that produce oral ulcers or erosions (e.g., vesicular stomatitis).
    e. **Therapeutic plan.** Therapeutic intervention is unnecessary. Good hygiene should be practiced to avoid secondary infections.

II. DENTAL CONDITIONS

A. **Observable changes in the teeth of ruminants.** A variety of inherited, congenital, and developmental conditions can affect the teeth of ruminants. Generally, therapy is only undertaken in valuable animals when the extraction of one or two affected teeth and supplemental feeding might prolong the animal's productive life.

1. **Staining. Porphyrinuria** stains the teeth of cattle reddish brown.

2. **Defective enamel formation. Osteogenesis imperfecta** causes defective enamel formation.

3. **Mottling. Fluoride toxicity (fluorosis)** damages the teeth prior to tooth eruption. The teeth appear eroded, mottled, and wear excessively.

4. **Excessive wear.** Mature animals of any species may be affected as a result of **abnormally abrasive diets** or **rations deficient in calcium.** The worn teeth prohibit proper prehension and mastication, resulting in weight loss (or diminished weight gain) and necessitating early cullage.

5. **Malpositioning and excessive rotation of the cheek teeth** may occur in goats secondary to **osteodystrophia fibrosa.**

6. **Broken teeth. Trauma** most commonly involves the incisor teeth.

B. **Dental conditions of sheep**

1. **Dentigerous cysts,** a developmental abnormality, occur most commonly in sheep. The incisors are usually encysted within the alveolar bone of the central mandible.

2. **Periodontal disease (periodontitis, alveolar periostitis)**
   a. **Clinical findings** include premature wear and breakage of teeth **(broken mouth),** painful mastication, and poor feed conversion or weight loss. Gingivitis is the primary lesion.
   b. **Etiology and pathogenesis.** A chronic bacterial infection (perhaps caused by *Bacteroides gingivalis*) leads to destruction of the periodontal membrane with resultant alveolitis, osteomyelitis, and bony lysis. The cause of the periodontitis is not

well defined; it may be multifactorial and related to either the accumulation of debris in the gingival sulcus or a mineral deficiency.

    c. **Therapeutic plan.** Antibiotics may be used to treat periodontal disease.

C. **Dental conditions of horses**

    1. Clinical findings

        a. Feed refusal or **selectivity in eating.** Grain is often preferred over hay, which has to be masticated more fully.

        b. Pain. Chewing is a slow process and the animal may toss his head in frustration. Food may be wadded in the mouth or expelled in masses **(quidding),** or grain may fall out of the mouth while the horse is eating. The animal may hold his head with the affected side of the jaw up. Performance animals may resist the bit or place unilateral tension on a line or rein.

        c. Weight loss may result from decreased feed intake or decreased digestibility of incompletely masticated feedstuffs. Whole-grain or long-stemmed fiber may be seen in the feces.

        d. Recurrent esophageal choke or **intestinal colic** may result from poor digestibility of the food or because water intake is decreased secondary to increased tooth sensitivity.

    2. Diagnostic plan

        a. The animal should be observed while eating, drinking, and working. In all cases, a **thorough oral examination** is necessary to identify the affected teeth and secondary mouth lesions. The animal should be sedated, and anesthesia may be necessary.

        b. In some cases, **radiographs** may be necessary.

    3. Specific conditions

        a. Ectopic teeth are incisors or cheek teeth that grow in an abnormal direction. They are thought to arise from injuries to the tooth bud and should be removed if they are causing problems for the animal.

        b. Supernumerary teeth are usually extra incisors; rarely, extra cheek teeth are seen. Any number of extra teeth, including whole rows, may be present. Supernumerary teeth are usually left alone unless they are causing problems.

        c. Wolf teeth are small, singular, vestigial premolars in front of the upper cheek teeth that may cause buccal lacerations or interfere with the bit. Occasionally, they are seen on the lower arcade. Because of their short root structure, they are easily extracted in the standing animal.

        d. Retained deciduous teeth are common.

            (1) Occasionally, incisors are retained if the permanent teeth erupt behind them. The retained incisor must be extracted.

            (2) More commonly, deciduous premolars are retained as **caps** over the erupting permanent tooth. The cap delays the eruption of the permanent tooth and acts as a hinge, trapping debris and causing buccal irritation. Caps can be removed by filing or with dental elevators or forceps.

        e. Sharp edges (points) develop on the buccal surface of the upper arcade of cheek teeth and the lingual border of the lower arcade. Points are most common in horses 2–5 years of age and occur when the enamel of the teeth wears unevenly as a result of friction between the narrow mandible and the wider maxillary arcade. These sharp edges can cause mucosal lacerations and may be removed by routine filing or floating.

        f. Infection

            (1) Etiology and pathogenesis

                (a) Infection can occur **secondary to trauma** or tooth fractures that extend into the pulp cavity.

                (b) Malocclusions, gingivitis, periodontitis, or **cementum defects** also predispose to infection.

                (c) A **patent infundibulum** allows material to enter the root canal, in many cases creating an **abscess.** An apical abscess in the mandibular bone looks like a normal eruption cyst, but radiographically it has the appearance of a proliferative osteomyelitis. An abscess of one of the last four cheek teeth in the upper arcade can cause **sinusitis.**

(2) **Therapeutic plan**

(a) **Medical therapy** is employed initially to attempt preservation of the tooth. Systemic penicillin (22,000 IU/kg twice daily by intramuscular injection) coupled with endoscopy and flushing of the maxillary sinus (if sinusitis is present) may be successful. Radiographic follow-up allows evaluation of the therapy.

(b) **Surgery** is often necessary to remove infected teeth and treat sinusitis or osteomyelitis. Horses do not shed infected teeth spontaneously.

g. **Malocclusions** or **abnormalities of the mouth** [e.g., **brachygnathism (parrot mouth), brachycephaly (sow mouth), sheer mouth, wave mouth, step mouth**] produce abnormal wear of the occlusal surfaces of the teeth, interfering with both performance and production. These defects may be breed-related. Many require routine dental attention to promote as much even wear as possible.

h. **Ameloblastoma** is the most common neoplasm of dental origin. The tumor, which arises from odontogenic epithelium, is invasive and results in bony degeneration.

 III. DYSPHAGIA

A. **Pharyngitis, laryngitis,** and **pharyngeal swelling** often occur together and concurrently with stomatitis.

1. **Patient profile and history.** Any animal can develop pharyngitis, regardless of age, breed, or gender. There may be a history of traumatic incident or administration of materials via dose syringe, speculum, balling gun, or orogastric intubation. Other historical findings depend on the causative agent.

2. **Clinical findings.** There is often an observable and palpable swelling in the pharyngeal or intermandibular region. There is reluctance or difficulty in eating and swallowing. There may be a mucopurulent nasal discharge and pain often causes the animal to hold the head and neck in extension. The regional lymph nodes may be enlarged and a spontaneous or easily induced cough may be present. The local pharyngeal problem may be accompanied by systemic signs (e.g., fever, tachycardia, tachypnea).

3. **Etiology and pathophysiology.** Pharyngitis may be an extension of stomatitis or, like stomatitis, it may be caused by physical, chemical, or infectious agents.

4. **Diagnostic plan.** A thorough oral examination is necessary to diagnose pharyngitis and determine its causes. Laboratory work, laryngoscopy, endoscopy, radiography, and ultrasonography may all be useful as diagnostic aids.

5. **Laboratory tests**

a. **Microbial culture and sensitivity testing** may be attempted from a swab of any discharges; however, because the upper alimentary and respiratory tracts are home to a variety of organisms, it may be difficult to interpret the growth of a mixed or contaminated population. Aspiration of abscesses percutaneously through properly prepared sites will yield more reliable results.

b. **Fine needle aspiration and cytologic interpretation** allows diagnosis of solid-core masses in the pharyngeal region.

c. **Hematologic work-up.** Hematologic changes may reflect inflammatory changes in the pharynx or a systemic disease.

6. **Differential diagnoses**

a. **Rabies** (in a domestic animal exhibiting dysphagia, hypersalivation, and mental changes)

b. **Respiratory diseases** [e.g., strangles, guttural pouch empyema, guttural pouch mycosis, viral respiratory disease, lymphoid follicular hyperplasia (LFH) in horses; calf diphtheria in cattle]

     c. Bacterial stomatitis (i.e., oral necrobacillosis, actinobacillosis)

  7. Specific conditions

    a. Mechanical injury

      (1) Etiology and pathogenesis. Trauma associated with the ingestion of foreign objects or administration of oral medications can lead to bacterial pharyngitis when organisms (e.g., *F. necrophorum*) secondarily infect the site.

      (2) Therapeutic plan. Measures include the following:

        (a) Penicillin (22,000 IU/kg twice daily intramuscularly)

        (b) Soft, palatable diets and free-choice water or supportive alimentation through a nasogastric tube (horses)

        (c) Nonsteroidal anti-inflammatory agents (NSAIDs) or corticosteroids to subdue inflammation and hasten return to normal function

    b. Pharyngeal phlegmon, a sporadic condition affecting adult cattle, produces an acute, deep-seated, diffuse, rapidly spreading cellulitis and inflammation of the oral mucosa and pharynx. The mortality rate is high in acutely affected animals.

      (1) Etiology and pathogenesis. It is not completely understood what causes pharyngeal phlegmon, but a mixed bacterial population is commonly found in the tissues of the head and neck.

      (2) Clinical findings include hypersalivation, lacrimation, fever, tachypnea, and tachycardia. There is marked swelling of the tissues of the head. The animal becomes completely anorexic and may die within 24 hours. In more chronic cases, pools of purulent debris build up in the subcutis, imparting a foul odor to the breath.

      (3) Therapeutic plan. Vigorous treatment, consisting of broad-spectrum antibiotics (e.g., trimethoprim–sulfamethoxazole) and anti-inflammatory agents, is required. Supportive care is also beneficial.

B. Pharyngeal obstruction

  1. Patient profile and history. There may be a history of foreign body ingestion or feeding on solid food objects (e.g., potatoes, turnips, whole cob corn, apples).

  2. Clinical findings include complete or intermittent dysphagia and the inability to swallow food, water, or both. The animal may make inspiratory noises, and the source of the obstruction may be palpable. Chronic obstruction will result in weight loss, dehydration, or both. Pharyngeal obstruction accompanied by esophageal obstruction will result in bloat in ruminants.

  3. Etiology and pathophysiology

    a. Congenital conditions may cause pharyngeal obstruction; however, this is rare.

    b. Foreign bodies may obstruct the pharyngeal lumen. Examples of foreign bodies include solid feedstuffs like potatoes, apples, or mangos, and nonedible objects, such as rocks, wood, or hard rubber. Pharyngeal obstruction as a result of foreign body ingestion occurs most commonly in mature cattle as a result of their indiscriminate eating habits.

    c. External masses (e.g., retropharyngeal lymph node adenopathies from infections or tumors) may impinge on the pharynx, displacing normal tissue and causing dysphagia.

      (1) In cattle, **actinobacillosis** or **lymphosarcoma** can cause external pharyngeal obstruction.

      (2) In horses, **strangles, guttural pouch disease,** and **lymphoid follicular hyperplasia** can cause dysphagia.

  4. Diagnostic plan. A **complete oral examination** is required. **Endoscopy** is valuable for visualizing the pharynx. Because small, highly portable instruments are available, this procedure can be used in many species under many circumstances.

  5. Laboratory tests. A leukogram may help confirm the presence of an inflammatory or invasive mass around the pharynx.

  6. Differential diagnoses include causes of pharyngeal paralysis (e.g., rabies) and other encephalitides or encephalopathies.

7. **Therapeutic plan**
   a. **Foreign body obstruction**
      (1) When the cause of the obstruction is a foreign body, the object can often be removed manually in a large enough patient. Sedation and the use of a wire loop may be required in some cases.
      (2) In more complicated cases, surgery followed by antibiotics and supportive care may be required; however, the prognosis is often poor because of the physical trauma sustained.
   b. **External masses.** The cause of the mass that is impinging on the pharynx must be identified and treated accordingly.

8. **Prevention.** Providing information to clients about principles of feeding management (e.g., appropriate chopping of tubers, gradual introduction to new feeds) may help minimize the number of foreign body obstructions.

C. **Pharyngeal paralysis**

1. **Patient profile and history.** Subjective and historical information may be of some value for determining the cause of pharyngeal paralysis and dysphagia. For example, the region may be endemic for rabies or the animal may have had access to moldy feed or toxic plants.

2. **Clinical findings.** In terms of the upper alimentary tract, the clinical findings will not be specific. Findings include dysphagia, ptyalism, and, possibly, regurgitation or abnormal vocalization if nerves other than the pharyngeal nerves are paralyzed as well.

3. **Etiology and pathophysiology.** Pharyngeal paralysis may result from a central or peripheral neurologic disorder; common causes include **rabies, botulism,** and **leukoencephalomalacia.**

D. **Esophageal obstruction.** In horses and sheep, esophageal obstruction is known as **choke.** In cattle with complete esophageal obstruction, the most significant clinical finding is the build-up of gas in the rumen; therefore, esophageal obstruction in cattle is discussed in Chapter 3 I B 1.

1. **Patient profile and history.** Esophageal obstruction may occur in any domestic animal on solid food but is most common in horses, sheep, and cattle.
   a. Choke is most common in older animals and is often associated with pelleted or dry feeds (e.g., beet pulp, oats, bran).
   b. There may be evidence of insufficient or inaccessible water (e.g., frozen or distant water supplies).
   c. There may be a history of administration of medicinal boluses.
   d. Greedy eaters, older animals with defective teeth, and young horses with erupting teeth are susceptible.
   e. Preexisting esophageal disease, previous episodes of choke, or trauma to the neck are predisposing factors.

2. **Clinical findings**
   a. **Early findings.** Animals will exhibit dysphagia, with extension of the head and neck. Coughing and retching may be accompanied by the discharge of food and frothy saliva from the nostrils. Anxiety, manifested by sweating and head-shaking, is common. If the esophageal mass is lodged in the cervical region, it may be palpable percutaneously.
   b. **Late findings** include depression and dehydration. The animal may repeatedly attempt to drink without success. Subcutaneous emphysema suggests esophageal rupture. Aspiration pneumonia, manifested clinically as tachypnea, harsh breath sounds, and fever, may occur with high cervical choke.

3. **Etiology and pathophysiology.** The esophageal diameter may be normal, narrowed, or dilated. Natural areas of esophageal narrowing are the anterior cervical region (in cattle and sheep), the midcervical region (in horses), the thoracic inlet, and the junction of the esophagus and gastric cardia.

      a. External esophageal compression may be brought about by enlargement of normal structures (e.g., **thymic lymphosarcoma**), compressive masses (e.g., **abscess**), or displacement of structures (e.g., **diaphragmatic hernia**).

      b. Lumenal obstruction may be the result of ingestion of solid objects (e.g., apples) or dry feed that was inadequately moistened. The latter cause is most common in horses.

      c. Defects in the esophageal wall (e.g., strictures from healed lesions, ulcers, or congenital or acquired diverticula) can lead to the development of the condition.

      d. Esophageal spasm has been implicated in some cases.

      e. Neuropathy. Certain neuropathies (e.g., equine protozoal myelitis, equine herpes virus I infection) may interrupt esophageal motility, leading to megaesophagus and esophageal obstruction.

4. Diagnostic plan. The diagnosis is often suspected on the basis of clinical inspection. A nasogastric tube (in horses) or an orogastric tube (in ruminants) can be used to ascertain the site of the obstruction. Endoscopic examination may clarify the diagnosis and offer a prognosis. Radiographic examination using contrast studies allows evaluation of the location and composition of the mass as well as esophageal integrity. (Iodinated organic iodide should be used as a contrast medium if either esophageal perforation or inhalation pneumonia is suspected.) Ultrasonography, fluoroscopy, or both may be warranted in some instances.

5. Laboratory tests. A hematologic work-up and blood chemistry are important adjuncts to diagnosis and can give some indication of prognosis.

      a. Packed cell volume (PCV), total serum protein (TSP), and blood urea nitrogen (BUN) evaluations provide information on the animal's hydration status.

      b. A leukogram should be requested to give an indication of any inflammatory reaction.

      c. Electrolyte analysis will reveal hyponatremia and hypochloremia in horses, as a result of the loss of large quantities of both sodium and chloride ion in equine saliva. These ion losses and attempts by the kidney to compensate will result in a transient metabolic acidosis followed by a metabolic alkalosis.

6. Differential diagnoses. The most common differentials for esophageal obstruction are listed in Table 1-3.

7. Therapeutic plan. This discussion focuses on the treatment of particulate matter (grain) choke in horses.

TABLE 1-3. Differential Diagnoses for Esophageal Obstruction

Neurologic disorders [e.g., rabies and botulism (all species), leukoencephalomalacia and yellow star thistle poisoning (in horses)]
Respiratory diseases in horses [e.g., lymphoid follicular hyperplasia (LFH), strangles, guttural pouch disease, laryngeal scarification following surgery]
Musculoskeletal diseases (e.g., fractured hyoid bone)
Plant toxicoses causing salivation in cattle (e.g., solanum, larkspur, bitterweed)
Mycotoxicoses causing salivation in cattle (e.g., red clover hay contamination with *Rhizoctonia leguminicola*)
Metabolic diseases in horses (e.g., eclampsia, hepatic encephalopathy, hypokalemia)
Oral cavity or pharyngeal foreign bodies
Extrapharyngeal masses in cattle (e.g., lymph node abscess, phlegmon)
Anaphylactoid reactions causing pharyngeal swelling
Dental disease
Congenital diseases, [e.g., persistent right aortic arch (PRAA), megaesophagus]

a. Hydraulic flush. All access to grain, hay, edible bedding, and water should be restricted. Warm water is instilled by gravity into the nasogastric tube, causing water and ingesta to flow out of the tube. Often, after a series of hydraulic flushes, the choke will be relieved and the nasogastric tube can be passed into the stomach. Occasionally, the mass can be forced into the stomach by the tube, but this should only be attempted with great care. Xylazine (0.5–1 mg/kg intravenously) is often used in horses to relieve anxiety, provide muscle relaxation, relieve esophageal spasm, and cause lowering of the head to guard against aspiration pneumonia.

   (1) If the hydraulic flush is not successful, another attempt can be made later. Often, a stubborn choke can be relieved by patience. A horse left without access to feed or water may also resolve the choke spontaneously.

   (2) If the choke persists for longer than 3 days, a hydraulic flush can be performed with the horse under anesthesia and in lateral recumbency. A cuffed endotracheal tube is placed in the trachea to prevent aspiration of material.

b. Other measures

   (1) Dioctyl sodium sulfosuccinate (DSS) is a wetting agent that may soften the mass. 10–15 ml of DSS are mixed with water and infused into the nasogastric tube. This treatment is contraindicated if aspiration of material is likely.

   (2) Suction. A ruminant stomach pump should be used only for suction, not for applying forceful hydraulic pressure against the mass.

   (3) Atropine (10–30 mg subcutaneously) has been recommended because of its ability to relax smooth muscle, although its efficacy may be limited in horses because of the significant amount of striated muscle in the equine esophagus. Side effects include intestinal colic, ileus, and drying of the mucous membranes.

   (4) Surgery. Surgical removal of a solid foreign body may be considered but chronic fistulation often develops as a result of poor healing.

c. Supportive therapy. With a readily resolved choke, supportive therapy is not necessary.

   (1) Feeding considerations. After the resolution of a long-standing choke, the horse should be held off feed for 2–3 days. Free-choice water should be available, and the horse should be gradually reintroduced to soft feed (mashes) and then a regular diet. Supplementary feeding of grain or pellet gruels via an indwelling nasogastric tube may be necessary in cases of esophageal perforation. Feed placed in an elevated position may help patients with compromised esophageal motility.

   (2) Broad-spectrum antibiotics should be considered if esophageal perforation is suspected or if the choke persists.

   (3) NSAIDs may be administered following resolution of the choke if esophageal irritation is suspected.

   (4) Intravenous fluids are necessary in cases of chronic choke.

8. Complications. Sequelae to choke include **esophageal perforation** and **cellulitis, esophageal fistula formation, acute mediastinitis** and **pleuritis, esophageal stricture, esophageal dilation (megaesophagus), recurrent choke,** and **aspiration pneumonia.** All of these complications carry an unfavorable prognosis. The animal should be monitored for 8 weeks after an incident of acute esophageal choke to check for stricture formation.

9. Prevention. Preventive measures include slowing down greedy eaters by feeding small amounts more often, wetting the feed, providing routine dental care, and ensuring that potable water is always available.

E. Esophagitis

1. Patient profile and history. Esophagitis is more common in companion animals and humans than in the large animal species. If esophagitis is suspected, there may be a history of consumption of irritant chemicals, the chronic retention of an esophageal foreign body, or trauma (e.g., perforation of the esophagus during nasogastric intubation). Other historical findings include upper gastrointestinal tract disease or chronic, low-grade abdominal pain.

2. **Clinical findings.** The signs of esophagitis may be similar to those of choke. Progression of esophagitis may result in an external fistula or extension through fascial planes, producing a cellulitis or thoracic inflammation and a corresponding deterioration of clinical signs.

   a. **Reluctance to eat, anorexia,** and **dysphagia.** Water consumption may or may not be impaired; therefore, hydration status is variable but weight loss is usually evident.

   b. **Pain** or **anxiety** may be apparent on swallowing and there may be pain, swelling, or crepitus over the site of the esophageal lesion.

   c. **Nasal regurgitation.** Esophageal spasm may cause the animal to regurgitate food mixed with saliva or blood through the nostrils.

   d. **Signs of aspiration pneumonia** (e.g., fever, tachypnea, tachycardia, harsh breath sounds) may be present.

3. **Etiology and pathophysiology**

   a. **Traumatic ulcerative esophagitis** may result when the prolonged presence of a foreign mass in the esophagus causes a pressure necrosis.

   b. **Corrosive esophagitis** may result from the ingestion or administration of corrosive materials. Agents that produce stomatitis (e.g., musculoskeletal counterirritants in horses) will also produce esophagitis.

   c. **Reflux esophagitis** occurs in simple-stomached animals and involves the retrograde movement of gastric or small intestinal fluids (e.g., acid, pepsin, bile salts) into the esophagus. Reflux esophagitis may occur with equine small intestinal obstruction, anterior enteritis, gastric ulcers, or gastric outflow problems.

4. **Diagnostic plan.** The diagnostic plan for esophagitis is similar to that for choke. After a thorough oral examination, a nasogastric tube (or orogastric tube in the case of ruminants) should be passed carefully into the stomach. Upon withdrawal, the tube should be examined for the presence of blood, ingesta, and saliva. Endoscopy and double contrast radiography are valuable adjuncts for determining the site and extent of the lesion.

5. **Laboratory tests** requested would depend on the etiology of the esophagitis.

6. **Differential diagnoses** are similar to those for choke (see Table 1-3).

7. **Therapeutic plan**

   a. **Specific conditions**

      (1) **Traumatic ulcerative esophagitis.** Intensive, conservative therapy may be necessary to remove a foreign mass. High dosages of broad-spectrum antibiotics may be necessary.

      (2) **Reflux esophagitis.** Gastric distention is treated by decompression via nasogastric intubation. A histamine$_2$ (H$_2$)-receptor antagonist such as cimetidine or ranitidine may be used to decrease gastric acid secretion.

      (3) **Esophageal perforations, strictures,** or **fistulas** may necessitate surgery.

   b. **Supportive therapy.** NSAIDs may be helpful. Solid food should be eliminated from the diet until healing has occurred, then solid foods should be introduced gradually. Supplemental feeding via nasogastric intubation may be necessary.

8. **Complications.** The sequelae to esophagitis may be similar to those of choke.

DIRECTIONS: Each of the numbered items or incomplete statements in this section is followed by answers or by completions of the statement. Select the ONE numbered answer or completion that is BEST in each case.

1. Which one of the following statements regarding vesicular stomatitis is true? Vesicular stomatitis:

(1) is confined to horses and occasionally swine.
(2) is unique in its clinical presentation.
(3) is a European disease that is chronic and circulates within herds.
(4) produces lesions that are confined to the mucous membranes of the mouth and nasal cavity.
(5) is hypothesized to be caused by a mutated plant virus spread by insects.

2. A major difference between foot and mouth disease and swine vesicular disease is that:

(1) foot and mouth disease is caused by a picornavirus.
(2) foot and mouth disease does not affect swine.
(3) swine vesicular disease is not reportable.
(4) swine vesicular disease virus can persist in processed meats.
(5) infection with swine vesicular disease is via the oral route.

3. Which statement regarding bluetongue is true? Bluetongue:

(1) causes disease in ruminants and horses worldwide.
(2) causes oral disease as well as coronitis and laminitis.
(3) is spread by ingestion or aerosol transmission.
(4) responds to broad-spectrum antibiotic therapy.
(5) causes disease only in animals less than 9 months of age.

4. A set of common dental conditions in domestic animals includes:

(1) dentigerous cysts in sheep, periodontal disease, caries.
(2) caps, caries, supernumerary molars.
(3) sharp edges (or points), supernumerary molars, caps.
(4) periodontal disease, dentigerous cysts in sheep, sharp edges (or points).
(5) supernumerary incisors, retained incisors, wolf teeth.

5. Which one of the following statements regarding pharyngitis of cattle is true?

(1) There may be a concurrent mucopurulent nasal discharge.
(2) Neurologic disease would not be a differential diagnosis.
(3) Bacterial culture will confirm the causative organism.
(4) Nonsteroidal anti-inflammatory agents are contraindicated.
(5) There is usually little indication of pain.

6. Which one of the following statements regarding pharyngeal phlegmon is true? Pharyngeal phlegmon is:

(1) caused by *Candida* species.
(2) a disease of low mortality but high morbidity.
(3) a cellulitis of the oral mucosa and pharynx.
(4) most common in milk-fed calves.
(5) responsive to oral astringents.

DIRECTIONS: Each of the numbered items or incomplete statements in this section is negatively phrased, as indicated by a capitalized word such as NOT, LEAST, or EXCEPT. Select the ONE numbered answer or completion that is BEST in each case.

7. All of the following statements regarding contagious ecthyma (contagious pustular dermatitis, orf) of sheep are true EXCEPT:

(1) It is common.
(2) It is usually diagnosed on the basis of clinical findings.
(3) It has zoonotic potential.
(4) It can be eliminated in a flock by the use of systemic antibiotics.
(5) It produces good immunity in individuals against subsequent infection.

8. Which one of the following statements regarding choke in horses is NOT correct?

(1) Sedatives are often used in acute equine choke to relieve esophageal spasm.
(2) Chronic or recurrent choke responds favorably to dietary management.
(3) Signs resembling dyspnea may predominate early in the course of the condition.
(4) Central nervous system (CNS) diseases should be included among the differential diagnoses when confronted with a case of possible choke.
(5) Many grain chokes respond favorably to gentle intraesophageal infusions of water.

1. The answer is 5 [I I 4]. Vesicular stomatitis virus affects many species including cattle. The disease appears similar to other vesicular diseases (e.g., foot and mouth disease) and is reportable to federal authorities. This disease is cyclical and seasonal in occurrence but is not enzootic in countries outside of tropical or subtropical climates. Lesions are found on the mucous membranes of the oral and nasal cavity but also on the feet and coronary band.

2. The answer is 1 [I I 5, 6]. Foot and mouth disease affects cloven-hooved animals including swine, and whereas it is caused by a picornavirus, swine vesicular disease is caused by an enterovirus. Swine vesicular disease, like foot and mouth disease, is reportable and can be transmitted through processed meats or other fomites via the oral route.

3. The answer is 2 [I I 8 b]. Bluetongue may cause oral disease, coronitis, laminitis, diarrhea, ocular changes, abortions and congenital defects in offspring. It is a viral disease of ruminants spread by biting flies or semen. Because it is a viral disease, bluetongue does not respond to antibiotics. The disease affects animals of all ages.

4. The answer is 4 [II B, C]. Common dental conditions of domestic animals include periodontal disease, sharp edges (or points), supernumerary incisors, dentigerous cysts, wolf teeth, and retained molars or caps. Less common conditions are dental caries, supernumerary molars, and retained incisors.

5. The answer is 1 [III A 2]. A mucopurulent nasal discharge and a cough may accompany cases of pharyngitis because dysphagia may cause pulmonary aspiration of feed. Pharyngitis is often accompanied by palpable swelling in the throat region, and the animal may hold its neck in extension and be reluctant to eat or swallow because of pharyngeal pain. There-fore, neurological disease (e.g., rabies) should be on the list of differential diagnoses. Bacterial culture does not necessarily confirm the causative organism in the case of bacterial pharyngitis due to the normal, mixed bacterial resident population of the pharynx. Nonsteroidal anti-inflammatory agents may hasten the response as inflammation is subdued.

6. The answer is 3 [III A 7 b]. Pharyngeal phlegmon is a deep-seated cellulitis of the oral cavity, head and pharynx. The cause is poorly understood, although bacteria are believed to be associated with the condition. It affects adult cattle sporadically. Mortality is high because this disease is difficult to treat and poorly responsive to any conventional therapy.

7. The answer is 5 [I I 9]. Contagious ecthyma (contagious pustular dermatitis, orf) cannot be eliminated in a flock of sheep by using systemic antibiotics. Antibiotics have no efficacy against the causative agent, a parapoxvirus that maintains persistence within a flock. Contagious ecthyma is a common disease that is usually diagnosed on the basis of clinical findings. It has zoonotic potential. Infection produces good immunity in animals that have been exposed to the virus.

8. The answer is 2 [III D]. Chronic or recurrent esophageal obstruction (choke) is likely to be attributable to internal or external esophageal stricture; therefore, dietary management (such as the feeding of slurries) is usually ineffective in the long term. Sedatives are often used in equine patients to relieve esophageal spasm in patients with acute choke. Signs resembling dyspnea may predominate early in the condition. Central nervous system (CNS) disorders must be ruled out when making the diagnosis. Many grain chokes respond favorably to hydraulic flush.

Chapter 2

Diseases of the Equine Gastrointestinal Tract

Timothy H. Ogilvie

I. **COLIC** is a nonspecific term referring to abdominal pain. In this chapter, its usage shall be restricted to gastrointestinal pain.

A. **Determining the severity of the colic.** Colic is usually sporadic in occurrence and may be mild or severe, acute or chronic. Repeated bouts in the same individual are not uncommon.

1. **Patient profile and history**
   a. Some intestinal problems that produce colic appear to be **age related.** For example, meconium impactions are restricted to neonatal foals, whereas feed impactions occur more frequently in older horses.
   b. An accurate history is essential in defining possible etiologies and pathophysiologies of medical colics. Retrospective information should include parasite-control measures, pasture size, and stocking rates. The use and work schedule for the horse should be explored, as should any changes in environment or feeding. A past and present medical history is important for diagnostic purposes as well as interpretation of presenting clinical findings.

2. **Clinical findings** (Table 2-1). A complete physical examination should be attempted in all cases of colic to determine the site and cause of gastrointestinal pain as well as ruling out conditions that mimic gastrointestinal pain. The examination should be performed without sedation in tractable patients. If sedation is necessary, it should be administered only after a complete general examination has been performed because sedation will affect clinically important findings.
   a. **Attitude.** Colics produce attitudinal changes in the horse. Mild colics (e.g., large and small colon impactions) cause slight to moderate depression. Colics producing severe depression and toxemia often result from strangulation obstructions, which are not medically manageable. Medical colics may produce severe pain and anxiety, as in the case of gastric dilatation. The horse will often continue to eat with mild colics.
   b. **Pain and anxiety** is manifested as straining, pawing, stretching, and sweating. It is important to determine if the pain is continuous or intermittent, static or changing in intensity, responsive or unresponsive to medication.
   c. **Temperature.** Rectal temperature readings are usually normal to slightly elevated with medical colics. **Subnormal temperatures** should alert the examiner to the possibility of terminal shock and toxemia. **High temperatures** are associated with infectious or septic conditions. Temperatures may be normal if there has been use of antipyretic drugs (e.g., dipyrone, phenylbutazone, flunixin meglumine).
   d. **Respiratory rate.** Respiratory rates usually increase in proportion to the amount of pain. Abdominal pressure creates a rapid, shallow respiratory rate and pattern. A metabolic acidosis associated with tissue devitalization causes an increase in the respiratory rate.
   e. **Evaluation of circulatory status**
      (1) **Pulse rates** reflect the nature of the colic. In the adult horse, the interpretation of the pulse rate is shown in Table 2-2.
      (2) **Pulse quality** should also be evaluated. A strong, full pulse (rather than a weak, thready pulse) is reflective of a mild and medically responsive colic.
      (3) **Capillary refill** is normal with medically responsive colics and increases with surgical colics (as a result of vascular compromise).
      (4) Normal **mucosal color** is reflective of normal circulatory status and mild or early colics. Congested mucous membranes indicate vascular compromise, fluid loss, or shock.

TABLE 2-1. Physical Findings Differentiating Mild (Medical) Colics From Severe (Surgical) Colics

Mild Colic	Severe Colic
Yawning	Rolling, thrashing, self traumatization
Straining as if to urinate	Depression, dullness
Bruxism, groaning	Labored breathing
Pawing ground	Distended abdomen
Looking at flank	Sweating
Getting up and down	Attempts at vomiting
Muscle tremors	
Possible sweating	

f. **Digestive system examination**
  (1) **Abdominal contour** is usually normal with medical colics. **Distention** is not a feature of serious small intestinal obstruction and most commonly is observed with large intestinal problems that are usually surgical in nature.
  (2) **Sharp molar teeth,** reflective of poor dental occlusion or improper husbandry, may predispose horses to impaction colics.
  (3) **Abdominal auscultation** should be carried out in a comprehensive, systematic way. Normal to increased **borborygmi** usually indicate a good prognosis for medical management. **Hypermotility** indicates early intestinal distention or enteritis. Hypermotility, which results from ischemia or longstanding intestinal obstruction, may also be an initial response to gut ischemia.
  (4) **Method of examination**
    (a) During an **esophageal examination,** use the largest tube possible and a gentle technique, being careful to avoid esophageal perforation. To retrieve reflux, the tube may be primed with a bolus of warm water and gravity flow or suction used. The pH and composition of any fluid should be determined. Low pH fluid (4–5) indicates a gastric source, whereas a higher pH (6–7) indicates that the fluid is from the small intestine. Previously administered medications may be found in the reflux (e.g., mineral oil).
    (b) A **rectal examination,** performed on patients of adequate size, is carried out in a systematic way, identifying normal and abnormal palpable structures. Feces may be present or absent in the rectum, a finding that is not indicative of the colic type. Firm and mucus-covered feces may point to an impaction colic. Sand in the feces is a special case of impaction colic.
  (5) **Abdominocentesis** often is performed as part of the initial database of colic evaluation. Either a **midline** or **paramedian site** is acceptable, and the technique is considered a **minor surgical procedure.**
    (a) A point 10–30 cm caudal to the xiphoid is chosen, and after the skin has been aseptically prepared and desensitized with a local anesthetic, either

TABLE 2-2. Interpretation of Pulse Rate*

Pulse	Rate (beats/minute)
Normal	30–39
Mild	40–59
Moderate	60–79
Serious	80–99
Severe	100+

* Foals will have relatively higher rates than adult horses.

TABLE 2-3. Laboratory Findings With Normal Equine Peritoneal Fluid

	Mean	Range
Total white blood cells ($\times 10^9$/L)	3	1–10
Neutrophils (%)	43	24–62
Lymphocytes (%)	20	4–36
Macrophages (%)	34	17–50
Eosinophils (%)	2	1–6
Red blood cells ($\times 10^{12}$/L)	0	. . .
Total protein (g/L)	0.1	0.05–0.15
Fibrinogen (g/L)	< 10	. . .
Specific gravity	1.005	1–1.015
Color	Yellow	. . .
Turbidity	Slightly cloudy	. . .

a disposable 18-gauge **hypodermic needle** or **blunt cannula** is used to penetrate the peritoneum. When using the blunt cannula, first a stab incision should be made through the skin with a scalpel blade to a depth of approximately 4 mm.

   (b) The tip of a **bitch catheter** or **teat cannula** is inserted through a gauze sponge, which absorbs surface blood. The catheter or cannula is then inserted through the incision.

   (c) Using firm steady pressure, the instrument is advanced into the **peritoneal cavity.** Usually a **final "pop"** is felt when the peritoneum is penetrated.

   (d) **Fluid** should be collected in two clear tubes, one sterile and one containing an anticoagulant, such as ethylenediaminetetraacetic acid (EDTA).

   (e) Results of **fluid analysis** should be normal with medical colics (Tables 2-3 and 2-4).

B. **Medically manageable colics**

   1. Meconium impaction

     a. Patient profile and history. Meconium passage may cause some degree of discomfort in newborn foals but is usually completed in 24–48 hours. Retention of meconium is the most common cause of colic in newborn foals.

TABLE 2-4. Gross Observation of Abnormal Peritoneal Fluid Samples

Fluid Samples	Indications
Flocculent fluid, no odor	Bacterial and toxic peritonitis seen in early infarctive disease
Serosanguineous, no odor	Leakage of RBCs, toxins, and bacteria from necrotic bowel into peritoneal cavity
Sanguinous, malodorous with fecal material	Associated with parietal pain
	Confirms presence of ruptured viscus
	Rectal tear
	Rarely, blood-tinged fluid is present
Frank blood in abdomen	Usually when blood vessel is entered or splenic parenchyma is penetrated
	Rarely neoplasms, such as hemangiosarcoma, may cause abdominal hemorrhage

RBCs = red blood cells.

    b. Clinical findings. There may be repeated attempts by the foal to defecate, which is indicated by straining with an arched back, tail swishing, and restlessness. Foals may develop a high meconium impaction, which is less obvious; signs of obstruction colic and abdominal distention take longer to develop.

    c. Diagnosis. Impactions usually occur in the colon and rectum and can be detected by digital examination. Radiographs are useful for demonstrating high impactions. Sonographic imaging also may be employed to evaluate bowel content, thickness, distention, and motility.

    d. Treatment. Enemas (mild soap and water or commercial types) usually are adequate. Refractory cases may require repeated enemas, intravenous fluids, and finally surgical exploration.

2. Large colon impaction

    a. Patient profile and history. This is one of the most common colics encountered in practice. Large colon impaction may be age-, feed-, or management-related and occurs with some repeatability in certain horses. Horses may have a history of dental problems, recent deworming, or feed or management changes.

    b. Clinical findings. The clinical findings are consistent with a medical colic. There is often slight depression and anorexia. There are no abnormalities of temperature, pulse, and respiration (TPR), but there is evidence of periodic visceral pain when the horse stretches and looks at its flank. There is decreased fecal output, and feces are small, firm, and covered with mucus. Fecal composition may indicate the nature of the impaction (e.g., grain, sand). **Rectal examination** may reveal the site and the degree of the impaction. For example, the pelvic flexure is a common site of large colon impactions. On **gastric intubation,** there is no reflux of stomach contents. **Abdominal auscultation** reveals a generalized decrease in borborygmi.

    c. Etiology and pathogenesis

      (1) Physical agents

        (a) Feed-related. Course roughage may predispose the horse to improper digestion of feedstuffs with a resultant impaction.

        (b) Water-related. Insufficient amounts of water create a dry ingesta prone to impaction.

        (c) Poor teeth. Similar to poorly digestible feeds, improper mastication causes some impactions.

      (2) Parasitic agents. Migrating larval forms of *Strongylus vulgaris* interfere with circulation and innervation of various parts of the large intestine, which affects gut motility and leads to impactions.

      (3) Extraluminal or intraluminal agents. Extraluminal events (e.g., abscesses, neoplasms, adhesions) or intraluminal masses (e.g., enteroliths) produce impaction colics. The majority of these, however, result in chronic, unresponsive colics that must be surgically managed.

    d. Diagnostic plan. The clinical findings often are enough to diagnose the condition of a large intestinal obstruction. The response to therapy also is a valuable diagnostic aid.

    e. Laboratory tests. Hematology and clinical pathology findings are normal. Abdominocentesis, although usually not warranted, yields fluid of normal characteristics.

    f. Differential diagnoses. Differential diagnoses to consider when presented with a large intestinal obstruction include early surgical colics (e.g., strangulating obstructions, nonstrangulating small intestinal obstructions), gastric ulcers, chronic salmonellosis, chronic liver disease (cholelithiasis), and urolithiasis.

    g. Therapeutic plan

      (1) Analgesics. Analgesics may be indicated if discomfort levels of the horse warrant. All of the following agents may be given intravenously or intramuscularly:

        (a) Flunixin meglumine: 1.1 mg/kg every 12 hours

        (b) Xylazine: 0.1–1.0 mg/kg as necessary

        (c) Butorphanol: 0.02–0.05 mg/kg as necessary

        (d) Detomidine: 0.005–0.03 mg/kg as necessary

        (e) Pentazocine: 0.3 mg/kg as necessary

    (2) Laxatives
        (a) Laxatives and **wetting agents** aid in softening the mass. The following substances are all oral medications:
            (i) Mineral oil: 2–4 L every 12 hours
            (ii) Dioctyl sodium sulfosuccinate (DSS): 10–20 mg/kg
            (iii) Bran mashes
        (b) Intravenous or **oral fluids** also may be employed to soften intestinal masses. Doses are empirical.
    (3) Surgery may be necessary if the condition persists, worsens, or if clinical signs become repetitive.
  h. Prevention
    (1) Revisits to the patient or a client's attention to clinical signs are necessary to judge the response to therapy. If repeated doses of analgesics are necessary to control the pain or if the pain increases in intensity or duration, the diagnosis of a primary medically responsive large intestinal impaction must be reassessed. A decision for surgery must be made early for the maximum probability of success.
    (2) Clients need to consider management changes in order to address the risk factors (e.g., feed types, feeding techniques, access to water, dental management, proper parasite control).

3. Distention colic (spasmodic or gas colic)
  a. Patient profile and history. This is a commonly diagnosed colic with similar subjective findings to other medical colics. Horses that crib (windsuck) often seem predisposed to distention colic.
  b. Clinical findings. As with other medical colics, there might be slight increases in TPR. On abdominal auscultation, there may be increased peristaltic activity, particularly between bouts of pain. Abdominal percussion may reveal tympanic sounds of intestinal gas. There will be minimal reflux on nasogastric intubation. Often during a rectal examination, bowel distended with gas is felt.
  c. Etiology and pathogenesis
    (1) Simple distention colics result from intestinal spasm or ileus. The intestine distends with fluid and gas cranial to the site(s) of spasm, causing visceral pain. **Peristalsis** may increase in the distended segments due to local myoelectrical stimulation.
    (2) The **initial cause** of the intestinal spasm or ileus may be related to the same risk factors associated with the development of simple obstruction colics (i.e., parasite migration, feed changes, management deficiencies).
    (3) As a **special case** of distention colics, horses that crib and swallow air cause gastric distention and pain.
  d. Diagnostic plan. The clinical findings should be compared with the degree of pain and response to therapy. Simple distention colics may appear similar to early cases of obstruction colics, strangulating obstruction colics, and nonstrangulating infarctions, which are more serious and may require surgical intervention.
  e. Laboratory tests. Laboratory values are not outside of normal ranges for this condition.
  f. Differential diagnoses. The following categories of colics and specific conditions are surgical in nature but early in their course may appear similar to a simple intestinal distention.
    (1) Nonstrangulating obstructions
        (a) Foreign bodies
        (b) Ascarid impactions (young animals)
        (c) Meconium impaction (foals)
        (d) Muscular hypertrophy of the ileum
        (e) Pedunculated lipomas
        (f) Abscesses
        (g) Adhesions
        (h) Neoplasms
    (2) Strangulating obstructions
        (a) Small intestinal volvulus

> (b) Strangulating lipomas
> (c) Intestinal entrapment—epiploic foramen entrapment, omental defects, mesenteric defects, nephrosplenic ligament entrapment, hernias (inguinal, umbilical, scrotal, diaphragmatic)
>
> **(3) Nonstrangulating infarctions**
> g. **Therapeutic plan.** Treat with analgesics, laxatives, and wetting agents similar to a large colon impaction.
> h. **Prevention.** Discuss treatment, management, and prevention in a similar way to other medical colics.

4. **Proximal enteritis (anterior enteritis, duodenitis)** is an idiopathic syndrome characterized by ileus and transluminal leakage of fluid into the gut. Horses with this condition exhibit moderate colic but marked depression. There are diminished gut sounds and copious gastric reflux.
   a. **Patient profile and history.** This disorder is seen primarily in adult horses. Proximal enteritis is not common in occurrence but is similar in appearance to a small intestinal obstruction, which presents as a surgical colic. There may be a history of recent grain engorgement or heavy grain feeding.
   b. **Clinical findings.** This colic is usually mild, but affected horses are extremely depressed.
      (1) A **fever** is often evident (38.5°C–40.0°C), and the heart rate is increased (60–120 beats/min). An elevated respiratory rate is caused by pain.
      (2) The horse may be **dehydrated,** with resultant signs of fluid volume depletion (e.g., dry and injected mucus membranes, increased capillary refill time, decreased skin elasticity).
      (3) **Gastric reflux** is invariably present with several liters being retrievable. The reflux is green-yellow with an alkaline pH (6–7) indicating small intestinal origin.
      (4) **Peristaltic sounds** are weak, and rectal palpation reveals a slightly distended small intestine. This distention does not increase over time. The course of the disease is 7–10 days.
   c. **Etiology and pathogenesis**
      (1) **Etiology.** Suggested causes include pancreatitis, clostridiosis, verminous arteritis, and gram-negative enteritis (e.g., salmonellosis).
      (2) **Pathogenesis.** The gastric reflux produces the pain associated with the condition. There is an associated **toxemia** with varying signs of shock, coagulopathy, laminitis, and renal dysfunction. **Postmortem findings** demonstrate inflammation and degeneration of duodenal intestinal mucosa. A fibrinopurulent exudate is present on the serosal surface. Lesions are less commonly found in the jejunum or at the pylorus.
   d. **Diagnostic plan.** The determination of a clinical diagnosis is challenging. A horse with mild to moderate pain, severe depression, and fever is more likely to have an enteritis than small intestinal obstruction. There is, however, gastric reflux in both instances. A small intestinal obstruction causes a progressive deterioration in clinical signs, whereas a proximal enteritis has a steadier course and pain that is relieved by nasogastric intubation.
   e. **Laboratory tests**
      (1) The packed cell volume (PCV) and total serum protein (TSP) are elevated, which indicates **dehydration.**
      (2) There is **hypokalemia** due to potassium sequestration in the small intestine.
      (3) There may be a **hypochloremic, metabolic alkalosis** due to HCl pooling in the stomach, but serum electrolytes are usually within normal ranges.
      (4) The **complete blood cell count (CBC)** may show a white blood cell picture indicative of an infective or inflammatory response.
      (5) Results of an **abdominocentesis** are nondiagnostic. There may be an increase in protein content of the abdominal fluid, but cellular components are usually normal.
   f. **Differential diagnosis.** Rule out small intestinal colics of a surgical nature (e.g., strangulating obstructions). Also, consider primary causes of enterocolitis (e.g., salmonellosis).

g. **Therapeutic plan.** The therapy remains empirical but needs to be aggressive. Removal of gastric fluid must be carried out by repeated or continuous nasogastric intubation. Large volumes of intravenous fluids (balance electrolytes or saline, depending on blood pH) should be administered. Pharmacologic agents include flunixin meglumine (0.25 mg/kg twice daily) and penicillin–gentamicin combination. It may also be necessary to treat concurrent disease (e.g., laminitis; see Chapter 13 III A 5). Therapy may need to be continued for up to 10 days before gastric reflux ceases and normal eating resumes.

5. **Flatulent colic (tympany, bloat, wind colic)**
   a. **Patient profile and history.** Adult horses are affected with this type of colic under conditions of recent stress or management changes. Histories might include any of the following:
      (1) Overfeeding on highly fermentable feed
      (2) Cold-water engorgement
      (3) Feeding while exhausted or overheated
      (4) Moldy hay or grain feed
      (5) Behavioral abnormalities (e.g., cribbing, greedy eaters)
      (6) Medication administration, such as atropine or broad spectrum antibiotics
   b. **Clinical findings**
      (1) Animals appear in **distress** and TPR is elevated out of proportion to other clinical signs.
      (2) **Abdominal distention** may be evident if gas is contained in the colon or cecum. Cecal tympany causes filling in the right paralumbar fossa, whereas bilateral abdominal distention occurs with large colon gas accumulation.
      (3) **Gastric distention** is not evident externally. Simultaneous auscultation and percussion may reveal the location of the distended viscus.
      (4) **Pain** and signs of colic accompany the visceral distention. Often, the **distended gut** is palpable per the rectum (excluding cranial viscera, such as the stomach). Passage of a nasogastric tube often relieves any gastric distention.
   c. **Etiology and pathogenesis**
      (1) Flatulent or tympanic colic results from **excessive gas accumulation** in the intestinal tract. The overdistention of viscera stimulates pain and pressure receptors, causing mild to severe colics. The severe forms mimic surgical colics.
      (2) **Gaseous distention** usually is caused by increased fermentation and gas production, air accumulation (e.g., as with cribbing), or ineffectual gastrointestinal tract motility, causing gas buildup.
      (3) Gas may accumulate anywhere along the gastrointestinal tract, resulting in some variation in the clinical findings.
   d. **Diagnostic plan.** This condition is diagnosed on clinical findings. It is important to note the disproportionate degree of pain relative to other findings that are absent (e.g., shock). This helps differentiate the condition as a medical colic.
   e. **Laboratory tests.** Laboratory findings are normal on hematology and abdominocentesis.
   f. **Therapeutic plan**
      (1) Employ **nasogastric intubation** to relieve stomach distention if this is the source of the colic. Treat with sedatives and analgesics (e.g., xylazine, butorphanol, pentazocine, detomidine). Administer mineral oil for its anti-fermentative properties.
      (2) If medical therapy is ineffective, **trocarization** of the cecum or colon may provide relief. This is a relatively radical therapy but may provide temporary relief until medical intervention can work to alleviate the problem. Trocarization must be carried out in an aseptic manner.
         (a) Determine the site of trocarization by simultaneous auscultation and percussion.
         (b) Block the site with local anesthetic, then use a number 15 scalpel blade to pierce the skin.
         (c) A 14-cm trocar is used to penetrate the abdominal wall and lumen of the bowel. Hold the trocar in place until gas is no longer free flowing.

(d) Inject 10–20 ml of antibiotic as the trocar is withdrawn, and place the horse on systemic antibiotics.

g. **Prevention.** The prognosis for uncomplicated cases of flatulent colic is usually favorable.

II. DIARRHEA.

II. **DIARRHEA.** The large intestine of the horse has tremendous water absorptive capabilities. Diarrhea (acute or chronic) results from large intestinal pathology or pathological changes to the small intestine that cause an overwhelming amount of fluid and ingesta to be presented to the large intestine.

A. **Acute diarrhea in adult horses**

1. **Salmonellosis**
   a. **Patient profile and history.** Salmonellosis is usually a sporadic disease in single animals unless in a referral center setting or in a barn or stable with frequent animal movement on and off premises. Salmonellosis infection may take various forms. The acute diarrheic form is most often seen in weanlings and young performance horses that are stressed following transport, shows, or surgery.
   b. **Clinical findings.** Clinical salmonellosis has a spectrum of clinical expression. The enteric form in the adult may be asymptomatic, mild, acute severe, or chronic.
      (1) **Mild infections** are associated with fever, anorexia, depression, and the production of poorly formed feces (cow-pie).
      (2) With **acute severe infections,** fever and depression is seen during the first 24–48 hours. Simultaneous with this is mild to severe abdominal pain. At this time, the condition can be confused with a surgical colic. Diarrhea begins sometime after the initial signs but may take 2–4 days to develop. Diarrhea is projectile, foul smelling, and persistent. Expression of diarrhea often is accompanied by improvement in the other clinical signs. Horses usually continue to eat, but in the case of anorexic animals, the prognosis for survival is poor.
      (3) The diarrhea may persist for 3–4 weeks, at which time horses will have experienced significant weight loss. Ventral edema caused by hypoproteinemia also may be a finding. Laminitis is a frequent sequela to salmonellosis.
      (4) A peracute form of enteric salmonellosis may occur; affected horses die within 6–12 hours.
   c. **Etiology and pathogenesis**
      (1) **Etiology.** *Salmonella typhimurium* is the isolate most commonly associated with equine diarrhea (60% of cases). The organism adheres to and invades the mucosa of the intestine. The development of enteritis is then dependent on factors such as the age of host, immune status, other stressors, and virulence of the organism strain.
      (2) **Pathogenesis**
         (a) Diarrhea and enteritis result from the effects of the bacteria and host inflammatory mediators (prostaglandins). There is an increased secretion of chloride, sodium, and water into the intestinal lumen via an increase in mucosal cell cyclic adenosine monophosphate (cAMP) content.
         (b) The characteristic fever and leukopenia are caused by the release of lipopolysaccharide endotoxin from the bacterial cell wall. White blood cells pool at the site of the infection, and protein leakage occurs across permeable intestinal vessel walls.
   d. **Diagnostic plan.** The diagnosis is based on clinical findings supported by laboratory confirmation.
   e. **Laboratory tests**
      (1) **Hematologic findings** are a neutropenia with a left shift and varying degrees of cellular morphologic changes (toxicity). The albumin fraction of the TSP is low, although the total protein may be elevated or normal due to dehydration. The PCV is elevated due to dehydration, and the horse will have a metabolic acidosis with electrolyte losses through the feces.

(2) **Fecal culture** for *Salmonella* may be unrewarding because of the dilution effect of diarrhea and the adherent nature of the bacteria to the intestinal mucosa. A rectal mucosal biopsy may enhance the likelihood of culturing the organism.

f. **Differential diagnoses** include equine monocytic ehrlichiosis, intestinal clostridiosis, antibiotic-induced diarrhea, proximal enteritis, and small intestinal obstruction.

g. **Therapeutic plan**

(1) Of primary consideration is **fluid replacement therapy,** with large volumes of alkalinizing fluids.

(2) The use of **antibiotics** is controversial and perhaps best restricted to bacteremic or septicemic manifestations of salmonellosis in foals. If antibiotics are used in the enteric form of the disease, those with gram-negative specificity are recommended (e.g., gentamicin, amikacin, trimethoprim–sulfa combinations). **Flunixin meglumine** is recommended for its anti-inflammatory effect.

(3) **Bismuth subsalicylate** is recommended as an intestinal protectant and antiprostaglandin. It turns the feces black.

(4) **Plasma transfusions** may be necessary in hypoproteinemic horses. **Heparin** may be used in cases of coagulopathies [e.g., disseminated intravascular coagulation (DIC)] associated with the disease.

h. **Prevention**

(1) Horses with diarrhea should be **isolated** in a separate barn if possible. Caretakers should wear dedicated and **protective clothing.** A **foot bath** should be used at the entrance to the facility. Manure from cases should be handled and disposed of in a secure and separate way. *Salmonella* species are zoonotic.

(2) In-contact animals should be cultured to identify fecal shedders. External sources of contamination (e.g., feed) should be examined particularly if multiple serotypes appear in several animals. Monitor stablemates for evidence of increases in body temperature or the appearance of lassitude. A total white blood cell count may be performed on suspect animals, and if a neutropenia is present (which often precedes clinical signs), isolation and therapy should be instituted.

(3) Most common **disinfectants** are effective against *Salmonella* species; however, sanitation is challenging because of the difficulty of removing all organic material. Recovered horses may become shedders, some chronically. However, shedding for more than 6 weeks is uncommon with most serotypes.

2. **Equine monocytic ehrlichiosis (acute equine diarrhea syndrome, Potomac horse fever)**

a. **Patient profile and history**

(1) First described in the United States Northeast, this disease is now evident throughout North America and has been recorded in Europe. It is seasonal in occurrence, with summer being the most common time of incidence. Any age group of animal may be affected, but the disease peaks in adult animals at age 12 years. It is most often found in Thoroughbred horses on pasture. Females are more at risk than males, and it is usually sporadic with single horses on any given farm.

(2) The owner may report a mild depression and anorexia followed by diarrhea.

b. **Clinical findings**

(1) Cardinal signs are anorexia, fever (39.5°C), injected mucous membranes, and depression. A profuse, watery diarrhea commences 24–48 hours after the onset of fever and lasts up to 10 days in the majority of animals. Mild abdominal pain with decreased borborygmi is evident.

(2) **Laminitis** may be a sequela in 25% of cases. Occasional horses may show injected mucous membranes, severe abdominal distention, and abdominal pain. Frequently, death ensues before diarrhea develops. Abortion may occur in pregnant mares.

c. **Etiology and pathogenesis.** *Ehrlichia risticii* is the etiologic agent. The organism has a predilection for mononuclear cells and is hypothesized to be spread by an arthropod vector.

d. **Diagnostic plan.** Indirect fluorescent antibody (FA) may be performed on serum collected at 1- to 3-week intervals. Serum should be separated promptly and submitted cool but not frozen because freezing lowers the antibody titre. A latex agglutination test has also been developed for diagnosis.

e. **Therapeutic plan.** Supportive care is essential, as with any acute enteritis. Tetracycline at 6.6 mg/kg administered intravenously once per day (if given 24 hours after the onset of fever) for 5 days results in a dramatic response. Diarrhea does not develop. Treatment with tetracyclines after the onset of diarrhea does not alter the course of the disease.

f. **Prevention.** Treatment is costly and often futile when full clinical signs develop. A vaccine is now available that seems to protect approximately 75% of horses.

3. **Colitis X**

   a. **Patient profile and history.** This is a sporadic disease associated with a history of recent stress in adult horses.

   b. **Clinical findings.** A short febrile period is followed by a normal to subnormal body temperature. There is marked tachypnea, hyperpnea, and depression. There is a rapidly developing, intense dehydration and occasional abdominal pain. The horse may die before diarrhea is evident.

   c. **Etiology and pathogenesis.** The causative agent is believed to be *Clostridium perfringens* type A. Clinical signs result from an enterotoxemia.

   d. **Diagnostic plan.** The condition usually is diagnosed post mortem.

   e. **Therapeutic plan.** Intensive therapy with massive quantities of isotonic saline and added bicarbonate is required to combat the dehydration and metabolic acidosis. Supplemental **potassium therapy** also may be necessary. Plasma transfusions may be warranted if hypoproteinemia is present. Flunixin meglumine and heparin also may be employed. **Antimicrobial therapy** may include penicillin–aminoglycoside or trimethoprim–sulfa combinations.

   f. **Prevention.** Little can be recommended to the client to prevent or treat this highly fatal, sporadic disease.

4. **Antibiotic-associated enteritis**

   a. **Patient profile and history.** There are anecdotal reports of enteritis in horses following antibiotic administration. **Tetracycline** is the antibiotic most often incriminated, but lincomycin, tylosin, and high doses of penicillin and erythromycin also have been associated with the disease. There also have been reports of diarrhea after the use of trimethoprim–sulfa drugs.

   b. **Clinical findings.** The frequency of enteritis associated with most of these drugs is low enough that they continue to be used when indicated. Typical signs of acute enteritis develop. Signs may subside rapidly when the antibiotics are discontinued.

   c. **Etiology and pathogenesis.** Antibiotics may upset the normal gut flora, allowing overgrowth by nonpathogenic or pathogenic bacteria. Pathogenic bacteria (e.g., salmonella, clostridia), when established, may have rapidly fatal consequences. Occasionally, chronic diarrhea has been seen in association with *Salmonella* isolated from the feces.

   d. **Therapeutic plan.** Discontinue the antibiotic use, and treat as other acute diarrheas.

5. **Intestinal clostridiosis**

   a. **Patient profile and history.** The disease affects horses that are most commonly over 1 year of age. The disease is sporadic and may be accompanied by the history of recent, severe stress. Although reported as a distinct condition, intestinal clostridiosis may be similar or identical to colitis X.

   b. **Clinical findings.** The disease is of peracute onset with profound depression, tachycardia, dehydration, and diarrhea, which is profuse and malodorous. Shock is evidenced by a rapid heart rate and cardiovascular compromise. Affected animals die within 24 hours of the onset of clinical signs.

   c. **Etiology and pathogenesis.** *C. perfringens* type A is the etiologic agent.
   d. **Laboratory tests.** *C. perfringens* counts may be performed on the feces. Laboratory findings are consistent with dehydration and circulatory collapse.
   e. **Therapeutic plan.** Massive **fluid therapy** is essential for any hope of success. Antibiotics are of little value, but penicillins may be employed as a logical choice for antibacterial therapy.

6. **Gastrointestinal ulceration [nonsteroidal anti-inflammatory drug (NSAID) toxicity]**
   a. **Patient profile and history.** Foals and young animals are extremely susceptible to NSAIDs. However, older horses occasionally are affected if the manufacturer's recommended dosages are grossly exceeded.
   b. **Clinical findings.** Diarrhea is an occasional clinical finding, but more commonly the condition is associated with recurrent abdominal pain, anorexia, and weight loss. Oral ulceration with excessive salivation may be evident. Dependent edema may be a finding.
   c. **Etiology and pathogenesis.** NSAIDs (e.g., phenylbutazone) produce **toxic side effects** if used in excess or in dehydrated horses. Organ systems most commonly affected include the gastrointestinal tract, kidneys, and hematopoietic system. Toxicity of the gastrointestinal tract results from depletion of protective prostaglandins (such as PE_2). These prostaglandins normally decrease gastric acid secretion and increase the protective layer of gastric mucosa. The agents also may produce vasoconstriction, resulting in devitalization and ulceration of mucosa along the entire intestinal tract. **Oral ulceration** is caused by the local irritative effect of the drug.
   d. **Diagnostic plan.** Diagnosis is based most often on clinical findings and a history of long-standing or overzealous use of phenylbutazone. The diagnosis may be supported by endoscopy of the stomach or double-contrast gastric radiography in foals and ponies. These techniques reveal ulceration of the glandular portion of the stomach.
   e. **Laboratory tests.** Laboratory tests may be helpful by revealing a hypoproteinemia and hypoalbuminemia from protein leakage across a reduced and devitalized gastrointestinal mucosa. Occult blood may be found in the feces, accompanied by a lowered hematocrit.
   f. **Therapeutic plan**
      (1) Discontinue all NSAIDs, and administer 1–2 g/100 kg of sucralfate orally four times daily and 6 mg/kg cimetidine orally, intravenously, or intramuscularly 2–3 times per day. Ranitidine may be substituted for cimetidine at 1–3 mg/kg orally twice daily or at 0.5 mg/kg intravenously twice daily. Plasma transfusions may be warranted in cases of severe hypoproteinemia.
      (2) Intravenous feeding or nasogastric intubation and alimentation may be necessary.
   g. **Prevention.** Phenylbutazone should be used with caution in ponies, younger horses, and dehydrated animals. Foals that are heavily parasitized or malnourished are extremely prone to toxic side effects.

7. **Fungal enteritis**
   a. **Patient profile and history.** Fungal enteritides are sporadic in occurrence.
   b. **Clinical findings.** The condition is indistinguishable from other acute diarrheas. Cases usually present with severe toxemia, profound dehydration, and severe, profuse, watery diarrhea.
   c. **Etiology and pathogenesis.** Fungal overgrowth of the gastrointestinal tract and lungs may occur due to immunocompromise or secondary to extensive antibiotic use.
   d. **Diagnostic plan.** There is little help for diagnosis. Fecal fungal elements occasionally may be found.
   e. **Therapeutic plan.** There is no known treatment.

B. **Diarrhea in nursing foals**

1. **Foal heat diarrhea**

a. **Patient profile and history.** Foals often develop diarrhea between 6 and 14 days of age. This may correspond with the dam's first postpartum estrus.

b. **Clinical findings.** The foal presents with soft to watery feces, but all other signs are usually within normal limits. There may be mild dehydration, but foals are generally alert with normal appetites. The condition is most often self-limiting in 2–3 days but may precede other diarrheas in the same foal.

c. **Etiology and pathogenesis.** The etiology of foal heat diarrhea is unknown but may be associated with a changeover of cell type as the intestinal mucosa of the neonate matures. Other postulated but less likely causes include hormonal or nutritional alterations in the mare's milk, coprophagia, *Strongyloides westeri* infestation, and alterations in intestinal microbiological flora.

d. **Diagnostic plan.** The diagnosis usually is based on clinical findings without the need for laboratory support.

e. **Therapeutic plan.** Therapy is dictated by the severity of the diarrhea. Uncomplicated cases may be treated with simple attention to nursing care, such as washing the perineum and applying petroleum jelly. If diarrhea persists beyond 3 days, treatment with 1–2 ml/kg bismuth subsalicylate four times per day orally and oral fluid replacement with commercial calf formulations should be considered.

2. **Nutritional diarrheas**

a. **Clinical findings.** Diarrhea may range from soft feces to very watery stool. Other clinical findings are usually normal, and the foal may have a normal attitude and appetite.

b. **Etiology and pathogenesis.** Diarrhea may develop secondarily to the following situations:

(1) **Ingestion of excessive amounts of milk.** This may occur with foals that are greedy eaters or when the mare and foal are reunited after a period of separation. Normally, a milk clot forms in the stomach within minutes of ingestion, and the whey advances to the small intestine in gradual amounts as the clot contracts. Overingestion can result in excessive amounts of whey entering the duodenum, overwhelming absorptive capabilities and creating an osmotic drive towards fluid accumulation in the gut.

(2) **Abnormal nursing.** Foals that ingest milk too rapidly or are fed by nasogastric tube experience decreased salivary secretion, which adversely affects milk dilution and clot digestion.

(3) **Sudden dietary changes**

(4) **Ingestion of fibrous material.** Grain, forage, mare's feces, or other fibrous material require digestion in the immature large intestine of the foal. This promotes indigestion and diarrhea.

(5) **Carbohydrate intolerance.** Young foals may have primary or secondary carbohydrate intolerance. Primary milk intolerance is relatively rare. Secondary carbohydrate intolerance results from an enteric infection, which causes an increase in mucosal cell turnover. More immature cells make up the absorptive cell component of the gut mucosa, decreasing the disaccharidase and absorptive activities in the mucosal brush border.

c. **Diagnostic plan.** The diagnosis is most often based on clinical findings and history. Diarrhea is usually self-limiting but may be unresponsive in the case of primary carbohydrate intolerance.

d. **Laboratory tests.** Laboratory findings are unrewarding. In the case of an unresponsive milk intolerance, a lactose tolerance test may be performed. Lactose is administered per os, and corresponding blood glucose levels are determined.

e. **Therapeutic plan**

(1) **Nursing care** may be the only therapy necessary in the case of short-lived diarrheas. Lactose intolerance presents a special case, in that continued exposure to a milk diet exacerbates the problem.

(2) **Elimination of milk** and **dietary replacement** with hand feeding of a commercial soy-based milk supplement may be necessary until the foal can be weaned back on whole milk. A commercial calf diarrhea oral replacement solution may aid in the recovery.

(3) A commercially available **lactase enzyme preparation** may be added to milk before feeding to partially digest lactose into its constituent monosaccharides.

3. **Antibiotic-related diarrheas**
   a. **Patient profile and history.** Oral antibiotics, such as aminoglycosides, may kill normal gut flora and predispose foals to diarrhea. Systemic antibiotics with an enterohepatic circulation (oxytetracycline, lincomycin, erythromycin) also have been shown to induce diarrhea.
   b. **Clinical findings.** Diarrhea may range from soft feces to very watery stool. The foal's appearance may range from systemically normal to significantly dehydrated with circulatory collapse.
   c. **Diagnostic plan.** The diagnosis is based on clinical signs, history, and response to therapy.
   d. **Therapeutic plan.** Stop antibiotic therapy. Oral administration of a slurry of fresh feces from an older horse may be beneficial in restoration of gut flora but is not proven for efficacy.

4. **Mechanical irritation**
   a. **Patient profile and history.** Young or older foals may be affected by consuming inordinate amounts of sand or dirt. Sand has an abrasive effect on the intestinal mucosa, resulting in enteritis and diarrhea. Also, physical impaction may result from the accumulation of sediment.
   b. **Diagnostic plan.** Demonstration of sand in the feces aids in the diagnosis. Sand can be seen by mixing feces with water in a rectal sleeve, then identifying and quantifying the gritty sediment.
   c. **Therapeutic plan.** Repeated therapy is necessary. Mineral oil may be used if an impaction is suspected. However, for elimination of sand over time, an agent producing fecal bulk is preferable. Bran, in the case of older foals, or psyllium hydrophylia muciloid is recommended at 0.5 kg/454 kg four times per day orally for days or weeks.
   d. **Prevention.** Foals or horses that actively eat soil are difficult to manage. Feeding from elevated mangers and ensuring adequate pasture cover may be effective in preventing further cases.

5. **Diarrhea caused by *Strongyloides westeri***
   a. **Patient profile and history**
      (1) *S. westeri* infestations occur when the foal ingests infective larvae in the dam's milk. The greatest number of larvae are shed 2–3 weeks postpartum. The prepatent period is 8–14 days.
      (2) It is speculated that diarrhea is associated with larval burdens. The larvae may cause intestinal mucosal damage and suppression of disaccharidase or polypeptidase production. However, foals with high fecal egg counts may have no evidence of diarrhea. Conversely, diarrhea may occur in foals with very low fecal egg counts. Thus, causation is speculative.
   b. **Diagnostic plan.** The diagnosis may be strengthened by the presence of *S. westeri* larvae in the mare's milk or the characteristic embryonated eggs in the foal's feces.
   c. **Therapeutic plan.** Various anthelmintics are effective against the adult parasites, including ivermectin at 200 μg/kg, thiabendazole at 50 mg/kg, cambendazole at 20 mg/kg, and oxibendazole at 10 mg/kg. The daily administration of cambendazole at 30 mg/kg to postparturient mares eliminates infective larvae in the milk for the duration of therapy.

6. **Bacterial enteric disease**
   a. **Patient profile and history.** The incidence of bacterial-induced diarrheas in foals is much lower than in other domestic species. Generally, if bacteria cause the diarrhea, there is a concomitant systemic disease. These systemic conditions (e.g., salmonellosis, *Actinobacillus equuli* bacteremia) are covered in Chapter 18.
   b. **Etiology and pathogenesis**
      (1) **Enteric colibacillosis** caused by *Escherichia coli* has been documented but is

of very low incidence. Normal foal management practices may limit the occurrence of this condition.

    (2) ***Clostridium perfringens* types A, B,** and **C** have been associated with enteritis and death in foals. ***C. difficile*** may be involved in the pathogenesis of acute enterocolitis or a more mild diarrhea.

  c. Differential diagnoses. Rule out causes of septicemia.

  d. Therapeutic plan. Treatment of bacterial enteric disease is as for neonatal calves [see Chapter 3 II B 3 a (6)].

7. Viral enteritis

  a. Patient profile and history

    (1) **Rotavirus** is a definitive cause of diarrhea in foals. Clinical signs occur in foals under 3 months of age. Diarrhea can occur in individual animals or in farm outbreaks. Rotavirus in foals produces a profuse watery diarrhea, and foals may become dehydrated, depressed, and anorexic. The diarrhea may last for days or weeks.

    (2) **Coronavirus** has been associated with diarrhea, but an etiologic relationship has not been established.

    (3) **Adenovirus** produces diarrhea as part of a severe clinical disease of combined immunodeficiency (CID) in Arabian foals.

    (4) Chronically affected foals become unthrifty as mucosal cell damage results in nutrient malabsorption.

  b. Etiology and pathogenesis. Enteric viruses produce gut pathology. Rotavirus is a prime example of gut pathology. The virus invades enteric mucosal cells, causing absorptive cell loss and compensatory crypt-cell hyperplasia with a resultant malabsorptive and hypersecretory diarrhea.

  c. Diagnostic plan. The virus is shed in greatest quantity early in the infection. Diagnosis depends on the demonstration of virus in the feces through electronmicroscopy, enzyme-linked immunosorbent assay (ELISA), or latex agglutination.

  d. Therapeutic plan. Treatment consists of nursing care and oral or intravenous fluids. Bismuth subsalicylate and lactobacillus culture may be administered orally. Total parenteral nutrition may be indicated if diarrhea is persistent.

  e. Prevention. Rotavirus persists in the environment and may be intermittently shed by carriers. The disease may occur under conditions of poor hygiene, overcrowding, or stress. **Vaccination** has not proven successful. Bovine colostrum, containing rotavirus antibodies, has provided some protection.

8. Cryptosporidiosis

  a. Patient profile and history. The disease occurs in foals less often than in calves but has been documented as a cause of diarrhea in foals 5 days to 6 weeks of age.

  b. Clinical findings. The diarrhea is of varying severity and self-limiting. *Cryptosporidium* species often act in concert with other agents, which complicates the clinical picture. Dehydration, anorexia, and weight loss all may accompany the diarrhea.

  c. Etiology and pathogenesis. The protozoan parasite, *C. parvum*, is ingested as a sporulated oocyst and matures through six major developmental stages. Some maturation events occur within the cells of the distal small intestine, cecum, and colon. Villous atrophy with malabsorption and diarrhea result.

  d. Diagnostic plan. The disease must be differentiated from other causes of neonatal diarrhea in foals.

  e. Laboratory tests. Fecal oocysts can be detected by the staining of fecal smears, fecal flotation, or immunofluorescence.

  f. Therapeutic plan. There is no known treatment for cryptosporidiosis, and animals are cared for symptomatically, with oral or intravenous fluids if necessary.

  g. Prevention. The transmission of infective oocysts is through a fecal–oral route. Therefore, hygiene and management changes may be warranted if a number of foals are affected. The disease is a zoonosis and is of particular concern in immunocompromised people. Proper personal hygiene is imperative when handling infective cases.

C. **Diarrhea in weanlings and yearlings**

1. **Parasite burdens**
   a. **Patient profile and history.** Intestinal parasites produce diarrhea and other clinical signs relative to the parasite. Intestinal parasites are ubiquitous and, under conditions of poor management techniques, produce serious problems.
   b. **Clinical findings.** The clinical findings with intestinal parasite infestation include diarrhea, poor weight gain, unthrifty appearance, colic, depression, inappetence, and occasional elevations in body temperature.
   c. **Etiology and pathogenesis**
      (1) *Parascaris equorum* has a prepatent period of 10–13 weeks and will cause diarrhea if present in large numbers. Foals ingest eggs from the environment, and migrating larvae induce inflammatory lesions in various viscera. The infection is very common in foals, but a natural immunity soon develops. Eggs are shed by infected animals and are highly resistant to the elements.
      (2) *Strongylus vulgaris* and *S. edentatus* induce diarrhea primarily by larval migration. The prepatent periods are 6 months and 11 months, respectively for the two parasites. Foals are infected by ingesting infective eggs while grazing contaminated pastures. *S. vulgaris* more commonly causes diarrhea.
   d. **Diagnostic plan.** Diagnosis depends on clinical findings, laboratory tests, and response to therapy.
   e. **Laboratory tests.** Fecal egg flotation aids in the diagnosis, although negative flotations in the face of significant worm burdens may be expected before the shedding of eggs by adult worms. Conversely, the presence of strongyle eggs in the feces of young foals may be caused by coprophagia.
   f. **Therapeutic plan**
      (1) For *P. equorum,* piperazine at 88 mg of base/kg is effective for the removal of adult worms. Foals should be dewormed at 8-week intervals to remove the adult worms before patency.
      (2) Several of the benzimidazoles, as well as pyrantel pamoate and ivermectin, are effective against *S. vulgaris* larvae.
   g. **Prevention.** An effective parasite-control program cannot be overemphasized. This should include deworming often and at regular intervals, pasture decontamination, and sound hygiene practices.

2. **Salmonellosis**
   a. **Patient profile and history.** *Salmonella* species, most commonly *S. typhimurium,* produce an acute diarrhea or septicemia in any age horse.
   b. **Diagnosis** and recommendations for **therapy** and control are the same as for the adult (see II A 1).

3. *Rhodococcus equi* **diarrhea**
   a. **Patient profile and history.** Affected foals range between 4–8 months of age, and there is usually a history of respiratory infection or *R. equi* isolation on the farm.
   b. **Clinical findings.** Feces have a variable consistency but are usually watery. Weight loss is common.
   c. **Etiology and pathogenesis**
      (1) The organism may be ubiquitous in the environment with many foals exposed; however, comparatively few foals develop clinical disease. **Route of infection** by *R. equi* is aerogenous [see Chapter 7 I A 2 b (2)]. Bacteria also may gain access via the oral route.
      (2) **Parasitic larval migration** may spread the bacteria through the lungs or colon, seeding down viscera with abscesses. Gastrointestinal disease may occur without primary lung involvement.
      (3) **Gastrointestinal signs** are referable to abscesses within the gastrointestinal wall or mesenteric lymph nodes.
   d. **Diagnostic plan.** A history of *R. equi* pneumonia on the premise aids in diagnosis, but a definitive diagnosis is difficult.
   e. **Laboratory tests.** Fecal staining and culture may reveal *R. equi;* however, the organism may be shed in the feces of normal foals. There may be an elevation in γ-globulins and fibrinogen, as well as a leukocytosis.

    f. Therapeutic plan. Extended therapy with erythromycin in combination with rifampin is recommended for the respiratory disease [see Chapter 7 I A 2 b (2) (f)].

    g. Prevention. The prognosis is poor to grave with intestinal disease caused by *R. equi.*

III. WEIGHT LOSS

A. Granulomatous enteritis (lymphocytic-plasmacytic enteritis)

1. **Patient profile and history.** This condition is relatively uncommon, sporadic in occurrence, and found in adult horses. There is no demonstrable breed or sex predilection. The history usually includes weight loss despite adequate nutrition and feed consumption.

2. **Clinical findings.** Diarrhea is infrequent, but thinness of the animal is evident. The horse may have ventral edema. Rectal examination may reveal a roughened, friable rectal mucosa, thick-walled intestines, and prominent mesenteric lymph nodes or abdominal masses.

3. **Etiology and pathogenesis**
   a. This condition appears to be an **immunologic phenomenon** that is poorly understood. It may present as a spectrum of inflammatory bowel disease in the horse. The bowel disease results in a malabsorption syndrome.
   b. **Agents** postulated to be involved in this immune-mediated condition include dietary constituents, cell wall components, infectious agents (e.g., mycobacteria), and internal parasites (e.g., *Strongylus vulgaris* larvae, cyathostomes).
   c. **Granulomatous changes** are most evident in the mucosa of the small intestine. Histological examination reveals infiltration of the lamina propria by mononuclear cells. Absorptive capabilities are compromised and protein leakage occurs into the lumen.

4. **Diagnostic plan.** The diagnosis is based on history, clinical findings, laboratory data, and the unresponsiveness of the condition.

5. **Laboratory tests.** There is marked hypoproteinemia and hypoalbuminemia. Occasionally, acid-fast organisms may be found in the feces or on rectal biopsy. Specific carbohydrate absorption tests (e.g., D-xylose absorption test) may show reduced absorption capabilities. Concurrent albumin loss may be measured by labeled albumin clearance into the feces (chromium 51).

6. **Therapeutic plan.** Therapy is not affective but is often attempted before a definitive diagnosis. Treatments include nutritional support, antiparasitasides, and corticosteroids.

B. Chronic eosinophilic gastroenteritis. This disease is similar in most respects to granulomatous enteritis and the resultant malabsorptive process. Differences include:

1. Incidence in younger horses

2. The excessive infiltration of eosinophils that is found throughout the gastrointestinal tract, associated organs, and skin

C. Lymphosarcoma

1. **Patient profile and history.** There is a wide age range of affected horses, but younger horses are more commonly affected.

2. **Clinical findings.** The clinical findings depend on the organ system involved, but if the gastrointestinal system is infiltrated by lymphocytes, the condition resembles other infiltrative diseases. If the skin or superficial lymph nodes are involved, the most obvious clinical finding may be cutaneous nodules.

3. **Etiology and pathogenesis.** No causative agent has been associated with this tumor in horses.

4. **Diagnostic plan.** The diagnosis is based on clinical findings, laboratory data, and the unresponsiveness of the condition.

5. **Laboratory tests.** Neoplastic lymphocytes may be found in a peripheral blood smear. A bone marrow aspirate or abdominocentesis may show neoplastic lymphocytes. There will be hypoproteinemia and hypoalbuminemia. Liver enzymes may be elevated with hepatic involvement.

6. **Therapeutic plan.** There is no treatment for this condition.

D. **Gastric ulceration/gastritis** (see II A 6)

E. **Parasitism**

1. **Patient profile and history.** Parasitism is one of the most common causes of weight loss and chronic diarrhea in horses. It should not be overlooked, particularly in younger animals. Parasitism is most clinically significant in the young, weak, or stressed animal. Management factors, such as overcrowding, inadequate nutrition, and neglecting pasture rotation, or parasite prophylaxis all greatly impact the internal parasite burdens. It is most commonly a disease of populations of horses. Poor thrift and recurrent abdominal pain (episodes of colic) may be historical findings in individual animals.

2. **Clinical findings.** The animal may present as thin with a poor haircoat. Diarrhea of varying degrees is a common finding. If a rectal examination can be performed, the anterior mesenteric artery may feel roughened or exhibit fremitus. Inappetence, anemia, and a low-grade fever also may be present to varying degrees.

3. **Etiology and pathogenesis**
   a. **Large strongyles** cause intestinal ischemia through the migration of larval forms within the walls of blood vessels supplying portions of the large intestine. Intestinal damage may also be caused directly, as larvae mature within the walls of the large intestine and cecum and emerge into the lumen. Ulceration and erosion of the cecum and colon also result from feeding of adult strongyles.
   b. **Cyathostomes (small strongyles)** cause less damage, except under the specific conditions of simultaneous maturation of many hypobiotic larvae. In this case, significant intestinal damage occurs with resultant diarrhea and rapid weight loss.

4. **Diagnostic plan.** The diagnosis is most often made on clinical signs and environmental and management history. Other horses on the premises often show evidence of harboring a parasite burden. For individual animals where verminous arteritis is considered, ultrasonography may be an aid to diagnosis.

5. **Laboratory tests**
   a. **Fecal egg counts** are the best diagnostic but may be negative if clinical signs are caused primarily by larval forms of the parasite(s). Egg counts are also affected by host immunity, species of parasite, and history of treatment.
   b. **Clinical pathology findings** of some help in individually affected animals include eosinophilia, an increase in β-globulins, and an abdominocentesis consistent with chronic abscessation (macrophages with ingested bacteria, eosinophilia, increased protein content, increased leukocytes).

6. **Therapeutic plan.** There are many effective, broad spectrum anthelmintics that may be used for large strongyle or cyathostome infestation.
   a. The **most common** and efficacious treatments are:
      (1) Ivermectin paste—0.2 mg/kg
      (2) Oxibendazole—10 mg/kg
      (3) Benzimidazoles plus piperazine
   b. For **migrating larval forms** of the strongyles producing verminous arteritis, the following treatments may be employed:
      (1) Ivermectin at 0.2 mg/kg and oxfendazole at 10 mg/kg in single doses

      (2) Fenbendazole—7.5–10 mg/kg daily for 5 days

      (3) Thiabendazole—440 mg/kg daily for 2 successive days

  7. Prevention. Prevention of heavy parasite loads revolve around recommendations that address pasture rotation, manure removal, and routine, effective deworming programs.

F. **Abdominal abscess**

  1. Patient profile and history. There are few subjective findings of diagnostic note. History and management factors may indicate parasitism as a possibility with secondary abscessation of vascular lesions.

  2. Clinical findings. Clinical findings are ill-thrift, fever of undetermined origin, and digestive disturbances (e.g., chronic abdominal pain, diarrhea, impaction colic).

  3. Etiology and pathogenesis. Agents such as *Streptococcus equi* and *S. zooepidemicus* may be seeded down in verminous tracts, invade the abdomen through hematogenous spread, or extend into the abdomen from the gastrointestinal tract. Abscesses and abdominal adhesions may affect bowel motility and produce signs of ill-thrift, diarrhea, fever, and inappetence.

  4. Diagnostic plan. Clinical findings are nonspecific.

  5. Laboratory tests. Laboratory findings may be helpful by revealing a leukocytosis, neutrophilia, and hyperfibrinogenemia. Protein electrophoresis may show an increased globulin fraction. Abdominocentesis exhibits an increase in leukocytes, protein, and bacteria. Culture of abdominal fluid is warranted to determine a pathogen.

  6. Therapeutic plan. Long-term antibiotic therapy is indicated. Surgical exploration may be warranted in select cases.

DIRECTIONS: Each of the numbered items or incomplete statements in this section is followed by answers or by completions of the statement. Select the ONE numbered answer or completion that is BEST in each case.

1. What is the most common cause of colic in newborn foals?

(1) Meconium impaction
(2) Atresia ani
(3) Atresia coli
(4) Ascarid impaction
(5) Gastric ulceration

2. Which one of the following statements regarding distention colics (also known as spasmodic colics) is true?

(1) They are accompanied by very high pulse rates.
(2) They are not at all similar in presentation to obstruction colics.
(3) They produce large quantities of gastric reflux.
(4) They cause reflex intestinal atony.
(5) They are seen with greater frequency in horses that swallow air.

3. Which statement regarding proximal enteritis is true? Proximal enteritis:

(1) causes signs of severe colic in affected horses.
(2) may be seen in horses with a recent history of grain engorgement.
(3) is best treated by observation.
(4) causes sequestration of large amounts of fluid in the large intestine.
(5) is seen primarily in juvenile horses (yearlings).

4. In horses, the diarrheic form of salmonellosis and equine monocytic ehrlichiosis differ in what way?

(1) Fever and depression is exhibited with equine monocytic ehrlichiosis but not with salmonellosis.
(2) Fluid replacement therapy is not necessary with equine monocytic ehrlichiosis.
(3) Laminitis is a frequent sequela to salmonellosis but not to equine monocytic ehrlichiosis.
(4) *Salmonella* organisms invade the intestinal mucosa, whereas *Ehrlichia risticii* invade mononuclear cells.
(5) *Salmonella* are readily isolated from the feces of horses with salmonellosis, whereas *Ehrlichia risticii* cannot be recovered.

5. Which statement regarding viral diarrheas in foals is true? Viral diarrheas in foals:

(1) do not produce changes to enteric cell morphology.
(2) can be prevented by vaccination.
(3) have been associated with infection by rotavirus, coronavirus, and adenovirus.
(4) are acute but very short-lived.
(5) are diagnosed by analysis of paired serum samples.

6. Abdominocentesis is often performed in horses with colic. Which one of the following statements is correct?

(1) Peritoneal fluid with normal cell counts and low protein levels will be retrieved in cases of early, pelvic flexure impactions.
(2) The collection of peritoneal fluid contaminated with ingesta confirms the presence of a ruptured viscus.
(3) The retrieval of frank blood on abdominocentesis indicates gastric ulceration.
(4) Peritoneal fluid can be obtained from most normal horses but should have a low total white blood cell (WBC) count and high protein level.
(5) Malodorous peritoneal fluid confirms the presence of acute diffuse nonseptic peritonitis.

7. Which one of the following sets of clinical signs would be compatible with a medically manageable equine impaction colic?

(1) A pulse of 56 beats/min, a capillary refill time of 5 seconds, and a rectal temperature of 36.7° C
(2) A capillary refill time of 2 seconds, a respiratory rate of 16 breaths/min, and a negative retrieval of fluids on gastric intubation
(3) Peritoneal surfaces that feel granular on rectal palpation, a respiratory rate of 36 breaths/min, and a negative retrieval of fluid on gastric intubation
(4) Increased borborygmi on abdominal auscultation, a capillary refill time of 5 seconds, and warm feet with an easily palpable digital pulse
(5) Anorexia, a rigid, splinted abdomen, and a pulse of 76 beats/min

---

DIRECTIONS: Each of the numbered items or incomplete statements in this section is negatively phrased, as indicated by a capitalized word such as NOT, LEAST, or EXCEPT. Select the ONE numbered answer or completion that is BEST in each case.

---

8. All of the following statements concerning proximal enteritis of horses are true EXCEPT:

(1) colic signs may be mild to moderate but the patient is often depressed and dehydrated.
(2) repeated or continuous gastric decompression is therapeutic.
(3) it is a condition usually found in foals or weanlings.
(4) this condition is very similar in presentation to a strangulating small intestinal obstruction.
(5) laminitis may be a complication of proximal enteritis.

9. Which one of the following agents is NOT thought to cause acute diarrhea in adult horses?

(1) Enterotoxigenic *Escherichia coli*
(2) *Ehrlichia risticii*
(3) *Clostridium perfringens* type A
(4) *Salmonella typhimurium*
(5) *Clostridium difficile*

10. All of the following statements comparing large intestinal impaction colics to flatulent colics in horses are true EXCEPT:

(1) both colic types may be feed related.
(2) both colic types may be relieved by treatment with mineral oil.
(3) clinical pathology findings are usually normal with both colic types.
(4) both colic types are seen more commonly in mature horses.
(5) both colic types are usually severely painful.

ANSWERS AND EXPLANATIONS

1. The answer is 1 [I B 1 a]. Meconium impaction is much more common than the congenital atresias in foals. Ascarid impaction and gastric ulceration may occur relatively frequently but in older foals.

2. The answer is 5 [I B 3 a]. Air swallowing results in pain due to gastric or small intestinal distention. This is not the only or most common cause of distention colic, but it will produce colic signs more frequently in horses with this vice. Distention colics do not result in major changes to vital signs or cause fluid reflux to accumulate in the stomach. Distention of intestinal segments usually result in a reflex hyperperistalsis in adjacent portions of the bowel. Distention colics may appear very similar to early obstruction colics or other more serious colics in early stages.

3. The answer is 2 [I B 4 a]. Grain engorgement or heavy grain feeding in adult horses is associated with the development of proximal enteritis. Colic signs are minimal with this condition but depression is significant. Treatment must be aggressive and consist of gastric decompression, large volumes of intravenous fluids, analgesics, and antibiotics.

4. The answer is 4 [II A 1, 2]. These organisms have predilection for different tissues even though resultant clinical signs may be similar. Both diseases cause horses to exhibit fever, depression, and often a subsequent laminitis. Both require aggressive fluid replacement therapy. *Salmonella* species often cannot be easily isolated from the feces of affected horses because of the dilution nature of the clinical diarrhea and the invasive nature of the organism.

5. The answer is 3 [II B 7]. Rotavirus causes diarrhea in foals, whereas coronavirus has been demonstrated in the feces of diarrheic foals and adenovirus involved with the diarrhea seen in foals with combined immunodeficiency. Viral diarrheas may be short or protracted in duration and have not proven to be preventable through vaccination. Diagnosis is usually via examination of the feces.

6. The answer is 1 [I A 2 f (5) (e); Table 2-3; Table 2-4]. Peritoneal fluid findings on abdominocentesis will be normal (i.e., normal cell counts, low protein levels) in patients with early pelvic flexure impactions (medical colic). Ingesta on abdominocentesis may indicate rupture of a viscus or penetration of the intestine by the needle or cannula. Gastric ulcers may bleed, but blood would be confined to the lumen of the gastrointestinal tract. Frank blood often indicates penetration of the spleen during the procedure. Malodorous peritoneal fluid on retrieval would suggest a septic process.

7. The answer is 1 [I A 2, B 2]. A pulse of 56 beats/min, a capillary refill time of 5 seconds, and a rectal temperature of 36.7°C would be the clinical findings most consistent with equine impaction colic, which is most commonly treated medically. The condition presents with normal vital signs and little reflux on nasogastric intubation. The impaction may be palpable per rectum. Generally, increased respiratory rates and capillary refill times are associated with surgical colics.

8. The answer is 3 [I B 4]. Proximal enteritis (anterior enteritis, duodenitis) is most common in adult horses, not foals or weanlings. The condition may be confused with a strangulating small intestinal obstruction. Continuous or periodic gastric decompression relieves the colicky signs and depression becomes the major finding. Dehydration is a reflection of gastric pooling of fluid and decreased fluid intake. Laminitis, a common complication of proximal enteritis, is believed to occur secondary to an endotoxemic state.

9. The answer is 1 [II A, B 6 b (1)]. Enterotoxigenic *Escherichia coli* causes neonatal diarrhea in many species and has been isolated from the feces of foals with diarrhea; however, its clinical significance is unproven in foals and it has not been shown to be cause of acute diarrhea in adult horses. *Escherichia risticii, Clostridium perfringens* type A, *Salmonella typhimurium*, and *Clostridium difficile* have been associated with diarrhea in adult horses.

10. The answer is 5 [I B 2, 5]. Large intestinal impactions are only mildly to moderately painful, whereas flatulent colics are very painful and may appear to be surgical in nature. Both colic types may be feed-related—an impaction of the large intestine may be related to improper digestion of feedstuffs, whereas a flatulent colic is often associated with grazing on succulent green feeds. Mineral oil can be beneficial in the treatment of both types of colics (i.e., it may coat an impaction, allowing for easier passage and it may act as an antifermentative in the case of flatulent colics). Clinical pathology findings are usually normal for both conditions and both conditions are most common in adult horses.

Chapter 3

Diseases of the Bovine Gastrointestinal Tract

Timothy H. Ogilvie

I. BOVINE FORESTOMACH AND ABOMASUM

A. **Indigestion.** The primary clinical signs for this condition are anorexia and ruminal changes characterized by hypomotility or occasionally hypermotility.

1. **Simple indigestion**
   a. **Patient profile and history**
      (1) Simple indigestion is a common disease in **dairy cattle** and less common in feedlot cattle and other ruminants. The condition is sporadic, usually affecting individual cows, but groups can be affected. This type of indigestion occurs more frequently in older cows, greedy eaters, or cows in advanced pregnancy.
      (2) There may be reported changes in the **feeding program** (i.e., quality, quantity, frequency) or other management changes. The owner might report that the cow is off feed and down in milk production. Feed refusal may have been progressive in that grain may have been refused first, followed by silage and hay.
   b. **Clinical findings.** The cow may be partially to completely anorexic. Vital signs [temperature, pulse, and respiration (TPR)] are normal to slightly elevated. The animal has a normal to mildly depressed attitude. Rumen motility may be normal but usually is slightly decreased in frequency and vigor. Feces may be normal in consistency or firm, and fecal output usually is reduced. Occasionally, the rumen is hypermotile, resulting in feces that are looser than normal.
   c. **Etiology and pathogenesis**
      (1) The condition is caused by a change in rumen fermentation resulting from a shift in feed quality, quantity, or presentation. Some **predisposing factors** in the development of the condition include:
         (a) Sudden changes of feed
         (b) Poor feed quality (e.g., moldy, spoiled)
         (c) Animal fatigue or stress (e.g., shipping)
         (d) Prolonged antibiotic therapy
         (e) Insufficient water
      (2) Any of the predisposing factors might change the **ruminal environment** necessary for fermentation and microbial degradation of feedstuffs. The rumen environment is composed of a mixture of proteins, carbohydrates, and fluid. Bacteria and protozoa act on these substances within an environment with a pH and temperature that is regulated by secretion and motility.
   d. **Diagnostic plan.** The history, lack of specific findings other than minor gastrointestinal changes, and a knowledge of the farm husbandry usually is sufficient to make the diagnosis. It is often a diagnosis by exclusion of other diseases, and the animal's recovery within 24–36 hours confirms the diagnosis.
   e. **Laboratory tests.** Laboratory tests ordinarily are not requested because all values usually appear normal. Occasionally, the cow may exhibit a "stress" leukogram. The rumen pH may be slightly alkaline (6–7) and show somewhat decreased protozoal activity. A mild metabolic alkalosis also may be present.
   f. **Differential diagnoses.** Other conditions to be considered would have clinical signs in addition to mild indigestion. These conditions include:
      (1) Traumatic reticuloperitonitis
      (2) Abomasal displacements
      (3) Vagal indigestion
      (4) Primary ketosis
      (5) Lactic acidosis
   g. **Therapeutic plan**

(1) Often, little if any therapy is necessary. Many owners diagnose the condition themselves, treating the animal with over-the-counter rumenatorics or providing good quality feed and water.

(2) **Rumenatorics** may contain nux vomica, capsicum, ginger, and tartar emetic. There is little need for rumen stimulants such as neostigmine. Cathartics, such as magnesium hydroxide (MgOH) or magnesium oxide (MgO), should be avoided because they exacerbate the mild metabolic alkalosis that may already be present. MgOH or MgO would be indicated if the rumen pH is below 5.5. If a primary cathartic is indicated, a better choice would be magnesium sulfate (500–1000 g orally).

(3) The **best treatment** is the provision of quality, long-stemmed hay and fresh water. The owner should monitor the animal's response and request a revisit 24 hours later if there is no improvement.

(4) If the animal does not respond within 24 hours, a clinical examination should be performed again. If the diagnosis is still simple indigestion, consider a rumen transfaunation with 1–2 L of fresh rumen juice. Before performing the transfaunation, clinicians may wish to adjust the rumen pH to physiological levels by administering alkalinizing agents (in the case of an acid rumen) or acidifying agents (vinegar 1–2 L orally) if the rumen pH is more than 7.

h. Prevention. For prevention of this condition, the client should be instructed to minimize sudden dietary changes and avoid damaged, spoiled, or contaminated feed.

2. Lactic acidosis (ruminal acidosis, acute grain overload, acute rumen impaction, rumen overload, D-lactic acidosis, grain engorgement, toxic indigestion, acid indigestion)

a. Patient profile and history

(1) Any ruminant is susceptible to lactic acidosis. **Dairy** and **beef cattle** seem to be most commonly affected possibly because of their representative numbers or husbandry and intensive production practices.

(2) Patient history includes access to **highly fermentable feed.** The offending substances are highly soluble carbohydrates such as finely ground grains (e.g., wheat, barley, corn), apples, pears, potatoes, bakery products, beets, whey, and brewers grain.

(3) There may be a history of poor feeding management or inconsistent concentrate feeding.

b. Clinical findings are variable and depend on the amount of feed consumed, feed composition, feed particle size, and previous adaptation of the animal to the ration. Clinical syndromes may vary from acute and severe to mild and similar to simple indigestion. A chronic form of lactic acidosis may also occur.

(1) **Acute severe cases**

(a) Clinical signs appear 12–36 hours after the feed is consumed. Symptoms include anorexia, lethargy, depression, muscle tremors, and ataxia.

(b) The animal is **dehydrated** (8%–12%), resulting in loss of skin turgor and a dull, sunken eye. There is severe ruminal **distention,** rumen stasis, and fluid splashy rumen contents. The animal may exhibit bruxism and grunting.

(c) **Body temperature** initially increases and then falls. There is tachycardia and a rapid, shallow **respiratory pattern.** Dairy cattle have a severe drop in milk production. The animal may appear **blind,** with a sluggish palpebral and eye preservation reflex.

(d) It may take 24 hours for **diarrhea** to develop, but the feces then appear foamy and liquid with an acid smell and a yellow-brown or grey color. The feces may contain undigested feed material (e.g., grain).

(e) The animal continues to deteriorate, becoming recumbent, comatose, and finally dying.

(2) **Subacute cases.** The pattern of clinical findings is similar to the acute cases but less intense.

(3) **Chronic cases**

(a) **Repeated episodes** of subacute rumen acidosis may be associated with herd problems of subclinical disease (e.g., laminitis, low-fat milk syndrome, liver abscesses, chronic rumenitis, chronic indigestion).

    (b) Individual episodes of indigestion appear mild and similar to simple indigestion or subacute indigestion. Animals appear bright and alert but with transient anorexia and decreased effective rumen motility. The rumen may be slightly distended. Feces are grey and porridge-like. Dairy cattle experience decreased milk production.

c. Etiology and pathogenesis

    (1) Normally, there is a balance of **cellulolytic** and **carbohydrate-using bacteria** within the rumen. The ingestion of excess carbohydrates or sugars promotes growth of lactic–acid-producing and -using bacteria within the rumen. Although lactate is used rapidly, the amount that accumulates plus the rapid fermentation of carbohydrates and the accumulation of volatile fatty acids (VFAs) drop the rumen pH. This decrease in pH kills rumen protozoa and microbes, including the initial lactate users. These organisms are replaced first by *Streptococcus bovis* and then by lactobacilli and gram-positive rods. The pH continues to fall with the further lactobacilli production of D- and L-lactic acid.

    (2) Finely ground feeds increase the surface area exposed to bacteria for fermentation. These feeds also decrease the amount of saliva secreted by the animal, which lessens the amount of buffer flowing into the rumen. Although both D- and L-lactic acid are absorbed through the rumen wall, only L-lactic acid can be metabolized by the ruminant, leaving the D-lactic acid to be eliminated. Therefore, D-lactic acid builds up and creates the systemic acidosis.

    (3) Feed fermentation, decomposition of the feed into very fine particles, and the lactic acid all increase the **rumen osmolality.** The accumulation of VFAs produce rumen stasis. Extracellular water flows into the rumen, producing rumen distention, diarrhea, and dehydration. These conditions lead to hypovolemia, circulatory collapse, metabolic acidosis, and death.

    (4) If the animal survives the initial bout of lactic acidosis, the high rumen acidity, hypertonicity, and corrosive nature of lactic acid produce a **chemical rumenitis.** This condition allows rumen-associated bacteria and fungi to invade the rumen wall and hepatic portal system.

    (5) Sequelae include rumen wall necrosis, hepatic abscess, and peritonitis. The release of toxins may produce laminitis, abomasal disorders, and cardiac, renal, and hepatic damage.

d. Diagnostic plan. The diagnosis often is determined based on clinical findings supported by a history of overeating or sudden dietary change. A sample of rumen fluid should be retrieved and analyzed.

e. Laboratory tests

    (1) Laboratory support is **rarely necessary** in acute cases where there is a reliable history. The most valuable laboratory aid is an evaluation of rumen content for subjective findings, pH, and protozoal activity.

    (2) The **rumen fluid** retrieved by orogastric intubation is milky grey and watery with an acid smell. The pH is variable, depending on time and diet, but it is diagnostic if less than 5.0. A wet mount shows no live protozoa. A Gram stain shows *Streptococci* with a predominant population of gram-positive rods and other mixed, mainly gram-negative, morphologic forms.

    (3) Hematologic work-up. A leukogram reveals a degenerative left shift. Hemoconcentration is evident on a packed cell volume (PCV). A chemistry panel shows an increase in blood urea nitrogen (BUN) and creatinine, hypocalcemia, hypomagnesemia, and hyperglycemia.

    (4) Urinalysis shows decreased volume, increased specific gravity, aciduria, and glucosuria (often a diagnostic indicator in sheep). If available, a **blood gas analysis** confirms a metabolic acidosis.

f. Differential diagnoses. Lactic acidosis may appear similar to many other septic or toxic conditions including:

    (1) Septic mastitis or metritis

    (2) Acute diffuse peritonitis

    (3) Parturient paresis

(4) Poisoning by lead, salt, arsenic, or nitrate
(5) Enterotoxemia
g. **Therapeutic plan.** It is often difficult to determine therapeutic intensity with acute lactic acidosis, particularly early on when the full range of clinical signs has not been manifested. Some guidelines for treatment follow.
  (1) There has been access to carbohydrates but the animal(s) has not shown clinical signs.
    (a) Prevent further access to feed, and offer free choice, good quality hay.
    (b) Exercise the animal(s) hourly for 12–24 hours to encourage movement of ingesta through the digestive tract.
    (c) Administer 1 g/kg of magnesium oxide, magnesium hydroxide, or sodium bicarbonate orally.
  (2) The animals show anorexia and depression within 6–8 hours of feed consumption.
    (a) Surgery. Perform a **rumenotomy** if the value of the animal warrants the procedure and if the case is still a good surgical risk. Tachycardia (greater than 140 beats/minute), dehydration, a subnormal body temperature, and severe depression indicate a poor prognosis for recovery. Couple surgery with fluid therapy for metabolic acidosis (e.g., Ringer's Lactate with sodium bicarbonate), and supply a rumen transfaunation. Other **supportive therapies** include calcium, thiamine, and nonsteroidal anti-inflammatory drugs (NSAIDs).
    (b) Recommend that the animal be slaughtered if economics do not dictate surgery and the animal will pass an antemortem and post-slaughter inspection.
    (c) Other treatments. Other less predictable or efficacious treatments include rumen lavage via rumen trocar, systemic or oral antibiotics to limit ruminal bacterial growth, and oral iodine-based disinfectants to kill rumen microbes. Because of the potential for a large number of animals to develop lactic acidosis simultaneously, the use of a large-diameter stomach tube (Kingman tube) to lavage the rumen may be both economic and beneficial.
  (3) Animals with chronic lactic acidosis. Individual animal treatment is often unsuccessful and usually not warranted. This is most commonly reflective of a herd problem and should be addressed in a preventive manner.
h. **Prevention**
  (1) Management strategies. Recommendations should revolve around ration and feeding management. Keep feed quality and practices consistent. Avoid abrupt changes and gradually adapt the rumen to concentrates. When introducing new concentrate or carbohydrate forms, prefeed animals with hay. Prevent accidental access to feeds by maintaining good animal holding facilities.
  (2) Feed content. Maintain a minimum **crude fibre content** of 14% of total digestible nutrients (TDN) for fattening cattle and 18%–22% for dairy cattle.

3. **Vagal indigestion (chronic or vagus indigestion, Hoflund's syndrome).** Vagal indigestion refers to a group of conditions that cause **forestomach outflow problems.** One possible cause of these problems is vagal nerve dysfunction, although this dysfunction has not been proven to be necessary or sufficient to cause the condition. The classifications of forestomach disturbances encompassed by vagal indigestion differ from author to author. Therefore, this section discusses the syndrome as a whole and delineates subtypes as necessary for diagnosis, therapy, and prognosis.
a. **Patient profile and history.** Although any ruminant may be affected, this type of indigestion is most common in **adult dairy cattle.** History may include mild but repeated bouts of transient indigestion with signs of anorexia, decreased milk production, mild bloat, weight loss, abdominal distention, and decreased amounts of manure. An episode of traumatic reticuloperitonitis (TRP) may be reported as an historical event.
b. **Clinical findings.** A **distended abdomen** is often a cardinal sign. The distention may be bilateral with gas distending the upper left flank, while fluid distends the

ventral right quadrant. The **rumen** is often hypermotile with frequent but weak contractions. The animal is often in poor condition. **Vital signs** are usually normal but occasionally, a bradycardia is evident (40–60 bpm).
- c. **Etiology and pathogenesis**
  - (1) Vagal indigestion is most often described as a **sequela** to **traumatic reticuloperitonitis,** although the syndrome is also associated with tumors (e.g., lymphosarcoma of the abomasum) and abomasal torsion.
  - (2) If **adhesive lesions** around the reticulum either interfere with vagal nerve function or the mechanics of reticular movement, then reticuloruminal cyclical activity and eructation waves are compromised, resulting in ruminal gas retention or free gas bloat. In this case, there are no other abnormalities, and the animal will improve transiently if the gas is removed via orogastric tube and recover fully if a rumen fistula is installed.
  - (3) If **failure of omasal transport** occurs, ingesta from the ruminoreticulum is not properly conveyed to the abomasum, and long (2–4 cm) fiber may be found in the manure. Fluid builds up in the rumen, and although acid–base status remains normal, the animal becomes mildly dehydrated. The prognosis for a return to function is guarded. The lesion causing the condition is either a functional or physical obstruction of omasal outflow. Examples of physical obstructions include ingested foreign bodies (baling twine, plastic bags, placenta) or space-occupying lesions (tumor).
  - (4) **Abomasal impaction** may be another manifestation of the syndrome and results from obstruction at the pylorus with conditions such as lymphosarcoma. This impaction also may occur secondary to abomasal torsions, where it is postulated that abomasal stretching and visceral compromise impairs gastric motility. The abomasum becomes distended with hard ingesta. A hypochloremic, metabolic alkalosis results due to reflux and pooling of gastric chloride ion in the rumen. This "chloride trap" makes it unavailable for reabsorption in the proximal small intestine.
  - (5) **Primary abomasal impaction** may occur in **beef cattle** on a coarse roughage diet with limited access to water and in calves suffering from abomasal trichobezoars or phytobezoars. These conditions are not usually considered as part of the vagal indigestion syndrome.
  - (6) The final manifestation of the syndrome is **chronic indigestion associated with advanced pregnancy.** The gravid uterus may occupy enough abdominal space that it interferes with forestomach outflow. It may also exacerbate reticular adhesions or abomasal outflow restrictions, resulting in ruminal distention. The prognosis with this condition is often fair to good following parturition.
- d. **Diagnostic plan**
  - (1) The set of clinical signs, chronicity, and continued lack of response to any treatment for simple indigestion is usually sufficient to diagnose vagal indigestion. The presence of a metabolic alkalosis often implicates the abomasum in the syndrome but this is not invariable.
  - (2) **Differentiation** of the causes may depend on findings on exploratory laparotomy; however, mixed conditions do occur and lesions are not invariably present. The poor response to interventive therapy with many of these cases often makes a morphologic diagnosis unnecessary.
- e. **Differential diagnoses.** It is often necessary to rule out simple indigestion and many other causes of decreased fecal output and abdominal distention (e.g., abomasal displacement, hydrops). Vagal indigestion is often a diagnosis of exclusion.
- f. **Therapeutic plan**
  - (1) **Surgical exploration** is often used in valuable animals as an aid to diagnosis and therapy. In cases of free gas bloat, the creation of a rumen fistula often enables a return to ruminal function while the underlying lesion heals. Indwelling rumen trocars have been used to relieve the bloat but are less reliable than surgery. The prognosis for vagal indigestion involving omasal or abomasal dysfunction is relatively poor, so **slaughter** should be considered as an option in these cases.
  - (2) In cases where exploratory surgery has been performed, **further surgical intervention** depends on findings. Foreign bodies (in the abomasum or fore-

stomach) should be removed, abscesses adherent to the reticulum can be drained into the reticulum, and softening agents (e.g., mineral oil) can be instilled into the abomasum by an orogastric tube directed through the omasal–abomasal orifice intraruminally.

(3) **Supportive therapies** include:
(a) Rumen transfaunation (repeated treatments may be necessary)
(b) Supportive feeding either by rumen fistula or an indwelling nasogastric tube that has been placed into the abomasum at surgery
(c) Intravenous fluids
(d) Calcium salts intravenously or subcutaneously
(e) Potassium chloride at 30–60 g orally twice a day
(f) Exercise

g. **Prevention.** There is little that can be done to prevent vagal indigestion. However, if chronic reticular adhesions indicate that traumatic reticuloperitonitis may be occurring in a herd, it would be good to administer magnets to breeding-age heifers as a preventive. Other measures to prevent foreign body or feed impactions from occurring should be implemented by decreasing access to indigestible substances (e.g., rope, twine, plastics).

4. **Abomasal impaction**
a. **Patient profile.** Primary abomasal impaction occurs most commonly in **beef cattle** and is most often seen in **pregnant cows.**
b. **Clinical findings.** Animals present with anorexia, scant feces, variable dehydration, and moderate abdominal distention. The distended, hard abomasum may be palpated in the lower right abdomen.
c. **Etiology and pathogenesis.** The pathogenesis is most commonly one of excessive intake of poor quality roughage at times of increased energy needs (i.e., pregnancy, winter months). Mechanical obstruction by a foreign body or pyloric mass is another cause. Obstruction results in excessive accumulation of rumen chloride, causing a metabolic alkalosis. A progressive starvation ensues.
d. **Diagnostic plan.** The diagnosis is based on clinical findings. The condition appears similar to vagal indigestion but is often a herd problem. Laboratory information helps narrow the diagnostic possibilities. Exploratory surgery confirms the condition.
e. **Laboratory tests** show metabolic alkalosis, hypochloremia, hypokalemia, and hemoconcentration.
f. **Therapeutic plan**
(1) By the time clinical signs develop, treatment usually is unrewarding. **Slaughter** of meat animals may provide some economic return.
(2) Measures undertaken for selected individuals include induction of parturition, surgery, softening agents per os, and supplemental nutrition. However, rarely are these heroic measures effective.
g. **Prevention.** Recommendations for prevention include provision of adequate amounts of nutrition for maintenance and pregnancy, particularly in the cold winter months. Nutritional counseling may be necessary for owners trying to maintain cattle on low-input regimens. The importance of good quality drinking water should not be overlooked.

B. **Bloat (ruminal tympany)**

1. **Acute bloat.** Acute or sudden-onset bloat can be divided into two types: **frothy bloat** and **free gas bloat.**
a. **Patient profile and history.** Bloat occurs more commonly in cattle than other ruminants, and certain individual cattle may be more susceptible than others.
(1) **Frothy bloat** is often associated with **dairy cows** that recently have been turned out on new-growth, lush pastures (e.g., alfalfa, clover). Several animals may be affected. Feedlot cattle can also develop frothy bloat when more than 50% of their ration is being consumed as concentrate.
(2) **Free gas bloat** is associated with a history of feeding whole or only partially chopped solid feeds (e.g., potatoes, apples, turnips).

b. **Clinical findings.** Animals present with severe abdominal distention and increased TPR. The distention initially is restricted to the left dorsal abdominal quadrant, but in severe cases the right flank will also distend. The rumen may be hypermotile or hypomotile. Animals have excessive salivation and are anxious. Animals will mouth-breathe, become recumbent, and quickly die.

c. **Etiology and pathogenesis**
   (1) **Frothy bloat** is associated with **legume consumption.**
      (a) It is thought that the fine, thin leaf structure of certain varieties of legumes coupled with tender growth (early or late season) allows for more rapid bacterial degradation and intraruminal particle suspension. Chloroplast released from the legume leaf forms monomolecular foams that trap gas bubbles. These foams have great surface tension and are highly stable.
      (b) The result is that **small gas bubbles** do not coalesce, the cardia or the forestomach cannot be cleared of this foam, and the animal is unable to eructate.
      (c) A **stable froth** can also be formed in feedlot animals consuming a primarily **finely ground grain** diet. In this case however, a mucoprotein slime stabilizes the foam. This foam is stable at a low pH created by lactate and VFA production. Salivation is decreased because of the fine grind of the diet, which also lessens intraruminal buffering.
   (2) **Free gas bloat** may have a variety of causes. The most common cause is **intraesophageal obstruction** with solid objects, such as apples or potatoes. Extraesophageal masses may also cause the build up of intraruminal gases. Abscesses caused by perivascular injections, *Hypoderma lineatum* reactions, and cervical neoplasia can all constrict the esophagus. Certain postures or diseases also can produce a functional free gas bloat. Examples include milk fever and tetanus. Moderate free gas bloat also may be a finding in vagal indigestion (see I A 3).

d. **Diagnostic plan.** An accurate history and the passage of an orogastric tube rapidly determines whether the condition is one of abdominal distention resulting from the accumulation of ruminal free gas or froth. If the tube cannot be passed, then the likely diagnosis is free gas bloat due to esophageal obstruction. If the tube can be passed but ruminal gas is not readily forthcoming, then frothy bloat is likely. Remove the tube and look at its end for evidence of froth. A reading of the foam pH further defines the type of frothy bloat; a feedlot bloat should have a pH of less than 5.5.

e. **Differential diagnoses.** If the diagnosis is not one of bloat, other causes for abdominal distention to rule out include ascites, acute diffuse peritonitis, and hydrops.

f. **Therapeutic plan**
   (1) **Acute bloat** is one of the **true medical emergencies** in bovine practice. Animals can die rapidly and many may succumb before the owner is aware of the problem, particularly if cattle have been turned out to new pasture for an unobserved length of time. In the case of **free gas bloat,** lethal ruminal pressures also build up very rapidly.
   (2) With **frothy bloat,** pass an orogastric tube and administer an oil to reduce the surface tension of the foam and allow the gas bubbles to coalesce. Either mineral oil at 1 L/100 kg orally or dioctyl sodium sulfosuccinate (DSS) in peanut oil at 17–66 mg/kg orally may be used (150–600 ml/450 kg animal). The treatment should be satisfactory and sufficient if the animal is still standing and not showing evidence of respiratory or cardiac failure. If the animal is in a deteriorating clinical condition, an **emergency rumenotomy** is warranted.
   (3) With **acute free gas bloat due to an intraesophageal mass,** the orogastric tube may force the obstruction into the reticulum. Should this not occur, trocarization of the rumen and either an indwelling trocar or fistula is placed to allow continued escape of gas while the mass softens and hopefully moves along. Post-surgical penicillin (22,000 IU/kg twice daily intramuscularly) should be used. Many masses block the esophagus just posterior to the pharynx. These can often be retrieved manually or with the aid of a wire loop to snare the object.

g. Prognosis
  (1) The prognosis for most cases of **frothy bloat** is favorable if intervention is rapid. A simple indigestion may occur secondary to treatment, and the animal should be fed good quality hay as a major component of its diet for 1–2 days. Animals that have undergone emergency rumenotomies may develop cellulitis or peritonitis, but these occurrences are infrequent.
  (2) The prognosis for **acute free gas bloat** is excellent if the offending object can be removed. If the object must be left in place to be swallowed, then **complications** include sequelae to trocarization or rumen fistulation as well as secondary esophageal stricture development.

h. Prevention
  (1) The prevention of **frothy bloat** may take many forms and several combinations including:
    (a) If legumes are fed, select cultivars of bloat-producing forages that are less likely to ferment quickly.
    (b) Feed dry roughage to animals before turning them out on legume pastures.
    (c) Allow only 20 minutes initially of grazing on lush legume pastures.
    (d) Feed antifoaming materials (poloxalene at 1–2 g/50 kg once daily; ionophore drugs such as monensin at 1 mg/kg once daily or lasalocid at 1.32 mg/kg once daily in nonlactating cattle).
    (e) Provide for slower introduction or less heavy feeding of concentrates if feedlot bloat becomes a problem.
  (2) The prevention of **free gas bloat due to esophageal choke** becomes a matter of cutting up feed objects in smaller sizes, slowing down greedy eaters by feeding hay first upon initial introduction, or introduction of the material gradually.

2. Chronic free gas bloat (see I A 3)

C. Hyperresonance

1. Left displacement of the abomasum (abomasal displacement, twisted stomach)
  a. Patient profile and history
    (1) Left displacement of the abomasum (LDA) is most common in **middle-aged, high producing dairy cows** but may be seen in other situations and classes of cattle. This condition is rare in other ruminants but may occur in ruminating calves. It is a sporadic disease of individual animals, but the prevalence may be relatively high in some herds.
    (2) Cattle are often in **early lactation** on a **high concentrate, low roughage diet.** Total mixed rations with short fibre lengths and silage-based rations seem to predispose cattle to the condition. There is often a concurrent disease, such as metritis, mastitis, or hypocalcemia.
  b. Clinical findings
    (1) Vital signs are normal to slightly elevated unless there is concurrent disease.
    (2) Appearance. The animal may have a slab-sided appearance or the last two ribs on the left may be sprung with a hollow left paralumbar fossa. In some cases, there may be a slight filling of the left paralumbar fossa directly behind the last rib.
    (3) Feces. There are decreased amounts of pasty manure or small amounts of diarrhea.
    (4) Rumen contractions are normal to slightly decreased. There may be tinkling sounds heard while auscultating the rumen. The animal exhibits total to moderate anorexia and may be ketotic. A **"ping"** is evident on simultaneous auscultation and percussion of the abdomen usually along a line drawn from the left tuber coxae to the left elbow.
    (5) On **palpation** of the left paralumbar fossa, the rumen is not palpable, but the dilated abomasum occasionally may be felt. Rectal examination may be relatively normal except for a smaller than normal, medially deviated rumen.
    (6) Calves with LDA exhibit quite an extensive left flank distention, with gas and fluid sounds on auscultation.
  c. Etiology and pathogenesis

(1) The **abomasum** is firmly attached at its cranial end to the omasum, but the fundus and pylorus are relatively freely moveable, being held only by the greater and lesser omentum. The abomasum continually generates gases (CO_2, methane, nitrogen) and secretes HCl and enzymes, which are passed into the duodenum by abomasal contractions (1–2/min).

(2) **High concentrate, low roughage diets** are thought to cause increased VFA production in the rumen, leading to an increase in VFAs in the abomasum, increased gas production in the rumen, and accumulation in the abomasum. This diet also may cause decreased stimulation to rumination, decreased salivation, and an increased rate of passage of ingesta, all resulting in decreased abomasal motility and increased gas production.

(3) **Other factors** that are postulated to reduce abomasal tone or motility are hypocalcemia, concurrent diseases through inflammatory mediators (endotoxin and interleukin-1), and lack of exercise. With reduced abomasal motility (atony) or increased gas accumulation, the abomasum distends and may rise dorsally out of place on the left or right side of the animal.

(4) **During late gestation,** it is thought that the gravid uterus pushes the rumen cranially and dorsally, and the abomasum pushes to the left. After parturition, the abomasum moves further left into the void, creating the displacement. This may be more likely in deep-bodied, large cows; thus, a breed or genetic predisposition has been postulated.

(5) **Abomasal displacements in calves** tend to occur at a time when the calf is changing from a monogastric to a ruminant. The pathogenesis is unknown and it is a rare event compared with cattle.

d. Diagnostic plan. It is a relatively straightforward diagnosis in animals that fit the subjective and clinical picture. The diagnosis becomes more suspect in nontraditional animals (calves) or when the ping is transient, recurring, or faint.

e. Laboratory tests

(1) **Clinical pathology tests** are nondiagnostic for the condition but can be helpful, particularly in cases when a ping is not readily auscultable. There may be mild hypocalcemia, hypoglycemia, hypokalemia, ketonemia, ketolactia, and ketonuria.

(2) **Liptak test.** Because other distended viscera produce a ping and may mimic LDA, it is sometimes of value to aspirate fluid percutaneously from just below the most ventral location of the ping. This is known as the Liptak test. Analysis of the fluid retrieved aids in identifying the viscus. If the pH of the fluid is less than 5 and has no evidence of protozoa, it is most likely from the abomasum. If the fluid has a pH of more than 6, it is most likely from the rumen.

f. Differential diagnoses. If LDA is indeed the diagnosis but no ping is auscultable, the condition may be confused with ketosis or simple indigestion. Other conditions that may produce a left-sided abdominal ping and mimic LDA are rumen atony with a gas cap and pneumoperitoneum.

g. Therapeutic plan

(1) **Medical (nonsurgical) management** of the condition is unreliable and usually unsuccessful. However, steps may be taken to treat concurrent disease (e.g., metritis).

(2) **Physical intervention.** Rolling the cow to replace LDA may be undertaken as a temporary treatment in cases where economics do not favor surgery or in cases where the owner wishes to gain some time before salvage. The procedure involves casting the animal into right lateral recumbency, bringing her to dorsal recumbency, rocking her gently back and forth while kneading the ventral abdomen, rolling the cow to her left side, and allowing her to rise. This seems to reposition the abomasum, but a majority of cases recur.

(3) **Surgical intervention** provides for a good to excellent prognosis for a return to economic potential. The following techniques have similar success rates, and choice of technique is a matter of preference or familiarity.

(a) Left flank abomasopexy

(b) Right flank omentopexy

(c) Right paramedian abomasopexy

(d) Right paramedian percutaneous toggle pin (bar suture) fixation
h. Prevention
    (1) Management strategies. Many clients tend to live with the problem of LDA as a trade-off because they are satisfied with herd production levels, happy with their feeding management [e.g., total mixed ration (TMR), corn silage], or content with their herd genetics (i.e., large, high-producing cows). The best advice if a client wishes to decrease the incidence of the disease is to incorporate more long-stemmed fiber in the ration, provide exercise for stabled cows, feed animals more frequently with the ration divided, and limit postpartum diseases (e.g., milk fever, metritis).
    (2) For the **individual cow** with LDA, most farmers are able to diagnose the condition themselves after seeing a few cases. However, these clients may need to be reminded that prompt correction of the condition returns the cow to a more economic production unit faster.

2. Right displacement of the abomasum (RDA)
  a. Patient profile and history (see I C 1 a)
  b. Clinical findings are similar to LDAs, but the ping is on the right side. In the case of a large distention of the abomasum, the displaced viscus may be felt per the rectum.
  c. Etiology and pathogenesis (see I C 1 c)
  d. Diagnostic plan. The diagnosis is based on clinical findings. An aspirate of fluid from within the viscus (e.g., a Liptak test) may be beneficial for diagnosis.
  e. Differential diagnoses. Other conditions that produce a right-sided ping include:
    (1) Colonic gas
    (2) Gas in the rectum
    (3) Cecal dilation
    (4) Cecal torsion
    (5) Abomasal torsion
    (6) Pneumoperitoneum
    (7) Physometra
  f. Therapeutic plan
    (1) Medical management may be attempted with smooth muscle stimulants, but surgery is the treatment of choice. Some sources think that surgery should not be delayed because the RDA might progress to an abomasal torsion/volvulus. Rolling the cow is contraindicated in RDA cases because an abomasal torsion/volvulus may result.
    (2) Surgery is either a right flank omentopexy or a right paramedian abomasopexy.

3. Right abomasal volvulus (right torsion of the abomasum, abomasal torsion)
  a. Patient profile and history. Subjective findings are similar to LDA and RDA, although in many cases, an abomasal volvulus may occur in animals other than the early postpartum cow. Sudden agalactia and anorexia are indications.
  b. Clinical findings
    (1) Appearance. The animal is markedly **depressed** and may show bruxism or grunting. There may be some evidence of **pain** or discomfort, such as treading, but this condition is not as painful as other intestinal accidents.
    (2) A **high-pitched ping** is evident over a large area on the right side from the eighth rib to the paralumbar fossa. Fluid may be succussed within the dilated viscus. The cow will be **dehydrated** as evidenced by a skin tent and sunken eye. Tachycardia is evident (usually 100 bpm), and the pulse is weak.
    (3) There is complete **rumen stasis** possibly with a mild bloat on the left from a gas cap. Feces are scant. There may be only mucus in the rectum, and occasionally, with a concurrent abomasal ulcer, there may be melena.
    (4) Rectal examination. The **volvulus** often can be palpated rectally in the right abdomen. RDA can progress to a volvulus by either a clockwise or counterclockwise twist (when viewing the animal from the side). A **torsion** can occur around the long axis of the abomasum. Various combinations can be found. If twisted long enough or to a large enough degree, the abomasum becomes con-

gested, hemorrhagic, and infarcted due to occlusion of gastric circulation. As the organ becomes devitalized, the cow goes into shock and dies.

(5) **Acid–base changes** accompany an abomasal volvulus.

    (a) In the **early condition,** abomasal outflow of HCl is compromised, and reflux occurs into the rumen. The rumen effectively traps H^+ and Cl^- ions. K^+ ions are lost in the urine in deference to H^+-ion retention, creating in total a hypochloremic, hypokalemic, metabolic alkalosis.

    (b) In the **advanced condition,** a metabolic acidosis may be found related to the state of shock of the animal.

(6) Occasionally, the **omasum** is involved in the abomasal volvulus (omasal–abomasal volvulus), which increases the gravity of the prognosis.

  c. **Etiology and pathogenesis.** Dilation is thought to precede torsion of the volvulus and is hypothesized to be caused similarly to LDA and RDA. Mechanical events may cause torsion in the volvulus of the distended abomasum.

  d. **Diagnostic plan.** Diagnosis of the condition is based on clinical findings and laboratory tests. A Liptak test is helpful in determining the affected organ.

  e. **Laboratory tests**

(1) Laboratory findings that support the diagnosis include:

    (a) An aspirate of a low pH fluid from the viscus

    (b) A toxic leukogram to varying degrees

    (c) A metabolic alkalosis (in late stages, a metabolic acidosis)

    (d) Evidence of dehydration and prerenal uremia [PCV, total protein (TP), BUN]

    (e) A paradoxical aciduria as K^+ ions are excreted in the face of whole-body, H^+-ion deficiency

(2) As the plasma anion gap increases, the prognosis for recovery decreases.

  f. **Differential diagnoses.** It is necessary to rule out other causes of abdominal pings that result in an animal's sick appearance. Conditions to be ruled out include:

(1) Cecal volvulus/torsion

(2) Mesenteric root torsion

(3) Small intestinal obstructions

(4) Acute diffuse peritonitis

  g. **Therapeutic plan**

(1) **Immediate surgical intervention** coupled with **fluid therapy** is indicated.

    (a) **Surgical approaches** are a right flank omentopexy or a right paramedian abomasopexy.

    (b) **Intravenous fluids** include isotonic sodium chloride and dextrose for volume expansion (likely 20–80 L), followed by a slow drip of potassium chloride (1 mEq/kg/hour), sodium chloride, and dextrose. Balanced electrolyte solutions are indicated for shock and metabolic acidosis.

    (c) Other **supportive treatments,** depending on the case, include antibiotics, corticosteroids, and NSAIDs.

(2) **Salvage** instead of surgery may be indicated if dictated by economics and if the animal will pass antemortem and post-slaughter inspection. The systemic involvement of the animal often dictates against this.

  h. **Prognosis.** The prognosis for an animal depends on the degree of abomasal compromise determined at surgery. In some cases that recover, abomasal torsion is associated with the subsequent development of vagal indigestion.

4. **Cecal dilation or cecal volvulus**

  a. **Patient profile and history**

(1) Cecal dilation and cecal volvulus are conditions that occur most commonly in **mature dairy cattle** in the first 2 months postpartum. These conditions are more common in the winter months and show no breed predisposition.

(2) The farmer reports that the cow is partially to completely **anorexic** with a drop in milk production. The herd ration is often a high grain diet rich in carbohydrates such as corn silage or high-moisture corn. It may be fed as a total mixed ration (TMR). The clinical signs usually are reported as moderately

progressive and not sudden in onset unless a dilation has converted into a torsion, in which case signs deteriorate rapidly.

b. Clinical findings

   (1) Cecal dilation. With a cecal dilation, the **vital signs** are usually normal. The animal may tread, indicating mild pain. Feces may be somewhat loose and decreased in amount. The right paralumbar fossa may be slightly distended, and a **ping** is auscultated in the right flank caudal to the site for RDA. Rumen motility is decreased in rate and strength. **Rectal examination** confirms the diagnosis, as the apex of the cecum will be felt at the pelvic inlet.

   (2) Cecal volvulus. A cecal volvulus offers more dramatic clinical signs than a cecal dilation. The **pulse** is elevated, and there is complete agalactia, rumen atony, and absence of manure. The cow exhibits **abdominal pain** by shifting hind-end weight, kicking at the abdomen, and frequent lying down and rising. The right paralumbar fossa may be distended. A **ping** can be elicited over a larger area than with a simple cecal dilation, and fluid, splashing sounds may be heard. **Rectal examination** reveals a distended cecal body (the apex has been twisted and directed cranially).

c. Etiology and pathogenesis

   (1) The **pathogenesis** of cecal distention is thought to be similar to abomasal displacements. It is believed that cecal organisms metabolize carbohydrates that have escaped upper gastrointestinal microbial degradation. VFAs, methane gas, and CO_2 are all produced. The VFAs inhibit cecal motility, and the gases accumulate, producing distention. Cecal dilations are thought to precede torsions.

   (2) When distended, the cecum may then rotate clockwise or counterclockwise (when viewed from the right). The amount of rotation determines the degree of vascular embarrassment of the organ and the severity of resulting clinical signs.

d. Diagnostic plan. The diagnosis usually is made on the basis of clinical signs and rectal findings.

e. Laboratory tests

   (1) Laboratory results usually are normal for simple **cecal dilation.** Animals with **cecal volvulus** often have a hypochloremic, hypokalemic, metabolic alkalosis. Other laboratory values reflect varying degrees of vascular compromise and shock.

   (2) To **differentiate** cecal volvulus from abomasal volvulus, it may be helpful to perform a Liptak test. The pH is higher (more than 6) with cecal fluid than with abomasal fluid.

f. Differential diagnoses

   (1) For **cecal dilations,** rule out conditions such as abomasal displacement, ketosis, simple indigestion, and colonic gas.

   (2) Cecal volvulus may appear similar to abomasal volvulus, traumatic reticuloperitonitis, mesenteric root torsion, and gastrointestinal accidents (e.g., intussusceptions).

g. Therapeutic plan

   (1) Simple cecal dilations are treated conservatively.

      (a) Diet and exercise. The roughage component of the diet should be increased and forced exercise employed to increase gastrointestinal motility. Calcium salts are used occasionally to treat low-grade hypocalcemia and increase digestive tract motility.

      (b) Surgery. Cecal dilation can be a chronic or recurrent condition. Surgery may be used with some success in these cases.

   (2) Cecal volvulus requires **surgical intervention.** The cecum is approached through the right flank. The cecum is decompressed, and ingesta is removed from both it and the adjacent colon. Recovery is usually good with uncomplicated cases. If part or all of the cecum is devitalized, a partial or complete typhlectomy is necessary. **Fluid replacement** is also recommended to correct the metabolic alkalosis (sodium chloride, potassium chloride, and dextrose).

h. Prognosis. Depends upon amount of devitalization.

D. **Bleeding ulcers and erosions.** Blood in the feces of ruminants may be frank (visible and either red or black) or occult (unseen). Frank red blood is indicative of lower intestinal origin, whereas dark blood is from higher in the gastrointestinal tract and has been digested by proteolytic enzymes. Occult blood is from minor bleeding of insufficient amount to cause a change in character of the feces.

1. **Type I**
   a. **Patient profile and history.** Individual animals suffering from a primary disease process may develop abomasal erosions and ulcers. **Dairy cows** and **weaning age calves** seem to be most susceptible. The owner usually notices only the primary disease process (a septic process such as acute mastitis, or an abomasal condition such as LDA or RDA). In calves, the history may be one of poor growth and appetite disturbances.
   b. **Clinical findings**
      (1) There may be **no clinical signs** of abomasal erosions or ulcers. The lesions may only be evident at slaughter of a normal animal or necropsy of an animal dying from a primary disease process.
      (2) Alternatively, the clinical signs of a primary disease may be accompanied by **signs of abomasal erosion** or ulceration. These signs include:
         (a) Dark, fluid feces with mild, chronic abdominal pain
         (b) Periodic bruxism
         (c) A capricious appetite
         (d) Intermittent fecal occult blood
   c. **Etiology and pathogenesis.** The ulcers in an individual are usually multiple and small. Possible factors contributing to the development of ulcers include:
      (1) **Hyperacidity.** Gastric acid secretion may be stimulated by histamines, high VFA levels, calcium, or stress.
      (2) **Corticosteroids,** which lower mucosal cell resistance
      (3) **Direct trauma** from fiber (straw, low-quality roughage) or foreign bodies (hairballs in calves)
      (4) **Abomasal distention,** resulting in the tearing of mucosa and exacerbation of the lesion by exposure to HCl
      (5) **Pasture grazing** and associations with rainfall, fertilization, and forage growth
      (6) **Unknown factors,** such as endotoxins and mediator substances (e.g., interleukins)
   d. **Diagnostic plan.** Clinical findings and the demonstration of positive fecal occult blood provide the diagnosis. Fecal blood is best discovered by the use of tablets which test for occult blood.
   e. **Therapeutic plan**
      (1) In the case of **adult ruminants,** the primary disease and erosions are self-limiting.
      (2) In **younger animals,** treatment usually is not attempted; however, the owner should pay attention to providing a diet composed of more easily digestible roughage.
      (3) **Laxatives,** such as mineral oil, may be used in the case of concomitant foreign bodies (e.g., hairballs). Alternatively, **surgery** may be necessary.
   f. **Prevention.** The erosions and ulcers are self-limiting when the primary disorder has been corrected.

2. **Type II**
   a. **Patient profile.** These ulcers occur in **adult cattle** usually within 2 months of parturition and are commonly associated with a concurrent abomasal disease (e.g., LDA).
   b. **Clinical findings.** The animal may die suddenly or present with dark, tarry stools (melena). The cow will be anemic, as evidenced by pale mucous membranes, tachycardia, and weakness.
   c. **Etiology and pathogenesis.** The pathogenesis of bleeding ulcers is speculated to be similar to type I ulcers; however, the ulceration involves a major blood vessel, resulting in blood loss. **Lymphosarcoma** of the abomasal wall is also a primary cause for erosion and invasion of major abomasal blood vessels.

d. Diagnostic plan. Diagnose the condition based on clinical findings and laboratory support. A test on the feces confirms the presence of blood.

e. Laboratory tests. With significant blood loss, the PCV and TSP is decreased. The anemia is characterized as a blood-loss anemia. If there is concurrent abomasal disease, there may be a hypochloremic, hypokalemic, metabolic alkalosis. The leukogram may support a diagnosis of lymphosarcoma in the case of abomasal involvement.

f. Differential diagnoses. Blood in the feces may come from any of several sources. The distinction must be made between dark blood and bright red blood.

(1) A duodenal ulcer presents with fecal blood.

(2) Tumors other than lymphosarcoma may bleed (e.g., squamous cell carcinoma of the stomach).

(3) With vena caval thrombosis in cattle, pulmonary abscesses may develop, which erode pulmonary blood vessels in the lung. Blood is coughed up and swallowed, resulting in fecal blood and a positive test finding.

(4) Salmonellosis, coccidiosis, and rectal lacerations all present with red blood in the feces.

g. Therapeutic plan

(1) Therapy is attempted if lymphosarcoma has been ruled out as a cause of the ulcer. With lymphosarcoma, humane destruction is recommended.

(2) **Supportive therapy**

(a) For gastric ulcers, therapy includes **oral astringents, antacids** (magnesium oxide at 225 g four times a day for an adult animal), and **protectants** (e.g., stat, kaolin, pectin).

(b) **H$_2$-receptor antagonists** and **sulfate disaccharides,** although efficacious in monogastrics, rarely are employed in large ruminants because of ruminal dilution and cost.

(c) **Propantheline bromide** (30 mg four times daily in an adult cow) may be recommended to decrease vagal tone.

(d) A **blood transfusion** is necessary if the animal's PCV is less than 14% and if the heart rate is more than 100 bpm.

(e) **Hematinics** may be used (iron, cobalt, B vitamins), and **broad-spectrum antibiotics** are often employed.

(3) **Bleeding ulcers** are often singular. **Surgical extirpation** of the ulcer may be considered if bleeding continues and a tumor has been ruled out as the cause. Usually, ulcers are not visible from the serosal surface. Therefore, an abomasotomy is required to locate the ulcer.

h. Prognosis. The prognosis for survival is variable for non–tumor-related abomasal ulcers. Cows respond well to blood transfusions. Lymphosarcoma-associated ulcers carry a grave prognosis.

i. Prevention (see I D 1 f)

E. **Anterior abdominal pain.** Anterior abdominal pain in the mature ruminant usually manifests itself as a set of common clinical findings. There is an obvious painful response when manual pressure is applied to the cranial portion of the ventral abdominal wall, triggering an audible grunt, noticeable tensing of the neck muscles, or tensing of the ventral abdominal wall. A short groan or grunt may also occur spontaneously when an animal stands or walks downhill.

1. Traumatic reticuloperitonitis (TRP, hardware disease, traumatic gastritis, traumatic reticulitis)

a. Patient profile and history. In North America, the condition is most common in **adult dairy cattle** and is sporadic in nature. The owner describes a cow that experiences an abrupt drop in milk production and exhibits partial to complete anorexia.

b. Clinical findings

(1) **Acute local peritonitis.** Animals in the **early stages** of TRP are reluctant to move and appear "tucked-up." There may be extension of the neck and an arching of the back. The cow may stand with its elbows abducted and hind feet in the gutter to alleviate the abdominal pain. The triceps muscles often tremble.

    (a) Vital signs. Cows may have a shallow, catchy respiratory pattern and a decreased abdominal component to the cycle. The temperature and pulse rate are usually elevated (39.5 °C–40.5 °C and 80–90 bpm, respectively). Usually, the cow is dull and depressed.

    (b) On **gastrointestinal examination,** the clinician finds a decrease in rumen motility or complete atony. The feces of affected animals are scant, firm, dry, and mucus covered.

    (c) Rectal examination reveals a small, firm-feeling rumen. The animal may grunt with pain as the viscera are pressed forward.

    (d) Manipulative tests may be of value in localizing the pain. Cows normally ventroflex when pinched over the withers. Cows affected by TRP will not ventroflex and may grunt with resentment of the procedure. Percussion over the xiphisternum with a closed fist, lifting under the thorax with a board held by a person on either side of the animal or pressure applied by a knee to the ventral thorax may all elicit the same grunt.

(2) Chronic and local peritonitis. The acute clinical signs may abate and be replaced by signs of a more chronic process 24–48 hours after the onset of TRP. Animals appear rough and in poor condition. The vital signs may be normal. Gastrointestinal function is depressed, but signs are usually nonspecific. Demonstrable pain is usually not a hallmark of the local peritonitis with chronic TRP.

c. Etiology and pathogenesis

  (1) Foreign bodies. Cattle are relatively indiscriminate eaters. Pointed, metallic foreign bodies (e.g., nails, wire) may be consumed on pasture or with the ration. The foreign body is deposited in the reticulum and penetrates the reticular wall, usually in an anterior direction. Ruminal fluid and bacteria follow the track of the foreign body and enter the peritoneal cavity, producing an acute, localized peritonitis.

  (2) Sequelae to reticular penetration by the foreign body include:

    (a) Resolution of the infection with or without medical intervention. The foreign body may "fall back" into the reticulum and the animal "walls-off" the infection site (acute local peritonitis). The bovine has a tremendous ability to isolate infections by fibrous tissue formation.

    (b) Acute diffuse peritonitis. The infection cannot be controlled by the previous inflammatory processes, and a fatal infection ensues.

    (c) Traumatic hepatitis or splenitis. Movement of a foreign body may occur in a direction other than directly cranial, resulting in the involvement of associated abdominal tissues, most commonly the spleen or liver.

    (d) Pericarditis, pleuritis, or **pneumonia** resulting from perforation of the diaphragm

    (e) Chronic peritonitis. A result of fibrous tissue production may be the formation of reticular adhesions and mechanical interruption of rumen motility (see I A 3).

    (f) Fatal hemorrhage due to great vessel perforation (rare)

    (g) Diaphragmatic hernia caused by the weakening of the diaphragm (rare)

d. Diagnostic plan

  (1) The condition is most often diagnosed through the combination of a thorough **physical examination** and **laboratory tests.** Ancillary aids to diagnosis may include the use of radiology, a metal detector, or a compass to determine if a magnet is present in the reticulum.

  (2) An **abdominocentesis** is warranted if the diagnosis is equivocal or requires confirmation. It should be performed 3–4 cm to the right of the midline and 5–7 cm cranial to the foramen of the subcutaneous abdominal vein. Other reported sites for abdominocentesis include a point 10 cm to the right of the umbilicus, on the midline just caudal to the umbilicus, or cranial to the udder under the right flank fold.

  (3) An **exploratory rumenotomy** and/or **laparotomy** may be both diagnostic and therapeutic.

e. Laboratory tests

(1) Hematologic work-up. The complete blood cell count (CBC) usually reveals a neutrophilia with or without a leukocytosis. A left shift will be present. The serum total protein (TP) is elevated because of an increase in the γ-globulin fraction. Fibrinogen levels are elevated (7–9 g/L). A mild hypocalcemia may be found on clinical chemistry. Note that either very early or chronic cases may have normal clinical pathology findings.

(2) The following findings on **abdominal fluid analysis** support a diagnosis of acute local peritonitis:

    (a) A cell population comprised of 40% neutrophils

    (b) Significant proportions of immature, toxic, or degenerative neutrophils

    (c) Bacteria contained within neutrophils

(3) The **differential cell counts** on a CBC and **cellular morphology findings** on abdominocentesis are most significant in forming a diagnosis because normal ranges of both cell numbers and fibrinogen may overlap with values found in cases of TRP (or other causes of acute local peritonitis).

  f. Differential diagnoses. Conditions that need to be ruled out include:

    (1) Simple indigestion

    (2) Rumen acidosis

    (3) Displaced abomasum

    (4) Abomasal ulceration

    (5) Liver abscess

    (6) Pyelonephritis

  g. Therapeutic plan

    (1) Management strategies. Keep the animal confined in a headgate for 10 days. The front end of the cow may be elevated slightly (20 cm) on a bedding pack. A magnet should be administered orally if there is no evidence or history of one being previously administered.

    (2) Antibiotics should be administered according to labeled dosages. Penicillin or broad-spectrum antibiotics may be used. Balanced, isotonic solutions containing added calcium may be administered if the animal is dehydrated.

    (3) A **rumenotomy** should be considered to remove the penetrating object(s) if conservative management fails and economics warrant surgical intervention.

  h. Prevention of the condition includes administration of magnets to heifers when confirmed pregnant, passing the dairy ration component of the diet over magnets before feeding, and critical attention to pasture or dry-lot management to eliminate sources of foreign bodies (e.g., nails, wire).

2. Perforating abomasal ulcers with localized peritonitis. Abomasal ulcers may perforate the serosa, producing an **acute local peritonitis.** These may be referred to as type III ulcers (instead of bleeding ulcers).

  a. Patient profile and history. Abomasal ulcers in mature ruminants most commonly occur in association with concurrent diseases (e.g., LDA), recent parturition, heavy lactation, and grain or pasture grass feeding.

  b. Clinical findings. Clinical signs resemble those of TRP (see I E 1 b). However, the pain is localized to the right side of the xiphoid. Careful palpation and ballottement is required to determine this distinction. Bleeding into the gastrointestinal tract rarely seems to accompany a perforated abomasal ulcer.

  c. Etiology and pathogenesis (see I D 2 c).

  d. Laboratory tests. Laboratory data are similar to the acute local peritonitis of TRP (see I E 1 e). There may be an associated hypochloremic metabolic alkalosis if ulcers are concurrent with LDA.

  e. Differential diagnoses. Consider other causes of acute local peritonitis on a list of differential diagnoses (e.g., TRP). Also consider conditions that may appear to mimic anterior abdominal pain, such as:

    (1) Liver abscess

    (2) Pericarditis

    (3) Pleuritis

    (4) Endocarditis

(5) Musculoskeletal conditions (e.g., degenerative joint disease, vertebral body diseases, laminitis, tetanus)

f. **Therapeutic plan**
  (1) **Management strategies.** Provide stall rest, and feed only good quality hay for 10–14 days. If ketosis becomes a problem, add coarse calf grain to the ration.
  (2) **Antibiotic therapy** should be provided as for TRP [see I E 1 g (2)]. Antacid therapy, H_2-receptor blocking agents, and mucosal protectants may be recommended.
  (3) If medical therapy is unsuccessful, **surgical intervention** with removal of adhesions and resection of the ulcer(s) may be employed in valuable animals.

g. **Prognosis**
  (1) The prognosis for **abomasal ulceration** is usually good; however, it worsens if the lesion is in the abomasal fundus because a pyloric stricture with digestive outflow obstruction may occur. Also, an acute local peritonitis is less likely to be controlled in late pregnancy because of the pressure of a large, gravid uterus. The inability of an animal to control and localize a peritonitis results in an acute diffuse peritonitis with almost invariably fatal consequences.
  (2) Occasionally, animals suffer from a **chronic, relapsing peritonitis** if adhesions break down and release bacteria or their products into the abdominal cavity.

h. **Prevention** (see I D 1 f)

II. BOVINE INTESTINES

A. Gastrointestinal pain (colic)

1. **Adult cattle**
   a. **Patient profile and history.** Most colics are caused by either a malposition of a gastrointestinal tract component or other causes of acute obstruction to outflow. Surgery is the treatment of choice.
   b. **Clinical findings**
     (1) **Appearance and vital signs.** The animal exhibits a painful abdomen by treading, kicking at the abdomen, stretching, and frequently lying down and rising. The pulse and respiratory rates are elevated. Auscultation of the abdomen reveals absence of both ruminal and intestinal motility. With abomasal or upper intestinal obstruction, the abdomen is slightly distended, and splashing sounds can be elicited by succussion in the lower right quadrant.
     (2) On simultaneous auscultation and percussion, **pings** may be evident over distended viscera having a fluid/gas interface. The pings may differ in intensity, location, pitch, and area of auscultation, depending on the source of the distention.
     (3) On **rectal examination,** the rectum is usually empty except for a thick, tenacious, dark red mucus. Insertion of the arm may cause pain or vigorous straining. The examiner may be able to palpate distended or displaced bowel or tight mesenteric bands.
     (4) The animal may be **dehydrated** or in **shock.** The more proximal the lesion in the gastrointestinal tract, the more rapid the deterioration of the patient.
   c. **Etiology and pathogenesis**
     (1) The **pathogenesis** of abomasal torsion/volvulus and cecal torsion/volvulus seems to follow the same course of events as simple dilatations. However, twisting of the dilated viscus on either its horizontal or vertical axis results in digestive outflow obstruction and venous vascular occlusion.
     (2) The **risk factors** or causes of other intestinal accidents are less clearly understood and less easily studied because of their sporadic nature.
     (3) **Intestinal accidents**
       (a) **Indications** include persistent abdominal pain, elevated heart and respiratory rates, abdominal distention, absence of feces in the rectum, and the presence of a gas-filled viscus or distended loops of intestine.

(b) Intestinal accidents that involve the **abomasum** or **intestinal tract** and produce a common subset of clinical findings include:
- **(i)** Right abomasal volvulus
- **(ii)** Small intestinal intussusception
- **(iii)** Mesenteric torsion
- **(iv)** Intestinal incarceration
- **(v)** Cecal dilatation/volvulus
- **(vi)** Stricture of the colon
- **(vii)** Colonic obstruction (e.g., enterolith)
- **(viii)** Colonic constriction (e.g., fat necrosis)

d. Diagnostic plan. Perform a thorough physical examination. The presumptive diagnosis is confirmed by surgery.

e. Laboratory tests. Laboratory information is seldom available in time to be of value in the diagnosis.
- **(1) Hematologic work-up.** Shock and dehydration is supported by an increased PCV, increased TP, and a high BUN (prerenal uremia). High duodenal obstruction or abomasal volvulus produces a hypochloremic, hypokalemic, metabolic alkalosis. Leukopenia and/or neutropenia is found with devitalization of infarcted intestine.
- **(2) Abdominocentesis findings** may be variable but often show increased red blood cells, increased leukocytes, and bacteria indicative of devitalized bowel.

f. Therapeutic plan. If the animal is to be successfully treated, a decision to perform surgery should be made early and the patient vigorously supported by fluid therapy.

2. Calves

a. Patient profile and history. Most frequently, abdominal pain (colic) in calves is caused by conditions of gastrointestinal origin.

b. Clinical findings are variable depending on the site of involvement, duration of the condition, and degree of vascular compromise of the viscus. Common signs of colic include frequent lying down and rising, kicking of the abdomen, bruxism, and stretching.

c. Etiology and pathogenesis. Acute abdominal pain is of sporadic incidence and often associated with congenital problems of the gastrointestinal tract of young calves. Some conditions may be hereditary.

d. Diagnostic plan. A thorough clinical examination is necessary to determine the most likely source of the pain. Ancillary tests include radiography and contrast studies, gastric intubation, rectal probe (for anal or colonic atresia), and ultrasonography.

e. Differential diagnoses
- **(1)** Causes to be ruled out include:
  - **(a)** Intestinal atresia
  - **(b)** Atresia coli
  - **(c)** Atresia ani
  - **(d)** Abomasal dilatation
  - **(e)** Abomasal torsion
- **(2) Other causes** of abdominal distention must be ruled out including bladder rupture and intestinal fluid pooling with neonatal calf diarrhea.

f. Therapeutic plan. Generally, therapies include surgery and fluid therapy for responsive conditions.

B. Diarrhea

1. Acute diarrhea in adult cattle

a. Bovine virus diarrhea (BVD)
- **(1) Patient profile and history.** The majority of animals affected are young cattle (8 months to 2 years of age) often housed in an intensive management environment (e.g., beef feedlot, dairy freestall housing). There is a variable incidence of clinical disease (usually low). Several animals in the herd may show clinical signs.

(2) Clinical findings. The clinical findings may range from inapparent to acute, severe, enteric disease.
  (a) Clinically inapparent disease is widespread. Serologic evaluation may reveal 60%–80% of animals exposed and seropositive.
  (b) Mild enteric disease may be seen in a large number of animals and presents as mild transient diarrhea, inappetence, depression, and fever. Cattle recover in a few days.
  (c) Acute enteric disease presents as fever, profuse watery diarrhea, dysentery, and tenesmus. Discrete oral erosions are present (or may develop within 7 days of diarrhea), and the animal may salivate excessively. Peracute cases may die without evidence of diarrhea. This has also been described as a **hemorrhagic syndrome** in cattle.
  (d) Clinical signs referable to other body systems include mucopurulent nasal discharge, lacrimation, corneal edema and central corneal opacity; coronitis with interdigital erosions, and reproductive or congenital diseases. Abortions and stillbirths in immunologically negative heifers or cows have been associated with the viral infection, as has the birth of weak calves.
  (e) Chronic enteric disease (see II B 2)
(3) Etiology and pathogenesis
  (a) BVD is caused by a pestivirus of the ***Togaviridae*** family. Calves acquire passive immunity through colostrum of previously infected dams. This passive immunity wanes in 3–8 months. Following an outbreak of BVD, a herd tends to be free from clinical BVD for several years. With addition of seronegative replacement animals, herd immunity diminishes so that a herd is again susceptible to infection.
  (b) The pathogenesis of **acute, fatal, enteric disease** may involve one of two processes.
    (i) Infection by a particularly virulent biotype (BVD Type 2)
    (ii) If the fetus is infected by a noncytopathic virus in a BVD-negative dam before 125 days gestation, the calf is immunotolerant to the BVD virus with persistent viral infection and shedding. Subsequent exposure of this animal to a cytopathic virus (likely a mutant of the noncytopathic biotype) results in an acute and fatal infection (**mucosal disease**).
(4) Diagnostic plan. Clinical findings that are helpful in the definitive diagnosis include diarrhea, shallow oral erosions, central corneal opacity, and interdigital erosions.
(5) Laboratory tests. In individual animals, evidence of leukopenia, seroconversion, virus isolation, and polymerase chain reaction (PCR) are helpful for diagnosis. Note that animals that are immunotolerant and suffering from mucosal disease may not seroconvert. Herd serology may aid in diagnosis, as will necropsy of affected animals.
(6) Differential diagnoses. Conditions to be ruled out include bovine malignant catarrh, rinderpest, and salmonellosis.
(7) Therapeutic plan
  (a) Mild cases. Therapy is not necessary in cases of mild disease and of little help with severe enteric disease. Treatment is of no value in mucosal disease.
  (b) Severe cases. When therapy is attempted in severe cases, treatment consists of fluid therapy, oral astringents, and systemic antibiotics to control secondary infections.
(8) Prevention
  (a) Isolation of clinically ill animals from naive animals may limit the spread in the case of a herd outbreak.
  (b) Vaccination may be practiced with either killed or modified live viruses. Modified live virus vaccines have been limited to nonpregnant animals in their use because of possible induced abortions. It is unsure if this is related to the vaccine virus, vaccine virus reversion, or vaccine

contamination. Beef calves should be vaccinated between 6 and 8 months of age and dairy cattle vaccinated annually.

b. Bovine malignant catarrh (BMC, malignant catarrhal fever)

(1) Patient profile and history. The condition is usually sporadic and found in single animals, although occasionally herd outbreaks occur. In North America, the history invariably includes contact with sheep (usually at lambing time). In Africa, history includes contact with wildebeest.

(2) Clinical findings

(a) **High fever** with **tachycardia** accompanies profuse diarrhea and dysentery. Other signs include anorexia, agalactia, mucopurulent nasal discharge, dyspnea, and lymphadenopathy.

(b) **Ocular changes** include a peripheral corneoscleral opacity that spreads centripetally, ocular discharges, eyelid edema, and blepharospasm.

(c) **Neurological signs** may be seen including incoordination, nystagmus, muscle tremors, head pressing, paralysis, and convulsions.

(d) **Chronic disease** produces eczematous lesions around the perineum, prepuce, axillae, and horns. Sloughing of the skin from the teats and vulva is found in **acute cases.**

(e) **Labeling.** This variety of clinical pictures has resulted in labeling the disease by its presenting form (i.e., alimentary form, head and eye form, neurological form, skin form).

(3) Etiology and pathogenesis

(a) BMC is a generalized infection of the **primitive mesenchyme.** Necrosis and proliferation of vascular adventitia (vasculitis) yields epithelial erosions, keratoconjunctivitis, and encephalitis. Lymph node enlargement is caused by atypical proliferation of T lymphocytes.

(b) Clinical disease occurs only in cattle, deer, and buffalo. **Sheep** and goats in North America and **wildebeest** in Africa transmit the virus, although neither of these hosts develop clinical signs. **Alcelaphine BMC virus** (BHV-3) is the wildebeest-associated agent. A yet unidentified **herpesvirus** (sheep-associated herpesvirus) is the North American agent. The sporadic nature of the condition makes studying the disease or determining etiologies difficult.

(4) Diagnostic plan. Diagnosis of the condition is aided by the history (association with hosts), sporadic nature of the condition, and uniqueness of the clinical findings.

(5) Laboratory tests

(a) **Hematologic work-up.** Animals exhibit an early leukopenia followed by a leukocytosis. There are inflammatory changes of the joint fluid and cerebrospinal fluid.

(b) **Serological conversion** occurs with the African disease but has not been demonstrated with the North American disease. Virus isolation remains difficult.

(c) **Postmortem examination** remains the definitive diagnostic tool.

(6) Therapeutic plan. Therapy is unrewarding and animals will die in spite of supportive care.

c. Rinderpest

(1) Patient profile and history. This disease is confined to the Middle East, Asia, and tropical Africa where it is enzootic. It affects all ruminants and emerges in outbreaks.

(2) Clinical findings

(a) **Acute cases.** A high fever precedes by a few days other clinical signs such as anorexia, agalactia, and lacrimation. Oral and nasal inflammation soon is followed by the development of coalescing necrotic ulcers. Other signs follow including hemorrhagic and purulent lacrimation, skin lesions, diarrhea, dysentery, and dehydration. In an immunologically naive population, many cattle die acutely, most succumb within 7–10 days and few survive.

    (b) **Subacute** and **chronic forms** of the disease occur in more resistant populations and survival rates are higher.

  (3) **Etiology and pathogenesis.** Rinderpest virus is a paramyxovirus spread by animal excretions. Close animal contact is necessary because the virus does not survive for long periods outside of the host. The virus has a high affinity for lymphoid tissue and alimentary mucosa, where it replicates and produces the focal necrotic stomatitis and enteritis. A strong antibody response is generated.

  (4) **Diagnostic plan.** Diagnosis is based on clinical findings, history, and postmortem lesions.

  (5) **Laboratory tests**

    (a) **Leukopenia** and **lymphopenia** occur in affected animals. Postmortem findings are highly suggestive in populations at risk.

    (b) **Viral antigen** may be detected in several excretions and will confirm the diagnosis. **Serology** is of less value because of the acuteness of the condition in many cases.

  (6) **Differential diagnoses.** Other diseases that cause oral lesions and diarrhea must be ruled out. It is equally important to differentiate this disease from others that produce similar oral lesions without diarrhea (e.g., foot and mouth disease).

  (7) **Therapeutic plan.** There in no known treatment for this virus.

  (8) **Prevention.** Vaccination programs are successful, and many have lead to the eradication of the disease. Total eradication requires regulatory measures ensuring vaccination of herds and limitations on movements of nomadic populations.

d. Salmonellosis

  (1) **Patient profile and history.** This disease occurs worldwide and is seen in all ages, species, and breeds of animals. There is often a history of stress (e.g., recent shipment, parturition).

  (2) **Clinical findings**

    (a) **Vital signs and diarrhea.** There is an initial fever followed by a subnormal temperature. The heart and respiratory rates are elevated. There is a severe, watery, hemorrhagic diarrhea with mucus, fibrin casts, and blood clots. There is frequently evidence of abdominal pain (groaning, kicking at the flank), and pregnant animals may abort.

    (b) The disease has been described as one of three syndromes: septicemia, acute enteritis, and chronic enteritis. The main presenting syndrome in cattle is the **acute enteritis.**

  (3) **Etiology and pathogenesis**

    (a) The **most common species** isolated worldwide is *Salmonella typhimurium,* although a variety of *Salmonella* species can cause disease. *S. dublin* has a more patchy distribution but is the most common isolate in Europe.

    (b) The most common **source of infection** is environmental and feed contamination. Any domestic or wild species of animal or bird can act as a source of infection.

    (c) *S. typhimurium* causes sporadic, occasionally fatal disease. Infected adults are carriers for short periods of time so that the disease incidence usually subsides when the source of infection is removed.

    (d) *S. dublin* is particularly well adapted to cattle, which may act as a reservoir for outbreaks. Continued excretion of the organism may occur for years after exposure.

    (e) **Route of infection.** After oral inoculation with the bacteria, salmonella invades the intestinal wall and progresses to localize in the mesenteric lymph nodes. Development of disease then depends on the immune status and age of host, virulence of the organism, and stresses on the animal. In susceptible animals exposed to a virulent species, septicemia and bacteremia occur. A carrier state may develop in survivors. Diarrhea occurs due to enteritis and the elaboration of an enterotoxin, which causes an increased secretion of sodium, chloride, and water into the gut lumen.

  (4) **Diagnostic plan.** Clinical findings together with laboratory test results usually are sufficient for diagnosis; however, fecal culture results may be negative even with diarrhea.

- **(5) Laboratory tests**
  - **(a) Clinical pathologic findings** reflect a profound toxic state and an inflammatory condition. Anemia from blood loss may be seen.
  - **(b) Fecal culture** is the best diagnostic test but may need to be repeated several times for success. Organisms may not be present in the feces for up to 2 weeks after commencement of diarrhea because of the dilution effect of the diarrhea. Culturing a rectal mucosal biopsy increases the likelihood of successfully isolating the organism in an affected animal.
- **(6) Differential diagnoses.** Other conditions that appear similar to enteric salmonellosis include winter dysentery, coccidiosis, general toxemia, and arsenic or superphosphate fertilizer toxicities.
- **(7) Therapeutic plan**
  - **(a) Early, aggressive treatment** with broad-spectrum or selective antibiotics is necessary for successful therapy. **Extralabel use** of these antibiotics requires restrictions on meat and milk use from treated animals. Examples include:
    - **(i) Trimethoprim–sulfa:** 25 mg/kg intramuscularly twice per day
    - **(ii) Gentamicin:** 2 mg/kg intramuscularly three times per day
    - **(iii) Amikacin:** 7 mg/kg intramuscularly three times per day
  - **(b) Oral** or **intravenous fluids** are necessary in amounts calculated for replacement and ongoing losses. Oral astringents and protectants (e.g., bismuth subsalicylate) and parenteral nonsteroidal anti-inflammatory agents (e.g., flunixin meglumine) may be employed.
- **(8) Prevention**
  - **(a) Recovered animals** (whether from treatment or naturally) may excrete the organism and expose herdmates for significant lengths of time. Treatment and isolation procedures must take this into account.
  - **(b) Management strategies.** Seek to remove sources of contaminated food, litter, and water. *Salmonella* organisms may infect humans, so hygienic precautions should be taken.

- **e. Winter dysentery**
  - **(1) Patient profile and history.** This disease commonly occurs in young adult, housed dairy cattle in the winter months. Diarrhea is most severe in lactating and pregnant animals and is rare in bulls and steers. Diarrhea is often related to a feed change, a change in housing, or sudden, significant temperature shifts.
  - **(2) Clinical findings**
    - **(a) Herd.** This disorder causes an outbreak of diarrhea involving the majority of animals in the herd. There is an accompanying drop in milk production. The condition may persist in the herd for up to 2 weeks.
    - **(b) In individual animals,** the TPR is usually normal. There is a nasolacrimal discharge and a cough, both of which precede the diarrhea. The diarrhea is projectile and hemorrhagic and lasts from a few hours to a week. The animal may demonstrate abdominal pain, have increased intestinal sounds, and become dehydrated and weak.
  - **(3) Etiology.** The cause is considered to be a bovine coronavirus.
  - **(4) Diagnostic plan.** The clinical picture and subjective findings along with response to therapy are enough to establish a diagnosis.
  - **(5) Laboratory tests.** Individual animals have a mildly elevated hematocrit and total plasma protein value. Direct electron microscopy and an enzyme-linked immunosorbent assay (ELISA) may be applied to the feces to demonstrate the virus. Acute and convalescent serum samples reveal seroconversion to coronavirus.
  - **(6) Therapeutic plan.** If necessary, animals may be treated with oral or intravenous fluids and oral intestinal protectants (e.g., kaolin).
  - **(7) Prevention.** Even with care regarding disinfection and attempts at isolation, the disease will run its course through the herd.

f. Arsenic toxicosis

 (1) Patient profile and history. Recent exposure to arsenicals (e.g., ectoparasite sprays, arsenic-based herbicides, arsenic-based wood preservatives) may be deduced from the history. The owner may report sudden death of an individual or group of animals.

 (2) Clinical findings

  (a) Animals may experience acute, subacute, or chronic signs referable to arsenic poisoning. With the acute toxicosis, cattle experience abdominal pain, diarrhea, dehydration, regurgitation, muscular tremors, convulsions, and death within 4–6 hours of showing clinical signs.

  (b) Other signs may involve the central nervous system (CNS; see Chapter 11).

 (3) Etiology and pathogenesis. Ingested inorganic arsenic causes inactivation of sulfhydryl groups in tissue enzymes. Tissues that are most susceptible are the alimentary tract, liver, kidney, spleen, and lung. In the gastrointestinal tract, this condition causes extensive capillary damage, hemorrhage, necrosis, and sloughing of the intestinal mucosa.

 (4) Diagnostic plan. Clinical findings and history are important, but diagnosis relies on laboratory confirmation.

 (5) Laboratory tests. Urine and hair samples are suitable antemortem specimens for arsenic analysis. Postmortem confirmation is best supported by liver arsenic levels.

 (6) Therapeutic plan

  (a) An attempt should be made to absorb the enteric arsenic with **activated charcoal** at 1–4 g/kg orally. Cattle are also treated with **sodium thiosulfate** at 15–30 g in 200 ml H_2O intravenously followed by 30–60 g orally, four times daily. Treatment should be continued until recovery occurs.

  (b) British antilewisite (BAL), also called dimercaprol, may be used but is less effective against inorganic salts than the organic forms. Intravenous fluid therapy is warranted in dehydrated animals.

 (7) Prevention. Limit exposure to arsenicals.

g. Toxemia. Toxemia, such as peracute coliform mastitis or toxic metritis in cattle, often are accompanied by diarrhea. The pathogenesis may be an effect of endotoxemia or caused by stress-related ulcers.

2. Subacute to chronic diarrhea in young and adult cattle

 a. Chronic parasitism. This condition is common, but diarrhea due to parasitism is relatively infrequent. Chronic wasting is the obvious sign, and of the parasites affecting the bovine abomasum and small intestine (e.g., *Ostertagia, Cooperia, Trichostrongylus, Nematodirus*), *Ostertagia* infestation produces the diarrhea.

  (1) Patient profile and history. Several young (6 months to 2 years) animals often are affected in a herd. There is a history of persistent diarrhea and weight loss.

  (2) Clinical findings. There is diarrhea without odor, mucus, or blood. Emaciation, dependant edema, and poor growth also may be signs of infection.

  (3) Etiology and pathogenesis

   (a) Type I. Infective (third-stage) larvae are ingested, molt to fourth-stage larvae, and penetrate the abomasal glands, causing hyperplasia of the mucus-secreting cells. This nodular hyperplasia may be discrete or confluent, presenting as a "moroccan-leather" appearance on necropsy. Mucosal layer destruction results in protein leakage.

   (b) Type II. Fourth-stage larvae enter the mucosal glands and remain there, causing little or no damage (a pretype condition). Type II disease occurs when larvae emerge, producing marked cellular hyperplasia. This emergence occurs at various times of the year in different countries. Abomasal pH rises due to a loss of parietal cells and failure of the conversion of pepsinogen to pepsin. Anorexia and plasma protein leakage cause hypoproteinemia. Diarrhea is constant and weight loss is rapid.

  (4) Diagnostic plan. Clinical findings, environmental findings, and investigation of management practices may indicate a parasite burden.

(5) Laboratory tests. Fecal egg counts are diagnostic, however, they may need to be repeated in the case of hypobiotic larvae.

(6) Therapeutic plan. Deworm in the event of any parasite load. Ivermectin and levamisole continue to be the drugs of choice (ivermectin for the hypobiotic state).

(7) Prevention. Reduce pasture or drylot contamination through management of stocking densities, pasture rotation, and routine anthelmintic treatment.

b. Chronic BVD

(1) Patient profile and history. The age range of affected cattle is usually 6 months to 2 years. There may be a history of a previous outbreak of BVD in the herd with the recovery of most animals. A few animals may have remained stunted with intermittent diarrhea, lameness, or both. There may be a history of recurrent bacterial infections (e.g., pneumonia).

(2) Clinical findings. Animals appear stunted with a rough, dry haircoat. Oral examination reveals the occasional erosion with blunted oral papillae. Crusty or erosive dermatitis is present at the commissures of the mouth, medial canthus of the eye, around the perineum, scrotum, coronary band, bulbs of the heels, and in the interdigital cleft. The animal may be lame. Diarrhea is intermittent or continuous.

(3) Etiology and pathogenesis. Cattle previously exposed to a noncytopathic strain of BVD virus in utero (before 125 days gestation) are immunotolerant to the BVD virus and are incapable of mounting a humoral antibody response when subsequently challenged with the virus. They are chronically infected with the virus, continue to excrete antigen, but remain negative by serum neutralization tests.

(4) Diagnostic plan. Diagnosis may be based on clinical findings, virus isolation or PCR for viral nucleic acid, and necropsy findings.

(5) Therapeutic plan. Therapy is useless and salvage should be considered as a realistic option.

(6) Prevention. Recommendations for control are as presented in II B 1 a (8).

c. Coccidiosis

(1) Patient profile and history. Subjective findings with this disease are similar to conditions predisposing to parasitism (i.e., overcrowded housing conditions, management practices that encourage fecal–oral spread of organisms). Groups of young animals are affected in a seasonal pattern depending on region of the country.

(2) Clinical findings. The cardinal signs are diarrhea (with mucus and blood) and tenesmus. Anemia also may be a finding, and some cattle may have nervous signs (see Chapter 11). Cattle often are unthrifty in appearance. Clinical syndromes may vary from peracute cases to inapparent infections.

(3) Etiology and pathogenesis

(a) Causative organisms are *Eimeria zuernii* and *E. bovis* in the large intestine and *E. ellipsoidalis* in the small intestine.

(b) Infestation occurs through the ingestion of sporulated oocysts from the environment. Oocysts are resistant to most environmental conditions. Multiple-species infections are quite common, and disease seems to be more prevalent in stressed or undernourished animals.

(c) Route of infection. Sporozoites are released from the ingested oocytes and invade the endothelial cells of the small intestine. Asexual schizonts develop, mature, and release merozoites through rupture of the endothelial cells. This cycle repeats itself in the large intestine followed by the sexual life cycle of macrogametocyte and microgametocyte production. These stages of the life cycle also produce intestinal mucosa destruction. Fertilization of the gametocytes produce oocysts, which are shed coincident with the development of diarrhea and dysentery. The prepatent period (and development of diarrhea) may be 15–20 days.

(4) Laboratory tests. Oocysts are seen in the feces 2–4 days after the onset of dysentery. Therefore, clinical signs may be present without demonstrable oocysts. *Coccidia* may be found in the feces of normal calves, so laboratory data must correlate to clinical findings. Direct fecal smears and fecal flotations are the most common laboratory tests used.

  (5) Therapeutic plan

  (a) Individual treatment. Coccidiosis is a **self-limiting disease** but causes death in severely affected animals. Clinical signs subside when the multiplication stages have passed. Most coccidiostats suppress early first-stage schizonts; therefore, treatment of clinical disease with coccidiostats is of limited value. Other **supportive care** for the individual animal (e.g., fluid therapy) may be warranted under certain circumstances.

  (b) Herd treatment. Mass medication, decreasing stocking densities, and removing feed and water from ground level are all treatment strategies used in a herd outbreak. **Medications** include sulfaquinoxaline at 2.72 mg/kg orally daily for 3–5 days and amprolium at 10 mg/kg orally for 5 days.

  (6) Prevention. Avoid undernutrition, overcrowding, and feeding from ground level. Coccidiostats may be efficacious and necessary under conditions that do not allow for management alterations. Control medications include sulfaquinoxaline, amprolium, decoquinate, monensin, and lasalocid.

d. Chronic salmonellosis. Salmonellosis in adult cattle usually presents as an acute, explosive, mucohemorrhagic diarrhea (see II B 1 d). However, when salmonellosis has become enzootic, chronic diarrhea and unthriftiness may be observed.

e. Johne's disease (paratuberculosis)

  (1) Patient profile and history. This disease occurs in adult dairy cows and beef cattle older than 2–3 years of age. There is a breed disposition, with Shorthorn, Angus, and Channel Island dairy breeds being over-represented. This may be an effect of historical numbers possibly related to breed popularity, similar to the way Holsteins are affected now.

  (2) Clinical findings. Early clinical disease presents as intermittent or continuous watery or "pea-soup" diarrhea associated with stress (e.g., parturition). Vital signs are normal, and appetite is good to excellent. Emaciation becomes progressive, and milk production decreases. Terminal signs include profound emaciation, profuse watery diarrhea, and dependent edema.

  (3) Etiology and pathogenesis

  (a) The disease is caused by ***Mycobacterium paratuberculosis.*** The infection is contracted principally by the ingestion of feedstuffs or water contaminated by animals that are fecal shedders. Nursing calves may ingest the organism off the dam's udder. Calves born to clinically affected cattle may be infected in utero.

  (b) Age of infection. Animals are most susceptible to infection as calves (less than 30 days of age), and most animals with the disease are infected before 4 months of age. However, clinical disease develops 2–5 years later.

  (c) Age of shedding. Animals may become fecal shedders 15–18 months before the development of clinical signs. Some animals are shedders without ever becoming clinically affected. The organism may be persistent in suitable soils.

  (d) Route of infection. Following oral ingestion, *M. paratuberculosis* localizes in the small intestine and associated lymph nodes. The bacteria multiply, and the animal either becomes resistant, a shedder, or a clinical case. Animals that are infected older than 6 months of age apparently are able to mount an effective immune response and develop resistance.

  (e) Disease progression. In those animals in which the organisms multiply unchecked, there develops a granulomatous enterocolitis initially around the ileocecal valve. The enterocolitis spreads, and a malabsorption syndrome results with a protein-losing enteropathy. There is a compensatory increase in protein synthesis by the liver, but eventually hypoproteinemia occurs with signs of edema.

  (4) Diagnostic plan. Clinical signs alone are not reliable for a diagnosis. Laboratory tests confirm the diagnosis. Postmortem examination of a specifically sacrificed animal is the most reliable diagnostic tool.

  (5) Laboratory tests

(a) **Fecal culture** is the most reliable and frequently used diagnostic test for infection in individual cattle. DNA probes and fecal culture by radiometric technique are also available and considered valuable diagnostic tools.

(b) **Serological tests** offer some value in determining herd status of infection but often must be carried out as a series of tests. Problems with sensitivity and specificity are common. These tests include complement fixation test (CFT), agar gel immunodiffusion test (AGID), and ELISA (the least costly and most accurate serological test).

(c) **Other tests.** Tests for **cell-mediated immunity** vary in their reliability. The intradermal and intravenous johnin tests are available. **Lymphocyte immunostimulation** tests are also available, of which some are highly reliable.

(6) **Therapeutic plan.** Therapy is as yet unwarranted because response to treatment with medications (e.g., streptomycin, isoniazid, clofazimine) is only transient.

(7) **Prevention**

(a) **Methods of herd management.** The disease may be kept in check on a herd basis by test and slaughter methods. Removal of reactor or culture-positive animals and their offspring is necessary. This needs to be combined with improved hygienic practices, which decrease the fecal–oral spread of the organism. Calves must be removed from the dams at birth and reared separately. The herd should be maintained as a closed herd or replacement animals purchased from known Johne's-free herds.

(b) **Problems with herd management.** The disease may be effectively eliminated from a herd, but the management changes required are intensive, rigorous, and expensive. Because of the inaccuracies in diagnostic tests, there is as yet no test and slaughter program that effectively eliminates all carriers. Therefore, the only effective method of elimination is one of repopulation of a new environment with unexposed or known negative animals.

(c) **Vaccination.** If local legislation permits, vaccination of calves may provide protection against clinical disease and reduce the rate of spread of infection. A major complication of a vaccination program is that vaccines are positive to the tuberculin test for bovine tuberculosis.

f. **Bovine leukosis (enzootic bovine leukosis).** Bovine leukosis is of major significance, but the gastrointestinal effects are of limited importance to the overall clinical picture and health management of the disease.

(1) **Patient profile and history.** The disease is seen most commonly in adult dairy cows. History related to gastrointestinal signs includes intermittent diarrhea.

(2) **Clinical findings.** The clinical signs depend on the degree and specificity of organ involvement. Many of the following forms often occur concurrently, resulting in the term **adult multicentric lymphosarcoma.**

(a) **Digestive form**—capricious appetite, persistent or intermittent diarrhea, melena

(b) **Lymph node form**—superficial, palpably enlarged lymph nodes

(c) **Cardiac form**—muffled heart sounds due to hydropericardium, dyspnea due to hydrothorax, jugular vein engorgement, brisket edema, and bottle jaw

(d) **Nervous form**—posterior paralysis

(e) **Respiratory form**—upper respiratory noise and dyspnea

(f) **Ocular form**—exophthalmos

(3) **Etiology and pathogenesis**

(a) The **pathogenesis** of the various forms is covered under the appropriate systems. Gastrointestinal signs are a result of tumor growth in the abomasal wall. Ulceration and gastrointestinal bleeding follows.

(b) **Etiology.** Enzootic bovine leukosis is caused by the bovine leukemia virus (BLV), a type-C retrovirus. Infection with the virus is common, but the development of solid tissue tumors is less common, depending on host genetic and environmental factors. Persistent lymphocytosis and bovine lymphosarcoma are manifestations of the endemic form of bovine leukosis. The usual incubation period between infection and development of clinical signs is 4–5 years.

    (c) Horizontal transmission via blood or contaminated instruments, which transmit infected lymphocytes, is thought to be the most common method of infection. Therefore, insect bites, surgical instruments, rectal sleeves, and contaminated needles have all been implicated in viral transmission.

    (d) Vertical transmission is possible through contaminated semen as is **transplacental exposure** to the virus during gestation. There is a familial tendency in the development of disease, indicating the possibility of a **genetic predisposition.**

  (4) Diagnostic plan. The diagnosis of bovine lymphosarcoma as causative for gastrointestinal disease relies on definitive tests, necropsy or exploratory laparotomy with abomasotomy. Clinical findings of diarrhea with palpably enlarged lymph nodes or other multicentric expressions increase the level of suspicion.

  (5) Laboratory tests. Laboratory tests that support a diagnosis include abdominocentesis demonstrating exfoliated, abnormal lymphocytes; serology (AGID, radioimmunoassay, ELISA, protein immunoblot test); persistent lymphocytosis; and solid tumor biopsy.

  (6) Therapeutic plan. There is no known treatment for this disease.

  (7) Prevention. Disease may be controlled or eradicated.

    (a) Control is based on a test and segregation practice. Animals are tested and divided into positive and negative groups, and they are distinctly separated in terms of housing and management. In one such scheme, AGID tests are used on a herd basis every 3 months and reactors removed to the positive group until reactors are no longer found. Testing is then used every 6 months until all animals have been negative for four successive tests. Replacement animals must be test negative on two separate occasions and quarantined for 60 days before the second test.

    (b) Eradication is effective but costly. Infected animals are identified by AGID. Seropositive animals are culled. This process is repeated every 30–60 days until the herd tests clean. Testing is then carried out every 6 months until four sequential negative herd tests allow the herd to be declared BLV free.

    (c) Several procedures help limit the spread of infection within herds including:

      (i) Feeding colostrum to newborn calves from BLV-free animals

      (ii) Housing calves in individual hutches

      (iii) Control of insect vectors

      (iv) Dedication of blood-bearing fomites to individual use (e.g., rectal sleeves, needles)

      (v) Disinfection of veterinary instruments

      (vi) Embryo transfer

g. Abdominal fat necrosis

  (1) Patient profile and history. Although uncommon, this condition is most prevalent in obese Channel Island cattle (Jersey, Guernsey). Often sporadic in occurrence, the disease has been associated on a herd basis with cattle grazing heavily fertilized, fescue pastures.

  (2) Clinical findings

    (a) Clinical signs include diarrhea or findings reflective of intestinal obstruction (i.e., anorexia, treading, stretching, bruxism, lowered fecal output, abdominal distention).

    (b) Rectal examination reveals large, irregularly-shaped masses associated with the kidneys, small intestine, and colon. Rectal stricture may be evident. Dystocia may occur secondary to the abdominal masses.

  (3) Etiology and pathogenesis. Fat deposits in the body are modified by a coagulative necrosis. This process is associated with over-conditioning in individuals or linked to high nitrogen levels in fescue pastures on a herd basis. The fat deposits harden and interfere with gastrointestinal function.

  (4) Diagnostic plan. Diagnosis is based on rectal examination and necropsy.

      (5) Therapeutic plan. There is no approved treatment for this disorder, although the condition may resolve if the animals are taken off an offending pasture. Iso-prothiolane has shown experimental efficacy. Salvage is recommended.

  h. Primary copper deficiency

    (1) Patient profile and history. The condition usually occurs in young adult cattle (1–3 years) that graze on sandy or peat soils. The condition presents as a herd problem. There is no breed predisposition.

    (2) Clinical findings. In clinically evident cases, animals are consistently poor in appearance with persistent diarrhea. Occasional depigmentation is evident around the eyes. Lameness may be evident as is anemia, decreased milk production, or occasionally sudden death. CNS signs (e.g., incoordination, paresis) occur in lambs (see Chapter 11).

    (3) Etiology and pathogenesis. Copper may be inadequate in the diet because of soil deficiency or unavailability. Lack of copper limits the cytochrome oxidase system through decreased production of ceruloplasmin. Failure of these enzyme systems result in the many manifestations of copper deficiency.

    (4) Diagnostic plan. The diagnosis may be supported by laboratory data (generated from herd-level sampling) and response to treatment.

    (5) Laboratory tests. Plasma and tissue (liver, hair) copper levels are low, but interpretation may be difficult because of wide variations in values for individual animals. Anemia is evident on a CBC. The diet may be analyzed for copper levels.

    (6) Therapeutic plan

      (a) Oral dosing of 4 g of copper sulfate for young animals and 8–10 g of copper sulfate for mature cattle weekly for 3–5 weeks is recommended. **Controlled-release boluses** are also available, but absorbed amounts may be less than desirable. **Copper oxide fragments** are available for oral dosing and may be the most reliable and efficacious method of supplementation.

      (b) Injectable copper treatments may provide advantages over oral forms in terms of ease in administration and rapidity of results.

    (7) Prevention. Treatment must be followed by oral maintenance. Oral dosing weekly with 5 g/adult or dietary supplementation in the mineral mix is recommended. Salt licks containing 2% copper sulfate should be adequate. Dietary modification to ensure 10 parts per million (ppm) copper as measured in the dry matter of the final ration is also adequate. Top dressing of the pasture with copper sulfate at a rate of 10 kg/ha may be employed.

  i. Secondary copper deficiency (molybdenum toxicity)

    (1) Patient profile and history. This deficiency affects young adult dairy cows and beef cattle grazing pastures high in molybdenum or sulfates.

    (2) Clinical findings. The clinical picture is as in primary copper deficiency, but anemia is not as common. Diarrhea (watery, yellow-green to black feces passed without straining) is more common than in primary copper deficiency.

    (3) Etiology and pathogenesis. Molybdenum reacts with sulfides in the rumen to produce thiomolybdates. The subsequent formation of copper–thiomolybdate complexes renders the copper unavailable. Soil levels of less than 3 ppm molybdenum are considered safe, whereas offending soils are frequently in the 10–100 ppm range.

    (4) Diagnostic and therapeutic plans. Diagnosis and treatment are as for primary copper deficiency (see II B 2 h). The removal of sulfates from drinking water may have a positive effect.

    (5) Differential diagnoses. Rule out parasitism.

    (6) Prevention centers around removing copper-complexing agents (e.g., sulfates) from the diet and water source.

3. Diarrhea in neonates

  a. Enterotoxigenic *Escherichia coli* **(ETEC)**

    (1) Patient profile and history. Diarrhea is a common occurrence in young calves of all breeds. Diarrhea due to *E. coli* occurs often at less than 5 days of age but can be seen in older neonates (up to 2 weeks).

(2) **Clinical findings.** Diarrhea is watery and profuse, leading to depression, weakness, dehydration, and anorexia. Terminally, there are signs of shock resulting from hypovolemia and electrolyte imbalances. Mild cases may recover spontaneously in a few days, whereas severe cases may result in death in as little as 8 hours (sometimes without external evidence of diarrhea).

(3) **Etiology and pathogenesis**

    (a) **Pathogenesis.** ETEC adhere to the intestinal epithelium via pili, which usually possess the K-99 antigen. When adherent, ETEC produces a heat stable toxin (ST). This results in a secretory diarrhea (loss of fluid and electrolytes), mediated by cyclic guanosine monophosphate (cGMP). The ST leaves the glucose (glycine)-Na^+ transport system intact but interferes with the Ca^{++}-mediated Na^+ Cl^- co-transport system.

    (b) In addition to the bacteria, **contributing factors** to the development of diarrhea include:

        (i) Intensive management conditions (e.g., overcrowding, communal feeding)

        (ii) Synergism with other diarrhea-producing agents (e.g., rotavirus)

        (iii) Ingestion of insufficient quantities or substandard quality of colostrum

(4) **Diagnostic plan.** Clinical findings must be supported by a laboratory diagnosis to allow appropriate recommendations to be made regarding herd prevention.

(5) **Laboratory tests**

    (a) **Fecal** or **intestinal culture** reveal ETEC often based on polyclonal antibody testing. ELISA test kits for demonstration of the K99 antigen are also available.

    (b) For the **individual calf,** laboratory findings show varying degrees of acidemia, hypoglycemia, and hypokalemia. Clinical pathology findings are reflective of hemoconcentration (e.g., elevated BUN and hematocrit). Total protein levels may be normal if hypoproteinemia is coincident with dehydration.

(6) **Therapeutic plan**

    (a) **Antibiotics.** Diarrhea caused by ETEC is often **self-limiting** without antibiotic therapy if vigorous supportive care is instituted early. However, antibiotics often are used with success in the field (e.g., sulbactam–ampicillin, trimethoprim–sulfas, gentamicin). Part of this rationale is because of the difficulty of accurately differentiating between septicemic colibacillosis and diarrhea due to ETEC.

    (b) **Supportive care** for the individual calf is an absolute necessity. Oral replacement solutions are efficacious early in the course of the disease. Later, it becomes necessary to replace lost fluids and electrolytes intravenously.

        (i) **Oral replacement solutions** work on the principle of an intact glucose absorption mechanism in the gut. Sodium is absorbed via coupling to glucose, and water is dragged along the osmotic gradient.

        (ii) Replacement solutions **contain** sodium chloride, sodium bicarbonate, and an energy source (e.g., glucose). The oral agents should be nursed by the calf in small quantities frequently, based on replacement needs and ongoing losses. It is not necessary to take calves completely off milk, but decrease quantities and alternate with electrolyte feedings. Do not feed oral electrolytes and milk simultaneously as this may interfere with milk clot formation in the abomasum.

        (iii) In calves more than 8% dehydrated, **intravenous replacement** and alkalinizing solutions are necessary. Isotonic $NaHCO_3$ (1.3%) is often administered in conjunction with balanced electrolyte solutions (0.85% sodium chloride) and isotonic dextrose (5%).

    (c) **Other therapies** include nursing care to keep the calf warm and dry and intestinal protectants (e.g., kaolin–pectin combinations, bismuth subsalicylate). There is no evidence that anticholinergics or oral antibiotics influence the course or magnitude of the diarrhea.

(7) **Prevention.** Total prevention of this condition is usually an unrealistic goal. A control program is built on the principles of reduction of exposure of neonates through hygienic and management practices, provision of adequate colostrum, and vaccination of the dam or calf. Many of these practices are difficult to fully achieve and require creative modifications, depending on the numbers of animals and the population at risk (i.e., dairy, beef, or veal calves).

b. **Rotavirus diarrhea**

(1) **Patient profile.** Rotavirus causes diarrhea in all breeds of calves from 5 to 7 days up to 3 weeks of age. This virus often is found in mixed infections with ETEC and cryptosporidia.

(2) **Clinical findings.** Clinical findings in pure rotavirus infections are diarrhea, dehydration, and anorexia. The condition may last for a few days, and recovery is usually uneventful. Combined infections with other pathogens (e.g., *E. coli*) result in a clinical picture of undifferentiated neonatal diarrhea indistinguishable from ETEC or combined enteric pathogens.

(3) **Etiology and pathogenesis**

(a) The condition is caused by one of several strains of RNA rotavirus. The virus attacks absorptive cells at the tips of the villi of the small intestine. Loss of these mature epithelial cells results in malabsorption (lactase washout), osmotic diarrhea, dehydration, electrolyte loss, and acidosis.

(b) Intestinal regeneration and epithelial cell function return to normal within approximately 7 days, although normal growth rates for the calf may take 10–21 days to return.

(4) **Diagnostic plan.** Accurate diagnosis depends on laboratory confirmation.

(5) **Laboratory tests.** The virus may be isolated from fresh feces or intestine. Tests that should be performed include electronmicroscopy, immunofluorescence, latex agglutination, and ELISA.

(6) **Therapeutic plan.** The treatment is as for ETEC or undifferentiated neonatal diarrhea [see II B 3 a (6)].

(7) **Prevention**

(a) **Management strategies.** The principles of control are the same as for undifferentiated neonatal diarrhea—limit exposure to the organism, ensure colostral intake, and increase specific antibody levels by vaccination of the calf or dam.

(b) **Vaccination** of calves has given less than satisfactory results in field studies. For vaccination of the dam to provide protection to the calf, it must occur at a time of colostrum production, and continued feeding of milk or colostrum with high antibody titers during the times calves are susceptible to infection is necessary. This may require management changes in veal or dairy operations.

c. **Coronavirus diarrhea**

(1) **Patient profile.** Coronavirus causes diarrhea in beef or dairy calves under a variety of management practices. The age range of infected calves is generally 5–20 days.

(2) **Clinical findings.** Clinical findings are similar to other cases of neonatal diarrhea, with the exception that flecks of frank blood may be seen in the feces of coronavirus-infected calves.

(3) **Etiology and pathogenesis.** Coronavirus replicates in and damages the villus epithelium of both the small and large intestines. The crypt cells also are damaged, which results in a longer rejuvenation time for cell repair and replacement. Loss of epithelial cells results in malabsorption, maldigestion, and diarrhea.

(4) **Diagnostic plan.** Diagnosis is based on confirmatory laboratory tests as in rotavirus infection [see II B 3 b (4), (5)].

(5) **Therapeutic plan and prevention.** Therapy and prevention is as for rotavirus infection, with the added caveat that calves with coronavirus diarrhea take longer to recover because of crypt cell destruction. Convalescence may be pro-

longed and weight loss significant. Attention to nutritional supplementation may be necessary.

d. Cryptosporidiosis diarrhea

   (1) Patient profile and history. Neonatal dairy or beef calves are affected.

   (2) Clinical findings

   (a) The **clinical signs** are indistinguishable from other causes of neonatal diarrhea. Calves are usually 1–3 weeks of age. Tenesmus may be a feature of the condition as is weight loss and the persistence of the diarrhea.

   (b) Appearance. Severe dehydration, weakness, and recumbency are not characteristic of uncomplicated cases of cryptosporidiosis.

   (3) Etiology and pathogenesis

   (a) The causative agent is the protozoan parasite, ***Cryptosporidium parvum.*** Infective oocysts are ingested and develop through six stages within the lower small intestine, large intestine, and cecum. The parasite produces villus atrophy, impairment of digestion, and absorption with a resultant mild diarrhea in uncomplicated cases. The organism is frequently seen in combination with other agents that cause neonatal diarrhea. This increases the severity of the diarrhea and the clinical effect on the calf.

   (b) The **prepatent period** is 2–7 days, and sporulated oocysts may be passed for 3–12 days in the feces.

   (4) Diagnostic plan. Diagnosis depends on laboratory confirmation.

   (5) Laboratory tests. Fecal oocysts may be detected by fecal floatation, direct staining of fecal smears, immunofluorescence, or ELISA.

   (6) Therapeutic plan

   (a) Medical therapy. Diarrhea with uncomplicated cases of cryptosporidiosis is self-limiting. However, there is no recommended or specific treatment for cryptosporidiosis. On an experimental basis, the anticoccidial agent **halofuginone** has been used with some success at 60–125 μg/kg orally for 7 days.

   (b) Supportive therapy. Other treatments are supportive and similar to treatments of all diarrheas (e.g., warmth, oral or intravenous fluids, milk feeding in small quantities several times daily, oral protectants).

   (7) Prevention

   (a) The only control at present is to **limit exposure** of calves to the organism. Procedures used include:

   (i) Segregation of infective calves

   (ii) Separation of feeding utensils

   (iii) Manure removal

   (iv) Disinfection of the environment with 5% ammonia or chlorine–dioxide-based disinfectants

   (b) Clients should be warned that *C. parvum* is a **zoonotic agent** and causes diarrhea in humans. The condition has serious implications in immunocompromised individuals.

e. Giardiasis

   (1) Patient history and etiology. *Giardia* (e.g., *G. duodenalis*) has been recovered in feces of diarrheic calves. Its etiological significance is yet to be proven because infection occurs experimentally, but clinical signs do not develop.

   (2) Clinical findings and therapeutic plan. A syndrome is described of *Giardia*-associated, chronic, pasty diarrhea lasting for 2–6 weeks. Growth is depressed. Fenbendazole at 11 mg/kg has shown efficacy against this parasite.

   (3) *Giardia* species cause disease in humans, so a **zoonotic potential** exists when calves are excreting the organism.

f. Salmonellosis

   (1) Patient profile and history. Salmonella usually affects calves older than 10–14 days of age.

   (2) Clinical findings. Three syndromes have been described in calves 10 days to 3 months of age. These syndromes are:

   (a) Peracute—sudden death, neurological signs (opisthotonos, convulsions), or gastrointestinal signs (abdominal pain, diarrhea).

      (b) Acute—fever, anorexia, depression, diarrhea, and dehydration. Diarrhea progresses from watery to mucus/epithelial casts to hemorrhagic feces.

      (c) Chronic—loose feces with poor growth rates and ill-thrift

(3) Etiology and pathogenesis. *Salmonella dublin* and *S. typhimurium* are the most common *Salmonella* isolates. The pathogenesis of the diarrhea is similar to that described for salmonellosis in the adult [see II B 1 d (3)]. A bacteremic form also may exist.

(4) Diagnostic plan. Diagnosis is supported by laboratory findings and farm history.

(5) Laboratory tests. Necropsy and culture findings of feces or intestinal contents confirm the diagnosis. Repeated culture attempts may be necessary to isolate the organism from feces.

(6) Therapeutic plan and prevention. Therapy and prevention are as for the adult [see II B 1 d (7), (8)].

g. Clostridial diarrhea

(1) Patient profile and history. This type of diarrhea may be reported as an outbreak in rapidly growing, vigorous, nursing calves. It is more commonly reported as a disease of older calves or sheep.

(2) Clinical findings. Sudden death may be the most common presentation. Less acute disease may present as abdominal pain, distention, and hemorrhagic enteritis.

(3) Etiology and pathogenesis

      (a) *Clostridium perfringens* normally is found in the intestinal tract and may proliferate at times of abrupt feed changes or overfeeding of carbohydrates. Enterotoxins (alpha, beta, epsilon, and iota) produced by the various organism types produce the clinical signs.

      (b) *C. perfringens* **type A** produces a hemorrhagic enteritis in Europe.

      (c) *C. perfringens* **type B** causes diarrhea in many types of neonates in Europe, South Africa, and the Middle East.

      (d) *C. perfringens* **type C** causes hemorrhagic enteritis of calves in North America.

      (e) *C. perfringens* **type E** causes necrotic hemorrhagic enteritis but is rare.

(4) Diagnostic plan. A tentative diagnosis may be made based on subjective and clinical findings but requires laboratory confirmation.

(5) Laboratory tests. Necropsy and/or mouse inoculation with intestinal contents and neutralization studies with specific antitoxin confirm the diagnosis.

(6) Therapeutic plan. Therapy with antibiotics (penicillin) and hydration support may be attempted but are rarely successful because of the peracute nature of the disease. Similarly, specific antitoxin therapy is rarely available.

(7) Prevention. Active immunization of the dam may be employed using toxoids appropriate for the serotype. Vaccination of the dam before parturition (6–8 weeks) imparts protection to the calf in the colostrum.

h. Dietary causes of diarrhea

(1) Patient profile

      (a) Amounts of liquid feed. Dairy calves should be fed fresh colostrum at the rate of 10% body weight (BW) per day for the first 3 days. This should be divided into two or three feedings. Following this, calves may be fed milk or milk replacer at 8%–10% BW/day not to exceed 2 L/feeding. Overfeeding in total or at any given feeding may result in diarrhea. In a cold climate, the total amount of milk fed may need to be increased to 12%–14% BW/day.

      (b) Type of liquid feed. Satisfactory performance can be achieved with the use of colostrum, whole milk or milk-based milk replacers.

            (i) Colostrum may be collected from mature cows and stored by freezing, refrigeration, fermentation, or through the addition of chemical preservative. Colostrum is diluted 2:1 or 3:1 with water before feeding.

            (ii) Milk replacers should be milk-based as plant proteins and starches are not well digested by the neonatal calf. Maldigestion of these ingredients results in poor growth rates and diarrhea. Milk replacers should also contain 10%–20% fat, which is an energy source and limits diarrhea.

(c) **Method of feeding.** Feeding via nipple feeder or open bucket in neonates causes no significant differences in health or growth rates. An exception to this is veal calves described as **"rumen drinkers"** where older calves (5–6 weeks) ingest milk from buckets directly into the rumen. This results in recurrent ruminal tympany/fluid distention, inappetence, poor growth rates, and the production of clay-like feces.

(2) **Clinical findings and therapeutic plan.** The clinical signs are caused by ruminal hyperkeratosis and intestinal villous atrophy. Treatment includes conversion to nipple pail nursing or weaning onto roughage diets.

i. **Infectious bovine rhinotracheitis** may cause diarrhea in young calves as part of a systemic infection (see Chapter 6 II B 6 a).

j. **Bovine viral diarrhea** is discussed in II B 1 a.

k. **Prolonged antibiotic therapy.** Prolonged oral antibiotic therapy may predispose calves to intestinal overgrowth of pseudomonas, proteus, or fungi. Intractable diarrhea may result.

STUDY QUESTIONS

DIRECTIONS: Each of the numbered items or incomplete statements in this section is followed by answers or by completions of the statement. Select the ONE numbered answer or completion that is BEST in each case.

1. What conditions should be included on a list of differential diagnoses for diarrhea in a calf younger than 1 week of age?

(1) Enterotoxigenic *Escherichia coli* (ETEC) diarrhea, coronavirus diarrhea, rotavirus diarrhea

(2) Salmonellosis, clostridiosis, primary disaccharidase deficiency

(3) Primary disaccharidase deficiency, rotavirus diarrhea, ETEC diarrhea

(4) Coronavirus diarrhea, salmonellosis, coccidiosis

(5) Giardiasis, transmissible gastroenteritis (TGE), clostridiosis

2. Which one of the following statements regarding traumatic reticuloperitonitis (TRP) is correct?

(1) Therapy should include antibiotics and confinement.

(2) TRP is least common in mature dairy cows.

(3) Left paramedian abdominocentesis should be attempted to diagnose peritonitis.

(4) Affected animals go off feed abruptly but continue to produce milk at 75% of the normal production level.

(5) Affected animals often stand with their hind feet elevated to relieve the acute pain.

3. A veterinarian is called to see a 5-year-old Jersey cow. She has been fresh for 2 months and was treated for hardware disease by the owner shortly after calving. She is now milking at a level that is 50% lower than would be anticipated and is selectively inappetent, preferring roughage to her concentrate ration. The owner has been treating her with rumenatorics for 2 weeks, but has seen no response to therapy. Physical examination reveals a distended abdomen with mild gaseous distention of the left paralumbar fossa and succussible fluid in the lower right abdominal quadrant. The cow is passing scant, pasty feces and appears to be thin and mildly dehydrated. The cow exhibits four weak rumen rolls per minute but is not chewing her cud. Her heart rate is 30 bpm. The most probable diagnosis is:

(1) chronic bovine virus diarrhea (BVD).
(2) simple indigestion.
(3) acute localized peritonitis.
(4) vagal indigestion.
(5) Johne's disease.

Questions 4–5

In January, a veterinarian is called to evaluate a herd of Holstein cows that are housed indoors. Eighty percent of the milking cows have developed acute, profuse, diarrhea over the last 12–24 hours. Occasionally, the feces are bloody and mucoid. The milk production in the herd has decreased by 50%. The cows are fed an 18% protein dairy ration and alfalfa-timothy hay. A new source of grain was introduced in the last 3 days. Other animals (virgin heifers and bulls) are normal, although they are fed a similar diet. Physical examination reveals that some of the animals are mildly dehydrated. The vital signs are normal and no other abnormalities are detected. Complete blood cell counts (CBCs) and biochemistry profiles obtained from several clinically affected cows are essentially normal except for increases in the packed cell volume (PCV) and total protein (TP).

4. What is the most likely diagnosis?

(1) Bovine virus diarrhea (BVD)
(2) Salmonellosis
(3) Winter dysentery
(4) Arsenic poisoning
(5) Rotavirus diarrhea

5. What is the appropriate next step?

(1) Treat all affected animals with potentiated sulfonamides, flunixin meglumine, and oral or intravenous fluids.
(2) Treat all affected animals with broad-spectrum antibiotics and intestinal protectants.
(3) Treat all affected animals with oral charcoal and systemic British antilewisite (BAL).
(4) Run serologic tests to confirm the diagnosis.
(5) Wait for the disease to run its course. Supportive care (e.g., fluid therapy and astringents) is indicated for dehydrated animals.

DIRECTIONS: Each of the numbered items or incomplete statements in this section is negatively phrased, as indicated by a capitalized word such as NOT, LEAST, or EXCEPT. Select the ONE numbered answer or completion that is BEST in each case.

---

6. All of the following are true statements regarding grain overload in sheep EXCEPT:

(1) administration of oral magnesium oxide to sheep not showing signs of shock and dehydration is one correct form of therapy.
(2) absorption of both D- and L-lactate occurs, but only the D-lactate causes acidemia.
(3) this condition occurs when gram-positive rods overgrow normal rumen flora.
(4) emergency surgery will allow salvage of animals that are convulsing and in shock.
(5) the severity of clinical signs depends on the amount and particle size of the ingested grain.

7. Which one of the following statements is NOT correct regarding calves born to cows 3–9 months after an episode of bovine virus diarrhea (BVD) in a nonimmune population?

(1) The calves may be born with mucosal disease that is unresponsive to therapy.
(2) The calves may be born with cerebellar disease.
(3) The calves are immunotolerant to the BVD virus but they are incapable of mounting an antibody response to it.
(4) The calves are chronic shedders of the BVD virus.
(5) The calves may appear normal or suffer from ill thrift.

8. All of the following statements concerning bovine malignant catarrh (BMC) are true EXCEPT:

(1) BMC occurs sporadically and is usually spread from cow to cow.
(2) BMC causes a vasculitis and atypical proliferation of lymphocytes.
(3) BMC causes lymph node enlargement.
(4) BMC causes a panophthalmitis. Corneal opacity usually begins peripherally and spreads centrally.
(5) BMC is frequently accompanied by nervous system signs.

9. All of the following are suspected pathophysiologies of left displacement of the abomasum (LDA) EXCEPT:

(1) reduction in abomasal motility due to hypocalcemia.
(2) reduction in abomasal tone through stabling and lack of exercise.
(3) reduction in abomasal motility from toxins released during concurrent disease.
(4) reduction in abomasal motility due to a decrease in volatile fatty acid (VFA) production.
(5) reduction in abomasal motility due to an increased dietary concentrate:roughage ratio.

ANSWERS AND EXPLANATIONS

1. The answer is 1 [II B 3]. Included on a list of differential diagnoses for diarrhea in a calf younger than 1 week of age would be entero-toxigenic *Escherichia coli* (ETEC) diarrhea, coronavirus diarrhea, and rotavirus diarrhea. Salmonellosis, clostridiosis, and coccidiosis are usually a cause of diarrhea in older calves. Primary disaccharidase deficiency has not been reported in calves. *Giardia lamblia*, although recoverable from the feces of some calves with diarrhea, is unproven as a cause of neonatal calf diarrhea. Transmissible gastroenteritis (TGE) is a disease of swine.

2. The answer is 1 [I E 1]. Traumatic reticuloperitonitis (TRP, hardware disease, traumatic gastritis, traumatic reticulitis) is most common in mature dairy cows. Clinical signs include an abrupt drop in milk production (to less than 50% of normal) and odd postures (e.g., the animal may stand with its hind feet in a gutter in an attempt to relieve diaphragmatic reticular pressure). A right, not a left, paramedian approach is recommended to collect peritoneal fluid for laboratory analysis. Conservative therapy entails confinement and administration of antibiotics; rumenotomy may be necessary if conservative management fails and economics warrant surgical intervention.

3. The answer is 4 [I A 3]. The clinical findings suggest vagal indigestion. The history may include mild but repeated bouts of transient indigestion with signs of anorexia, decreased milk production, mild bloat, weight loss, abdominal distention, and decreased amounts of manure. The animal may have experienced an episode of traumatic reticuloperitonitis (TRP) in the past. Chronic bovine virus diarrhea (BVD) is seen in young animals with diarrhea, a stunted growth pattern, and lameness. Simple indigestion resolves within a few days. Acute local peritonitis (while perhaps the initial cause of this chronic disease) would have resolved. Intractable diarrhea is the most evident complaint and finding in animals with Johne's disease.

4–5. The answers are: 4-3, 5-5 [II B 1 e]. The most likely diagnosis is winter dysentery.

The subjective findings (e.g., housed cattle, month) support a diagnosis of winter dysentery. The cows present as essentially normal, except for an explosive outbreak of diarrhea. These findings eliminate salmonellosis and arsenic poisoning from the list of differential diagnoses. Rotavirus has not been demonstrated as an etiologic agent for diarrhea in adult ruminants. A virulent virus serotype responsible for bovine virus diarrhea (BVD) would cause similar, but more severe, clinical findings (e.g., severe dehydration).

A bovine coronavirus is the etiologic agent of winter dysentery. Treatment consists of supportive care and waiting for the disease to run its course. Antibiotics are unnecessary and ineffective. British antilewisite (BAL) is a treatment for arsenic toxicity. Serologic studies would be of no value for diagnosis.

6. The answer is 4 [I A 2]. In a convulsing animal in shock as a result of grain overload, surgery is not economically warranted because these animals have a poor prognosis for recovery. Lactic acidosis resulting from grain overload occurs when gram-positive rods overgrow the normal rumen flora. Absorption of both D- and L-lactate occurs, but only D-lactate causes acidemia. The severity of the clinical signs depends on the amount and particle size of the grain ingested; finely ground feeds are associated with more severe clinical signs. Administration of oral magnesium oxide to sheep not showing signs of shock and dehydration is one appropriate therapy.

7. The answer is 1 [II B 2 b]. Calves that have been exposed to the bovine virus diarrhea (BVD) virus in utero are not born with mucosal disease; rather, they may develop a fatal mucosal disease sometime later after being exposed to a cytopathic form of the virus. Affected calves are immunotolerant to the virus but are unable to mount a humoral antibody response against it. Affected calves may appear normal at birth, or they may suffer from ill thrift. Affected calves are chronic shedders of the BVD virus.

8. The answer is 1 [II B 1 b]. Bovine malignant catarrh (BMC) occurs sporadically and is caused by a wildebeest-associated virus (in Africa) or a sheep-associated virus (in North America). The virus is not known to be spread cow-to-cow. Disease outbreaks are often associated with ewes lambing near cattle. BMC causes vasculitis, atypical proliferation of lymphocytes, panophthalmitis, and lymph node enlargement and is frequently accompanied by nervous system signs.

9. The answer is 4 [I C 1]. High dietary concentrate:roughage ratios increase the production of volatile fatty acids (VFAs). VFAs are known to decrease intestinal motility; it is hypothesized that this leads to gas build-up within the abomasum and eventual displacement of the left abomasum. It is thought that abomasal tone is also negatively affected by low serum calcium levels, circulating toxins, and lack of exercise in deep-bodied cows.

Chapter 4

Diseases of the Porcine, Ovine, and Caprine Gastrointestinal Tract

Timothy H. Ogilvie

I. **PORCINE GASTROINTESTINAL TRACT**

A. **Stomach. Gastric ulcers** may be found at any production stage in swine.

1. **Clinical findings** include:
   a. Sudden death resulting from perforation of a major blood vessel or acute, diffuse peritonitis
   b. Melena
   c. Anemia
   d. Poor growth

2. **Etiology and pathogenesis.** Risk factors for the development of gastric ulcers include finely ground feed, wheat feeds, and stressors (e.g., concurrent disease, competition for social status). Also, there has been an association made with vitamin E and selenium deficiency.

3. **Diagnostic plan.** The diagnosis is often made on necropsy or through clinical signs.

4. **Laboratory tests** confirm anemia and blood in the feces.

5. **Therapeutic plan.** Treatment often is not carried out in individual animals. Affected animals may be culled. If warranted, treatment may follow similar courses as with other monogastrics (i.e., antacids, mucosal protectants, H_2-receptor blocking agents). Note that with H_2-receptor blocking agents, such as cimetidine, extra-label use is required.

B. **Intestines**

1. **Diarrhea in neonatal swine**
   a. **Enterotoxigenic** *Escherichia coli* **(ETEC)**
      (1) **Patient profile and history.** ETEC is a common cause of acute diarrhea in newborn piglets and can be a significant cause of diarrhea up to weaning age.
      (2) **Clinical findings.** The condition presents as acute diarrhea (nonhemorrhagic) with dehydration, anorexia, weakness, and, in advanced cases, signs of shock and death caused by hypovolemia and acidemia.
      (3) **Etiology and pathogenesis**
         (a) Many strains of ETEC are causative (more than 300 strains with varying combinations of O, K, and H antigens). **Risk factors** include poor hygiene, poor quality or insufficient colostrum, weak piglets at birth, and low herd immunity.
         (b) **Route of infection.** Enterotoxigenic strains of *E. coli* adhere to the mucosa of the small intestine, proliferate, and elaborate an enterotoxin, which causes the secretory diarrhea. Adherence to the small intestinal mucosa is achieved through any of several bacterial surface pili (K88, K99, 987P). Secretion is mediated through bacterial enterotoxins (heat-stable toxins, heat labile toxins, or both), which act on intact intestinal mucosa. These toxins increase the secretion of fluids and electrolytes to the gut lumen through activation of cyclic guanosine monophosphate (cGMP) or cyclic adenosine monophosphate (cAMP) systems. Absorptive capabilities of the mucosal cells remain intact.
      (4) **Diagnostic plan.** Diagnosis is based on clinical signs, response to therapy, and laboratory confirmation.
      (5) **Laboratory tests** include:
         (a) **Fecal culture** and *E. coli* identification using a pooled antigen antiserum

   (b) Histopathology of intestinal sections revealing gram-negative bacteria attached to relatively healthy-looking intestinal mucosa

  (6) Therapeutic plan. This condition is readily responsive if correct therapy is initiated early and encompasses the entire litter. Treatment includes:

   (a) Antibiotics with a therapeutic index for gram-negative infections (e.g., trimethoprim–sulfas)

   (b) Free-choice oral **electrolyte solutions**

  (7) Prevention

   (a) Management strategies. Improvements in hygiene should be recommended and a system of "all-in, all-out" movement of swine groups implemented if possible.

   (b) Vaccination. Immunity of sows (particularly gilts) may be improved through vaccination with an *E. coli* bacterin or early exposure to farrowing room flora.

   (c) Antibiotics may be used prophylactically in litters during an outbreak.

 b. Transmissible gastroenteritis (TGE)

  (1) Patient profile and history. This disease, which is common in North America, presents in two forms: endemic (or mild) and epidemic. The epidemic form causes explosive outbreaks in neonatal piglets with high morbidity and mortality. The condition can be devastating to producers, both economically and psychologically.

  (2) Clinical findings

   (a) Epidemic form. There is acute diarrhea with vomiting, dehydration, and death.

   (b) Endemic form. There is chronic diarrhea late in the nursing period or in the weaner pig population. Although mortality is low, growth retardation is significant. Diarrhea is sporadic.

  (3) Etiology and pathogenesis. The epidemic and endemic forms are caused by separate and distinct **coronaviruses.**

   (a) The **epidemic form** results from severe enteric damage caused by the coronavirus. There is villus atrophy, resulting in compromised gut function, malabsorptive and osmotic diarrhea, severe dehydration, and death. If death does not ensue, piglets recover as the enterocytes mature to cover the villus (5–7 days).

   (b) With the **endemic form,** the pathogenesis is similar to the epidemic form but less pronounced.

  (4) Diagnostic plan. The diagnosis is aided by clinical findings, infection profile, and unresponsiveness to therapy. Laboratory tests are confirmatory.

  (5) Laboratory tests include intestinal histopathology, virus isolation from the feces or intestine, immunofluorescence of tissue, and serology.

  (6) Therapeutic plan. Neither form of TGE is responsive to antibiotics or supportive treatment.

  (7) Prognosis

   (a) Mortality. With the epidemic form, virtually all piglets die within a one-month age cohort (2 weeks prepartum to 2 weeks old at the time of infection).

   (b) Normal production resumes approximately 1 month after infection.

   (c) Herd immune response may be hastened by feeding the fecal content of infected pigs to sows who have yet to produce colostrum and farrow.

  (8) Prevention

   (a) Management strategies. The herd should be closed and new introductions farrowed offsite. Biosecurity prevents the entry of pigs or fomites (e.g., birds, rodents, visitors). The virus may disappear over time.

   (b) Vaccination may be beneficial in an area where prevalence is high. Both killed and modified live virus vaccines are available.

 c. Rotavirus. This condition is similar to the endemic form of TGE (see I B 1 b). Rotavirus infection in pigs is similar to the same infection in other species (see Chapters 2 and 3). Vaccination lessens the effect of infection.

 d. Hemagglutinating encephalomyelitis virus (HEV, vomiting and wasting disease)

- **(1) Patient profile and history.** This disease produces vomiting and weight loss in nursing pigs. There may be acute encephalomyelitis. Infection is global, as evidenced by serological findings. Outbreaks occur with high morbidity and mortality.
- **(2) Clinical findings.** Vomiting is the major gastrointestinal tract sign followed by emaciation and dehydration. Diarrhea is not usually a finding. Wasting, over time, is followed by death.
- **(3) Etiology and pathogenesis.** The condition is caused by a coronavirus. In the case of encephalomyelitis, the virus may be isolated from the central nervous system. The pathogenesis of the vomiting and wasting component is unclear. There may be a central cause for the gastrointestinal tract signs or a local effect of the virus on the stomach.
- **(4) Diagnostic and therapeutic plans.** The diagnosis is based on histopathologic findings. There is no treatment for this condition.
- **(5) Prevention.** The disease runs its course in 2–3 weeks, and herd immunity is good.
- **e. Coccidiosis**
  - **(1) Patient profile and history.** Coccidiosis is common in young pigs. It is a disease of high morbidity and low mortality.
  - **(2) Clinical findings.** Commonly, a profuse diarrhea occurs after piglets are 1 week of age. There is no blood or mucus evident. Piglets may become anorexic and dehydrated. The diarrhea may persist for 3–5 days, and within a herd, the course may be chronic where there is continuous movement of animals on and off the premises.
  - **(3) Etiology and pathogenesis.** *Isospora suis* is the causative coccidian parasite. Similar to other coccidia, sexual and asexual life cycles occur in the intestinal tract. Asexual reproduction in the small intestinal mucosa produces villus atrophy and destruction of villus epithelial cells.
  - **(4) Diagnostic plan.** Diagnosis depends on the laboratory findings.
  - **(5) Laboratory tests** include the demonstration of significant numbers of oocytes in the feces, histopathology of the small intestine, direct smears of intestinal contents, or combinations of these techniques. Diarrhea may occur before patency of infection, during biphasic peaks of patency, or after oocyte production has waned. Consequently, detection of oocysts may be difficult and require necropsy confirmation, evaluation of the feces of littermates, or both.
  - **(6) Therapeutic plan.** Treatment during clinical disease is of little value.
  - **(7) Prevention**
    - **(a) Environmental conditions.** The infection creates most problems under conditions that allow for environmental contamination and transfer of infective oocysts. Oocysts are difficult to kill. Housing pigs on dirt or cracked concrete floors provides suitable conditions for maintenance of the organism in the environment. Wet floors encourage chilling of the piglet and infection by oocysts.
    - **(b) Preventive procedures** include maintenance of a dry environment, raising piglets on slatted floors to reduce the fecal–oral spread, or resurfacing floors to eliminate cracks.
- **f. *Clostridium perfringens* enteritis**
  - **(1) Patient profile and history.** This condition is seen most commonly in nursing pigs but may occur in animals up to 10 weeks of age. The disease is most common in western North America.
  - **(2) Clinical findings.** *C. perfringens* type C produces an acute, hemorrhagic diarrhea in suckling pigs, which rapidly results in death. In older (even weaned) pigs, a more protracted, nonbloody diarrhea is found and results in a lower mortality. *C. perfringens* type A has been reported to produce diarrhea and poor growth rates.
  - **(3) Etiology and pathogenesis.** The clostridial organisms are soil borne and enter the animal through the oral route. Attachment to the intestine and proliferation occurs with the production of a β-toxin (*C. perfringens* type C), which is

responsible for the necrosis of the intestinal mucosa and the development of clinical signs.

(4) Diagnostic plan. Diagnosis is based on laboratory findings.

(5) Laboratory tests include necropsy findings, histopathology, and intestinal tract smears. Culture of intestinal contents is inconclusive because *Clostridia* make up much of the natural gut flora.

(6) Therapeutic plan. Treatment is unrewarding and should be reserved for very early cases. Penicillins may be used.

(7) Prevention. Vaccination with a type-specific or multi-spectrum toxoid is recommended.

2. **Diarrhea in feeder pigs**
   a. **Swine dysentery**
      (1) Patient profile and history. This disease is endemic in many operations and very costly to the economic production of pork. It is most common in the 7- to 16-week age group.
      (2) Clinical findings. There is a mucohemorrhagic enteritis with anorexia, dehydration, and poor growth rates in affected pigs. The disease may be of high morbidity and moderate mortality. The condition may last 3–4 weeks in untreated animals. A chronic diarrhea may result in some pigs.
      (3) Etiology and pathogenesis. The causative organism is *Serpulina hyodysenteriae*. It invades colonic crypts and produces an erosive colitis, resulting in colonic malabsorption, diarrhea, dysentery, and the mucoid feces seen clinically.
      (4) Diagnostic plan. The diagnosis is confirmed by laboratory findings.
      (5) Laboratory tests include dark field microscopy or stained fecal smears, fecal culture, and identification via fluorescent antibody staining or slide agglutination. Serological tests may aid in the identification of carrier pigs.
      (6) Differential diagnoses include salmonellosis, proliferative enteritis, spirochetal diarrhea, and hog cholera.
      (7) Therapeutic plan
         (a) Effective treatments include any of the following drugs at labeled dosages and routes of administration. However, relapses may occur. Treatment is usually administered to all animals in the group by water medication. Individual animals may require selective treatment if dehydrated and anorexic.
         (b) **Medications** include tylosin, dimetridazole, ronidazole, lincomycin, tiamulin, and carbadox.
      (8) Prevention. If the disease is present, there are two management responses.
         (a) Live with the condition through continuous medication to control the clinical expression.
         (b) Eradicate the organism through depopulation and repopulation. **Depopulation** may be carried out in two ways:
            (i) One radical method includes the removal of all pigs coupled with disinfection of the premises and restocking with known disease-free hogs.
            (ii) All pigs may be mass-medicated simultaneous with premise disinfection, serial depopulation of pigs, and restocking with disease-free pigs.
         (c) **Management strategies.** Either system will eliminate the disease but must be followed by fastidious hygiene and biosecurity to restrict the entrance of the organism via carrier pigs, rodents, or manure-contaminated fomites.
   b. **Spirochetal diarrhea.** This condition is similar to swine dysentery but may be found in clean herds. It is caused by an unknown spirochete (*Spirochaeta innocens* variety). The infection produces a mild postweaning diarrhea with weight loss. It responds to medication in a way similar to swine dysentery [see I B 2 a (7)].
   c. **Nonspecific colitis.** This condition is also similar to swine dysentery but is not associated with a demonstrable pathogen (see I B 2 a). This condition may be associated with high-protein or pelleted feeds and may respond to a feed change.
   d. **Postweaning coliform gastroenteritis**

(1) Patient profile and history. This condition affects pigs from a few days to 2 weeks post weaning. Morbidity may approach 100%, but the mortality is usually moderate.

(2) Clinical findings. A few pigs may be found dead, and within a few days, most remaining pigs in the group are showing signs of diarrhea, skin discoloration, anorexia, and a marked loss of condition. The course of the disease is usually 7–10 days.

(3) Etiology and pathogenesis

    (a) The condition is caused by one of several serotypes of **ETEC.** Colonization and proliferation of the *E. coli* in the small intestine produces the clinical signs.

    (b) The **pathophysiological development** of diarrhea is similar to ETEC in neonatal piglets [see I B 1 a (3)]. However, there are a variety of associated **risk factors** for this condition including:

        (i) Concurrent infection with rotavirus

        (ii) Stressors (mixing, weaning)

        (iii) Loss of lactogenic immunity

        (iv) Normal intestinal villus turnover

(4) Diagnostic plan and laboratory tests. Necropsy results coupled with intestinal tract culture findings are confirmatory.

(5) Differential diagnoses include salmonellosis and swine dysentery.

(6) Therapeutic plan. Mass medication of all pigs in the group is essential. Water medication is best with one of many broad-spectrum antimicrobials. Electrolytes should be offered in the drinking water.

(7) Prevention. Recommendations for control are empirical and unproven, although many producers will prophylactically medicate growing pigs and introduce feed changes or other sources of stress gradually.

e. Salmonellosis

    (1) Patient profile and history. This disease may occur in a septicemic or enteric form.

    (2) Clinical findings

        (a) With **septicemia,** there is sudden death or **terminal signs** of septicemia including cyanosis, subcutaneous petechial hemorrhages, and recumbency with convulsions.

        (b) The **enteric form** presents as diarrhea with occasional signs of pneumonia or encephalitis. A chronic diarrhea with resultant poor growth, rectal strictures, or both may develop.

    (3) Etiology and pathogenesis. The septicemic form is most commonly caused by *Salmonella choleraesuis,* whereas the enteric form yields cultures of *S. typhimurium.* The pathogenesis is as for other species with salmonellosis (see Chapters 2 and 3).

    (4) Diagnostic plan and laboratory tests

        (a) The **septicemic form** is almost invariably fatal, and diagnosis is based on necropsy, histopathology of intestinal tissue, and culture and sensitivity of intestinal contents and tissues (e.g., lymph nodes).

        (b) The **enteric form** is diagnosed on postmortem. Culture of the feces of live pigs may be attempted but is subject to the same drawbacks as fecal culture in horses or ruminants.

    (5) Therapeutic plan. Enteric or broad-spectrum antimicrobials may be used with limited success even in the enteric form.

    (6) Prevention. The occurrence of the disease is lessened by attention to hygiene and group movements of pigs through barns to allow for periodic disinfection of premises.

f. Porcine proliferative enteropathy (PPE)

    (1) Patient profile and history. This condition affects pigs from weaner age through to young adults. As with other disorders, this condition affects hogs that are intensively raised in confinement. This condition may be seen more often in minimal disease (specific pathogen-free) facilities and appears worldwide.

(2) Clinical findings

(a) There may be **sudden death** and **hemorrhagic diarrhea** in older feeder pigs (gilts and boars). This manifestation of the disease is called **porcine hemorrhagic enteropathy.**

(b) PPE is most commonly seen as diarrhea, anorexia, and ill thrift in growing pigs. Pigs are afebrile but suffer from chronic, intermittent diarrhea.

(3) Etiology and pathogenesis. Older literature associates the condition with *Campylobacter mucosalis.* The clinical syndromes are now associated with a new pathogen, *Lawsonia intracellularis.* The pathogenesis is not well understood, but affected animals develop a regional ileitis, hypertrophic terminal ileum, and hemorrhagic and necrotic enteritis with the passage of blood in acute severe cases.

(4) Diagnostic plan and differential diagnoses. Clinical findings are helpful in differentiating this condition from postweaning coliform gastroenteritis. Postmortem examination is the method of choice for diagnosis.

(5) Therapeutic plan. Treatment is often not undertaken in individual animals but could be attempted by using macrolides (lincomycin, tylosin). Control with medicated feeds and management changes is variable.

g. **Intestinal parasites.** Enteric parasites are common and impact productivity in feeder barns.

(1) *Trichuris suis*

(a) Clinical findings. Clinically, the signs of swine **whipworm** infestation may appear similar to swine dysentery (see I B 2 a).

(b) Diagnostic plan. Diagnosis is by fecal floatation of worm eggs and by postmortem evaluation.

(c) Therapeutic plan. Dichlorvos anthelmintics are therapeutic.

(d) Prevention. Eggs are very resistant in the environment, and attention to hygiene is necessary to prevent ongoing infestations.

(2) *Ascaris suum*

(a) Patient profile and clinical findings. Roundworms are common in growing pigs. They cause growth impairment at high infestation rates and are associated with some cases of respiratory disease caused by the larval migration patterns through the lungs. The larvae also produce "white-spotted liver lesions" caused by hepatic migration during maturation.

(b) Diagnostic plan. Diagnosis is based on fecal floatation findings or slaughter checks of viscera (liver).

(c) Therapeutic plan and prevention. Treatment and control is based on hygiene and regular, strategic anthelmintic usage: sows 7 days before farrowing, and feeder pigs at 50 kg or every 3 weeks. Improvements in hygiene limit direct fecal–oral exposure of infective eggs.

(3) *Hyostrongylus rubidus*

(a) Patient profile and etiology. *Hyostrongylus* causes anemia, poor growth, and diarrhea in feeder pigs because of a parasitic gastritis. In older animals, this worm has been associated with "thin sow syndrome."

(b) Clinical findings. Animals may carry heavy infestations without showing clinical signs.

(c) Diagnostic plan. Diagnosis is made by clinical findings and fecal egg identification.

(d) Therapeutic plan and prevention. If this parasite is suspected of causing problems, regular deworming with levamisole or dichlorvos is warranted.

(4) *Oesophagostomum*

(a) Patient profile. This is the nodular worm of the large intestine that produces inflammatory nodules in the colon, cecum, and rectum.

(b) Clinical findings. There are few clinical signs expressed with infestation unless concurrent infections with intestinal pathogens occur (e.g., *Salmonella* species).

(c) Diagnostic plan. Diagnosis is based on necropsy or fecal floatation.

(d) Prevention of this and other gastrointestinal parasites include improving hygiene, removing manure, feeding above floor level, and other ways of limiting the fecal–oral spread of parasite eggs.

II. OVINE AND CAPRINE GASTROINTESTINAL TRACT

A. Diarrhea

1. **Salmonellosis**
   a. **Patient profile and history.** This disease is seen in young lambs or adults with a recent history of stress (e.g., shipping, parturition).
   b. **Clinical findings.** There may be a sudden onset of fever, depression, and diarrhea with fibrin and blood. Abortion may be seen within the flock.
   c. **Etiology and pathogenesis.** *Salmonella dublin* or *S. typhimurium* are usually isolated. Pathogenesis is similar to other species of host (see Chapters 2 and 3).
   d. **Diagnostic plan, therapeutic plan, and prevention.** These plans are identical to those in other species (see Chapters 2 and 3).

2. *Clostridium perfringens* **type C**
   a. **Patient profile.** This infection occurs in lambs and kids less than 3 weeks of age.
   b. **Clinical findings and etiology.** Proliferation of *C. perfringens* type C in the intestine causes elaboration of a β-toxin, which causes an acute hemorrhagic enteritis in affected animals.
   c. **Diagnostic plan, therapeutic plan, and prevention.** These plans are similar to those of the neonatal calf (see Chapter 3).

3. *Clostridium perfringens* **type D (pulpy kidney disease, overeating disease, enterotoxemia)**
   a. **Patient profile.** This infection is seen in young, rapidly growing animals on a high plane of nutrition.
   b. **Clinical findings.** Various clinical pictures are described, but clinical signs are apparent only early in the course of the disease.
      (1) **Sudden death** is the most common presentation.
      (2) **Neurological signs** are observed before death.
      (3) **Transient diarrhea in sheep** occurs early in the course of the fatal disease; diarrhea may be a finding.
      (4) **Persistent diarrhea in goats** is a specifically different syndrome of clostridial enterotoxemia. Diarrhea is chronic with weight loss. Feces contain flecks of mucus and blood.
   c. **Etiology and pathogenesis**
      (1) **Sheep.** Pulpy kidney disease results from the proliferation of *C. perfringens* type D in the small intestine. The bacteria release a number of toxins, including the ϵ toxin. This toxin causes vascular and nervous system damage.
      (2) **Dairy goats** are often fed a high-energy ration during lactation, predisposing them to intestinal clostridiosis. This condition may take the form of acute disease with sudden death or produce a more chronic diarrhea and wasting form of disease.
   d. **Diagnostic plan and laboratory tests**
      (1) **Sheep.** In lambs, the history, clinical findings, and necropsy findings are diagnostic. In adult sheep, pulpy kidney disease must be differentiated from rabies, acute lead poisoning, hypomagnesemic tetany, pregnancy toxemia, and louping-ill (see Chapter 11).
      (2) **Goats.** Fecal collection for toxin identification (mouse bioassay) is necessary for accurate diagnosis.
   e. **Therapeutic plan**
      (1) **Feed.** Treatment is centered on decreasing the energy component of the ration. This advice may run counter to the objectives of the owner.
      (2) **Vaccination** with *C. perfringens* type D toxoid is effective in decreasing the severity of the disease but does not eliminate it in the face of high-energy rations. Vaccination every 6 months may be warranted. Local reactions occur at the vaccination sites.

4. *Clostridium septicum* **(braxy)**
   a. **Patient profile.** This infection occurs in sheep sporadically in North America.

    b. Clinical findings. Sudden death is the most common presentation. Early signs include anorexia, fever, abdominal pain, and distention.

    c. Etiology and pathogenesis. Braxy is an infectious abomasitis-toxemia of sheep caused by *C. septicum*. Bacteria or spores are introduced through breaks in the abomasal mucosa, proliferate and cause death through the systemic absorption of toxins. Infection occurs only in the winter months and is associated with consumption of frozen feeds.

    d. Diagnostic plan. The diagnosis is made by isolating *C. septicum* from the typical inflammatory lesions of the abomasum or from necropsy specimens.

5. Intestinal helminthiasis

    a. Patient profile. This condition is common in sheep and should not be overlooked or underemphasized. Lambs and kids are affected more than adults.

    b. Clinical findings

        (1) The **clinical hallmarks** of infestation are weight loss, poor growth, diarrhea, and edema.

        (2) Other signs include poor feed conversion, wasting, and eventually death of the host. Sudden death may be the presenting problem with *Haemonchus contortus* infestation. Not all parasites produce the entire range of clinical signs.

        (3) *Haemonchus* and *Bunostomum* species feed off of blood with resultant **anemia.**

    c. Etiology and pathogenesis. Infective eggs and larvae are ingested usually at pasture and mature in various areas of the gastrointestinal tract. An exception to this is the tapeworm, which requires an intermediate host in their life cycle. This host (an orbatid mite) is ingested by the ruminant. The total effect of a heavy parasite burden is more significant in the young than in the mature animal.

        (1) Abomasum—*Haemonchus contortus, Ostertagia circumcincta* and *O. trifurcata, Trichostrongylus axei*

        (2) Small Intestine—*Trichostrongylus* species, *Nematodirus* species, *Bunostomum* species, *Cooperia* species, *Strongyloides papillosus, Moniezia* species, *Thysanosoma* species

        (3) Large Intestine—*Oesophagostomum* species, *Chabertia ovina, Trichuris* species

    d. Diagnostic plan and laboratory tests. Diagnosis depends on the demonstration of fecal larvae, fecal flotations and egg counts, necropsy, and intestinal worm counts.

    e. Therapeutic plan and prevention. Parasite control strategies for most sheep-rearing areas in North America include:

        (1) Prelambing treatment. This treatment of ewes is critical to prevent the occurrence of a periparturient rise in the fecal egg counts. Treatment with a product effective against hypobiotic larvae is essential (e.g., levamisole, ivermectin). The usual management strategy dictates a winter treatment in northern climates to prevent maturation of worms and eventual seeding down of the pastures in the spring.

        (2) Creation of safe pastures

            (a) Lambs **raised indoors** in a relatively parasite-free environment may be turned out onto virgin pastures without anthelmintic treatment. The only indoor risk of infestation is from *Coccidia* or *Strongyloides papillosus*.

            (b) Regrowth pasture after harvested crops generally can be considered as safe. Pastures previously grazed by cattle or other species are generally safe for sheep and goats because of the limited cross-infection between species.

        (3) Deworming. In the spring, deworming of animals prevents the summer buildup of parasite eggs and larvae. A regimen of 4–8 treatments should be considered at 3-week intervals throughout spring and summer.

        (4) Treat and move. A single treatment followed by movement to a safe pasture limits reinfestation.

        (5) Anthelmintic agents

            (a) Levamisole given at 7.5 mg/kg orally and **ivermectin** given at 0.2 mg/kg orally are highly efficacious for the control of sheep parasites.

      (b) Thiabendazole, piperazine, and **phenothiazine** may still be used but have a narrower spectrum of activity or suffer from parasite resistance patterns.

6. **Coccidiosis**
   a. **Patient profile.** Coccidiosis can occur in any sheep or goat but is most significant in the young. Clinical signs are not expressed in animals until 2–3 weeks of age and are most common in lambs 1–4 months of age.
   b. **Clinical findings.** There is a severe, watery diarrhea that lasts for 1–2 weeks. The diarrhea may be hemorrhagic. Also evident are dehydration, weakness, anorexia, and death as the disease progresses.
   c. **Etiology and pathogenesis.** *Eimeria arloingi* and *E. ovina* are the most commonly diagnosed coccidial pathogens. The pathogenesis is similar to bovine coccidiosis (see Chapter 3).
   d. **Laboratory tests.** The diagnosis is confirmed by the demonstration of large numbers of *Coccidia* oocysts in the feces. Also, lambs will be hypoproteinemic and anemic.
   e. **Therapeutic plan and prevention**
      (1) **Sulfamethazine** at 30 mg/kg daily is added to the drinking water. Lambs and kids are treated at 3–4 weeks of age for 7 days. This is repeated in 3 weeks. Treatment may need to continue in 3-week cycles until weaning in some flocks or herds.
      (2) **Monensin** may be added to the ration at 5–7.5 g/ton of total pelleted ration. Feeding of this medicated ration should continue until 3 weeks post weaning.
      (3) **Lasalocid** is effective at 25 mg/kg of feed or 2–5 mg/kg body weight/day. It may also be fed as a ground salt at .75%.
      (4) **Amprolium** may be used on kids or lambs 2 weeks of age at 50–60 mg/kg for 10 days. Thiamine deficiency may result from the use of this product (see Chapter 11).
      (5) **Decoquinate** is an excellent preventive and may be mixed at home. It should be used at 5 mg/kg. It should be introduced at 2 weeks of age and fed for 1 month or longer. Older animals may be offered salt with 2 kg of 6% decoquinate premix in 45 kg of salt.

7. **Toxicities.** As with cattle, toxic agents (e.g., lead arsenate, copper sulfate, superphosphate fertilizers) may cause gastrointestinal signs (see Chapter 3).

8. **Dietary disturbances.** Nutritional diarrheas are common in lambs turned out onto lush pastures or introduced to high-energy rations. These conditions (mainly diarrheas) are self-limiting and are prevented by more gradual introduction to the ration. Occasionally, symptomatic treatment may be necessary if the diarrhea is severe.

B. **Chronic weight loss** in sheep or goats may result from the involvement of any one of several body systems. Differential diagnoses include: primary undernutrition, secondary undernutrition, parasites (ectoparasites and endoparasites), infectious diseases (Johne's disease, pseudotuberculosis, chronic pulmonary disease, chronic degenerative joint disease), chronic renal disease, other chronic disease.

1. **Paratuberculosis (Johne's disease)**
   a. **Patient profile and history.** Goats are affected more commonly than sheep and are usually 1 year of age or older before showing clinical signs. The onset of clinical signs coincides with stress (parturition, heavy lactation, environmental or managemental changes).
   b. **Clinical findings.** Animals with this disorder exhibit chronic, progressive weight loss, a capricious appetite, and lethargy and weakness. The haircoat or wool is poor and breaks easily. Diarrhea and submandibular edema may occur terminally.
   c. **Etiology and pathogenesis.** *Mycobacterium paratuberculosis* is the causative organism. Transmission is oral, and ingested organisms localize in the gastrointestinal tract and adjacent lymph nodes. The organisms may remain dormant for extended periods of time.
   d. **Diagnostic plan** depends on the laboratory findings.
   e. **Laboratory tests**

    (1) There is **hypoproteinemia** and **hypoalbuminemia** along with a mild anemia and hypocalcemia. It is also common to find a concurrent heavy parasite burden on **fecal floatation examination.**

    (2) Reliable tests. Many diagnostic tests suffer the same deficiencies as in the bovine (see Chapter 3). However, there are some reliable tests.

      (a) Fecal culture is the most reliable indicator of infection.

      (b) In the goat, the **agar gel immunodiffusion (AGID) test** has a sensitivity that approaches fecal culture and is a useful test for subclinical infection.

      (c) Cold or modified complement fixation tests are the **serological tests** of choice in sheep.

    (3) Histological examination of mesenteric and intestinal lymph nodes of affected sheep with acid fast stains are diagnostic.

  f. Therapeutic plan and prevention. Treatment is impractical, and elimination efforts revolve around depopulation, either complete or selective via fecal culture. Prevention requires maintenance of a closed herd or flock.

2. Visceral caseous lymphadenitis (CLA)

  a. Patient profile and history. Goats and sheep are subject to this disease, and there may be a history of recent shearing or dipping (sheep) or other recent animal contacts. Draining abscesses may also be evident in the flock.

  b. Clinical findings

    (1) Superficial lymph node abscess may be found in the case under examination or in the flock (see Chapter 16 V D 2). In the case of visceral CLA, there are no pathognomonic clinical signs, simply insidious and progressive **weight loss.** Emaciation may occur over weeks or months and may not be visible on heavily fleeced or haired animals. Body surface palpation may be necessary to adequately evaluate flesh cover.

    (2) Concurrent bloat, dysphagia, or **vagal indigestion** may be seen. Other body systems may be involved with signs referable to the respiratory tract, central nervous system (CNS), or mammary gland.

  c. Etiology and pathogenesis. *Corynebacterium pseudotuberculosis* is the causative organism and resides in manure and soil. The gram-positive organism invades the body through both abraded and intact skin. It migrates and causes abscesses in both deep and superficial lymph nodes. Superficial lymph node abscesses, if present, are readily visible and palpable.

  d. Diagnostic plan and laboratory tests. Visceral caseous lymphadenitis is difficult to diagnose. Laboratory findings that are helpful in defining the condition include:

    (1) A possible leukocytosis with a normal lymphocyte to neutrophil ratio

    (2) A possible hyperfibrinogenemia and hypergammaglobulinemia

    (3) Hypoproteinemia secondary to decreased appetite and possible malabsorption

    (4) Recovery of organism or signs of chronic peritonitis on abdominocentesis

    (5) Detection of serum antibodies on paired sera submitted for enzyme-linked immunosorbent assay (ELISA)

  e. Therapeutic plan and prevention. Exploratory abdominal surgery may be attempted in a valuable animal but is of limited value. Control is as for CLA (see Chapter 16 V D 2 f).

3. Abomasal emptying defect in Suffolk sheep

  a. Patient profile. This condition is seen specifically in Suffolk sheep and is hypothesized to be breed-related.

  b. Clinical findings include anorexia, chronic weight loss, and abdominal and abomasal distension.

  c. Therapeutic plan and prevention. Treatment is ineffective, and there are no recommended preventive procedures.

STUDY QUESTIONS

DIRECTIONS: Each of the numbered items or incomplete statements in this section is followed by answers or by completions of the statement. Select the ONE numbered answer or completion that is BEST in each case.

1. Salmonellosis and pulpy kidney disease of lambs are similar in what way?

(1) There may be a sudden onset of diarrhea.
(2) Sudden death is the most common presentation.
(3) Chronic diarrhea with flecks of blood is a common presentation.
(4) Diagnosis is based on fecal culture.
(5) Eating frozen feeds increases the risk of disease.

2. Which statement regarding intestinal nematode parasites of sheep is true?

(1) They are of greatest clinical importance in adults.
(2) They cause the most problems in animals raised indoors or in feedlots.
(3) They may cause anemia and diarrhea.
(4) They are ingested as mature, egg-laying adults.
(5) They live primarily in the large intestine.

3. Which of the following statements regarding porcine proliferative enteropathy (PPE) is true? PPE:

(1) is seen most often in association with pneumonia.
(2) is a congenital disease in piglets.
(3) causes sudden death and encephalitis.
(4) is diagnosed best on postmortem examination of clinically diseased pigs.
(5) occurs in range pigs with heavy parasite burdens.

4. Which one of the following statements regarding visceral caseous lymphadenitis (CLA) is true?

(1) It affects only the gastrointestinal system.
(2) It is transmitted mainly through aerosolization.
(3) It may produce a hyperfibrinogenemia.
(4) It is restricted to sheep.
(5) It is caused by *Mycobacterium paratuberculosis*.

5. Which statement regarding gastric ulcer in swine is correct? Gastric ulcers in swine:

(1) are seen only in adult pigs.
(2) are most common in free-ranging pigs.
(3) are more common with coarse diets.
(4) may present with signs of sudden death or poor growth.
(5) cause diarrhea.

6. Which statement describing coliform bacteria that cause diarrhea in neonatal pigs is true?

(1) They are usually from a single strain.
(2) They elaborate an enterotoxin.
(3) They disrupt absorption capabilities of the small intestine.
(4) They cause a hemorrhagic diarrhea.
(5) They do not attach to enterocytes.

7. Transmissible gastroenteritis (TGE) and hemagglutinating encephalomyelitis (HEV) disease in swine differ in what way?

(1) TGE causes diarrhea, whereas HEV presents as vomiting and emaciation.
(2) Morbidity and mortality due to HEV infection is low compared to TGE.
(3) HEV occurs in weaner pigs, whereas TGE is a disease of nursing pigs.
(4) TGE is caused by a coronavirus and HEV, by a rotavirus.
(5) HEV is responsive to treatment, whereas TGE is not.

8. Coccidiosis causes which one of the following clinical signs?

(1) Bloody diarrhea in market age pigs
(2) Bloody diarrhea in nursing piglets
(3) Few clinical signs in swine
(4) Little morphologic change to intestinal cells
(5) Profuse diarrhea in young pigs

9. Successful management strategies to limit the production losses due to *Serpulina hyodysenteriae* include which of the following herd procedures?

(1) One week of oral antibiotics followed by increased attention to biosecurity of the premises

(2) Depopulation followed by premise disinfection and restocking with disease free stock

(3) Ten days of mass water medication followed by oral electrolytes

(4) Individual medication of sick animals followed by increased biosecurity of the premises

(5) Decreased fiber in the diet followed by medication of any remaining sick animals

1. The answer is 1 [II A 1, 3]. Both salmonellosis and pulpy kidney disease cause diarrhea, but pulpy kidney disease causes this only early in disease because death soon ensues. Sudden death is not a common feature of salmonellosis. Chronic diarrhea may occur with salmonellosis or in goats with clostridial enterotoxemia but not with pulpy kidney disease. Fecal culture of *Salmonella* organisms is disappointing because of the dilution factor associated with the diarrhea and because the organism attaches to the enterocyte. Toxin analysis, not bacteriology, is necessary to diagnose pulpy kidney disease. Frozen feed consumption is associated with braxy.

2. The answer is 3 [II A 5 b]. Intestinal parasites in sheep may cause anemia, poor growth, diarrhea, edema, and weight loss. Parasites are of greatest clinical significance in young animals raised on pasture where infectious eggs or immature larvae are ingested off of or near blades of grass. Parasites may be harbored throughout the gastrointestinal tract.

3. The answer is 4 [I B 2 f (4)]. Porcine proliferative enteropathy (PPE) affects pigs after weaning and is best diagnosed by sacrificing affected pigs for necropsy. Pigs confined to minimal disease (specific pathogen-free) facilities are most commonly affected. Pathology includes a regional ileitis and hypertrophic terminal ileum, resulting in the clinical signs of diarrhea and poor growth performance.

4. The answer is 3 [II B 2 d]. Clinical pathology often reveals a hyperfibrinogenemia with this deep-seated infection. Other systems (e.g., respiratory) may be affected by the enlargement and abscessation of visceral lymph nodes. The organism (*Corynebacterium pseudotuberculosis*) is transmitted mainly through skin trauma of goats and sheep. *Mycobacterium paratuberculosis* is the causative agent of Johne's disease.

5. The answer is 4 [I A 1]. Clinical signs with gastric ulceration in swine are melena, sudden death, anemia, or poor growth rates. Diarrhea is not a common finding. Risk factors include finely ground diets and crowded conditions. Growing pigs are at greatest risk.

6. The answer is 2 [I B 1 a (3) (b)]. Enterotoxigenic *Escherichia coli* (ETEC) elaborate an enterotoxin that causes gut mucosa cells to secrete excess fluid and electrolytes. However, absorptive characteristics of the cells are maintained. There are many pathogenic stains of this organism that adhere to the enterocytes by bacterial surface pili. The diarrhea may be frothy, white, or brown but is not hemorrhagic.

7. The answer is 1 [I B 1 b (2), d (2)]. Both transmissible gastroenteritis (TGE) and hemagglutinating encephalomyelitis virus disease (HEV) are diseases of high morbidity and high mortality. Both occur in nursing pigs, although TGE may occur in weaner pigs as well. Both are caused by coronaviruses, and neither is responsive to treatment.

8. The answer is 5 [I B 1 e (2)]. Coccidiosis (infection with *Isospora suis*) causes a profuse diarrhea in young pigs. The diarrhea is not bloody, although the coccidian parasites cause atrophy and destruction of villus epithelial cells.

9. The answer is 2 [I B 2 a (8)]. *Serpulina hyodysenteriae* is the causative organism of swine dysentery. Correct management procedures to limit the effects of disease in an infected population include continuous mass medication of all pigs or depopulation followed by disinfection of the premises and restocking with disease-free animals. This must then be followed by increased attention to hygiene and biosecurity measures to prevent reintroduction of disease.

Chapter 5

Hepatobiliary Diseases

Jeanne Lofstedt

I. INTRODUCTION

A. General principles

1. **Hepatic disease versus hepatic failure.** Multisystemic diseases (e.g., endotoxemia, hypoxemia) and toxic insults often cause hepatic disease without causing hepatic failure. Affected animals generally do not exhibit clinical signs of liver dysfunction and do not require specific therapy to support the liver. Hepatic disease in these patients is recognized by abnormally high serum hepatic enzyme activities or microscopic examination of the liver.

2. **Acute versus chronic disease.** Distinguishing acute liver failure from chronic liver failure on the basis of clinical signs alone may be difficult. The onset of signs in patients with acute liver failure is sudden and dramatic whereas patients with chronic liver failure usually have a history of chronic weight loss and anorexia prior to developing signs of acute disease. Because signs indicating chronicity can be missed, a liver biopsy is required to differentiate between acute and chronic liver failure.

3. **Hepatocellular versus cholestatic (obstructive) disease.** Liver failure, accompanied by icterus, is produced by two major mechanisms: primary hepatocyte damage (hepatocellular disease) or primary cholestasis (cholestatic disease). Cholestasis may be caused by canalicular dysfunction (intrahepatic cholestasis) or blockage of the large bile ducts.

B. Diagnosis of hepatobiliary disease. Physical examination and laboratory findings in large animals with liver failure are often similar regardless of the cause of disease.

1. **Clinical findings**
   a. **Dermatologic signs**
      (1) **Icterus (jaundice)** results from bilirubin deposition in tissues of animals with hyperbilirubinemia. Hyperbilirubinemia in liver failure is caused by failure of uptake, conjugation, or excretion of bilirubin.
         (a) Icterus is common in horses with acute liver failure and variably present in horses with chronic liver failure. Anorexia or fasting can cause icterus in horses with normal liver function.
         (b) Biliary obstruction is the most likely cause of icterus in ruminants.
      (2) **Photodermatitis.** Phylloerythrin, produced by bacterial degradation of chlorophyll, is normally excreted in the bile. In patients with cholestasis, phylloerythrin accumulates in the systemic circulation and binds to the skin, where it acts as a photodynamic agent, causing erythema and necrosis of nonpigmented skin following exposure to sunlight.
      (3) **Pruritus,** attributed to the accumulation of bile salts in the skin, has been reported on occasion in horses with liver failure.
   b. **Neurologic signs. Hepatic encephalopathy** is a clinical syndrome that occurs secondary to liver failure and is characterized by abnormal mental status.
      (1) The pathophysiology is incompletely understood, but contributing factors include hypoglycemia, hyperammonemia, a decrease in the branched chain:aromatic amino acid ratio, and increased concentrations of mercaptans, sulfur-containing amino acids, and short-chain fatty acids in the plasma.
      (2) Clinical signs are often subtle and behavioral changes may only be obvious to the owner. Overt signs may include depression, incoordination, aimless wandering, head pressing, stupor, or coma. Frequent yawning and pharyngeal or laryngeal collapse with severe inspiratory dyspnea have been reported in

TABLE 5-1. Laboratory Findings in Hepatocellular and Cholestatic Liver Disease

Parameter	Hepatocellular Disease	Cholestatic Disease
Total bilirubin	Increased	Increased
Direct (conjugated) bilirubin	Mild to moderate increase	Marked increase
Indirect (unconjugated) bilirubin	Moderate increase	Normal to mild increase
Urine bilirubin	Normal to mild increase	Marked increase
Urine urobilinogen	Normal to slight increase	Absent (complete bile duct obstruction)
Alkaline phosphatase (AP)	Mild increase	Marked increase
γ-Glutamyl transferase (GGT)	Mild to moderate increase	Moderate to marked increase
Aspartate aminotransferase (AST)	Mild to moderate increase	Normal to mild increase
Sorbitol dehydrogenase (SDH)	Mild to moderate increase	Normal to mild increase

horses with hepatic encephalopathy. Excessive vocalization and tenesmus may be a feature of this neurologic syndrome in cattle.

c. Gastrointestinal signs

(1) **Weight loss** is a common but nonspecific finding in large animals with chronic liver disease. Anorexia and failure of hepatic metabolic functions likely contribute to the weight loss.

(2) **Diarrhea,** a common finding in cattle with chronic liver disease, has been attributed to increased hydrostatic pressure associated with portal hypertension. Because of the low fat content of the herbivore diet, steatorrhea is an unlikely cause of diarrhea in herbivores with liver failure.

(3) **Tenesmus,** followed by rectal prolapse, is observed in some cattle with liver disease. Hepatic encephalopathy, diarrhea, and intestinal edema secondary to portal hypertension are thought to be predisposing factors.

(4) **Ascites** is a common finding in cattle with hepatic cirrhosis, but is rarely reported in horses. Portal hypertension, and possibly hypoalbuminemia, lead to ascites.

(5) **Fecal color change** is unlikely in mature herbivores with biliary obstruction because chlorophyll contributes to fecal color. However, in suckling herbivores, fecal color is attributed to the presence of stercobilin (a bilirubin metabolite) and biliary obstruction can result in light feces.

(6) **Recurrent subacute abdominal pain** has been reported in horses with liver failure, particularly those with cholelithiasis.

d. Hematologic signs

(1) **Bleeding diathesis.** Coagulopathy leading to hemorrhage (e.g., epistaxis, prolonged bleeding from venipuncture sites) may accompany severe terminal liver failure and is caused by inadequate hepatic synthesis of clotting factors (I, II, V, VII, IX, and X). If liver disease causes decreased bile flow to the intestines, absorption of fat-soluble vitamins, including vitamin K, will be impaired. Vitamin K_1 is required by the liver for the production of factors II, VII, IX, and X.

(2) **Hemolytic crisis.** A terminal hemolytic crisis, attributed to increased red blood cell (RBC) fragility, has been reported in horses with liver failure.

2. Laboratory tests. Laboratory studies can help distinguish hepatocellular and cholestatic liver disease (Table 5-1).

a. Liver enzyme studies

(1) **γ-Glutamyl transferase (GGT)** is predominantly associated with the cell mem-

branes of hepatocytes and biliary epithelial cells. Other sources of GGT in horses are the pancreas and the renal tubular epithelium. However, because pancreatic disease is rare in horses, and renal disease causes an increase in urine but not serum GGT activity, increased serum GGT activity can be considered fairly specific for hepatocellular and cholestatic liver disease.

    (a) Hepatocyte necrosis causes an increase in GGT activity due to leakage of this enzyme from the hepatocyte; therefore, GGT activity is almost always increased in large animal patients with **acute** or **chronic hepatocellular disease.**

    (b) Cholestasis causes the greatest increase in GGT activity; the exact mechanism of this increase is not known, but it is usually attributed to increased production.

(2) Alkaline phosphatase (AP) activity can be used to evaluate the status of the liver, but this enzyme is not liver-specific. In addition to the hepatobiliary membrane, other tissues that may contribute to increased serum AP activity include bone, intestinal tissue, and placental tissue. In horses, GGT has been shown to be a better indicator than AP of hepatobiliary and cholestatic liver disease.

    (a) AP activity is usually increased in horses with **chronic liver failure.**

    (b) In the presence of cholestasis, there is increased production and release of AP, possibly mediated through the action of bile salts. Concurrent increases in AP and GGT activity are the expected finding in large animal patients with **biliary obstruction.**

(3) Dehydrogenases [e.g., **sorbitol dehydrogenase (SDH), lactate dehydrogenase (LDH), glutamate dehydrogenase (GDH)**] are found in hepatocytes. Activity of these enzymes is usually increased with **acute hepatocellular damage,** but is often normal to below-normal in patients with chronic liver failure.

b. Serum bilirubin assessment. Hyperbilirubinemia in large animals can result from hemolysis, cholestasis, or hepatocellular disease. In horses, fasting commonly causes hyperbilirubinemia.

    (1) Animals with hepatocellular disease will have increases in both conjugated and unconjugated bilirubin, with unconjugated bilirubin showing the greatest increase.

    (2) In animals with significant biliary obstruction, the magnitude of increase in conjugated bilirubin is usually greater than the magnitude of increase in unconjugated bilirubin. Horses are the exception to this rule; in this species, a conjugated serum bilirubin level that is greater than or equal to 25% of the total bilirubin indicates bile duct obstruction. Bilirubinuria, in the absence of hemolysis, is also indicative of bile duct obstruction.

c. Bile acid concentration. Bile acids are synthesized in the liver from cholesterol. They are present in high concentrations in the portal circulation, are extracted by the liver with high efficiency (greater than 90%), and are transported via the biliary tree. An elevated bile acid concentration has high specificity for diagnosis of liver disease, but cannot be used to differentiate between hepatocellular and obstructive disease.

    (1) Hepatocellular disease. Bile acid concentrations are increased in patients with hepatocellular disease as a result of decreased extraction from the portal circulation.

    (2) Obstructive liver disease. Bile acid concentrations are increased in patients with obstructive liver disease as a result of decreased biliary excretion.

d. Dye excretion tests. Sulfobromophthalein and indocyanine dyes can be used to assess hepatobiliary transport. Because these dyes are difficult to obtain, serum bile acid measurements have replaced dye excretion tests for evaluation of liver function in large animals.

e. Miscellaneous laboratory assessments

    (1) Serum prothrombin time (PT). The serum PT may be increased as a result of decreased synthesis of clotting factors in patients with liver failure.

    (2) Plasma triglyceride concentration. The plasma triglyceride concentration may be increased in horses and cattle with hepatic lipidosis.

(3) Plasma ammonia concentration. The plasma ammonia concentration may be increased due to decreased conversion of ammonia to urea in the liver. The degree of elevation of the plasma ammonia level is poorly correlated with the severity of the hepatic encephalopathy.

(4) Glucose level. Hypoglycemia due to anorexia, decreased hepatic glycogen stores, and decreased hepatic gluconeogenesis occurs in large animals with liver failure.

(5) Plasma protein level. The liver produces most plasma proteins, including albumin and α and β globulins. Hypoalbuminemia is uncommon in patients with liver failure, but decreased α and β globulin concentrations have been reported in horses with chronic liver failure. In contrast, γ globulin concentrations are increased due to chronic antigenic stimulation.

3. **Other diagnostic modalities**
   a. **Hepatic ultrasound.** Ultrasound examination of the liver is used to diagnose hepatomegaly, cholelithiasis (with or without biliary dilatation), and space-occupying lesions in the liver.
   b. **Percutaneous liver biopsy** is used to determine the presence and cause of liver disease.
      (1) Procedure. Samples may be obtained blindly or with ultrasound guidance and should be placed in formalin for histology and appropriate media for bacterial culture.
      (2) Contraindications. The procedure is relatively safe, provided that the coagulation profile is normal. A liver biopsy should be avoided when liver abscesses are suspected.

C. **Treatment of hepatobiliary disease.** Supportive care is most appropriate in patients with acute hepatic failure because the liver has a tremendous regenerative capacity. Treatment of patients with chronic liver failure is generally unrewarding because regeneration is restricted by fibrosis that bridges lobules. Supportive medical therapy may entail the following measures:

1. **Management of hepatic encephalopathy**
   a. **Sedation.** Restless or convulsing animals should be sedated. **Xylazine** (0.5–1.0 mg/kg) and **diazepam** (0.05–0.4 mg/kg) are effective sedatives in most patients; drug dosages may have to be adjusted because most sedatives and anticonvulsants are metabolized by the liver.
   b. **Minimization of the production or absorption of toxic metabolites**
      (1) Mineral oil is used to decrease absorption of toxic protein metabolites produced by enteric bacteria.
      (2) Lactulose (0.3 ml/kg orally once every 6 hours) can be used to decrease ammonia absorption from the gut, and **neomycin** (10–100 mg/kg orally once every 6 hours) may be given to decrease the production of ammonia by intestinal microflora. However, these two treatments are costly and may cause diarrhea.
      (3) Diet. Proper dietary management is crucial. A diet that provides 30–40 kcal/kg body weight (BW) in the form of low-protein, high-energy feeds rich in branched-chain amino acids (e.g., milo, sorghum, beet pulp) has been recommended for all horses with liver failure, but particularly those with signs of hepatic encephalopathy.
         (a) A mixture of two parts beet pulp and one part cracked corn in molasses fed at 2.5 kg/100 kg BW/day is usually divided into six or more feedings.
         (b) Oat or grass hay should be substituted for high-protein alfalfa or legume hay.

2. **Intravenous fluid therapy.** 5% Dextrose (2 ml/kg/hour) should be used for the first 24 hours in patients that are hypoglycemic or exhibiting signs of hepatoencephalopathy. If fluid therapy is to be continued for more than 24 hours, 2.5%–5% dextrose in lactated Ringer's solution should be substituted. In anorexic patients, potassium chloride can be added to fluids at a rate of 20–40 mmol/kg.

TABLE 5-2. Recommended Oral Dosages of Corticosteroids for Patients with Chronic Active Hepatitis

Day	Dosage
1–3	1.5 mg/kg twice daily
4–6	1.0 mg/kg twice daily
7–11	1.0 mg/kg once daily
12–16	0.5 mg/kg once daily

3. **Vitamin supplementation**
   a. **Vitamin K₁** (40–50 mg/450 kg BW subcutaneously once weekly) is indicated to prevent coagulopathies.
   b. **Vitamin B₁** and **folic acid** may also be administered once weekly.

4. **Antimicrobial therapy.** Ideally, antimicrobial therapy should be based on culture and sensitivity results. Empiric therapy for suppurative cholangitis usually includes the administration of a β lactam and an aminoglycoside, or trimethoprim–sulfamethoxazole. Metronidazole should be added if anaerobic infection is suspected.

5. **Therapy for chronic active hepatitis.** A variety of diseases can cause chronic active inflammation of the liver.
   a. **Corticosteroids.** Administration of corticosteroids may benefit patients with chronic active hepatitis. A recommended dosage schedule is given in Table 5-2.
   b. **Colchicine.** Theoretically, colchicine will reverse hepatic fibrosis, but the efficacy of this drug in horses is not known.

II. HEPATOBILIARY DISEASES OF HORSES

A. Hepatobiliary diseases of adult horses

1. **Serum hepatitis (Theiler's disease)** is a complication of equine-origin biologic administration [e.g., tetanus antitoxin (TAT)].
   a. **Epidemiology.** Sporadic cases, epidemics, and seasonal (early summer and fall) patterns have been described. Even in epidemics, the morbidity rate is low, ranging from 2%–18% for inoculated horses. The mortality rate is high, approximately 66%.
   b. **Patient profile and history**
      (1) **Patient profile.** Lactating mares appear to be at highest risk due to the practice of administering TAT at parturition. Foals rarely develop the disease, even when treated with the same batch of TAT used to treat the dams.
      (2) **History.** Affected horses usually present with a history of neurologic signs 4–10 weeks after the administration of equine-origin biologics.
   c. **Clinical findings.** Signs of acute hepatic failure (e.g., photodermatitis, hepatic encephalopathy, icterus, inappetence, pica, yawning) are commonly observed. Fever may occur in 50% of patients.
      (1) Weight loss, ventral edema with jugular pulsations, and severe dyspnea were reported as atypical signs in one outbreak.
      (2) Subclinical disease characterized by increases in serum enzyme activity has been documented in TAT-treated mares and foals.
   d. **Etiology**
      (1) A **viral agent,** similar to the hepatitis B virus that affects human beings, is the proposed but unproven cause of serum sickness. Affected horses that had not been previously inoculated usually have had contact with treated horses, suggesting contact transmission.

       (2) Theiler's disease has also been attributed to a **type III (immune complex–mediated) hypersensitivity reaction.**

    e. Diagnostic plan

       (1) History and clinical findings. Icterus and neurologic dysfunction, coupled with a history of recent administration of TAT or another equine-origin biologic, suggests a diagnosis of serum hepatitis.

       (2) Liver biopsy. Histologic examination of liver samples obtained antemortem or postmortem usually reveals moderate to severe hepatocellular degeneration throughout the lobule, with the most severe changes occurring in the centrilobular and zona intermedia regions.

    f. Therapeutic plan. Supportive medical therapy is the key to treating horses with serum hepatitis, but the mortality rate is high. Recovery in treated horses may take 4–21 days. Survivors of postvaccinal epidemics have no clinical evidence of lasting hepatic disease.

    g. Prevention. Vaccination of the mare with tetanus toxoid 30 days before parturition is a safer approach to tetanus prophylaxis than the routine use of TAT in recently foaled mares and foals.

2. Pyrrolizidine alkaloid (PA) toxicosis can occur when horses graze contaminated pastures or hay. PA-containing plants are unpalatable and will only be consumed by horses if growth is so heavy that the toxic plants cannot be separated from normal forage, or if pastures are overgrazed. The plants remain toxic in hay, including pelleted and cubed products, and silage.

    a. Patient profile and history. Horses and cattle are equally susceptible to PA toxicosis, whereas sheep and goats are quite resistant. Because signs are often delayed, liver failure may not be recognized until 1 year or more after the contaminated feed source has been removed.

    b. Clinical findings. Clinical signs of PA toxicosis are those described for liver failure and commonly include weight loss, icterus, and hepatic encephalopathy. Photodermatitis and diarrhea are occasionally seen.

    c. Etiology and pathogenesis

       (1) Etiology. Plants containing PA include *Senecio, Amsinckia, Crotalaria,* and *Heliotropium.*

       (2) Pathogenesis. Following gastrointestinal absorption, the PAs are carried via the portal circulation to the liver and **metabolized by hepatic microsomal enzymes** to more toxic **pyrroles.**

          (a) The pyrroles may cause cross-linking of DNA and an antimitotic effect; hepatocytes that cannot divide become megalocytes as cytoplasm expands without nuclear division.

          (d) Pyrroles also cause centrilobular and periportal hepatocellular necrosis. Ultimately, severe hepatocellular fibrosis and biliary hyperplasia ensue.

    d. Diagnostic plan

       (1) Serum biochemical profile. In acute cases, dehydrogenase activity is increased. GGT and AP activity is consistently increased. Increased concentrations of bile acids and direct and indirect bilirubin are also seen. Hypoalbuminemia and clotting abnormalities occur terminally.

       (2) Liver biopsy will reveal a triad of **fibrosis, bile duct proliferation,** and **megalocytosis,** which is almost pathognomonic for PA toxicosis, although similar changes have been reported in cases of aflatoxicosis. Modest hepatocellular changes and bile duct hyperplasia indicate a fair prognosis; extensive fibrosis bridging portal areas implies a guarded prognosis.

    e. Therapeutic plan. There is no specific treatment for PA toxicosis. Affected horses should be removed from contaminated pastures.

       (1) Horses with overt clinical signs of liver failure usually die within 5–10 days.

       (2) Supportive therapy is indicated for horses with mild signs and reversible liver lesions.

    f. Prevention

       (1) PA toxicosis is prevented by avoiding exposure of horses to contaminated hay or pasture. The growth of *Senecio* can be controlled by cultivation or herbicide spraying.

(2) Sheep, which are more resistant to poisoning, are sometimes used to graze *Senecio*-infested pastures.

3. Cholelithiasis
  a. Patient profile and history
    (1) Patient profile. The mean age of affected horses is 11 years (range, 5–23 years). No breed or sex predilection has been reported.
    (2) History. Affected horses are presented with a history of repeated bouts of mild abdominal pain over periods of up to 1 year.
  b. Clinical findings. Recurrent abdominal pain and fever spikes, accompanied by weight loss and icterus, are characteristic clinical signs. Signs of hepatic encephalopathy have been reported in a few affected horses.
  c. Etiology. The etiology of cholelithiasis in horses is not known. Bacterial infection ascending from the duodenum to the common bile duct, leading to bile stasis, has been proposed as a cause. *Salmonella* has been cultured from the biliary tree of some affected horses.
  d. Diagnostic plan
    (1) Hematologic work-up. Hematologic findings in horses with biliary obstruction usually include leukocytosis with neutrophilia, hyperproteinemia, and hyperfibrinogenemia.
    (2) Serum biochemical profile. Common serum biochemical abnormalities reported in affected horses include marked increases in serum activity of cholestatic liver enzymes (i.e., GGT, AP) and moderate increases in dehydrogenase activity. Conjugated hyperbilirubinemia and bilirubinuria are also seen.
    (3) Abdominocentesis. Because recurrent colic occurs in horses with cholelithiasis, abdominocentesis is usually performed. Peritoneal fluid in affected horses may be orange-tinged, increased in volume, and have cytologic findings that suggest chronic active inflammation.
    (4) Ultrasonography can assist with antemortem diagnosis of cholelithiasis. Typical findings are hepatomegaly, marked dilatation of bile ducts, and hyperechoic areas (choleliths), which cause acoustic shadowing.
    (5) Liver biopsy, with samples submitted for bacteriology and culture, is a useful ancillary diagnostic test in equine patients with cholelithiasis.
      (a) Although histologic findings are nonspecific, they can provide useful prognostic information; extensive periportal fibrosis, bile duct proliferation, biliary stasis, and hepatocyte necrosis usually indicate a poor prognosis.
      (b) Bacterial culture and sensitivity results can be used to guide antimicrobial therapy.
  e. Therapeutic plan
    (1) Supportive therapy should be employed in horses with signs of liver failure.
    (2) Antimicrobial therapy is indicated to treat secondary bacterial cholangitis. Because enteric bacteria are most commonly involved, penicillin and an aminoglycoside or penicillin and trimethoprim–sulfamethoxazole are indicated.
    (3) Cholelith removal
      (a) Cholelithotripsy and **choledochotomy** have been attempted, but poor surgical outcomes are common because of extensive hepatic fibrosis, multiple unremovable stones throughout the hepatobiliary tree, secondary choleperitoneum, and postoperative *Salmonella*-induced colitis.
      (b) Bile acid therapy, used to dissolve choleliths, has not been employed in horses because dissolution of calculi takes many months and most calculi in horses are not composed of cholesterol, a requirement for the effectiveness of bile acid therapy.
  f. Prevention. There are no specific recommendations for the prevention of cholelithiasis because the predisposing factors have not been identified.

4. Hyperlipidemia is a disorder of lipid metabolism.
  a. Patient profile and history
    (1) Patient profile. Hyperlipidemia occurs primarily in ponies and donkeys. Although the disease is uncommon in horses, it has been recognized with some frequency in miniature horses. Mares in late gestation or early lactation are

more frequently affected than stallions or geldings. Animals that are in good to obese condition seem to be predisposed to the disease.

(2) **History.** Many equids with hyperlipidemia have a history of recent stress (e.g., transportation, inclement weather, changes in diet).

b. Clinical findings

(1) Initial clinical signs include inappetence, lethargy, reluctance to move, and incoordination and weakness. Mild intermittent abdominal pain and decreased intestinal motility and fecal output are common findings. Diarrhea develops terminally. Prior to death, most affected animals exhibit neurologic signs. The interval between the first appearance of signs and death is usually less than 10 days.

(2) Other variable and nonspecific findings include pyrexia, tachypnea, icterus, congested mucous membranes, and ventral subcutaneous edema.

c. Etiology and pathogenesis

(1) **Etiology.** The theory that hyperlipidemia occurs solely as a complication of a primary disease process has recently been refuted. Concurrent disease has only been identified in one third of cases. Examples of such diseases include intestinal parasitism and other gastrointestinal disorders, hyperadrenocorticism, laminitis, and metritis.

(2) **Pathogenesis.** In hyperlipidemia, lipolysis of adipose tissue is induced by activation of **hormone-sensitive lipase** during times of negative energy balance or stress. However, the lipolysis is unregulated because of resistance of the hormone-sensitive lipase to the inhibitory action of insulin. Insulin resistance is induced by factors such as breed, obesity, pregnancy, and lactation.

(a) Unregulated lipolysis results in the release of **free fatty acids** into the circulation in amounts that overwhelm the liver's oxidative ketogenic capacities. The excess free fatty acids are esterified to **triglycerides** in the liver, which are subsequently secreted as **very low-density lipoproteins (VLDLs).** Therefore, patients with hyperlipidemia have increased plasma triglyceride and VLDL concentrations.

(b) Circulating triglycerides and VLDLs are hydrolyzed by **lipoprotein lipase,** which is located in capillary endothelium of adipose tissue, skeletal, and cardiac muscle.

(i) Free fatty acids released from the hydrolyzed triglycerides are used as an energy source in muscle or stored in adipose tissue as triglycerides.

(ii) Direct uptake of VLDLs into the peripheral tissues by cells or the reticuloendothelial system may explain the fatty infiltration of organs identified in affected equids at necropsy.

d. Diagnostic plan

(1) **Plasma triglyceride assessment.** The plasma of severely affected equids is lipemic, with a milky appearance. Plasma triglyceride concentrations commonly exceed 400 mg/dl.

(2) **Serum biochemical profile.** Other biochemical findings include hypoglycemia, metabolic acidosis, evidence of liver failure (e.g., increased serum liver enzyme activity, hyperbilirubinemia, hyperammonemia, prolongation of the PT), and azotemia. Laboratory findings should be interpreted with care because lipemia can interfere with some clinical chemistry tests.

e. Therapeutic plan

(1) **An attempt should be made to treat any underlying disease.**

(2) **The energy balance should be corrected and maintained.**

(a) **Diet.** Highly palatable feedstuffs (e.g., newly cut grass, leafy hay, rolled grains, or meals with added molasses) should be offered. Enteral feeding of slurries made from alfalfa cubes, or pelleted hay and electrolyte solutions, should be administered via nasogastric tube 4–8 times per day in anorectic patients.

(b) **Intravenous fluid therapy.** In patients with compromised gastrointestinal function, 5% dextrose should be administered as a constant intravenous infusion at a rate of 1–2 ml/kg/hour; balanced electrolytes should be added if fluid therapy is continued for more than 24 hours.

(c) **Appetite stimulants.** Anabolic steroids and vitamins may be used as appetite stimulants and to assist hepatic function. Glucocorticoids are contraindicated because they induce the activity of hormone-sensitive lipase.

(d) **Reduction of energy drain**

    (i) **Abortion** is an option in pregnant mares with hyperlipidemia; however, retained fetal membranes and laminitis are likely sequelae.

    (ii) **Weaning.** Foals should be weaned from lactating mares with hyperlipidemia.

(3) **Plasma lipid concentrations should be lowered.**

(a) **Exogenous insulin** (30–80 IU protamine zinc insulin administered intramuscularly twice daily) is used to inhibit the activity of hormone-sensitive lipase. Insulin should be used in conjunction with oral or intravenous glucose to promote the esterification of fatty acids in adipose tissue. However, insulin resistance may render this treatment ineffective.

(b) **Heparin** (100–200 IU intravenously twice daily) has been employed in an attempt to lower triglyceride concentrations by increasing the activity of lipoprotein lipase. However, recent research has shown that lipoprotein lipase activity is near maximum in ponies with hyperlipidemia, so heparin may act only to increase the risk of coagulopathy.

f. Prevention

(1) Attempts should be made to reduce stress and prevent obesity in susceptible animals.

(a) Exercise and controlled feed intake may improve insulin sensitivity in ponies and reduce the risk of hyperlipidemia.

(b) Feed intake of animals being transported should be closely monitored and high-quality, energy-rich concentrates should be provided during transportation.

(c) Drastic weight reduction programs for conditions such as laminitis should be avoided in at-risk equids.

(2) Due to the rapid progression of the disease, owners of at-risk animals should be advised to seek immediate veterinary attention for animals that are lethargic and anorectic.

5. Other disorders. The following disorders are uncommon causes of hepatic failure:

a. Chronic active hepatitis

b. Hepatocellular and cholangiocellular carcinomas

c. Bacterial cholangitis (caused by *Salmonella* infection)

d. Hepatic abscess

e. Parasite migration

f. Chronic hepatotoxicosis resulting from exposure to aflatoxins, kleingrass, or alsike clover

g. Overzealous steroid administration

B. **Hepatobiliary diseases of foals**

1. Tyzzer's disease

a. Patient profile and history

(1) **Patient profile.** Tyzzer's disease is observed in foals 7–42 days of age.

(2) **History.** Usually there is a history of sudden death. The client may describe a foal that is in shock and exhibiting neurologic signs.

b. Clinical findings. The disease has a short clinical course (hours to 2 days); sudden death without clinical signs is common. If there are clinical signs, they are nonspecific and include depression and anorexia that rapidly progress to recumbency, seizures, and coma. Foals may be hypothermic or febrile (temperatures can range from 39°C–41°C) and marked icterus develops terminally.

c. Etiology. Tyzzer's disease is caused by *Bacillus piliformis*, a gram-negative, spore-forming, motile bacillus.

d. Diagnostic plan

(1) **Laboratory studies.** Clinical pathologic data are nonspecific and include marked increases in liver-derived serum enzyme activity, marked hypoglycemia, and neutropenia or neutrophilia.

(2) **Postmortem examination.** Findings include severe icterus, generalized petechiation, and marked hepatomegaly. The cut surface of the liver usually contains multiple scattered foci of necrosis 1–2 mm in diameter. *B. piliformis* is difficult to culture. A diagnosis is usually confirmed by demonstrating long, slender bacilli in silver-stained formalin-fixed liver sections.

e. **Therapeutic plan.** Suspected early cases may respond to treatment, but the prognosis for recovery is generally poor. **Intravenous antimicrobial therapy** with penicillin and an aminoglycoside and **supportive treatment for acute liver failure** are recommended.

f. **Prevention.** There are no specific control measures for this sporadic disease. Because the dam may be the source of infection, subsequent foals should be closely monitored for signs of disease.

2. **Ferrous fumarate poisoning (toxic hepatic failure).** Foals that received a microorganism inoculum containing ferrous fumarate before nursing developed liver failure at 2–5 days of age. Hepatic encephalopathy, marked hyperbilirubinemia, hyperammonemia, and prolongation of the PT were consistent findings in affected foals. Postmortem examination of affected foals revealed small, reddish-brown livers with evidence of massive hepatocellular necrosis. The nutritive supplement containing this iron preparation is no longer available.

3. **Other disorders.** The following disorders are occasionally associated with hepatic failure in foals:
   a. Congenital equine herpesvirus 1 infection
   b. Septicemia *(Actinobacillus equuli)* infection
   c. Endotoxemia
   d. Perinatal asphyxia
   e. Portocaval shunts
   f. Biliary atresia
   g. Administration of parenteral nutrition (associated with cholestasis and hepatic disease)
   h. Gastric ulcers and duodenitis in older foals (associated with duodenal strictures leading to bile stasis and secondary cholangitis)
   i. Hepatic abscesses (possibly as a sequela of septic omphalophlebitis)

III.   HEPATOBILIARY DISEASES OF RUMINANTS

A. Hepatobiliary diseases of adult ruminants

1. **Hepatic abscesses**
   a. **Patient profile and history**
      (1) **Patient profile.** Ruminants of all ages, breeds, and sexes may be affected. Liver abscesses are common in dairy and beef cattle fed diets high in carbohydrates and low in roughage. Approximately 40% of feedlot cattle may have liver abscesses; feedlot cattle 6–24 months of age are affected most often.
      (2) **History.** A history of rumenitis or reticuloperitonitis is common.
   b. **Clinical findings**
      (1) **Subclinical disease.** Most liver abscesses are incidental findings at postmortem. The only clinical sign may be the fact that the rate of gain is usually reduced by more than 3.5% in animals with subclinical disease.
      (2) **Clinical disease** is characterized by weight loss, anorexia, depression, and decreased milk production. Intermittent fever spikes can occur. Some cattle may be reluctant to move or lie down and experience pain when pressure is applied behind the right posterior rib cage.
      (3) **Clinical findings related to sequelae**

(a) **Caudal vena cava thrombosis** can occur following erosion of the caudal vena cava by a liver abscess, resulting in one of three clinical syndromes
  (i) **Sudden death** (due to septic shock following rupture of the abscess)
  (ii) **Epistaxis, hemoptysis,** and **anemia** caused by widespread pulmonary thromboembolism and rupture of an aneurism
  (iii) **Severe dyspnea** and **diffusely abnormal lung sounds** following nonfatal rupture of a pulmonary abscess
(b) **Bile duct occlusion.** Large abscesses may occlude the bile duct, leading to **icterus** and **photodermatitis.**
(c) **Diffuse peritonitis** following rupture of the abscess into the abdominal cavity

c. Etiology and pathogenesis
  (1) **Etiology.** The primary etiologic agent of hepatic abscesses in cattle is *Fusobacterium necrophorum*. Other bacterial etiologic agents include *Actinomyces pyogenes, Streptococcus, Staphylococcus,* and *Bacteroides.*
  (2) **Pathogenesis.** In cattle, erosion of the ruminal epithelium secondary to grain overload is thought to be the most common mechanism for *F. necrophorum* colonization of the liver.

d. Diagnostic plan
  (1) **Laboratory studies.** Findings supporting a diagnosis of liver abscess in cattle include **neutrophilia, hyperfibrinogenemia, hyperproteinemia,** and **hyperglobulinemia. Anemia** [evidenced by a decreased packed cell volume (PCV), RBC count, and decreased hemoglobin] may result from blood loss secondary to hemoptysis or from chronic inflammation. Serum liver enzyme activities are usually normal because abscesses are focal and encapsulated.
  (2) **Liver biopsy** is of little use for diagnosis because focal lesions are easily missed. Biopsies may cause rupture of an abscess and septic peritonitis.
  (3) **Ultrasound examination** can confirm the presence of hepatic abscesses.

e. Therapeutic plan. Long-term penicillin or tetracycline therapy is indicated for treatment of affected animals; however, affected cattle, particularly those with caudal vena cava thrombosis, have a very poor prognosis and are usually not treated.

f. Prevention
  (1) Gradually introducing concentrate feeding over a 3- to 4-week period and providing adequate amounts of coarse hay (1 kg/head/day), will reduce the incidence of hepatic abscesses in feedlot cattle.
  (2) Feeding a total mixed ration and long-stemmed hay (2.3 kg/head/day) with rumen buffers (e.g., sodium bicarbonate, magnesium oxide) may reduce incidence of liver abscesses in dairy cattle.
  (3) Antimicrobials can be added to beef cattle rations to decrease the incidence of liver abscesses (e.g., chlortetracycline at 70 mg/kg/head/day or oxytetracycline at 75 mg/kg/head/day).

2. Fascioliasis (liver fluke infestation)
  a. Patient profile. Liver flukes cause disease in cattle, sheep, and goats.
  b. Etiology and pathogenesis
    (1) **Etiology.** Fascioliasis in domestic ruminants is caused by the trematodes *Fasciola hepatica, Fasciola gigantica,* and *Fascioloides magna.*
      (a) *F. hepatica* occurs primarily in the Gulf Coast and western states.
      (b) *F. gigantica* is found in Hawaii.
      (c) *F. magna* occurs in the Gulf Coast states, Great Lakes region, and northwestern states where grazing domestic ruminants share pastures with deer, elk, and moose (natural hosts of the parasite).
    (2) **Pathogenesis.** All have an aquatic snail (limnaeid snails) as an intermediate host. The life cycle of *F. hepatica* and *F. gigantica* are similar; *F. magna* completes the full life cycle only in its natural hosts (deer, elk, moose).
      (a) Fluke eggs hatch in the water to **miracidia,** which develop through sporocyst, redia, and cercaria stages after the miracidia penetrate the snail intermediate host. **Cercariae** later emerge from snails, encyst as **metacercariae** on herbage, and are eaten by the final host.

(i) *F. hepatica* infestation occurs in livestock grazing low-lying swampy pastures, flood irrigation areas, and pastures adjacent to slowly moving streams. These habitats favor the propagation of the snails that act as the intermediate hosts for liver flukes. In the Gulf Coast states, warm, wet winters and springs favor massive proliferation of snails, hatching of fluke eggs, and development of cercariae. Most fluke transmission occurs between February and July; transmission ceases when summer heat and drought results in the death of snails and metacercariae. Mature egg-laying flukes, susceptible to flukicides, are present in the fall.

(ii) In the Pacific Northwest, fluke transmission may be delayed because freezing weather causes death of metacercariae and snails.

(b) Metacercariae encyst in the small intestine. Young flukes migrate through the gut wall and peritoneal cavity and reach the liver in 4–6 days. They migrate in the liver for 4–6 weeks, enter the bile ducts, and mature to egg-laying adults 10–12 weeks postinfection. *F. hepatica* can survive for many years in sheep and shed thousands of eggs per day; cattle develop resistance and usually eliminate flukes within 1 year.

(i) **Acute *F. hepatica* disease** is caused by invasion of the liver by massive numbers of immature flukes. Severe hepatic parenchymal damage and massive hemorrhage into the peritoneal cavity cause liver failure and severe blood loss anemia.

(ii) **Chronic *F. hepatica* disease** is attributed to activity of adult flukes in the bile ducts. Cholangitis, biliary obstruction, and biliary fibrosis are responsible for weight loss and icterus. Anemia and hypoproteinemia result from blood-sucking adult flukes.

(iii) ***F. gigantica*-induced disease.** The pathogenesis is similar to that of disease caused by *F. hepatica*.

(c) Anaerobic necrotic tracts produced by migrating liver flukes may trigger proliferation of latent *Clostridium novyi* or *Clostridium hemolyticum* spores. Exotoxins produced by these bacteria are responsible for black disease in sheep (see III A 3) and bacillary hemoglobinuria in cattle (see III A 4).

c. Clinical findings

(1) ***F. hepatica.*** Disease caused by *F. hepatica* infestation can be acute or chronic.

(a) **Acute disease** due to *F. hepatica* is common in sheep and goats, but rare in cattle due to natural and acquired immunity. Outbreaks last 2–3 weeks and signs include anorexia, depression, weakness, pale mucous membranes, dyspnea, ascites, abdominal pain, and dry feces. Acute fascioliasis causes high mortality in sheep.

(b) **Chronic disease.** Chronic fluke infestation causes significant production losses in cattle and sheep.

(i) Clinical manifestations in sheep include progressive weight loss, pale mucous membranes, intermandibular edema, ascites, and, occasionally, icterus.

(ii) Chronic disease is the only manifestation of fascioliasis in cattle. Reported signs include poor body condition, decreased milk yield, and anemia.

(2) ***F. gigantica*** infestation causes signs similar to those of *F. hepatica* infection.

(3) ***F. magna*** infestation causes acute, rapidly fatal disease in sheep and goats, and chronic disease in cattle as a result of unrestricted fluke migration. *F. magna* infestation is subclinical in cattle because flukes are rapidly encapsulated by fibrous tissue.

d. Diagnostic plan

(1) **Serum biochemistry and hematology.** Serum biochemical and hematologic findings include severe anemia, hypoalbuminemia, eosinophilia, and increased serum liver enzyme activity in acute disease. Chronic disease is characterized by anemia, hypergammaglobulinemia, and conjugated hyperbilirubinemia.

(2) **Fecal sedimentation** is the standard method for diagnosing *F. hepatica* infection in cattle. The technique is time-consuming and infections may be missed because low egg counts are common and immature flukes do not produce eggs. A new fecal test (Flukefinder®), based on the use of two sieves, is simple to perform in the field and reduces sample processing time.

(3) **Enzyme-linked immunosorbent assay (ELISA) tests** for serologic diagnosis of liver fluke infestation are being developed. These tests are limited by their low sensitivity and specificity and the difficulty of using these tests to differentiate between current infection and prior exposure.

(4) **Postmortem examination**
(a) Findings in **acute cases** include an enlarged hemorrhagic liver covered by fibrin strands, a large volume of serosanguinous peritoneal fluid, and excessive numbers of immature flukes (more than 1000) in the liver parenchyma.
(b) In **chronic cases,** the liver is small and fibrotic with more than 200 adult flukes in the bile ducts.

e. **Therapeutic plan.** Two drugs are available for treatment of fascioliasis in North America, and two experimental drugs (triclabendazole and netobimin) are being developed.
(1) **Clorsulon** (7 mg/kg orally) is a narrow-spectrum flukicide with no activity against gastrointestinal nematodes. Clorsulon is more than 99% effective against adults and 96% effective against late immature flukes.
(2) **Albendazole** (10 mg/kg orally) is a broad-spectrum flukicide, effective against both liver flukes and gastrointestinal nematodes. Albendazole is 75%–90% effective against adults and 33% effective against late-stage immature flukes.

f. **Prevention**
(1) Livestock should not be grazed in high-risk areas during periods of peak transmission. Snail habitats should be fenced or drained if possible.
(2) Molluscicides (e.g., copper sulfate) may be of value when applied to small snail habitats, but toxic effects on nontarget species is a problem.
(3) Flukicides should be used strategically.
(a) A summer treatment in the Gulf Coast states with a broad-spectrum flukicide (or a narrow-spectrum flukicide combined with an anthelmintic) will remove a high proportion of drug-susceptible mature and late-stage immature flukes and peak numbers of hypobiotic nematode larvae.
(b) Annual fall treatments are sufficient in the Pacific northwest because they will remove adult fluke burdens before the winter nutritional stress period.

3. **Black disease (infectious necrotic hepatitis)** occurs worldwide in areas where liver flukes are endemic and sheep are raised.
a. **Patient profile and history**
(1) **Patient profile.** Black disease affects sheep and, to a lesser degree, cattle.
(2) **History.** The chief complaint is of sudden deaths in the herd or flock.
b. **Clinical findings.** The usual clinical manifestation is sudden death. Affected animals show signs for only a few hours; the sudden onset of a fever (40°C–41°C) that rapidly progresses to hypothermia, signs of toxemia, and respiratory distress may be observed.
c. **Etiology and pathogenesis**
(1) **Etiology.** Black disease is usually caused by the interaction of *Clostridium novyi* type B bacteria and immature *F. hepatica* liver flukes.
(2) **Pathogenesis.** Spores of *C. novyi* present in normal liver may germinate when hepatic tissue is damaged by migrating immature liver flukes. (Other forms of liver damage, including biopsy, can also trigger the condition.) Sporulating bacteria produce potent necrotizing α and β toxins that damage the liver parenchyma, causing toxemia and death.
d. **Diagnostic plan.** Diagnosis is usually made at postmortem. There is evidence of recent liver fluke migration and toxemia (i.e., the presence of serosanguinous fluid in the thoracic cavity and pericardial sac and subendocardial and

subepicardial hemorrhages). Bacilli can be observed in necrotic tracts in the liver on histologic examination.

    e. Therapeutic plan. Therapy is not usually feasible, but affected animals can be treated with **intravenous fluids** and **massive doses of sodium penicillin** (44,000 U/kg intravenously every 6 hours). Specific antisera are not commercially available.

    f. Prevention. Control of fluke infection through pasture management and treatment of individual animals should be instituted together with vaccination against *C. novyi* type B. Vaccinations should be given in the late spring and early summer preceding the seasonal occurrence of black disease. In endemic fluke areas, cattle are vaccinated every 6 months.

4. Bacillary hemoglobinuria is an acute, highly fatal, toxemic infectious disease affecting cattle and, occasionally, sheep. It is caused by *Clostridium hemolyticum* (*Clostridium novyi* type D), a soil-borne anaerobe that, under hypoxic conditions, multiplies in hepatic tissue and produces a potent necrotizing and hemolytic exotoxin. Clinical signs include fever, hemoglobinuria, rapid death, and a large anemic infarct in the liver.

5. Hepatic lipidosis is associated with fat cow syndrome of dairy cattle (see Chapter 9 I G), pregnancy toxemia (protein energy malnutrition) of beef cattle (see Chapter 9 I H), and pregnancy toxemia in ewes and does (see Chapter 9 I F).

6. Hepatotoxicosis
    a. Aflatoxicosis
        (1) Patient profile. Aflatoxicosis affects cattle and small ruminants, although these animals are less susceptible than monogastric animals and poultry. Young animals are more susceptible than adults to the toxic effects of aflatoxins. Aflatoxicosis occurs in areas with high rainfall, humidity, and temperatures.

        (2) Clinical findings
            (a) Acute aflatoxicosis causes signs of liver failure resulting from hepatic necrosis.
            (b) Chronic aflatoxicosis is associated with reduced weight gain, poor feed conversion, and decreased milk production (as a result of aflatoxin's adverse effect on the rumen microflora). Affected animals also have an increased susceptibility to infection.

        (3) Etiology and pathogenesis. Aflatoxins are produced primarily by *Aspergillus* species in stored grains; these fungi can occasionally invade cereal crops prior to harvest if climactic conditions favor growth.
            (a) *Aspergillus flavus* is the primary producer of **four major aflatoxins (B_1, B_2, G_1, and G_2)** and several related compounds. Aflatoxin B_1 is the most abundant aflatoxin and is converted in lactating animals to aflatoxins M_1 and M_2, which are concentrated and secreted in milk. Aflatoxin M_1 is as toxic and carcinogenic as aflatoxin B_1, thereby posing a hazard to humans consuming contaminated milk.
            (b) Acute, massive exposure to aflatoxin causes hepatocellular necrosis through a direct toxic effect.

        (4) Diagnostic plan
            (a) Acute aflatoxicosis
                (i) Histopathologic evaluation of a liver biopsy sample or liver tissue obtained postmortem will reveal hepatocellular necrosis, hemorrhage, vacuolation, fatty infiltration, and megalocytosis.
                (ii) Laboratory studies. Serum liver enzyme activities are increased. Urine, milk, and blood may contain detectable levels of aflatoxin during acute exposure, and the toxin is readily detected in feed.
            (b) Chronic aflatoxicosis. It may be difficult to link subtle effects of growth suppression, poor feed efficiency, and impaired immune function to previous aflatoxin exposure, because contaminated feed that initiated chronic events may no longer be present and tissue residues may be too low to

be detected by routine methods. Therefore, chronic aflatoxicosis often goes undiagnosed.

(5) **Therapeutic plan.** Aflatoxicosis presents as a herd problem and intensive individual animal therapy is not practical.

(a) Suspect feed should be removed and a high-quality protein diet supplemented with vitamins A, D, E, K, and B complex should be provided to counteract the effect of aflatoxin on protein and vitamin utilization.

(b) There are no specific antidotes, but in acute cases of experimentally induced aflatoxicosis, goats treated with L-methionine (200 mg/kg orally every 8 hours) and sodium thiosulfate (50 mg/kg orally every 8 hours), had improved survival.

(c) Because animals exposed to aflatoxin may have compromised immune systems, clinical signs of infectious disease should be aggressively treated with antimicrobial therapy.

(6) **Prevention**

(a) Proper feed storage is indicated to prevent mycotoxicosis; the maximum safe moisture content of cereal grains is 14%. High-moisture grains can be stored by excluding air or adding preservatives (e.g., propionic acid).

(b) Aflatoxin-contaminated corn can be detoxified by treatment with ammonia, but this is a costly and impractical procedure.

(c) Aflatoxin-contaminated feed can be diluted with normal feed, but this practice is risky because even low levels of aflatoxin are potentially harmful.

b. **PA toxicosis** (see also II A 2). Signs of PA toxicosis in cattle include diarrhea, weight loss, a prolapsed rectum, ascites, and subtle neurologic signs. Icterus is uncommon. Calves are more susceptible to PA toxicosis than mature cattle.

c. **Copper toxicosis** is an acute, highly fatal hemolytic crisis affecting primarily sheep. It is associated with the sudden massive release of hepatic copper stores that have accumulated over a prolonged period as the result of excessive copper intake. Liver necrosis, which occurs secondary to copper accumulation, precedes the onset of hemolysis.

d. **Halothane toxicosis.** Halothane gas anesthesia is commonly used without complications in goats, but there have been two reports of presumed halothane toxicity causing massive hepatocellular necrosis and signs of hepatoencephalopathy a few days after administration of anesthesia.

B. Hepatobiliary diseases of calves, lambs, and kids

1. **Portosystemic anomalies** are rarely diagnosed in calves.

a. **Clinical findings.** Clinical signs include stunted growth and various episodic manifestations of hepatoencephalopathy.

b. **Diagnostic plan**

(1) **Laboratory studies.** Hyperammonemia, delayed sulfobromopthalein clearance, and increased bile acid concentrations, without alterations in serum liver enzyme activity, suggest a diagnosis of portosystemic shunt.

(2) **Liver biopsy.** The only abnormality on liver biopsy is mild periportal fibrosis.

(3) **Imaging studies.** Diagnosis is confirmed using **ultrasound** or **intraoperative mesenteric portography.**

c. **Therapeutic plan.** Successful surgical correction has been reported.

2. **Hepatic abscesses** in neonatal ruminants can be a complication of an umbilical vein abscess.

3. **Congenital diseases**

a. **Dubin-Johnson syndrome** is an autosomal recessive condition of Corriedale sheep characterized by a defect in biliary excretion of conjugated bilirubin and phylloerythrin.

(1) **Patient profile and history.** This syndrome affects 6-month-old Corriedale lambs on green feed.

(2) **Clinical findings** include anorexia, icterus, and severe photodermatitis.

(3) **Diagnostic plan**

       (a) **Laboratory studies.** Biochemical abnormalities include conjugated hyper-bilrubinemia and delayed sulfobromopthalein clearance.

       (b) **Liver biopsy** reveals brown to black granules in hepatocytes with normal hepatic architecture.

    (4) **Therapeutic plan.** Affected animals may survive if exposure to sunlight is avoided, but this approach may be impractical and affected lambs are usually culled.

    (5) **Prevention.** Selective breeding reduces the incidence of disease.

  b. **Gilbert's syndrome** is inherited as an autosomal recessive trait and is characterized by a failure of hepatic uptake of bilirubin and phylloerythrin. Renal failure accompanies this condition.

    (1) **Patient profile and history.** This syndrome affects 6-month-old Southdown sheep on pasture.

    (2) **Clinical findings.** Photodermatitis, without icterus, resulting in ulcerative lesions around the mouth and ears is the usual clinical presentation.

    (3) **Diagnostic plan**

       (a) **Laboratory studies.** Findings include unconjugated hyperbilirubinemia (exacerbated by fasting), delayed sulfobromopthalein clearance, and azotemia.

       (b) **Liver biopsy.** Histologic evaluation of liver biopsy specimens usually reveals no abnormalities.

    (4) **Therapeutic plan.** Affected sheep should be kept out of sunlight to prevent photodermatitis.

    (5) **Prevention.** Affected sheep and their dams and sires should not be retained for breeding purposes.

IV. HEPATOBILIARY DISEASES OF SWINE

A. Ascariasis

1. **Patient profile and history**
   a. **Patient profile.** Ascariasis affects young growing pigs up to 5 months of age.
   b. **History.** There is usually a complaint of poor growth.

2. **Clinical findings.** An occasional cough may be noted in pigs infected with ascarids. In rare cases of massive infestation, pigs exhibit severe dyspnea or die of acute hepatic insufficiency. Adult worms may be vomited; occasionally, intestinal obstruction and rupture or obstructive jaundice are seen.

3. **Etiology and pathogenesis**
   a. **Etiology.** Roundworms (*Ascaris suum*), the cause of ascariasis, are found in most swine-producing regions.
   b. **Pathogenesis**
      (1) *A. suum* begins its life cycle with eggs shed by adult worms. In warm conditions, infective second-stage larvae hatch from the eggs in 10–14 days. Ingested larvae penetrate the intestine and are carried via the portal circulation to the liver. Migration through the liver to the lungs is complete within 1 week. Within 2 weeks of ingestion, migration to the trachea is complete. Larvae are swallowed and develop to adults in the intestine. Egg production by adults commences 6–9 weeks post infection.
      (2) Larval migration through the liver leaves characteristic white foci of fibrosis. Initially, the liver lesions are caused by the migration of the larvae; subsequent exposure causes damage following an antigen–antibody reaction. Lesions generally heal 35 days after migration.
      (3) Immunity to roundworm infection develops first in the lungs, resulting in decreased lung larval counts. Liver and gut immunity take longer to develop. Under natural conditions, liver lesions occur until the pig weighs approxi-

mately 90 kg. In pigs older than 2 years, full gut immunity prevents larvae from reaching the liver.

4. **Diagnostic plan. Fecal flotation** can detect the presence of ascarid eggs in feces.

5. **Therapeutic plan. Ivermectin, levamisole,** and **pyrantel tartrate** are effective anthelmintics.

6. **Prevention.** Because exposure to ascarids during the growing phase may permanently affect growth rate and feed conversion and add 5%–13% to the cost of production to market, and liver lesions caused by ascarid migration create losses in the meat packing industry, prevention of disease is important.

   a. **Monitoring of ascarid burdens.** Annual examination of five to ten fecal samples from all categories of pigs is recommended. Liver inspection at slaughter can be used to monitor ascarid burdens on farms.

   b. **Disinfection of living spaces.** If pigs are confined to concrete pens, normal hygienic precautions will decrease the risk of ascariasis. Farrowing pens should be cleaned with a pressure sprayer.

   c. **Prophylactic anthelmintic therapy** may be indicated for piglets until they are weaned.

      (1) If sows are dewormed prior to being placed in a farrowing pen cleaned with a pressure sprayer, prophylactic anthelmintic treatment for piglets may not be required.

      (2) Periodic or continuous low level treatments with anthelmintics may be required if hygiene is poor.

   d. **Prevention of exposure.** Early weaning of piglets (at 3–4 weeks of age) will remove them from a potentially infective environment (*Ascaris* ova require 30–35 days to reach infectivity in a farrowing house environment).

B. **Hepatosis dietetica** occurs in rapidly growing pigs 2–16 weeks of age. It is caused by vitamin E and selenium deficiency. Lesions include subcutaneous edema, transudate in serous cavities, and hepatocellular necrosis with hemorrhage.

C. **Aflatoxicosis** (see also III A 6 a). Swine are more susceptible than cattle to the effects of aflatoxins. As with cattle, young swine are more susceptible than adults. The main target organ is the liver; affected pigs may die of acute liver failure or exhibit signs of ill thrift.

STUDY QUESTIONS

DIRECTIONS: Each of the numbered items or incomplete statements in this section is followed by answers or by completions of the statement. Select the ONE numbered answer or completion that is BEST in each case.

1. Which one of the following statements concerning liver failure in large animals is true?

(1) Pale feces suggest significant bile duct obstruction in suckling herbivores.
(2) Ascites is a common finding in horses with acute liver failure.
(3) A hemolytic crisis is a frequent complication of liver failure in ruminants.
(4) Hyperammonemia is the only metabolic alteration responsible for hepatic encephalopathy.
(5) Hypoalbuminemia is a consistent finding in horses and ruminants with liver failure.

2. Which one of the following is appropriate dietary management for an equine patient exhibiting signs of hepatic encephalopathy?

(1) Feeding high-quality alfalfa or legume hay
(2) Force feeding an alfalfa meal and cottage cheese slurry
(3) Withholding feed and administering 50% dextrose intravenously
(4) Feeding a mixture of beet pulp and cracked corn
(5) Feeding a bran mash with added mineral oil

3. Which one of the following statements pertaining to serum hepatitis (Theiler's disease) of horses is true?

(1) Serum hepatitis is caused by the hepatitis B virus.
(2) Serum hepatitis is most commonly diagnosed in lactating mares.
(3) Serum hepatitis is attributed to tetanus toxoid administration.
(4) Serum hepatitis is usually diagnosed in the winter months.
(5) Serum hepatitis is a disease with high morbidity and low mortality rates.

4. A veterinarian is called to a farm to examine a 5-year-old pony mare. The mare was bred 310 days ago and has been anorexic and depressed for 2 days. Recently, the owner restricted her feed intake because she was diagnosed as having laminitis. A jugular venous sample is obtained; the plasma has a milky appearance. What is the most likely diagnosis?

(1) Hyperlipidemia
(2) Pregnancy hypercalcemia
(3) Abdominal fat necrosis
(4) Pregnancy toxemia
(5) Tyzzer's disease

5. Which one of the following statements regarding pyrrolizidine alkaloid (PA) toxicosis in large domestic animals is true?

(1) Cattle are more resistant to PA toxicosis than are sheep and horses.
(2) Cattle, sheep, and horses are equally susceptible to PA toxicosis.
(3) Sheep are more resistant to PA toxicosis than are cattle and horses.
(4) Horses are more resistant to PA toxicosis than are sheep and cattle.
(5) Cattle, sheep, and horses are equally resistant to PA toxicosis.

6. Which one of the following statements regarding hepatic abscesses in feedlot cattle is true?

(1) They are a common cause of diffuse peritonitis.
(2) Common clinical manifestations include epistaxis and hemoptysis.
(3) The presentation is subclinical in most cases.
(4) They are a common cause of septic shock.
(5) They usually cause obstructive icterus (as a result of bile duct occlusion).

7. Inherited icterus and photosensitization have been reported in 6-month-old:

(1) Corriedale and Southdown lambs.
(2) Dorset and Corriedale lambs.
(3) Finn and Dorset lambs.
(4) Hampshire and Southdown lambs.
(5) Merino and Suffolk lambs.

8. Which one of the following treatments is contraindicated in a donkey suffering from hyperlipidemia?

(1) 5% Dextrose intravenously
(2) Anabolic steroids
(3) Insulin
(4) Glucocorticoids
(5) Heparin

9. Which one of the following anthelmintics will treat both *Ostertagia circumcincta* and *Fasciola hepatica* infestation in beef cattle?

(1) Albendazole
(2) Fenbendazole
(3) Clorsulon
(4) Ivermectin
(5) Morantel

DIRECTIONS: The numbered item in this section is negatively phrased, as indicated by a capitalized word such as NOT, LEAST, or EXCEPT. Select the ONE numbered answer or completion that is BEST.

10. Which one of the following is NOT hepatotoxic to large domestic animals?

(1) *Quercus*
(2) *Senecio*
(3) *Amsinckia*
(4) *Crotolaria*
(5) *Aspergillus flavus*

ANSWERS AND EXPLANATIONS

1. The answer is 1 [I B 1 c (5)]. Pale feces are a likely finding in suckling ruminants with biliary obstruction because stercobilin, a bilirubin metabolite excreted in the bile, is responsible for fecal color and would not be present in the feces of animals with significant biliary obstruction. Ascites is a common finding in cattle with hepatic cirrhosis, but is rarely reported in horses. A terminal hemolytic crisis, associated with increased red blood cell (RBC) fragility, has been reported in horses, but not in cattle, with terminal liver failure. A multitude of metabolic derangements contribute to the development of hepatic encephalopathy, not just hyperammonemia. Hypoalbuminemia is an uncommon finding in large animal patients with hepatic encephalopathy.

2. The answer is 4 [I C 1 b (3) (a)]. A high-energy, low-protein diet rich in branched-chain amino acids is recommended for horses with liver failure and signs of hepatic encephalopathy. A mixture of two parts beet pulp and one part cracked corn in molasses is often used. Feeding of a high-quality alfalfa or legume hay or force feeding an alfalfa meal and cottage cheese slurry would be inappropriate because both of these diets are high in protein. The goal is to limit protein consumption, because protein serves as a substrate for ammonia production by intestinal bacteria. Feed should not be withheld, and 5% (not 50%) dextrose should be administered. Higher concentrations of dextrose will cause glucosuria and dehydration. A bran mash diet is too low in energy to be offered as the primary feed source.

3. The answer is 2 [II A 1]. Lactating mares appear to be at higher risk for serum hepatitis (Theiler's disease) due to the common practice of administering tetanus antitoxin (TAT) postpartum. There is speculation that a virus, similar to the hepatitis B virus that affects humans, causes serum hepatitis in horses, but this theory remains to be proven. Serum hepatitis usually occurs 4–10 weeks after the administration of TAT, not tetanus toxoid. Serum hepatitis occurs most often in the summer and fall, and is characterized by low morbidity rates (2%–18%), but high mortality rates (greater than 60%).

4. The answer is 1 [II A 4]. Ponies in advanced gestation are prone to developing hyperlipidemia when fasted. The milky (lipemic) plasma supports this diagnosis. Pregnancy hypercalcemia, abdominal fat necrosis, and pregnancy toxemia do not occur in horses. Tyzzer's disease occurs only in foals.

5. The answer is 3 [II A 2 a]. Sheep are more resistant than cattle and horses to pyrrolizidine alkaloid (PA) toxicosis. For this reason, sheep are often used to graze pastures with PA-containing plants, which would be unsafe for cattle and horses.

6. The answer is 3 [III A 1]. Hepatic abscesses may occur in up to 40% of feedlot cattle and are usually an incidental finding at slaughter. Diffuse peritonitis, epistaxis and hemoptysis, septic shock, and bile duct occlusion leading to obstructive icterus are uncommon sequelae of hepatic abcessation in feedlot cattle.

7. The answer is 1 [III B 3]. Dubin-Johnson syndrome of Corriedale sheep and Gilbert's syndrome of Southdown sheep are hereditary diseases characterized by icterus and photodermatitis. Six-month-old lambs on pasture are affected.

8. The answer is 4 [II A 4 e]. Glucocorticoids are contraindicated in the treatment of a donkey with hyperlipidemia because they induce activity of hormone-sensitive lipase, which will further stimulate lipolysis. The administration of 5% dextrose, anabolic steroids, insulin, and heparin is appropriate, although the efficacy of insulin and heparin have been questioned.

9. The answer is 3 [III A 2 e (2)]. Albendazole is a broad-spectrum flukicide that is effective against liver flukes, such as *Fasciola hepatica* and nematodes, such as *Ostertagia circumcincta*. Fenbendazole, ivermectin, and morantel are not efficacious against liver flukes. Clorsulon is a narrow-spectrum flukicide that will eliminate liver flukes, but not gastrointestinal nematodes.

10. The answer is 1 [III A 6]. *Quercus* (oak) is nephrotoxic, not hepatotoxic. *Senecio, Amsinckia,* and *Crotolaria* contain pyrrolizidine alkaloids (PAs), which are hepatotoxic. *Aspergillus flavus* produces aflatoxin, which is also hepatotoxic.

Chapter 6

Diseases of the Upper Respiratory Tract

John Pringle

I. RHINITIS AND NASAL OBSTRUCTION

A. Rhinitis in horses

1. **Patient profile and history**
   a. **Acute rhinitis** in the horse is most commonly found in young horses and is associated with infectious (viral, bacterial) respiratory diseases. In such cases, the infection is accompanied by signs of equine rhinotracheitis (see II A 3 f).
   b. **Fungal infections (cryptococcosis, rhinosporidiosis)** also can cause rhinitis in the form of granulomatous, pedunculated masses. Cases are most common in the southern United States and are rare and sporadic. Tumors causing signs of rhinitis are uncommon in horses.

2. **Clinical findings.** Mucoid, mucopurulent, or blood-tinged nasal discharge is evident, as is inspiratory stridor if the nasal passages are markedly inflamed. In some cases, there may be decreased or unequal airflow from the nostrils, accompanied by malodorous air if necrotic processes are present.

3. **Diagnostic and therapeutic plans** (see II A 3)

B. Rhinitis and nasal obstruction in cattle

1. **Etiology and pathogenesis**
   a. **Causes** include **viruses, bacteria, fungi, allergens,** and masses (tumors). Rhinosporidium-like organisms produce polyps in the anterior nares.
      (1) **Allergic rhinitis** occurs mainly in Channel Island breeds, but it has been reported as a familial tendency in other breeds, occurring in spring and fall pollen seasons.
      (2) **Ethmoid carcinomas** are sporadic causes of nasal obstruction. Although there may be a familial tendency for occurrence, there is also a viral origin implicated in the genesis of these tumors. The tumors are suggested to be of moderate malignancy and can metastasize to the lymph nodes and lungs.
   b. **Pathogenesis.** Nasal obstruction may cause severe dyspnea, cyanosis, and stertorous breathing.

2. **Clinical findings**
   a. **Allergic rhinitis.** Signs include acute dyspnea and **sneezing,** accompanied by yellow-orange nasal discharge. Chronic cases present with multiple nodules in the anterior nares. Affected animals may rub their nasal cavities by pushing sticks or twigs up the nostrils, resulting in lacerations or foreign bodies in the nasal cavity.
   b. **Ethmoid carcinomas.** Signs include bulging facial bones, epistaxis, and dyspnea. The tumors are usually unilateral but can be bilateral, blocking both nasal passages. In these cases, open-mouthed breathing is often necessary. These tumors occur most often in older cattle, age 6–9 years.

C. Rhinitis and nasal obstruction in sheep and goats

1. **Patient profile and etiology.** Rhinitis and nasal obstruction in sheep and goats have primarily parasitic causes (e.g., *Oestrus ovis*) but can be sporadically caused by nasal tumors (e.g., adenopapillomas, adenocarcinomas) and viral infections or allergies, as in the other species. *Oestrus ovis* is the most common cause of nasal obstruction in sheep, but occasionally goats may also be affected.

2. **Clinical findings** include catarrhal to mucopurulent nasal discharge, sneezing, and difficult, snoring respiration.

3. Specific conditions
   a. *Oestrus ovis*
      (1) Etiology and pathogenesis
         (a) The fertilized females deposit larvae at the external nares during the summer and fall months. After hatching, young larvae crawl up the nasal cavity to the dorsal turbinates and frontal sinuses where they remain for several weeks to months before migrating to the nostrils and being sneezed out to pupate on the ground.
         (b) Irritation and secondary bacterial infection result in a purulent or mucoid nasal discharge, sneezing, low head carriage, and inspiratory dyspnea. Larvae can cause death in rare cases through secondary infections or encephalitis.
         (c) The presence of the adult fly attempting to larviposit on the nostrils can severely disrupt grazing; thus, the main effect of this parasite is production loss.
      (2) Diagnostic plan. A definitive diagnosis can be made if the larvae are seen in the nasal cavity; however, a careful search for foreign bodies in the nasal cavity should be made.
      (3) Therapeutic plan and prevention. Effective antibiotics include ivermectin (200 μg/kg) orally or rafoxanide 7.5 mg/kg (where available). Treatment should be administered in late summer to prevent buildup of heavy infestations. Winter treatment removes overwintering larvae.
   b. Miscellaneous causes
      (1) Allergic rhinitis
      (2) Bluetongue
      (3) Contagious ecthyma (see also Chapter 1 I I 9) usually is confined to the mouth and external nares but may spread to the muzzle and nostrils and, in rare cases, to the upper and lower respiratory tract, resulting in bronchopneumonia.
      (4) Nasal adenopapillomas are not uncommon in mature animals.
         (a) Enzootic nasal adenocarcinomas occur in sheep in the United States and Canada where the incidence in individual flocks suggests an infectious cause. A similar-appearing tumor is enzootic in goats in Europe, where extracellular retroviral-like particles have been observed. A similar tumor is only rarely reported in goats in North America.
         (b) Clinical findings include nasal stridor and dyspnea, with progressive anorexia. The tumor is only locally invasive and not metastatic. However, because of the location, death from asphyxiation or inanition usually occurs within 90 days from the onset of clinical signs.

D. Rhinitis in swine

1. Atrophic rhinitis
   a. Patient profile and history. This disease affects mostly young pigs but the residual anatomical defects persist for the life of the pig. The condition starts as an episode of acute rhinitis, followed by chronic atrophy of the turbinate bones.
   b. Clinical findings. This disease is characterized by shortening or distention of the snout, sneezing, nasal discharge, and epistaxis in growing pigs. Severe cases may exhibit impaired growth rates.
   c. Etiology and pathogenesis. There is substantial evidence to implicate *Bordetella bronchiseptica* as the inciting agent of the acute inflammation, followed by invasion of toxigenic strains of *Pasteurella multocida*. Up to 50% of finished pigs may have evidence of atrophic rhinitis. The true economic significance of atrophic rhinitis remains undetermined, as field studies have failed to show strong evidence of adverse effect on daily weight gains in growing pigs.
   d. Prevention has been attempted with early administration of antibiotics (e.g., tylosin, oxytetracycline, trimethoprim-sulfadoxine) in the early creep feed. Control has been aimed either at total eradication by depopulation or reduction of infection through mass medication or vaccination of pregnant gilts with *B. bronchiseptica* followed by *P. multocida* bacterins.

2. **Inclusion body rhinitis.** This common disorder is caused by a *β*-herpes virus but is fortunately a minor disease in young pigs. Occurrence is probably worldwide, clinically affecting piglets up to 10 weeks in age. Sneezing is the most prominent sign, often occurring in paroxysms following play fighting. There may be a mild serous nasal discharge, occasionally blood tinged, with all the piglets in the group affected. The clinical course is usually 2–4 weeks with no mortality. This virus is not implicated in the genesis of atrophic rhinitis.

3. **Swine influenza**
   a. **Patient profile and history.** This highly contagious disease is characterized by fever and watery ocular and nasal discharge in a high proportion of the herd.
   b. **Clinical findings and etiology.** The disease is caused by the type A influenza virus, possibly from an adaptation of the human influenza virus. Pigs also develop anorexia, prostration, and labored jerky breathing (thumps), accompanied by sneezing and a deep painful cough, often in paroxysms. Often, after 4–6 days, the signs rapidly abate.
   c. **Therapeutic plan and prevention.** There is no specific treatment, and although vaccines have been produced, the antigenic diversity of the virus may limit effective immunity.

4. **Necrotic rhinitis.** Otherwise known as **bullnose,** this disease is characterized by facial deformities and is often confused with atrophic rhinitis.
   a. **Patient profile and history.** This condition is most commonly seen in growing pigs that are raised in poor environments with heavy organic debris contamination.
   b. **Clinical findings.** Initially, there is cellulitis of the soft tissues of the nose and face with localized swelling that may interfere with respiration and mastication.
   c. **Etiology and pathogenesis.** *Fusobacterium necrophorum* is commonly isolated from the affected sites. If untreated, the inflammation spreads to the nasal bones and can cause facial deformity, toxemia, reduced appetite, and death.
   d. **Differential diagnosis.** The main differentiating feature of bullnose in comparison to atrophic rhinitis is the presence of soft tissue cellulitis, which is usually completely lacking in atrophic rhinitis.
   e. **Therapeutic plan and prevention.** Antibacterials, such as sulfonamides, are effective when treating young infected pigs and early stages of the disease. However, the aim should be the reduction of incidence, which is best managed by improved sanitation and disinfection of pens and elimination of any material that may cause mouth or head injuries (sharp edges on feeding troughs or waterers).

5. **Pseudorabies.** Some outbreaks of pseudorabies (**Aujeszky's disease)** may show signs of rhinitis.

II. ACUTE PHARYNGITIS, LARYNGITIS, AND TRACHEITIS

A. Pharyngitis, laryngitis, and tracheitis in horses

1. **Etiology**
   a. **Infectious agents** are the most common clinical causes of important diseases with predominately upper respiratory signs.
   b. **Noninfectious causes** are more sporadic and include irritation, pharyngeal abscess, foreign body, or retropharyngeal lymph node rupture.

2. **Clinical significance**
   a. **Decreased exercise tolerance.** It is often necessary to halt racing and showing activity in horses with upper respiratory tract infection.
   b. **Secondary infection.** These disorders predispose the horse to secondary bacterial infections of the lower respiratory tract. Only rarely do these viruses cause lower respiratory disease, with the exception of immunocompromised animals (see II A

3 e). Although viral respiratory disease commonly causes only transient mild pyrexia in most animals, it can be fatal in young animals.

3. **Specific conditions**
   a. **Equine influenza virus infection** is one of the most common causes of viral respiratory disease in horses older than 2 years.
      (1) **Patient profile and history**
         (a) Affected horses are primarily the young stock (age 2–3 years), but all ages are susceptible. Older horses usually have a milder infection or may show few signs other than a transient fever.
         (b) The disorder usually occurs as an **explosive outbreak** of respiratory disease in stables, but where immunity is strong, either from past exposure or vaccination, signs may be limited to several horses in a stable showing only fever or mild hindlimb edema. Less commonly there can be associated complications of myositis and myocarditis.
      (2) **Epidemiology**
         (a) A **hallmark** of this infection is its extremely **rapid spread** though a population of susceptible horses. In contrast to the shorter surviving human and swine types of virus, the equine type virus survives for up to 36 hours on fomites. This, combined with a short incubation period and a 3- to 8-day period of infectivity of affected horses, produces a rapid new infection rate.
         (b) Outbreaks often occur in spring and fall. **Risk factors** include:
            (i) A mixing of young horses, such as in the show or racing season
            (ii) An increased number of unvaccinated animals
            (iii) Stress caused by moving and crowding
         (c) The reservoir for this virus is unknown, but there may be inapparent carriers or vaccinated, asymptomatic carriers. Equine influenza is common in most countries, with the exception of Australia and New Zealand, where it has yet to be recorded.
      (3) **Etiology and pathogenesis**
         (a) The causative virus is a **myxovirus,** which is an RNA virus with two serologically distinct antigenic types (influenza A/equi 1 and A/equi 2). There seems to be no cross-species infection, and, as in most influenza viruses, the viruses are subject to antigenic drift. Thus, the commercially available vaccines, although affording protection, are seldom 100% effective.
         (b) Infection is initiated by **inhalation** or **contact** with nasal secretions from an infected animal. The virus can persist in an infected horse's secretions for up to 8 days, and the most common source of infection is coughed secretions.
         (c) After an **incubation period** of 1–5 days, the infection results in clinical signs, which reflect the epithelial inflammation of the respiratory tract. When the virus invades the respiratory epithelium, changes include hyperemia, edema, and cellular desquamation. Superficial erosions to the upper and lower respiratory tracts can occur with a loss of normal mucociliary clearance mechanisms, which provide at least transient potential for secondary bacterial invasion.
         (d) **Postinfection complications**
            (i) When the virus has cleared, the **respiratory epithelium** can take up to 3 weeks to fully recover to its normal state. This may be one reason that some horses continue to exhibit coughing for several weeks after apparent resolution of the infection.
            (ii) Associated but less common complications include myocarditis with arrhythmias (atrial fibrillation), secondary bacterial pneumonia, pleuritis, persistent cough, and exacerbation of underlying chronic obstructive pulmonary disease.
      (4) **Clinical findings**
         (a) The disease causes a **fever** (38.5°C–41°C) and a **dry hacking cough,**

which later turns moist and persists longer than the fever. **Nasal discharge** is watery when present but is seldom prominent.

    (b) Adenopathy. Although the **submaxillary lymph nodes** are not appreciably swollen, they are often painful to palpation in the early stages, which indicates the pharyngeal inflammation that occurs and may cause signs of dysphagia.

    (c) Other signs include dyspnea with or without exercise, systemic signs associated with infection (e.g., fever, inappetence, lassitude), or muscular stiffness and limb edema. In uncomplicated cases, the signs usually resolve completely within 3 weeks.

(5) Diagnostic plan and laboratory tests

    (a) On the routine **complete blood cell count (CBC),** there can be a leukopenia with distinct lymphopenia, but this is transient. For a definitive diagnosis, virus isolation is necessary.

    (b) Nasopharyngeal swabs must be collected in the first 48–72 hours of illness, beyond which viral culture is unlikely to be successful.

    (c) Serologic confirmation of infection relies on a rise in antibody titer in paired sera collected 3 weeks apart, with a positive finding based on a fourfold rise in hemagglutination inhibitor or serum neutralization titer.

    (d) For rapid diagnosis, a test based on direct **immunofluorescence** applied to nasopharyngeal smears also has been successful in investigating outbreaks.

(6) Differential diagnoses

    (a) Viral infections. This includes mainly the other upper respiratory viral infections (herpesvirus, rhinovirus, or adenovirus). Although equine viral arteritis (EVA) also can cause respiratory signs, these signs are often of secondary importance. Other signs, such as conjunctivitis, petechiation of mucous membranes, and limb and palpebral edema, are more prominent.

    (b) Bacterial infection by *Streptococcus equi* also can cause similar initial clinical signs, but generally the submandibular lymph nodes are obviously enlarged and painful.

(7) Therapeutic plan

    (a) As with most viral infections, there are few specific treatments available to hasten recovery. The main goal is to provide a **clean, stress-free environment** to allow the horse to recover from the infection.

    (b) For increasing the comfort of the horse, **nonsteroidal anti-inflammatory drugs (NSAIDs),** such as phenylbutazone, can be used to decrease fever and maintain the horse's appetite during the acute phase of the infection. However, disadvantages of this approach include:

        (i) The antipyretic action of NSAIDs might mask any fever due to secondary bacterial infection.

        (ii) Owners might return the horse to competition or work before the effects of the disease have fully abated.

    (c) Antibiotic treatment is appropriate if secondary bacterial infection is suspected or in high-risk animals, such as young foals. Ideally, the choice of drug should be based on culture results from transtracheal wash. In the absence of this, broad-spectrum antibacterials such as trimethoprim–sulfas can be administered, with a course when initiated of 5–7 days.

(8) Prevention

    (a) Vaccines. There are several manufacturers of killed-strain influenza vaccines, containing both A/equi 1 and A/equi 2. Manufacturers recommend two intramuscular injections several weeks apart initially, then revaccination annually.

    (b) Reaction to vaccination. Vaccinated horses should be rested for several days after vaccination because they are often reported to be "off" the day following injection. Horses develop a transient reaction to vaccination that may include mild fever, malaise, and pain at the injection site.

    (c) Frequency of vaccination. Vaccination results in at least partial immunity to disease, but not to infection. The duration of immunity from any of the vaccines is probably less than 1 year. Vaccination in the face of an **outbreak** may be beneficial if it can be done in advance of the spread of disease.

   (i) For **high-risk animals,** such as young horses in the show season, it is recommended to repeat vaccination every 3–4 months during the high-risk period.

   (ii) For **backyard horses** with no new additions, annual vaccination may not even be necessary for those horses older than 3 years.

   (iii) For **foals,** the usual recommendation is to begin vaccination between 2 months and 6 months. Some workers suggest that beginning vaccination at 30 days of age may decrease the incidence of foal pneumonia.

b. Equine viral rhinopneumonitis [equine herpesvirus (EHV) 4 and 1] infection

   (1) Patient profile and history. Rhinopneumonitis usually is most prominent in weanlings and yearlings that are experiencing periods of intermingling and stress. However, this disease can be seen in horses of all ages, with the presenting complaints being fever, conjunctivitis, and coughing.

   (2) Epidemiology

   (a) Carrier animals are often present in herds and serve to maintain the infection from year to year. The disease can be reactivated in periods of stress or by corticosteroid administration.

   (b) Rapid spread through a herd is associated with **high morbidity** and **low mortality rates;** the respiratory disease is generally mild. Outbreaks most commonly occur in fall and winter months, and 85% of respiratory outbreaks involving EHV in serologic surveys are attributed to EHV-4.

   (3) Etiology and pathogenesis

   (a) Etiology

   (i) The disease is caused by several differing strains of EHV, with **EHV-4** causing most of the outbreaks of respiratory disease in horses in any population at any time of the year.

   (ii) **EHV-1,** serologically related to EHV-4 by only 20% homology, has two subtypes. **Subtype 1** is associated with abortion. **Subtype 2,** while also abortogenic, can cause respiratory disease.

   (iii) **Neurologic disease** can also accompany EHV-1 infection, but the pathogenesis is poorly understood (see Chapter 11).

   (b) Pathogenesis

   (i) This highly infectious disease is **transmitted** by inhalation or contact with secretions (e.g., placenta, nasal secretions, aborted fetuses) containing infectious EHV particles. However, because the virus can survive from 15 to 45 days outside the animal in the environment, infections can occur in the apparent absence of an initiating case.

   (ii) The virus **rapidly proliferates** in the mucosa of the nasal, tonsillar, and pharyngeal regions, resulting in the rhinitis, pyrexia, and associated respiratory signs. Following this, there is a short-lived viraemia in which the virus is closely associated with circulating lymphocytes, from which the virus can be isolated. The virus is then transported to the tissues (e.g., lung, placenta, fetus, nervous tissues) and induces various subsequent organ damage.

   (iii) **Immunity.** The virus can be present in nasopharyngeal swabs for up to 10 days and can be shed spontaneously at times of stress in carrier animals. Immunity to these forms of herpesvirus is weak, and an animal can become clinically affected several times. Passive immunity in foals in the form of antibodies declines to zero by 180 days after birth. However, even the presence of virus-neutralizing antibodies are not necessarily an indication of resistance to infection, as cell-mediated immunity is a key feature of resistance to herpesvirus.

   (4) Clinical findings

   (a) The **respiratory signs** vary with the amount of exposure, animal age, and immunity. Signs are similar to those of influenza but are milder and more transient. As with influenza, younger animals most obviously are affected in an outbreak, whereas older animals may show few or no signs of respiratory disease.

    (b) The **most common findings** are pyrexia (39.5°C–40.5°C), conjunctivitis, serous nasal discharge, and a possible mild cough. The appetite of infected horses generally remains unaffected, and there may be slight enlargement of lymph nodes of the throat region.

    (c) The **clinical course** is usually 3–7 days, but some horses may cough for up to 3 weeks. Whereas some horses may undergo inapparent infection, very young foals can develop a primary interstitial pneumonia. Reinfection may occur within 4–5 months, but usually immunity from clinical infection lasts 6–12 months.

    (d) **Endoscopic examination** of the upper respiratory tract shows mild mucosal inflammations, consisting of rhinitis, pharyngitis, and lymphoid hyperplasia.

    (e) For respiratory disease caused by **EHV-1,** there may also be **abortions** up to 4 months later and possibly **neurologic disease** 8–11 days after respiratory infection on the same farm.

(5) Diagnostic plan. Respiratory disease accompanied by abortions, neurologic signs, or both is strong presumptive evidence of EHV-1 infection. However, where respiratory signs are the only abnormality, confirmation of infection can be either by acute and convalescent serology, or by virus isolation from nasal secretions, which is possible for up to 10 days.

(6) Laboratory tests. On the routine CBC, there is, as in most viral diseases, a nonspecific leukopenia and lymphopenia. Confirmation of the infection is best accomplished by collection of acute and convalescent titers, but virus isolation can be successful from nasal washing obtained in first few days of infection.

(7) Differential diagnoses. For problems that are solely showing signs of upper respiratory disease, the same considerations as for influenza are appropriate. These include equine **rhinovirus, adenovirus,** and **viral arteritis.** Bacterial infection by *Streptococcus equi* also can show similar initial clinical signs, but generally the mandibular lymph nodes are obviously enlarged and painful.

(8) Therapeutic plan. As for influenza and other upper respiratory infections, there is little specific treatment other than providing a clean, draft-free, low-stress environment and discontinuing work while the horse is allowed to recover.

(9) Prevention is with **vaccination.** Because the respiratory disease is sufficiently mild, a major goal of vaccination is the prevention of abortion. It is generally accepted that vaccination should be incorporated into routine health maintenance only when there is a known enzootic problem.

    (a) There are cell–culture-adapted **live viruses** that can be used safely for routine work in most breeding farms; however, the weakness is the brevity of immunity from this vaccine. Brood mares need to be vaccinated twice during the latter half of pregnancy, and its use in foals and yearlings requires, at the minimum, trimonthly boosters.

    (b) A **killed vaccine** is in wide use for protection against abortion due to EHV but should not be assumed to protect against respiratory signs.

    (c) To protect against the **respiratory form** of the disease, a modified live EHV-4 combined with a EHV-1 and influenza antigens is available. This vaccine is administered initially when a foal is 2–4 months of age, repeated in 4–8 weeks and then yearly until 2 years of age. Many clinicians recommend more frequent administration of these antigens in areas where the incidence of clinical disease is high.

c. Equine viral arteritis (EVA)

    (1) Patient profile and history. EVA, a disease seen in outbreaks on breeding farms, causes pregnant mares to abort. Serological evidence suggests a high prevalence of exposure (70%–90%) in Standardbreds, but Thoroughbreds have only a 2%–3% seropositive rate.

(2) **Etiology.** EVA is caused by an arterivirus similar to the agent that is implicated in porcine reproductive and respiratory syndrome. Virulence between strains varies, but there is little antigenic variation.

(3) **Clinical findings**

(a) This disease primarily causes **abortion,** with acute systemic illness including fever, limb edema, and respiratory signs. Abortion usually occurs within a few days of clinical onset of disease. This is in contrast to abortions caused by equine viral rhinopneumonitis, which occur much later after clinical disease.

(b) The **respiratory signs** are usually of secondary importance to the disease and include nasal and ocular discharge that is initially serous but can become purulent. There is a cough, nasal mucosal congestion, and in some horses, petechiation. In horses with pulmonary edema, dyspnea also may occur.

(4) **Pathogenesis.** Although outbreaks of the classic disease can occur, infections are commonly subclinical with sporadic abortions. Stallions can act as carriers, and there is an effective vaccine available for prevention where indicated.

(5) **Therapeutic plan and prevention**

(a) **Specific therapy** for this viral infection is not available, so treatment is only directed against secondary bacterial infection if respiratory signs are present.

(b) **Quarantine.** Because the virus is contagious, the quarantine of any infected horse returning from a racetrack, sale, or show may be necessary for up to 4 weeks.

(c) A currently available **modified-live virus vaccine** may be useful to control this disease on breeding farms.

d. **Equine rhinovirus (ERV) infection**

(1) **Etiology.** Infection with rhinovirus, equine rhinovirus-1 (ERV-1), is widespread, and most of the population of horses develop antibodies early in life. Infection with several types of rhinovirus (ERV-1, ERV-2, and ERV-3) is common, but only ERV-1 is clinically significant.

(2) **Clinical findings.** Although infection is often subclinical, horses with clinical signs exhibit low-grade fever, pharyngitis, pharyngeal lymphadenitis, and copious serous nasal discharge that becomes purulent in later stages. A cough may persist for 2–3 weeks.

(3) **Diagnostic plan.** Serum neutralization titers from acute and convalescent sera can establish a diagnosis. Alternatively, virus isolation may be attempted to allay concerns regarding more significant problems associated with influenza or rhinopneumonitis.

(4) **Therapeutic plan and prevention.** Because clinical disease is usually mild and self-limiting, there is little that needs to be done for treatment other than appropriate rest to allow recovery. Currently, there is no commercially available vaccine; however, planned exposure of young horses to infection has been recommended.

e. **Adenovirus infection**

(1) **Patient profile and history.** Adenovirus infection in the horse population appears to be widespread but is clinically of major importance in the **Arabian breed.**

(2) **Clinical findings.** Infection with adenovirus in adult horses generally does not cause any clinical disease. However, mild respiratory signs and transient softness of the feces may result in some cases. The exception to this usually mild infection is infection of immunocompromised foals, such as in failure of passive transfer or Arabian foals with inherited combined immunodeficiency (CID). Experimentally, this virus can cause a severe but nonfatal pneumonia, with the full scope of signs including conjunctivitis, coughing, nasal discharge, fever, dyspnea, and diarrhea. In Arab foals with CID, the pneumonia

is invariably fatal. There is hyperpnea, dyspnea, and adventitious sounds on auscultation of the lungs, suggestive of bronchopneumonia. Affected foals often have a poor hair coat, are depressed, and may have diarrhea.

    (3) **Etiology and pathogenesis.** Adenovirus infection is widespread in all ages of horses. Arabian CID foals develop fatal pneumonia and die, regardless of therapy. The virus attacks the upper and lower respiratory epithelium and leads to loss of epithelium with subsequent hyperplasia and interstitial pneumonia. Secondary bacterial bronchopneumonia also ensues, but these foals lack the ability to mount any defenses to recover from infection.

    (4) **Diagnostic plan.** For most horses, the infection is mild, and diagnosis can be made from a number of serologic tests or from identification of the characteristic intranuclear inclusion bodies in cells taken from conjunctiva or nasal mucosa.

    (5) **Laboratory tests and differential diagnoses**

        (a) In the case of an affected Arabian foal, it is important to exclude CID. Tests include the presence of lymphocytes above 1000 μl, and the presence of precolostral serum immunoglobulin M after 36 days of age.

        (b) Other viruses, including equine parainfluenza-3 (PI-3) virus and a reovirus, have also been recorded as viruses to be suspected in causing mild upper respiratory tract inflammation in horses but are of doubtful significance.

    (6) **Therapeutic plan and prevention**

        (a) For **adult horses,** there is no specific treatment other than as indicated for other mild upper respiratory infections.

        (b) **Foals** with failure of passive transfer are at increased risk of adenovirus infection because it is so prevalent in the horse population. These foals should receive plasma and, in high-risk situations, antibiotics.

        (c) Although an inactivated **vaccine** of apparent high immunogenicity has been produced against adenovirus in the horse, it has not had extensive field exposure.

  f. Noninfectious equine rhinotracheitis can be the result of pharyngeal abscess, foreign body, irritation from orally administered medication, or nasogastric intubation. These causes are far less common than infectious causes.

  g. Chronic pharyngitis. The most commonly managed chronic problem of the pharynx is **lymphoid hyperplasia (follicular pharyngitis),** as observed by endoscopy in performance horses. This abnormality does not appear to affect health but is suggested by some to affect athletic ability. This and other pharyngeal abnormalities, including structural or functional abnormalities of the soft palate or larynx, are in the realm of equine surgery.

B. **Acute pharyngitis, laryngitis, and tracheitis in cattle**

  1. Clinical findings. The common upper respiratory tract infections in cattle frequently have **nonspecific signs,** and an etiologic diagnosis based solely on clinical signs is not possible. The exception to this is infectious bovine rhinotracheitis (IBR), in which there can be characteristic nasal reddening, plaques, and conjunctivitis.

  2. Pathogenesis. Most of the incriminated bovine respiratory viruses are ubiquitous, and exposure and immunity are widespread. An important factor of these infections is the potential to **compromise normal pulmonary defense mechanisms** and allow colonization by bacteria that would normally be cleared. Therefore, although viral respiratory infections may not extend to the lower respiratory tract, secondary bacterial infection is the primary consideration in the management of both treatment and prevention.

  3. Diagnostic plan and laboratory tests. Specific etiologic diagnosis requires virus demonstration or isolation and identification and is seldom successful in later stages of the disease. To maximize the potential of an etiologic diagnosis, a routine **set of samples** should be obtained in outbreaks.

    a. From **live, acutely infected febrile untreated cattle,** nasal swabs or conjunctival scrapings are suitable for most viral isolation. Acute and convalescent serum samples also can be collected and screened for the suspected viruses, with a fourfold titer increase over 2–3 weeks proving active recent infection. For some viruses (e.g., bovine respiratory syncytial virus), immunofluorescence on lung lavage cells also has proven highly valuable.

   b. Necropsy of animals can be useful but is seldom rewarding in chronically ill, treated, or cull animals or those dead long enough to have undergone significant organ autolysis. In a field necropsy, tissues selected for virus isolation include conjunctiva, tonsil, pharynx, lung, lymph node, spleen, liver, kidney, small intestine, cecum, spiral colon, and rectum. These tissues require placement in appropriate viral transport medium, freezing, and transport by overnight courier to the laboratory.

4. Therapeutic plan

   a. Supportive care including ready access to feed and water and minimizing competition for feed and space is often all that is required.

   b. Antibiotic therapy for possible secondary bacterial infection can be instituted. Although glucocorticoids impair defense mechanisms and are contraindicated in IBR infections, NSAIDs (e.g., aspirin) may be beneficial in reducing fever and improving appetite. Therapy of individual animals is generally not as important as control of herd outbreaks.

5. Prevention. Vaccines are available for the more clinically important viruses and are often combined in a single product.

   a. Modified live virus of bovine cell origin for IBR vaccines should not be used in pregnant cows because these vaccines may cause vaccine virus shedding, infertility, and abortions. Potential stud bulls should be vaccinated with products containing the IBR antigen only at the owner's request.

   b. Products that are designed for **intranasal administration** of live vaccine stimulate strong local (immunoglobulin A) immunity and a rapid response, including local interferon.

   c. When considering the **young stock** in the herd, any early vaccination, such as is sometimes performed by administration of intranasal vaccines soon after birth, should be repeated after 6 months of age because the colostral immunity has waned by that time for most of these viruses.

   d. In **dairy herds,** annual or semiannual vaccination is recommended, as well as vaccinating any replacement animals 3–4 weeks before introduction.

   e. In **feedlot management,** because of high stress of transport and shipping, killed or at least inactivated vaccines may be appropriate, unless modified live viruses can be administered at least several weeks in advance of anticipated stress periods.

6. Specific conditions

   a. Infectious bovine rhinotracheitis (IBR), also known as bovine herpes virus-1 (BHV-1), is a highly infectious condition of worldwide distribution in cattle and some wild ruminants. Recent studies have revealed at least five major biotypes, which might explain the distinct clinical manifestations of this viral infection. The respiratory form is a common manifestation of infection in cattle and is usually restricted to upper respiratory signs, as uncomplicated IBR does not usually spread into the lungs.

   (1) Patient profile and history. BHV-1 can affect all ages of cattle, but those older than 6 months are most commonly affected, with animals in beef feedlots experiencing higher morbidity than dairy herds.

   (2) Epidemiology. The **morbidity** rate varies from 8% to 20%–30% in feedlots, but in herds of low immunity, morbidity can approach 100%. However, the case fatality rate is usually low at 1% or less. Where fatality rises to 10%, deaths are usually related to secondary bacterial bronchopneumonia (see Chapter 7).

   (3) Etiology and pathogenesis

   (a) Transmission. The α-herpes virus BHV-1 is transmitted via respiratory aerosol, semen, fetal fluids and tissues, and fomites.

   (b) After infection in the field, it appears there is an **incubation period** of 10–20 days, although experimentally this only lasts 3–7 days. The BHV-1 virus multiplies in nasal mucosa, causing rhinitis and tracheitis. Viral extension via the lacrimal duct causes conjunctivitis and, in some cases, corneal edema.

(c) **Route of infection.** From nasal mucosal infection, the virus travels up the trigeminal nerve, where it can establish latency or infect the central nervous system. The virus also can be transported by peripheral leukocytes to the placenta and transferred to the fetus, resulting in abortion.

(d) **Carriers**
  (i) The virus can persist and be discharged from the animal as a result of natural infection or live virus vaccination for at least 2 years.
  (ii) **Carrier states** are thought to occur in some cattle, and there also may be wildlife reservoirs of infection in wild ruminants.
  (iii) **Latent infections** occur with the virus presumably sequestered in the trigeminal ganglion, which can recrudesce during stress or corticosteroid administration.

(e) **Immunity** to BHV-1 is complex and requires both cell-mediated and humoral parts of the animal's defenses. Therefore, it follows that systemic antibody levels, as determined by the many serologic tests available, correlate poorly with protection against disease.

(4) **Clinical signs**
  (a) The **various clinical manifestations** of IBR include:
    (i) Upper respiratory inflammation with or without prominent conjunctivitis
    (ii) Venereal infections, such as infectious pustular vulvovaginitis (IPV) in cows and balanoposthitis in bulls
    (iii) Encephalitis
    (iv) Infertility
    (v) Abortion

  (b) With the **respiratory form** of IBR, there is a sudden onset of severe signs, including high fever (up to 42°C), anorexia, and severe hyperemia of the nasal mucosa.
    (i) **Necrotic plaques** appear as greyish foci of necrosis on the nasal mucosa just inside the nares, accompanied by a serous to mucopurulent nasal discharge.
    (ii) **Conjunctivitis** with a serous ocular discharge is also a common sign. Although this may sometimes be mistaken for infectious keratoconjunctivitis caused by *Moraxella bovis,* the lesions are confined to conjunctiva, which are reddened and swollen with no invasion and ulceration of the cornea.
    (iii) A **short, explosive cough** can accompany these signs but is not always present in outbreaks. If lactating dairy cattle are affected, there is also an accompanying dramatic fall in milk production.

  (c) **Duration of infection.** When restricted to respiratory signs, infection generally resolves in 10–14 days. Abortions can occur some weeks following clinical illness. The genital tract infections (IPV or balanoposthitis) can result in reproductive failure.

(5) **Diagnostic plan and differential diagnoses.** The classic signs of fever, nasal lesions, and bilateral conjunctivitis should suggest the respiratory form of IBR. Other possibilities include:
  (a) **Bovine respiratory disease complex (BRDC; shipping fever).** With BRDC, there is toxemia, abnormal lung sounds, and affected animals respond well to antibiotics.
  (b) **Bovine virus diarrhea/mucosal disease (BVD/MD).** With BVD/MD, there should be oral erosions and usually diarrhea in addition to nasal ulceration.
  (c) **Bovine malignant catarrh (BMC).** BMC exhibits similar signs to BVD/MD.
  (d) **Calf diphtheria.** This condition may resemble IBR with inspiratory dyspnea but usually has severe toxemia and necrotic oral and laryngeal lesions.
  (e) **Allergic rhinitis.** Although it resembles IBR, allergic rhinitis does not

result in fever and usually is accompanied by sneezing and a characteristic thick greenish orange nasal discharge.

   (6) **Therapeutic plan**

      (a) **Antibiotics.** Although of no direct effect against the viral infection, antibiotics such as oxytetracycline or sulfa drugs can be given to control against secondary bacterial tracheitis and bronchopneumonia. As most cattle recover uneventfully without antibiotics, this must be weighed against the cost of treatment and possible need for appropriate withdrawal periods of milk or meat.

      (b) **Management strategies.** As in other viral infections, it is important to aid recovery by **reducing stress** (e.g., crowding) and providing high-quality feed and access to water. In feedlot situations, this is best managed in a separate "sick pen" where competition for feed and space is reduced, and particular attention can be given to monitor for signs of onset of secondary bronchopneumonia.

      (c) **Glucocorticoids** are specifically contraindicated in this disease.

   (7) **Prevention**

      (a) There are several **effective vaccines** commercially available. Because the disease can occur unpredictably at any time and even in what seem to be closed herds, vaccination by either an intranasal aerosol of modified live vaccine or intramuscular modified live or inactivated vaccines is indicated.

         (i) The **intranasal vaccines** stimulate local as well as humoral immunity, and in addition to being safe for use in pregnant cows, can be used in the face of an outbreak because of stimulation of local interferon within 72 hours of administration. However, these vaccines are more labor intensive to administer and generally more expensive.

        (ii) **Intramuscular vaccines,** if not inactivated, can cause abortion and infertility. Thus, if used, they should be given to heifers and cows at least 2 weeks before breeding.

        (iii) Vaccination with **modified live products,** although stimulating a stronger immune response than that obtained from inactivated products, may result in shedding of the virus.

      (b) For those herds in which export of cattle or production of bulls for artificial insemination units is an economically important consideration, vaccination against BHV-1 is not advised because this may result in the rejection of animals for export or sale to bull studs.

  b. **Bovine adenovirus.** This virus often causes an inapparent infection, and although a potential cause of upper respiratory inflammation, it is relatively unimportant other than for its possible association with pneumonia, enteritis, or both in calves. Adenovirus may play a role in enzootic calf pneumonia (see Chapter 7). Adult cattle are the source for infection in calves. Latent infection with stress may result in recrudescence and viral shedding.

  c. **Bovine viral diarrhea (pestivirus, BVD).** Similar to adenovirus, BVD can result in mild, nonspecific clinical signs of respiratory infection. Although BVD virus is not a primary pathogen of the respiratory system, some affected animals do have oral lesions extending into the nasal cavity and signs suggestive of primary rhinitis. However, oral erosions and gastrointestinal signs such as diarrhea are usually striking and avoid confusion with uncomplicated rhinitis and upper respiratory tract infections. A main factor in the relationship of BVD virus to respiratory disease is the immunosuppressive effects of infection (see Chapter 7).

  d. **Parainfluenza-3 (PI-3)**

   (1) **Patient profile and history.** PI-3, a paramyxovirus, is a ubiquitous virus that can be recovered from normal and acutely ill cattle. The major importance of this infection is its potential link to pneumonia in calves (see Chapter 7) and bacterial bronchopneumonia in older cattle.

   (2) **Clinical findings.** Animals with uncomplicated infections have mild upper re-

spiratory disease with cough, serous nasal discharge, and fever. The clinical abnormalities are nonspecific for this infection.

(3) Pathogenesis

(a) The virus invades the respiratory tract and can infect pulmonary macrophages, which may permit viral replication and impair phagocytic function.

(b) PI-3 infection has been associated with concurrent viral infections (e.g., bovine respiratory syncytial virus) or *Pasteurella haemolytica* infection and serious pneumonia.

(4) Diagnostic plan. Acute and convalescent serology can establish the occurrence of recent infection, and the virus can be isolated from affected animals.

(5) Therapeutic plan and prevention

(a) As in the other mild upper respiratory infections, this is usually **self-limiting** and needs no treatment unless signs of pneumonia occur with secondary bacterial infection.

(b) There are a number of commercially available **vaccines** that contain this antigen. For calves, a modified live intranasal vaccine stimulates both nasal and humoral antibodies and appears effective against challenge exposure.

(c) The antigen is also commonly included in **multivalent vaccines** for prevention of undifferentiated bovine respiratory disease.

e. Bovine respiratory syncytial virus (BRSV)

(1) Patient profile and history

(a) Infection by BRSV can occur in any age of cattle, particularly in immunologically naive herds. Beef breeds may be more susceptible than dairy animals. There is generally rapid onset resulting from a short incubation period and rapid spread of the disease through the herd. Fall and winter are the most common times for disease.

(b) Although it causes upper respiratory signs (e.g., serous nasal discharge, cough), this viral infection is more important in its ability to invade the lung and cause viral pneumonia (see Chapter 7). A high percentage of North American cattle have serum antibodies to BRSV, indicative of widespread (greater than 80%) infection. Conversely, clinical disease is not nearly so common. The virus has a close antigenic relationship to sheep and goat RSV as well as human RSV.

(2) Clinical findings vary depending on the stage of the disease, primary or secondary.

(a) Primary stage. There is sudden onset of fever (40°C–42°C), nasal/lacrimal discharge, cough, hypersalivation, and decreased appetite. Tachypnea (more than 30 breaths/min) and abnormal lung sounds (i.e., increased bronchial tones, wheezes, fine crackles) also may be present, indicating viral invasion of the lungs. If infection occurs in lactating cows, there is a moderate but transient fall in milk production. A transient diarrhea also may occur. In this stage, clinical signs are usually mild and quickly resolve.

(b) Secondary stage. The term *secondary stage* arises from the clinical course of such animals often appearing after remission from an initial mild infection of BRSV and the suggestion that this manifestation may be a hypersensitivity reaction to the initial antigen, with involvement of immunoglobulin E (see Chapter 7).

(i) In the secondary stage, the disease produced is far more severe, with **profound dyspnea, anorexia,** and **open-mouth breathing** with froth at the muzzle. These animals are often unable to eat because of severe dyspnea. Some animals have subcutaneous emphysema over the trunk and submandibular edema.

(ii) Auscultation of the chest often reveals prominent crackles. These animals are clearly in respiratory failure.

(3) Pathogenesis. Despite considerable research efforts, the pathogenesis of BRSV infection remains poorly understood. Experimental infection has been difficult to achieve and, in most cases, results in only mild clinical disease with limited lesions.

(a) The virus infects respiratory tissues from the nasal cavity to the bronchi/bronchioles. Epithelial destruction follows and peaks at 5–7 days post infection but is usually mild and incomplete.

(b) The rapid **serologic response** (3 days) makes routine serologic testing sometimes nondiagnostic (titers already elevated at "acute" sample). There is usually a mild interstitial pneumonia with alveolitis, but this quickly resolves.

(c) The **secondary stage** of disease is **sporadic** in occurrence and may be caused by repeated infection, hypersensitivity, or possibly some alteration of host cell surface antigen in the lung. In these cases, there is a profound interstitial pneumonia with bronchiolitis and bullous emphysema likely caused by the intense respiratory effort.

(4) **Diagnostic plan and laboratory tests.** The clinical signs of this infection are seldom sufficiently specific to establish a diagnosis. Demonstration of the virus by culture of lung tissue is seldom possible in field cases. However, if the "acute" sample is taken very early in the course of the disease, blood samples may demonstrate seroconversion, and direct immunofluorescence on nasopharyngeal swabs or fresh lung tissue from a recently infected animal may provide a definitive diagnosis.

(5) **Therapeutic plan**

(a) The **primary stage** of infection usually warrants no treatment because it is mild, and animals quickly recover unassisted. Because of the potential for secondary bacterial invasion of the lung, prophylactic antibiotics may be indicated (see Chapter 7).

(b) Those cattle with the **secondary stage** may benefit from administration of antihistamines, corticosteroids, or both. It is extremely important in such cases to minimize respiratory stress and limit any need for exertion. Despite this, the case fatality rate in the secondary cases is high.

(6) **Prevention.** There are several BRSV vaccines available commercially, alone or in combinations with other respiratory viruses (modified live). These appear to be effective against experimental challenge and also in reducing the incidence of respiratory disease of nonspecific etiology in the field.

f. **Bovine malignant catarrh (BMC)** is an acute, highly fatal systemic disease of cattle characterized by nasal, ocular (keratoconjunctivitis), and gastrointestinal lesions. This disorder is included in consideration of the upper respiratory tract because it also causes a rhinitis that must be differentiated from other respiratory tract diseases.

(1) **Patient profile.** Any age, sex, or breed of cattle can be affected. Although individual animals usually are infected, BMC can also occur in outbreaks. The disease shows the greatest incidence in late winter, spring, and summer.

(2) **Clinical findings**

(a) There are **several clinical manifestation** of BMC, including the peracute, alimentary tract, and common "head and eye" forms. These forms appear to be gradations of the same disease.

(b) In the **head and eye form,** there is a sudden onset of fever (41°C–41.5°C), severe dyspnea with obstruction of the nasal cavities caused by exudate from the superficial erosions on the mucosa and mucopurulent nasal discharge. Also evident are ocular discharge, eyelid swelling, blepharospasm, and scleral congestion. These animals exhibit extreme dejection. Characteristic and distinguishing signs also include peripheral lymphadenopathy and severe oral erosions.

(3) **Etiology.** The clinical signs can be caused by two different infectious agents: the alcelaphine BMC virus (wildebeest-associated virus, AHV-1) or a sheep-associated BMC virus, probably similar to AHV-1.

(4) **Therapeutic plan.** The disease is almost invariably fatal and must be distinguished from the treatable and mild causes of upper respiratory infections of cattle, such as IBR, PI-3, and BRSV.

C. **Pharyngitis, laryngitis, and tracheitis in sheep, goats, and swine.** Although these conditions undoubtedly occur in sheep, goats, and swine, far less attention is given to these conditions in North American veterinary literature.

1. **Viral causes** of pharyngitis and tracheitis are similar to those in cattle (e.g., **respiratory syncytial virus** has been reported). A more common cause in the small goat herd or sheep flock is **traumatic pharyngitis,** caused by drenching or balling gun injuries as a result of owner-administered medications.

2. Pharyngitis in **swine** is reported in some outbreaks of **pseudorabies (Aujeszky's disease)** and is part of the manifestation of **anthrax** in this species.

III. LARYNGEAL OBSTRUCTION

A. **Equine strangles.** Strangles, also called horse distemper, occurs worldwide and historically caused major epidemics in cavalry horses. This remains an important disease of horses in developed countries because of the resulting disruption in management in brood mare or racing farms, time and expense of treatment, and unpleasant aesthetics of draining abscesses and purulent nasal discharges.

1. **Patient profile.** The disease affects horses less than age 5 or 6 years, although all ages can be susceptible. Foals less than 3 months are most often unaffected, probably because of colostral protection.

2. **Clinical signs**
   a. After an **incubation period** of 1–3 weeks, affected horses suddenly develop depression, complete anorexia, fever (39.5°C–40.5°C), and serous nasal discharge.
   b. The **nasal discharge** rapidly becomes copious and purulent, and horses show signs of severe pharyngitis and laryngitis, with reluctance to swallow and a soft, moist cough that appears painful. Possibly as a result of this pain, affected horses often stand with their head and neck extended and may appear dyspneic.
   c. For 3 or 4 days, the **lymph nodes** of the throat region enlarge and are hot, painful, and initially firm in consistency. The lymph node enlargement may be sufficiently severe to cause obstruction to swallowing, dyspnea, and, in severe cases, death by asphyxia. Within 10 days, the swollen lymph nodes begin to weep serum and develop a soft spot from which they rupture (usually externally) and drain thick yellow material. Occasionally, these nodes rupture and drain internally into the pharynx. Often, the horse shows an improved attitude when the lymph nodes rupture and drain.
   d. **Complications**
      (1) Most animals recover within 3–6 weeks, but there can be a number of secondary complications. These include **pneumonia** secondary to aspiration with internal rupture or extension into the guttural pouches, causing guttural pouch empyema.
      (2) **Very young foals** can develop **bacteremia** or **septicemia** with joint infections and generalized lymphadenopathy.
      (3) The most common complication is metastatic strangles, or **"bastard strangles,"** in which abscesses can spread to internal organ systems (i.e., lung, mesentery, spleen, brain) and cause subsequent localizing signs. Localized abscesses on the limbs can induce limb edema with the lower limb swelling three or four times its size. Finally, a delayed reaction due to immunologic sensitivity to the streptococcal protein can result in vasculitis, causing **purpura hemorrhagica.**

3. **Epidemiology**
   a. **Outbreaks** in susceptible animals often occur in cold wet weather, although movement and exposure to infected horses are also factors.
   b. The causative organism is **highly resistant** in the environment, lasting up to a

month outside the host. Thus, contaminated water or feed buckets, or even objects such as blankets, brushes, and tack can be the source of infection.

   c. The organism is known to persist in the pharynx of clinically normal, recovered horses for up to 8 months, and field experience suggests that such horses can be a source for new infections during this time.

4. Etiology and pathogenesis

   a. Strangles is caused by a β-hemolytic streptococcus, ***Streptococcus equi,*** which is present in the nasal discharges and draining abscesses of affected horses. This organism is not considered part of the normal nasal flora of the horse.

   b. The bacteria usually is **transmitted** by inhalation but can also be ingested. After **incubating** for 1–3 weeks, the organism causes acute pharyngitis and rhinitis. *S. equi* has M protein in its capsule, which is antiphagocytic and provides a means of avoiding normal defenses.

   c. From the mucosal surfaces, the organism moves by **lymph drainage** to local lymph nodes (submandibular and retropharyngeal) with subsequent abscessation at these sites.

   d. **Strong immunity** occurs immediately after infection and lasts 6 months to several years.

5. Diagnostic plan and laboratory tests

   a. In addition to clinical signs, **cultures** of nasal swabs or lymph node draining is key to diagnosis. Although other streptococcal species, such as *S. zooepidemicus,* also are readily found in nasal swabs and can give mild upper respiratory signs along with occasional lymph node abscessation, identification of *S. equi* is important because it requires rigorous control and quarantine measures.

   b. **Routine hematology** reveals neutrophilic leucocytosis, hyperfibrinogenemia, and anemia of chronic infection, but this is not specific to strangles.

6. Therapeutic plan

   a. Horses with **early clinical signs** (e.g., fever, anorexia, depression, pharyngitis, purulent nasal discharge)

      (1) **Procaine penicillin G** is the drug of choice administered at 22,000 IU/kg twice daily intramuscularly for 5 days or until all clinical signs are absent.

      (2) **Tetracyclines** are also effective but should be avoided because of the risk of inducing colitis.

      (3) **Trimethoprim-sulfadiazine** is an alternative to penicillin treatment, with its advantage being oral administration.

   b. Horses with **lymph node abscessation** require local treatment to enhance maturation and drainage of the abscesses.

      (1) **Hot packs** and poultices can be applied to the area of swellings several times daily. When the abscesses are mature, with the softening of a point of overlying skin, they can be lanced and flushed with 3%–5% povidone iodine.

      (2) **Parenteral antibiotics** given after abscess formation tend to prolong rather than arrest disease. However, some veterinarians suggest treating all affected horses to reduce the risk of more animals becoming ill.

   c. Horses recently **exposed to strangles** with yet no clinical signs may benefit from **antimicrobial therapy** (e.g., benzathine penicillin) at the time of exposure and every 2 days thereafter until the end of the outbreak. This may prevent seeding of lymph nodes with the organism.

   d. **Treatment for secondary complications**

      (1) For **bastard strangles,** long-term penicillin treatment (3–6 months) is required. Oral phenoxymethyl penicillin (110,000 IU/kg every 8 hours) is possible but very expensive. Thus, trimethoprim-sulfadiazine is usually the drug of choice.

      (2) **Purpura hemorrhagica,** being an immunologic disease, requires glucocorticoids (dexamethasone) and supportive treatment such as leg wraps for the limb edema (see Chapter 9).

      (3) **Guttural pouch empyema** is treated locally by flushing the affected pouches with saline through the pharyngeal opening, often with the use of indwelling catheters for repeated treatment.

7. **Prevention**
   a. **Management strategies**
      (1) From the onset of clinical signs, it is critical to **isolate** affected animals because this highly contagious infection can spread through many of the young stock. Isolation for at least 6 weeks after start of signs is suggested, but based on field experiences, some veterinarians strongly suggest 8 months is a safer time frame. Clearly this latter recommendation must have the full cooperation and understanding by the client.
      (2) Because of the highly resistant nature of the organism, it is also imperative to **thoroughly clean** and **disinfect** stalls and grooming and feeding equipment, and burn the bedding from infected animals.
   b. **Vaccination** against this organism provides only partial protection, with reduced severity and incidence of disease if and when it occurs.
      (1) Several commercial products are available and require a minimum of three doses at 2- to 4-week intervals, followed by annual boosters. Some products also induce muscle soreness and possible abscess formation, and for this reason vaccination should be administered in the pectoral muscles.
      (2) A vaccine containing a concentrated, purified M-protein extract of *S. equi* has been shown to reduce the rate of clinical disease by 50%.

B. **Laryngeal obstruction in cattle**

1. **Patient profile and history**
   a. **Adult cattle**
      (1) Adult cattle develop **acute** laryngeal obstruction most commonly as a result of laryngeal necrosis secondary to balling gun and drenching injuries. Laryngeal edema secondary to smoke inhalation also can result in signs of laryngeal obstruction.
      (2) **Chronic** laryngeal obstruction in adults is most often caused by retropharyngeal swelling, either from lymphadenitis or abscess, or a tumor in the throat latch region.
   b. **Calves,** particularly those between 3 and 18 months, most commonly develop laryngeal obstruction as a result of the **calf diphtheria** (oral laryngeal necrobacillosis).

2. **Clinical signs**
   a. Laryngeal obstruction causes characteristic **inspiratory dyspnea** and **stertor.** There is also apparent **excessive salivation** caused by the reduced willingness for the animal to swallow as a result of the dysphagia induced by laryngeal inflammation.
   b. There is **anorexia, depression,** and **fever** in calves with diphtheria and adult cattle with balling gun injuries that develop extensive cellulitis. In calves with diphtheria, there is invariably a characteristic foul necrotic odor to the breath.

3. **Etiology and pathogenesis**
   a. Inflammation of the larynx and pharynx depends on the inciting cause. For example, smoke inhalation may be a combination of chemical and thermal burn and, thus, be diffuse yet affect only the superficial mucosa.
   b. **Balling gun injuries** often extend into the interstitial tissues around the pharynx and have extensive cellulitis from contaminating oropharyngeal inhabitants.
   c. In **calf diphtheria,** the initial mucosal trauma from coarse feeds or shedding teeth allows invasion beyond mucosal tissues of *Fusobacterium necrophorum,* which is responsible for both the extremely foul odor to the calf's breath and severe toxemia.

4. **Diagnostic plan.** The clinical signs and history often are sufficient to provide a working diagnosis.
   a. **Oral examination** with a speculum or an endoscope via the nares provides ready assessment of most of the structures of the pharynx and larynx.
   b. For **balling gun injuries,** radiology of the pharyngeal region also can be valuable with the demonstration of gas or foreign matter in areas swollen with cellulitis.

5. Therapeutic plan

    a. Most conditions benefit from **parenteral antibiotics,** such as sodium sulfadimidine 150 mg/kg for 2–3 days or procaine penicillin 20,000 IU/kg intramuscularly twice daily for 5 days.

    b. In severely **dyspneic animals,** a **tracheostomy** should be performed as asphyxiation may occur before laryngeal swelling subsides.

    c. Those animals that are unable to swallow require **parenteral fluid therapy.**

    d. In cases of **balling gun injury** that are recognized at the time of occurrence and presumed to have caused extensive trauma, **emergency slaughter** should be considered as an economic alternative to treatment.

C. **Laryngeal obstruction in sheep, goats, and swine**

1. Patient profile and history. Similar sporadic causes of laryngeal obstruction as found in cattle also can occur in small ruminants. In sheep, there also have been outbreaks of laryngeal obstruction reported resulting from necrotic laryngitis, with *Fusobacterium necrophorum* isolated from lesions.

2. Clinical signs include laryngeal stenosis, causing the characteristic inspiratory dyspnea. Also, regional lymphadenopathy and lung abscessation are seen.

3. Therapeutic plan. Treatment is similar to that described for cattle. Laryngeal obstruction in swine is most commonly seen as a result of encroachment of regional subcutaneous abscesses or abscessed lymph nodes.

STUDY QUESTIONS

DIRECTIONS: Each of the numbered items or incomplete statements in this section is followed by answers or by completions of the statement. Select the ONE numbered answer or completion that is BEST in each case.

1. Which one of the following statements regarding viral respiratory disease in horses is true?

(1) Although equine viral arteritis (EVA) is associated with conjunctivitis, limb edema, and respiratory signs, subclinical infections are most common, with aborting mares acting as the main carriers of the virus.

(2) Equine rhinopneumonitis virus infection caused by equine herpesvirus-4 (EHV-4) results in fever, conjunctivitis, and cough, whereas equine herpesvirus-1 (EHV-1) is associated with late-gestation abortion and neurologic disease in addition to fever, conjunctivitis, and cough.

(3) In addition to fever and the acute outbreak of cough, equine influenza virus can cause limb edema, myositis, and conjunctivitis in affected horses.

(4) Painful submandibular lymph nodes are a characteristic of rhinopneumonia.

(5) In horses, clinical signs of viral infection are seldom pathognomonic, and finding evidence of seroconversion is the only method of identifying many viruses.

2. A growing pig shows acute nasal discharge and rhinitis, followed by shortening of the snout and turbinate atrophy. Which one of the following statements is true?

(1) Inclusion body rhinitis is a major factor in the turbinate atrophy noted.

(2) The changes to the snout are typical of necrotic rhinitis (bullnose).

(3) *Bordetella bronchiseptica* infection followed by *Pasteurella multocida* infection is the most likely cause of these clinical signs.

(4) Infection by type A swine influenza virus damaged the nares and was followed by *Fusobacterium necrophorum* infection of the turbinates.

3. Equine herpesvirus-4 (EHV-4) is recovered from a group of horses on a brood mare farm following an outbreak of upper respiratory disease. Which one of the following statements is correct?

(1) Vaccination against equine herpesvirus-1 (EHV-1) provides temporary but strong cross protection against EHV-4 infection.

(2) Most respiratory outbreaks in horses caused by herpesviruses are caused by EHV-4.

(3) Complications of EHV-4 infection include abortion and hind-end paresis.

(4) Differentiating EHV-4 infection from EHV-1 infection can be done using currently available serologic tests for specific antibodies.

4. A 3-week-old Arabian foal that has been receiving treatment for pneumonia dies and adenovirus is recovered from the lungs as the only pathogen. Which one of the following statements is true?

(1) Serum obtained from this foal immediately prior to death can be used to confirm an immunodeficiency in this foal.

(2) The presence of presuckle immunoglobulin M (IgM) against adenovirus confirms that this infection was present at birth.

(3) Adenovirus is unlikely to cause significant disease in non-Arabian foals.

(4) The other foals on the farm of similar ages should be vaccinated against adenovirus.

(5) Because secondary bacterial involvement was not found, a fungal pathogen should be suspected instead of a primary viral agent.

5. Inspiratory dyspnea and stertor are observed in an 8-month-old Hereford calf. The rectal temperature is 39.9°C, and the calf is depressed. Furthermore, a foul, necrotic breath odor is detected, and the calf appears reluctant to eat. What is the most likely diagnosis?

(1) Calf diphtheria caused by *Fusobacterium necrophorum*
(2) Balling gun injury sustained 24 hours ago
(3) Enzootic pneumonia complicated by lung abscessation
(4) A tooth root abscess with invasion by anaerobic bacteria
(5) Papular stomatitis or bovine virus diarrhea (BVD)

6. Absence of passage of air in one nostril is a specific finding that may suggest which one of the following?

(1) Ethmoid hematoma, in a horse with concomitant blood-tinged and malodorous nasal discharge
(2) *Oestrus ovis* infection, in a sheep with concomitant bloody nasal discharge from the affected nares
(3) Inclusion body rhinitis, in a pig with concomitant serous bilateral nasal discharge and sneezing
(4) Ethmoid carcinoma, in a cow with concomitant bilateral bloody discharge and bulging of the facial bones
(5) Granulomatous pedunculated masses caused by *Rhinosporidia* , in a horse with minimal to no concomitant nasal discharge

7. An owner reports the sudden onset of a harsh cough and bilateral ocular discharge in an 18-month-old steer. Other similarly aged animals in the herd are also similarly affected. Clinical examination reveals a rectal temperature of 40°C, a serous nasal discharge, swollen conjunctiva, and small necrotic plaques in the nares. What advice should be offered to the owner?

(1) The affected animals need to be isolated from the breeding herd because they may be a source of an infection that can cause cerebellar hypoplasia or immunotolerance in calves.
(2) To halt the spread of infection, an intranasal vaccine can be administered.
(3) Signs are typical for *Pasteurella* pneumonia; affected calves need to be placed on antibiotics.
(4) This is likely an upper respiratory virus but additional tests will be needed to identify it.
(5) Treatment should include broad-spectrum antibiotics because lung infection is likely to occur.

8. A yearling Standardbred filly is receiving treatment in a clinic for clinical signs of strangles. *Streptococcus equi* is cultured from the nasal cavity. The owner wants to know if she will be able to successfully bring the filly back to the riding establishment she operates. Of the following comments, which one is correct?

(1) A vaccine containing the antiphagocytic *S. equi* capsular antigen can be administered to the other horses to prevent them from developing the disease. Immunity is highly effective but short lived.
(2) This filly can spread the organism to the other horses for at least 6 weeks after her clinical signs resolve.
(3) Although isolation of this filly is important during the clinical stage, other horses at the riding school are likely to carry the organism as part of their normal flora, which can undergo rapid proliferation at times of high stress.
(4) This filly will have strong immunity as a result of clinical disease and thus is unlikely to develop the disease hereafter.

1. The answer is 2 [II A 3 b (3) (e)]. Equine viral rhinopneumonitis caused by equine herpesvirus-4 (EHV-4) and equine herpesvirus-1 (EHV-1) is associated with fever, conjunctivitis, and cough. In addition, EHV-1 infection may cause late-gestation abortion and neurologic disease. Stallions, rather than aborting mares, are the presumed carriers of the virus that causes equine viral arteritis (EVA). Although equine influenza may be associated with limb edema and myositis, conjunctivitis is not a recognized sign. Equine rhinopneumonia, a viral process, should not induce enlarged and painful lymph nodes; this sign is more consistent with *Streptococcus equi* infection. Some viruses can be cultured in the early stages; therefore, serology is not the only means of identifying some viruses.

2. The answer is 3 [I D 1 b]. Atrophic rhinitis often occurs after infection of *Bordetella bronchiseptica*, which causes acute inflammation. *B. bronchiseptica* infection is then followed by *Pasteurella multocida* infection. Inclusion body rhinitis can cause acute nasal discharge but is not thought to be a component of atrophic rhinitis. Necrotic rhinitis is a cellulitis in the soft tissues around the snout and is thought to be caused by *Fusobacterium necrophorum* infection.

3. The answer is 2 [II A 3 b (2) (b)]. More than 80% of respiratory outbreaks involving equine herpesvirus are associated with equine herpesvirus-4 (EHV-4). EHV-4 cannot be differentiated from EHV-1 using commonly available serologic methods. Equine herpesvirus-1 (EHV-1) has only 20% homology with EHV-4; therefore, vaccination against EHV-1 does not provide much protection against EHV-4. Abortion and hind-end paresis are complications associated with EHV-1 infection.

4. The answer is 3 [II A 3 e]. Adenovirus only causes severe disease in foals with combined immunodeficiency, such as that observed in some Arabian foals that lack the ability to produce their own immunoglobulins and are severely lymphopenic. The foal has no ability to produce its own immunoglobulin M (IgM); therefore, sera from the foal at this age will likely contain immunoglobulins present from the dam's colostrum. The other foals on the farm are unlikely to be at risk for such a severe, overwhelming infection because they probably are not immunodeficient. Adenovirus in this case can be the sole pathogen for pneumonia.

5. The answer is 1 [II B 6 a (5) (d)]. The inspiratory dyspnea, fever, and necrotic breath odor are characteristic signs of calf diphtheria. A balling gun injury sustained 24 hours previously would not be likely to produce an extremely necrotic breath odor so quickly. The breath odor of lung abscesses is consistent with that described here, but calves with enzootic pneumonia will not have dyspnea on inspiration. Dental problems would not be characterized by dyspnea. Papules and ulcers, not necrosis, are more likely to be associated with papular stomatitis or bovine viral diarrhea (BVD).

6. The answer is 4 [I B 2 b]. Clinical findings of ethmoid carcinomas in cattle include bulging facial bones and the discharge of blood from the nostrils. The bloody discharge should not have a notable odor. The discharge is not usually blood-tinged; it is blood. Clinical signs are usually minimal.

7. The answer is 2 [II B 6 a (7) (a) (i)]. The signs are typical of infectious bovine rhinotracheitis (IBR). An intranasal vaccine is available that can be used in the face of an outbreak because it stimulates the production of local interferon within 72 hours. The presence of the conjunctivitis and nasal plaques should allow the clinician to rule out bovine virus diarrhea and mucosal disease. An animal with *Pasteurella* pneumonia would not have the conjunctivitis and would be significantly depressed. In uncomplicated viral infections such as this one, antibiotics are not indicated.

8. The answer is 2 [III A]. Shedding of the organism that causes equine strangles (horse distemper), *Streptococcus equi*, can persist for 6 weeks or longer after the clinical signs of infection resolve; therefore, the filly is at risk of spreading the disease to other horses at the horse establishment. A vaccine is available, but the immunity is not strong and offers only partial protection. *S. equi* is not part of the normal flora in horses. Immunity does occur with infection but is not permanent.

Chapter 7

Diseases of the Lower Respiratory Tract and Thorax

John Pringle

I. DISEASES OF THE LOWER RESPIRATORY TRACT

A. Pneumonia in young animals

1. **Pneumonia in neonates.** Clinical signs of pneumonia in all species generally include fever, tachypnea or dyspnea, anorexia, and, particularly with bacterial involvement, depression. Accompanying these signs are a productive cough and a bilateral mucoid to mucopurulent nasal discharge. On chest auscultation, loud bronchial tones over the trachea and lungs are audible, with adventitious sounds (wheezes, crackles) over the lung fields.

2. **Pneumonia in foals.** Respiratory disease of foals can have a variety of causes, both infectious and noninfectious. Of these causes, the more important infectious diseases are discussed in this chapter.
   a. **Overview**
      (1) **Viral pneumonia**
         (a) **Patient profile and etiology.** The viral agents that result in signs of pneumonia in foals include the equine herpesviruses (EHV-1, EHV-4), influenza virus, and adenovirus. Pure viral pneumonia in foals is associated with immunocompromised, debilitated foals (e.g., failure of passive transfer, combined immunodeficiency, steroid therapy, poorly nourished foals). The main problem with these infections is the potential to predispose to more clinically serious secondary bacterial pneumonia.
         (b) **Clinical findings** are similar to those described for neonatal pneumonia because they are seldom specific for any one viral agent. In foals, the severity of pneumonia is often poorly correlated to chest auscultation findings. For the pathogenesis, diagnostic plans, and therapeutic plans for these agents, refer to Chapter 6.
      (2) **Bacterial pneumonia**
         (a) **Patient profile and etiology.** A variety of bacteria can be associated with pneumonia in foals.
            (i) *Streptococcus zooepidemicus* is the most common [see I A 2 b (1)].
            (ii) *Actinobacillus equuli* can cause pneumonia in older foals, whereas this organism causes septicemia and nephritis in very young foals.
            (iii) *Klebsiella pneumoniae* causes a severe pneumonia in septicemic foals, as do the *Salmonella* species in foals 2–3 weeks of age, in which other signs include diarrhea and arthritis.
            (iv) *Escherichia coli* can be a cause of embolic pneumonia secondary to septicemia.
            (v) *Bordetella bronchiseptica* has been a cause of bacterial pneumonia in foals, though it is usually not a primary pathogen.
            (vi) *Rhodococcus equi* is a specific pathogen for foals, with lung abscessation as the primary lesion [see I A 2 b (2)].
         (b) **Risk factors**
            (i) In the early stages of life, foals with **septicemia** usually have an associated bacterial pneumonia. Clearly, the elements that predispose to septicemia (e.g., problems with sufficient passive transfer) are key factors.
            (ii) **Older foals** are at risk to secondary bacterial pneumonia when they experience respiratory viral infection. In these cases, there is usually stress of transport and overcrowding, as may occur accompanying transport of the mare to be bred.

(iii) **Inadequate ventilation** (excessive dust levels, poorly cleaned stalls), **poor nutrition,** and **parasite migration** are thought to contribute to foals being predisposed to developing pneumonia, although these are not sufficient causes on their own.

b. **Specific conditions**

(1) *Streptococcus zooepidemicus* **pneumonia**

(a) **Patient profile and history** is variable because the organism is an opportunistic pathogen in horses of all ages and ubiquitous in their environment.

(b) **Clinical findings.** Signs include tachypnea, anorexia, depression, fever, abnormal lung sounds, and possibly a cough. None of these signs are specific for *S. zooepidemicus* infection. However, this organism can cause lymph node abscessation, in contrast to the other opportunistic bacteria, and could resemble *S. equi* infection in the early stages before signs of pulmonary involvement.

(c) **Etiology and pathogenesis**

(i) **Etiology.** *S. zooepidemicus* is a normal inhabitant of the equine upper respiratory tract and does not normally invade intact mucous membranes. Any of several stressors (e.g., poor air quality, inadequate ventilation, damage to respiratory epithelium by viral infections) to the normal respiratory defenses may predispose this organism to spread to the lungs.

(ii) **Pathogenesis.** Acute infections result in severe fibrinopurulent bronchopneumonia with hemorrhage, whereas less fulminant infections cause abscesses in the lungs, lymph nodes, and occasionally in the pleura (pyogranulomatous pneumonia).

(d) **Diagnostic plan and laboratory tests**

(i) A **transtracheal aspirate** aids diagnosis and rapidly directs specific treatment. Typically, there are gram-positive cocci noted in the fluid recovered, which is evidence of *Streptococcus* involvement. Thus, while awaiting culture of the organism, treatment can then be selected against this family of organism.

(ii) **Thoracic radiographs** (used for foals only because these are not usually available for adult horses) can confirm the presence of pneumonia and may detect lung abscesses, which require far more prolonged treatment.

(iii) **Hematology** usually reveals leukocytosis and increased fibrinogen, but these changes are not specific for this infection.

(e) **Therapeutic plan**

(i) **Penicillin** is the drug of choice for *S. zooepidemicus* infections. If the clinical signs are marked (indicating fulminant infection), foals should be started on intravenous medications, such as **sodium** or **potassium penicillin** (20,000 IU/kg intravenously every 6 hours). For less severe clinical signs, affected foals (and adult horses) respond well to **procaine penicillin** (20,000 IU/kg intramuscularly every 12 hours).

(ii) An **alternative treatment** is **trimethoprim-sulphadiazine** (30 mg/kg orally every 12 hours). Treatment should continue well beyond resolution of clinical signs. Treatment effectiveness should be monitored using blood work and serial chest radiographs.

(f) **Prevention.** Because there are 13 serotypes of *S. zooepidemicus,* there is no vaccine available. Therefore, preventive measures include attention to hygiene and reduction of stress, particularly in the neonatal period. For older foals and even adult horses, adequate rest and a stress-free environment following respiratory viral infection should be ensured for at least several weeks.

(2) *Rhodococcus equi* **pneumonia**

(a) **Patient profile and history.** This is an infectious respiratory disease of foals usually 4 months or younger that is usually sporadic in occurrence on any one farm. *R. equi* is an opportunistic bacterium that appears to infect the foal when maternal antibody levels are waning and viral infections impair defense mechanisms. Affected foals can have a prolonged course of chronic respiratory signs or exhibit a sudden onset of severe respiratory distress that can be rapidly fatal.

(b) Epidemiology

  (i) Foals between the ages of 1 and 3 months are most commonly affected, but the onset of signs can range from age 2 weeks to 6 months. The disease is rare in adult horses and occurs only in immunocompromised animals.

  (ii) There appears to be an increased incidence during the hot, dry months of summer, which may be attributable to the increased spread of soil- and fecal-born organisms in dusty conditions. During these dry conditions, the risk of infection can be reduced if the foals are put onto grass pasture. Morbidity is low, but the case fatality rate is high if left untreated.

(c) Clinical findings. The signs of disease appear to vary with the age at which foals become affected.

  (i) Young foals affected after 1 month of age often have acute signs of illness with fever, respiratory distress, anorexia, and, in some cases, swollen joints.

  (ii) Older foals can develop serious lesions in the absence of marked clinical abnormalities, which then begin to manifest as a persistent cough and a progressive increase in respiratory effort at rest, with crackles and wheezes audible over the chest. These foals often suckle normally and have no fever during such disease progression, but they become emaciated. In some foals, diarrhea may follow or accompany the respiratory signs, but nasal discharge and lymph node enlargement in the throat region are absent.

  (iii) Other clinical signs can include arthritis in one or several joints and uveitis, both presumed to be immune mediated. In foals with these signs, the slow development of apparent pneumonia masks the severity of underlying pulmonary disease; therefore, it is prudent to suspect *R. equi* infection in a foal with nonresponsive pneumonia.

(d) Diagnostic plan and laboratory tests. Although clinical signs are usually suggestive of pneumonia, it is important to establish an etiologic diagnosis in the case of *R. equi* infection for appropriate treatment and advice on prognosis. **Transtracheal aspirate** cytology and culture, along with **thoracic radiography,** are the most valuable diagnostic tests.

  (i) On **transtracheal wash,** there are usually large numbers of neutrophils, and the bacteria (often intracellular) can have a characteristic "Chinese letter" appearance. Culture of the sample should be positive for *R. equi*, but in those foals that have been treated with antibiotics, there may be no bacterial growth.

  (ii) Radiography. Classically, **"cotton-puff abscesses"** of the lung are present on chest radiographs, although the radiographic image can also consist of diffuse pulmonary infiltration and air bronchograms with hilar lymphadenopathy.

  (iii) Blood work. A complete blood cell count (CBC) and fibrinogen level, although not definitive for *R. equi*, are useful for monitoring the course of the inflammatory process. Affected foals usually show a neutrophilic leukocytosis with hyperfibrinogenemia, accompanied by anemia of chronic disease. The fibrinogen response can also be used as a guideline for response to treatment.

  (iv) Serologic tests have been of limited value because although foals with pulmonary infection caused by *R. equi* show seroconversion to this organism, normal foals in the first few months of life can also show seroconversion as a result of intestinal colonization by the organism.

(e) Etiology and pathogenesis

(i) Etiology. *R. equi* is a gram-positive pleomorphic rod isolated from the soil and feces of normal horses. Although it causes disease in horses, it also can cause cervical abscesses in swine and abscesses in the intestinal and pulmonary lymph nodes of cattle. Because of the ubiquitous nature of the organism, most foals are exposed to infection, but only a few develop disease. The organisms can survive in moist soil for periods longer than 1 year. In some farms where *R. equi* pneumonia appears endemic with multiple cases each year, there is likely a bacterial load in the environment.

(ii) The **route of infection** is not definitively known, but most evidence supports aerosolization or inhalation of soil-derived bacteria. An alternate route suggested is ingestion and intestinal colonization with subsequent hematogenous spread.

(iii) Pathogenesis. When the bacteria reach the lung, they induce a suppurative **pyogranulomatous bronchopneumonia** with characteristic abscessation. Abscessation occurs because *R. equi* are able to survive within macrophages. This ability to live and multiply within phagocytes results from failure of phagosome–lysosome fusion and also from the lack of a superoxide anion response in the equine pulmonary macrophage following ingestion of *R. equi*.

(iv) Parasite migration through lungs may contribute to development of disease. **Other disease manifestations** include nonseptic arthritis, ulcerative colitis, hepatic and splenic abscesses, vertebral abscesses, and uveitis.

(f) Therapeutic plan. Because the underlying process is a pyogranulomatous reaction, attributes of the selected antibacterial treatment should include good distribution and activity in lungs, adequate penetration into thick caseous abscesses, and penetration into cells to act on bacteria within macrophages and neutrophils.

(i) Rifampin (5–10 mg/kg orally every 12 hours) with **erythromycin estolate** (25 mg/kg orally every 6 hours) is the combination of choice. The erythromycin may cause a transient diarrhea but is usually self-limiting and abates on temporary withdrawal of the drug.

(ii) Treatment should be continued for at least 30 days. The fibrinogen concentration can be used as a guide for efficacy, a reduction signaling treatment effectiveness. Follow-up chest radiographs can be helpful in determining the response to treatment.

(iii) If foals have periodic serum biochemical tests during treatment, enzyme elevations suggestive of cholestasis may occur but can be expected with use of these drugs.

(g) Prevention. Because the organism is ubiquitous in the foals' environment, it is difficult to control.

(i) Minimizing exposure. With the increased risk associated with dusty environments, exposure can be minimized by maintaining the mare and foal on **grassy paddocks** or pasture. The pasture management technique of **routine disposal of feces** may also decrease exposure.

(ii) Administration of hyperimmune serum. As yet, there is **no effective vaccine** for use against this disease. However, recent studies indicate that administering **hyperimmune serum,** obtained from mares that were given an autogenous vaccine, to foals at risk did limit the severity of disease produced by experimental challenge. Additionally, field studies have shown that administration of hyperimmune serum to foals in their first month of life has resulted in a significant reduction in the disease incidence. Unfortunately, vaccination of the dam to boost the specific colostrally transferred passive immunity has not been met with similar positive results.

(3) *Pneumocystis carinii* **pneumonia.** *P. carinii* is an ubiquitous sporozoan that causes interstitial pneumonia in immunocompromised humans. This opportunistic pathogen is associated invariably with other organisms and has occurred in foals with *R. equi,* in immunocompromised foals (e.g., combined immuno-deficiency), or in foals taking corticosteroids on a long-term basis. Although clinical signs reflect a bacterial bronchopneumonia, this disease is usually diag-nosed postmortem.

3. **Enzootic pneumonia in calves**
   a. **Patient profile and history.** This disease occurs almost exclusively in calves raised indoors. Therefore, enzootic pneumonia is found mainly in dairy herds. Although this disorder can occur as early as the first week of life, this disease is most com-mon in calves between 2 and 5 months and up to 1 year of age. Fall and winter are the times it is most often observed. Poor air quality is a contributing factor to infection.
   b. **Clinical findings**
      (1) Affected calves in the acute stage have a moderate **fever** (40°C–40.5°C) and a **harsh, hacking cough** that is easily induced by pinching the trachea.
      (2) **Tachypnea** and **dyspnea** are often present, with increased bronchial tones audi-ble over the cranial lung fields suggestive of lung consolidation. Crackles and wheezes at the periphery of areas of consolidation may also be audible, sug-gesting bronchiolitis.
      (3) Calves are usually alert unless there is a significant bacterial component to the pneumonia, in which case the fever may be higher.
   c. **Etiology and pathogenesis.** At approximately 2 months of age, calves' immunity to respiratory infection (a combination of waning colostral immunity and the slow de-velopment of an independent response) is at its lowest point. This may be a key reason that most of the calf pneumonia problems caused by infections begin to ap-pear at this age.
      (1) **Infection** may begin as a viral respiratory infection, which may resolve or be-come complicated by a variety of bacteria, mycoplasmal organisms, or both (multifactorial).
         (a) **Viral agents** include parainfluenza-3 (PI-3), bovine respiratory syncytial virus (BRSV), and bovine viral diarrhea (BVD), of which PI-3 and BRSV ap-pear the most significant. BRSV is increasingly implicated as a major fac-tor in the genesis of enzootic pneumonia. Unless there is secondary com-plication by bacteria, the disease is generally an interstitial pneumonia affecting the cranial lung lobes. Other viruses of cattle (e.g., rhinoviruses, adenoviruses, reoviruses) are not considered important.
         (b) **Mycoplasmal organisms,** including *Mycoplasma bovis, M. dispar, M. bovi-rhinis,* and *Ureaplasma,* also are found in many cases of enzootic pneu-monia.
            (i) These organisms inhabit bronchiolar epithelium; thus, they cause cili-ary destruction and changes in mucus composition as goblet cells pro-liferate and mucus hypersecretion occurs.
            (ii) The **classic pathology** attributed to mycoplasmal infection in these calves is peribronchial lymphocytic cuffing of the bronchioles. It ap-pears that the adult cattle act as mycoplasma carriers and transfer the organisms by aerosol up to several meters' distance to calves.
         (c) **Bacterial agents** involved in this pneumonia include many of the organ-isms that can be found in the pharyngeal region of normal calves, includ-ing *Pasteurella haemolytica, P. multocida,* and *Actinomyces pyogenes. Chlamydia* species also have been involved in some mixed infections. In-volvement of these secondary agents results in purulent secretions accumu-lating in the airways and eventually the formation of microabscesses, bron-chiectasis, or both. The **pathology** that occurs is a consolidation of cranial, middle, and accessory lobes with bronchiolitis and alveolitis, with varying degrees of consolidation and suppuration depending on the numbers and type of bacterial involvement.
      (2) **Environmental factors**
         (a) The infectious agents are seldom able to induce pneumonia in calves with-

out the added stress of **poor** or **absent ventilation** in the housing areas for the calves.

    (b) Colder weather often precipitates problems when the producers try to prevent the calf housing temperature from dropping by reducing fresh air circulation. Consequently, there is increased humidity in the ambient air of the calves, which allows pathogen multiplication. This is compounded by a high pathogen density developing with the lack of fresh air to dilute the ambient air.

    (c) Another factor of adverse air quality is the increased exposure to **noxious gases** (e.g., ammonia) that can adversely affect mucociliary clearance.

  (3) Management factors include the crowding and mixing of various age groups that frequently occurs with indoor housing, particularly in older barns.

d. Diagnostic plan and laboratory tests

  (1) Clinical signs of pneumonia are the main mode of diagnosis. Attempts can be made at virus isolation or viral serology, but these efforts are often unrewarding and unlikely to change the methods of management of the problem.

  (2) Laboratory studies. For the individual calf, a **transtracheal aspirate** can be performed. **Cytology findings** of increased numbers of degenerate neutrophils with numerous intracellular bacteria implicate secondary bacterial involvement. In these cases, bacterial culture and sensitivity may aid in guiding antibiotic treatment of the calf. A CBC indicates changes of leucocytosis and hyperfibrinogenemia where bacteria are involved.

  (3) Radiography. For calves that have a prolonged course of pneumonia and respond poorly to antibiotics, **thoracic radiographs** may identify processes such as abscessation or bronchiectasis, indicating a poor prognosis.

e. Therapeutic plan. Acutely affected calves often respond well to antibiotics, unless the infection is purely viral, as can occur in some BRSV infections.

  (1) Although many of the commonly available antibiotics for cattle can be used, drugs that are effective against the mycoplasmas, such as **tylosin tartrate** (10 mg/kg intramuscularly daily for 3–4 days) or **oxytetracycline** (10 mg/kg intramuscularly daily for 3–4 days), provide appropriate coverage against the spectrum of possible organisms involved.

  (2) More recently, **flunixin meglumine** (2.2 mg/kg intravenously every 24 hours for 2–3 days) also has been advocated as an adjunct treatment because it may reduce lung inflammation in these calves.

f. Prognosis. In chronically debilitated calves that may have extensive lung damage, including abscessation, the prognosis for full recovery is poor, and therapy may not be cost-effective.

g. Prevention

  (1) Vaccines. The commonly available vaccines against the viral pathogens are of questionable value, as colostral immunity usually interferes with adequate response at the time of administration.

  (2) Management strategies

    (a) For producers with major problems, **individual outdoor calf hutches** are highly recommended because they provide optimal ventilation and a level of isolation from older cattle.

    (b) Producers with less severe problems can reduce the incidence of enzootic pneumonia with attention to adequate ventilation in the calf barn, which removes pathogens, noxious gases, and excess moisture.

    (c) Adequate colostral feeding also may prevent enzootic pneumonia because survival of calves with respiratory disease has been directly correlated with serum immunoglobulin G levels.

4. Pneumonia in lambs and kids is similar to that in adult sheep and goats (see I B 3).

5. Pneumonia in piglets

  a. Etiology. Pneumonia in piglets can be caused by viruses, including pseudorabies, swine influenza (see Chapter 6), and the recently described **porcine reproductive and respiratory syndrome (PRRS).**

  (1) PRRS, also known as porcine endemic abortion and respiratory syndrome,

blue-eared pig disease, swine infertility and respiratory syndrome, and origi-
nally "mystery disease of swine," was first recorded in the United States in
1987 and is thought to be caused by the Lelystad virus in Europe and a similar, if not identical virus, in North America. Since being reported in the United
States, this virus has been recorded in Canada and several countries in Europe.
   (2) **Transmission** appears to be airborne because even well-managed and isolated
       herds can become infected.
   b. **Clinical findings**
       (1) **Adults.** Signs include anorexia and fever lasting several days, after which there
           may be mid- to late-term abortions with large mummified fetuses or partially
           autolysed fetuses, increased percentages of stillbirths, and weak piglets. This
           period of reproductive problems is followed or accompanied by severe respira-
           tory disease in nursing or weaned piglets.
       (2) **Piglets.** Signs include dyspnea, polypnea, and decreased growth. The abdo-
           men, ears, or vulva may appear bluish (hence the name blue-eared pigs). In a
           litter, up to 50% have anorexia, 30% show respiratory distress, 10% have
           fever, and only 5% show cyanosis. Morbidity in weanling pigs can be as high
           as 30%, with mortality of 5%–10%.
   c. **Diagnostic plan and laboratory tests.** There are several serologic tests available to
       detect seroconversion to the virus, but because of the possible widespread infec-
       tion, the serodiagnosis should be based on a herd rather than on a sample from an
       individual animal. There are no characteristic lesions in the aborted or stillborn pig-
       lets or in the sows. Piglets will have a proliferative and necrotizing pneumonia
       and, in some cases, a purulent bronchopneumonia.
   d. **Differential diagnoses.** This disease needs to be differentiated from other condi-
       tions that cause abortion, stillbirths, and weak piglets, such as pseudorabies, par-
       vovirus, leptospirosis, and the encephalomyocarditis or hog cholera viruses.
   e. **Therapeutic plan and prevention.** Because there is no specific treatment available,
       control is the main focus. There is not sufficient data available for understanding
       the methods of transmission, but restricting the movement of pigs from affected to
       unaffected areas has slowed the spread.

B. **Pneumonia in growing and mature animals**

1. **Equine bacterial pneumonia**
   a. **Patient profile and etiology.** Pneumonia in the adult horse is not common and is
       usually secondary to upper respiratory virus infection [see I A 2 b (1)] or occurs
       after stressful events (e.g., shipping), in which case it often develops into pleuritis
       (see I E).
   b. **Diagnostic and therapeutic plans.** The guidelines given for foals are used, with the
       exception that chest radiographs are not obtained because they are not readily
       available for monitoring progress in the adult horse.

2. **Bovine respiratory disease complex (shipping fever, pneumonic pasteurellosis)**
   a. **Patient profile and history.** This disease can affect cattle of any age, breed, or sex.
       However, because of current management practices, this condition occurs primar-
       ily in young cattle between the ages of 6 and 18 months. Characteristically, the dis-
       order follows a stressful event (e.g., shipping, mixing in sales), occurring 2–14
       days later, and is one of the major causes of morbidity and mortality in feedlot cat-
       tle in North America.
   b. **Clinical findings**
       (1) Affected cattle are **depressed,** usually **anorexic,** and have rapid shallow respira-
           tions with a **weak, productive cough.** Early signs of the depression may be sim-
           ply a failure to stretch freely when encouraged to rise. **Fever** is often as high
           as 41°C, and examination of the penmates may reveal fever in animals that
           otherwise appear clinically normal.
       (2) In the **early stages** of the disease, lung sounds only consist of increased breath
           sounds. In the **advanced stages,** crackles and wheezes become readily audi-
           ble, and there may be pleural friction rubs in some animals. A mucopurulent

nasal discharge, crusty nose, and ocular discharge may appear, along with a gaunt appearance to the abdomen after several days of not eating.

c. Etiology and pathogenesis

(1) Etiology

(a) This disease is a fibrinous pneumonia caused by ***Pasteurella haemolytica*** (biotype A, serotype I) and, less commonly, *Pasteurella multocida* or *Hemophilus somnus*. Experimentally, these organisms alone do not produce disease without massive doses or manipulation of the host with viral pathogens or severe stressors.

(b) In naturally occurring disease, the associated **stressful events** are numerous and include weaning, transportation, sudden changes in climatic conditions (e.g., temperature, humidity), inadequate or irregular feeding, water deprivation, crowding, dehorning, castration, and vaccination. Respiratory viral infection can be a factor, but in many outbreaks of naturally occurring disease, there is no preceding viral infection.

(2) Pathogenesis. *P. haemolytica* and *P. multocida* are normal inhabitants of the bovine upper respiratory tract. With the stressors, these organisms are able to colonize and proliferate in the lower respiratory tract. *P. haemolytica* stressors are associated with increased numbers and virulence of the strain found in the pharynx of cattle. Because this organism appears as the predominating agent in this disease syndrome, most investigation into pathogenesis has focused on *P. haemolytica.*

(a) *P. haemolytica* has **four virulence factors** that interact to produce disease: fimbriae, polysaccharide capsule, endotoxin, and leukotoxin.

(i) The **bacterial fimbriae** enhance the colonization and proliferation of bacteria in the upper respiratory tract.

(ii) The **polysaccharide capsule** inhibits complement-mediated serum killing as well as phagocytosis and intracellular killing of the organism.

(iii) **Endotoxin** is directly toxic to the bovine endothelium and greatly modifies cardiopulmonary hemodynamics. Also, it can alter bovine leukocyte functions.

(iv) **Leukotoxin** is a species-specific cytotoxin against ruminant leukocytes and platelets, acting as a pore-forming cytolysin.

(b) Transmission. Cattle either have the bacterial organisms in their nasopharynx or become infected by aerosol from other cattle. However, the disease does not appear to be contagious in the way it affects the individual.

(c) Route of infection

(i) With increased proliferation of the bacteria in the nasopharyngeal region and increases in virulence type, *P. haemolytica* is allowed to colonize the airways of the lung. The presence of *P. haemolytica* (lipopolysaccharide) attracts neutrophils to the lung as a normal defense mechanism.

(ii) Although local immunity such as immunoglobulin can be protective, some forms of systemic immunity can actually enhance intrapulmonary pathology of *Pasteurella* infections, possibly because of opsonization (immunoglobulin G) effect.

(iii) *P. haemolytica* produces an exotoxin during log phase growth that is cytotoxic for ruminant neutrophils and macrophages. Therefore, the increased bacterial phagocytosis induced by opsonization may merely cause increased cell death of the very cells (neutrophils and macrophages) that are intended for defense. Also, release or "spilling" of the cytotoxic contents of these cells can contribute to lung damage.

(iv) The pathology that results is a severe fibrinous pneumonia with increased capillary permeability, thrombosis, and coagulation necrosis. Bacterial cell death, which releases endotoxin (lipopolysaccharide), probably contributes to these changes. In contrast to earlier theory, viral involvement is not an essential component of this disease.

d. Diagnostic plan and laboratory tests

(1) Clinical findings of rapid onset of high fever, depression, and rapid, shallow, often guarded breathing, combined with a stressful event is usually sufficient for a tentative diagnosis.

(2) Laboratory analysis is seldom warranted with individual cases and is not diagnostic for shipping fever.

  (a) Blood work. Predictably, there is a leukocytosis on the **CBC,** but there also can be leukopenia if endotoxemia is a major component. Hyperfibrinogenemia is usually present (greater than 7 g/L).

  (b) A **transtracheal aspirate** yields septic, degenerate tracheal exudate containing gram-negative rods and often *Pasteurella* species on culture.

  (c) If **nasopharyngeal swabs** are taken, *P. haemolytica* can be cultured, but there appears to be poor correlation of antimicrobial sensitivities between isolates from the nasopharynx versus the lung. Therefore, these samples should not be used to guide the choice of antibiotic for the treatment of acute cases.

e. Therapeutic plan

  (1) Antimicrobial treatment. Early treatment of acutely affected cattle with almost any of the commonly available antimicrobials (e.g., oxytetracycline, trimethoprim-sulfadoxine, penicillin, sulfonamides) is highly effective.

  (a) Surprisingly, a single-dose treatment in early stages is often sufficient, but severely affected cattle should be treated daily for 3–5 days.

  (b) Delayed or **irregular treatment,** inappropriate dose, or premature termination of therapy in some cattle can result in **increased mortality.** Cattle with more than 50%–60% pulmonary consolidation generally respond poorly and frequently relapse. These animals may be individuals that were not detected in the acute stage or were not adequately treated early in the course of the disease.

  (2) In addition to antimicrobial treatment, sick cattle should receive **adequate shelter** and **good nutrition,** particularly when the management system in place encourages crowding and competition for feed and water space.

  (3) Response to treatment

  (a) Antimicrobial-resistant strains of *P. haemolytica* have been appearing and, with resistance being plasmid mediated, may significantly increase the incidence of poor response to treatment.

  (b) To assess adequate response to treatment, the **rectal temperature** should be used as a guide. A positive response is the abatement of fever within 48 hours of treatment.

f. Prevention. Because this disease is so clearly linked to stressful events, a great deal of the prevention can be managed by avoiding or lessening the impact of known and preventable stressors.

  (1) Preconditioning. The best example of stressful events is the practice of weaning calves simultaneously with castration, dehorning, and vaccination. By performing some of these procedures at a separate time, such massive stress can be lessened. This management method, called preconditioning or backgrounding, vaccinates and processes (castrates, dehorns, implants) calves before weaning, all of which should occur 3 weeks to 1 month before shipping. There are many variations of the timing and order of these preventive measures. However, the financial benefit to the producer is less clear, and unless a premium is paid for these calves at sale, the extra cost and effort may not be worthwhile.

  (2) Vaccination against shipping fever has been a main focus of prevention but has not been particularly effective until recently.

  (a) Where **respiratory viral agents** (e.g., IBR, PI-3, BRSV) are involved, the use of such antigens in vaccines may be beneficial when they are administered at least several weeks before weaning and shipping. Also, there has been evidence that vaccination with live products at the time of stress may increase morbidity or mortality.

  (b) Progress has been made in creating vaccines against the pathogenic effects of **P. haemolytica.** Recently, a vaccine was produced to stimulate immunity against the exotoxin or leukotoxin that is produced as a major part of the pathogenicity of *P. haemolytica*. This vaccine appears to protect against pulmonary disease in experimental models of disease but is less effective in field use. Current evidence from field trials suggests that this vaccine at best only marginally reduces the morbidity and mortality.

(3) Chemoprophylaxis. Another tact taken to reduce the morbidity and mortality of shipping fever is the administration of antibiotics at the time of stresses or upon arrival at a feedlot.

(a) Drugs used include long-acting oxytetracycline (LA200, 20 mg/kg) or tilmicosin (micotil, 10 mg/kg subcutaneously). Such treatment is presumed to be effective by postponing the bacterial invasion of the lung, so that the infection is usually less severe and less likely to result in relapses.

(b) Medication in **feed** or **water** has been used also, but both these approaches can give a false sense of security, reducing scrutiny of the cattle's health and leading to more advanced cases occurring before diagnosis. Also, with the current consumer concern regarding drug use in animals that are intended for human consumption, such practices can create problems for the image of the industry.

3. Ovine and caprine bacterial pneumonia
a. Pasteurellosis

(1) Patient profile and history. Outbreaks are often associated with sudden changes in environment or climate (e.g., when a flock of sheep is exposed to inclement weather shortly after shearing).

(2) Etiology and pathogenesis

(a) Etiology. As in cattle, *Pasteurella haemolytica* is the most common cause of bacterial infections of the respiratory tract in sheep and goats. However, the resulting diseases are not the same as those in cattle.

(i) There are **two major biotypes: biotype A,** which causes primarily pneumonia, and **biotype T,** which causes primarily acute septicemia in younger animals. Each biotype contains several serotypes.

(ii) *P. haemolytica* is commonly found in the **nasal passages** and **tonsils** of apparently healthy sheep. Several serotypes may be present at one time, but during outbreaks of respiratory pasteurellosis, one serotype usually predominates in both the upper and lower portions of the respiratory tract. The nasal carriage rate of *P. haemolytica* varies throughout the year and appears to increase as ewes approach parturition. Although *P. haemolytica* may occasionally cause mastitis in ewes, it is not often found in colostrum.

(b) Predisposing factors. Although *P. haemolytica* can be a primary pathogen in young lambs, older animals require predisposing factors for the occurrence of disease.

(i) In lambs, prior viral infection by such viruses as PI-3, followed in 4–7 days with *P. haemolytica* infection can produce pneumonia that is similar to naturally occurring cases.

(ii) Adenovirus has also been incriminated as predisposing to naturally occurring and experimentally occurring pneumonia.

(iii) Other factors, such as exposure to **inclement weather, transportation,** and **poor nutrition,** are also predisposing factors.

(c) Pathogenesis. These factors combine to allow proliferation of the resident bacteria in the upper respiratory tract and invasion of the lung, where virulence factors, such as polysaccharide and leukotoxin (the specific cytotoxin against the ruminant leukocytes), cause extensive pulmonary damage.

(3) Clinical findings. Clinical disease is usually most severe in young lambs and kids, particularly with biotype A, which can cause a rapidly fatal septicemia.

(a) If **detected early,** affected lambs or kids appear dull and become prostrate before death in a matter of hours. Sick animals are often unobserved until the final stages of the disease.

(b) In the older animals, **signs of respiratory disease** are observed, with dyspnea, slight frothing at the mouth, cough, and nasal discharge. These signs are accentuated when the herd or flock is moved and affected animals fall behind the rest. Fever (greater than 40.5°C), depression, and anorexia also accompany these signs.

(4) Diagnostic plan and laboratory tests. Clinical signs of pneumonia are usually sufficient for a provisional diagnosis. There is little reported on the use of clinical pathology for assisting with a diagnosis. In outbreaks, there will likely be some mortalities on which **necropsy** can be performed.

   (a) Changes generally include marked consolidation of the cranial and middle lobes with a distinct demarcation between affected and unaffected lungs. Extensive fibrinous pleuritis, pericarditis, and in more chronic cases, abscess formation in the lung, also may be present.

   (b) For **biotype A septicemia,** there is often subcutaneous hemorrhage over the neck and thorax, with edematous lungs and subpleural ecchymosis, but pneumonia is not a feature. There is ulceration and necrosis of the pharynx and esophagus, as well as the occurrence of small necrotic areas on the tips of the abomasal mucosal folds.

   (c) The organism can usually be isolated in large numbers from tonsils, lung, liver, and the ulcerated areas of the intestinal tract.

(5) Therapeutic plan. The choice of **antibiotic therapy** in lambs is based on etiologic probability. *P. haemolytica* is the most likely pathogen, and the choice of drugs available includes penicillin, ampicillin, tetracyclines, trimethoprim-sulfonamides, and triple sulfas.

   (a) Although not all strains of biotype A are sensitive to penicillin, almost all strains are sensitive to **oxytetracycline,** which makes it a suitable first-line drug of choice. An additional advantage is that these drugs are effective against *Chlamydia* and most *Mycoplasma* species.

   (b) Long-acting tetracyclines can be effective, particularly because they can reduce the stresses of handling (only one or two injections are needed); however, tetracyclines are irritating when administered intramuscularly.

(6) Prevention

   (a) Vaccination with autogenous and commercial bacterins has not been effective in controlling disease. Specific serotypes or "protective" antigens may be absent from these products.

   (b) Prophylactic antibiotics

   (i) Feed medication with chlortetracycline or chlortetracycline with sulfamethazine has been evaluated as a preventive for pneumonia in range lambs but has met with equivocal results.

   (ii) Sulfonamides have been recommended as a preventive for baby lamb pneumonia by intermittent medication of the drinking water of ewes before lambing.

   (c) Management strategies

   (i) Avoid overcrowding by providing a minimum of 14 square feet per pregnant ewe and a minimum of 4–5 square feet for each lamb.

   (ii) The producer should consider **prelambing shearing,** which has an advantage in that housed animals with access to the outdoors are not carrying a high moisture content in their fleeces; thus, the humidity of the barn is lower. Shorn ewes will also seek shelter at lambing, reducing the risk of hypothermia due to exposure in newborn lambs. However, adequate shelter from wind and rain does need to be provided for the shorn ewes.

   (iii) During shearing, young sheep should be shorn first, and any cuts should be disinfected and clippers blades sterilized to reduce the risk of spreading *Corynebacterium pseudotuberculosis.* Additionally, avoid dipping or spraying for external parasites if there is any sign of cold wet weather approaching.

b. Other bacterial causes of pneumonia in sheep and goats

   (1) *P. multocida, Streptococcus* **species,** *Escherichia coli,* **and** *Haemophilus* species may be present in ovine and caprine pneumonia. These bacteria are usually secondary invaders. *S. typhimurium* and *S. dublin* cause diarrhea and abortion in sheep and goats. Respiratory signs may be seen initially.

(2) ***Francisella tularensis*** infection can result in acute illness manifested by high fever, prostration, diarrhea, and respiratory signs, including nasal discharge and coughing. Diagnosis is confirmed by the isolation of the causative agent, the presence of *Dermacentor andersonii,* and a die-off of rodents in the area.

4. Porcine pneumonia. Although individual pigs can be affected with pneumonia on a sporadic basis, there are two forms of infectious respiratory problems that plague the swine industry: **enzootic pneumonia** and **pleuropneumonia.**

a. Enzootic pneumonia

(1) Economic implications. Enzootic pneumonia consistently ranks as the most economically important disease in finishing pigs in North America. Enzootic pneumonia occurs worldwide and has a particularly high incidence in intensive rearing operations. In infected herds, the morbidity rate is highest during the growing period, but the case fatality rate is low. The main adverse effects of this disease include an increase in the need to treat clinical illness caused by secondary bacterial pneumonia and the reduction in feed efficiency and average daily gain for getting the pigs to market.

(2) Clinical findings. The most common form of the disease, as observed in endemically infected herds, begins at 3–10 weeks of age and is insidious in onset.

(a) Initially, the only clinical abnormality is **cough** in a small proportion of the piglets. This increases such that most animals in the pen show persistent cough, which is particularly obvious at times of activity, such as feeding, and can continue through the entire growing period. The cough is dry and hacking, but signs of respiratory embarrassment are rare, and there is no fever or diminished appetite.

(b) Those pigs that develop signs of pneumonia usually have **secondary invasion** of the lungs by *Pasteurella* species or other bacteria. Clinical signs of disease become less obvious with increasing age.

(3) Etiology and pathogenesis

(a) Etiology. The disease is caused by the primary initiator *Mycoplasma hyopneumoniae* (or *suipneumonia*) with *Pasteurella multocida* as a common secondary invader of the lung. *M. hyopneumonia* appears to be host specific, inhabiting the respiratory tract of pigs and surviving in the environment for only a short time. Other pathogens can cause similar pathologic lesions, but this organism appears to be the primary cause of enzootic pneumonia in pigs.

(b) Pathogenesis

(i) Piglets are infected by the mycoplasmal organism early in life, likely from the sow, but also possibly from airborne particles from other pigs.

(ii) *M. hyopneumonia* causes peribronchiolar lymphoid hyperplasia and mononuclear accumulation in the lamina propria, resulting in obliteration of the bronchial lumen. Also, the bronchial mucous glands undergo hypertrophy, and there is hypertrophy of the type II alveolar epithelial cells and progressive loss of cilia on the bronchial mucosa, decreasing the defenses against secondary bacterial infection.

(iii) These damages heal on their own, but if secondary bacterial invasion occurs, more severe pathology occurs, including bronchopneumonia and pleuritis. These complications also cause decrease in feed efficiency and average daily gain.

(4) Diagnostic plan and laboratory tests. The gross and microscopic findings on the lungs of pigs affected with enzootic pneumonia are not pathognomonic; thus, a positive diagnosis requires **culture** of *M. hypopneumoniae* from tissues. However, a negative result can often occur because the organism is difficult to culture and is readily overgrown by other nonsignificant organisms, such as

M. hyorhinis. A **fluorescent antibody test** or an **enzyme-linked immunoperoxidase technique** may help demonstrate the organism in tissues.
(5) **Therapeutic plan.** Treatment is usually restricted to **individual pigs** showing acute respiratory distress, which, being of a secondary bacterial nature, should respond to most broad-spectrum antibiotics.
   (a) There is no effective treatment that eliminates infection by *M. hyopneumonia.* However, antibiotics such as **tylosin tartrate** (50 mg/kg) and **tiamulin** (10 mg/kg) orally for 10 days can reduce pulmonary lesions.
   (b) **Other antibiotics** show activity against this mycoplasma, including tetracyclines and the newer fluoroquinolones, such as ciprofloxacin.
(6) **Prevention.** Because *M. hyopneumonia* infects only pigs and transmission requires close pig-to-pig contact, its spread can be limited or even eradicated from a herd.
   (a) **Eradication** is the most satisfactory method of control but requires depopulation of the herd, followed by repopulation with pigs from specific pathogen-free (SPF) herds. Such pigs are commercially available, having been raised in special units populated with the progeny of Caesarian-derived piglets.
   (b) **Separation. Less successful methods** involve isolating the farrowing area for sows believed free of infection from the rest of the herd, and raising the piglets separately. Alternatively, newborn piglets can be treated with antibiotics effective against *Mycoplasma* species and removed to isolated premises, with subsequent serologic testing of the breeding herd and culling of seropositive animals. These techniques are far less successful than complete repopulation with disease-free pigs.
b. **Contagious pleuropneumonia**
   (1) **Economic implication.** This disease is of major economic importance, is worldwide in occurrence, and appears to be increasing in prevalence with the more intensive swine operations.
   (2) **Patient profile and history.** The disease is predominately found in growing pigs, from ages 2 to 6 months.
   (3) **Clinical findings**
      (a) The disease is characterized by rapid onset and a short course of **severe dyspnea,** the passage of blood-stained foam from the mouth, and a high case-fatality rate.
      (b) **Clinical course.** The disease can be **peracute, acute,** or **chronic,** depending on the immune status, and each form is reasonably well defined. The clinical course of the disease in a herd can last several weeks, with new acute cases occurring as chronically affected animals develop a generally unthrifty appearance.
         (i) In **peracute cases,** the only sign is sudden death in pigs that may be close to market weight.
         (ii) In **acute cases,** severe respiratory distress is observed along with an exaggerated abdominal component (thumps), a reluctance to move, anorexia, and a fever up to 41°C.
         (iii) In more **chronic cases,** there is fever and anorexia, but the respiratory distress is less severe and a persistent cough develops.
   (4) **Etiology and pathogenesis**
      (a) **Etiology.** The condition is caused by *Actinobacillus pleuropneumonia* (formerly known as *Hemophilus pleuropneumonia*), a highly contagious organism that is not isolated from normal porcine respiratory tissues but persists in chronic lesions in the lungs of recovered and apparently healthy pigs, which provide the source for continued infection.
      (b) **Pathogenesis**
         (i) It is thought that natural **transmission** occurs by the aerogenous route, with the source of infection being a subclinically infected or recovered pig. Outbreaks appear to occur in pigs that lack immunity and are overcrowded or subjected to recent stressors, such as large

fluctuations in temperature, recent transportation, or problems with ventilation in the barn.

    (ii) When the organism begins to multiply in the lung (within hours of infection), there is rapid development of **pulmonary edema** and diffuse neutrophilic bronchiolitis and alveolitis. There are also marked vascular effects, which result in infarcts in the lung, thrombosis, and hemorrhage. A hemorrhage, in turn, may result in the pleural inflammation. Pigs appear to die of septic shock.

  (5) Diagnostic plan and laboratory tests. The clinical signs in growing pigs of rapid onset and sudden death associated with respiratory signs provides a presumptive diagnosis. Culture at necropsy confirms the infection, and there is a reliable serological test to assess recent infection in the live animals.

  (6) Therapeutic plan. Antimicrobial treatment, with drugs such as tetracyclines, spectinomycin, or penicillin, can reduce mortality and improve daily gain in affected pigs. However, the animals treated often continue to remain infected with the organism. Therefore, combined with the peracute losses not possible to prevent, the overall clinical response to treatment can be disappointing.

  (7) Prevention

    (a) Depopulation followed by **repopulation** with uninfected pigs is the only effective control method for this infection. The all-in, all-out system of feeding and marketing pigs can help by reducing the introduction of new stock to the herd.

    (b) Management practices that can reduce the impact of this disease should emphasize the raising of weaned pigs in pens that are separate from the older stock in the herd.

    (c) Vaccination is effective in reducing mortality, but vaccinated animals can still be carriers. A major problem plaguing the production of an effective vaccine is the large number of serotypes of *Actinobacillus pleuropneumonia*, against which effective serotype-specific vaccines incorporating all the important antigens have yet to be produced.

C. **Parasitic pneumonia**

  1. Equine parasitic pneumonia

    a. Lung worms

      (1) Patient profile and history. The donkey is the natural host of the equine lungworm *Dictyocaulus arnfieldi*. Horses become infected when they graze pastures with infected donkeys or previously contaminated pastures. The common complaints include a persistent cough, increased respiratory rate, and forced expiration in horses. Donkeys usually show no signs even with heavy infestation.

      (2) Clinical findings. The predominate clinical sign is a chronic cough. Horses are afebrile, and their appetites are unaffected.

      (3) Etiology and pathogenesis. The larvae migrate through the gut wall and are carried hematogenously to the lungs.

        (a) In the **donkey,** the larvae mature in the bronchi and lay eggs. The eggs are coughed up and swallowed.

        (b) In the **horse,** the maturation of the larvae in the airways is retarded, and the worms remain immature; thus, the infection does not become patent. Lung pathology is limited to the caudal lobes. There is epithelial hyperplasia with an increase in size and number of goblet cells. Grossly, there are areas of overinflation, mucous exudate, and coiled worms.

      (4) Diagnostic plan and laboratory tests. Clinical signs of lungworm infestation must be differentiated from chronic obstructive pulmonary disease (COPD).

        (a) Clinical suspicion. Exposure to donkeys on pasture is suggestive of lungworm infestation, and although this infestation is not patent in horses and is fecal Baerman-negative, it may be useful to perform **fecal sedimentation** on any closely housed donkeys.

        (b) A **transtracheal aspirate** shows neutrophils and eosinophils, and **bronchoalveolar lavage** may recover intact lungworms.

    (5) Therapeutic plan. Anthelmintics, such as **fenbendazole** (30 mg/kg) or **ivermectin** (200 μg/kg orally), are effective treatment. Animals may initially worsen with treatment because of the death of larvae causing an intense inflammatory response. Therefore, affected horses may benefit from concurrent treatment with anti-inflammatory agents, such as **nonsteroidal anti-inflammatory drugs (NSAIDs), or a glucocorticoid.**

    (6) Prevention. Donkeys should be treated with appropriate anthelmintics, and pastures should be rotated. In temperate regions, the parasites are unable to survive during winter on pasture. Most routine broad-spectrum anthelmintic regimens for intestinal parasites also control lungworms in horses.

  b. Parascarid migration in foals

    (1) Patient profile and history. This disease occurs in foals and weanlings, with cough as the main complaint.

    (2) Clinical findings. Signs consist of a transient episode of coughing accompanied by a mucopurulent nasal discharge. Throughout the episode, the rectal temperature remains normal, and there is seldom sufficient damage in the lungs to cause a noticeable increase in the respiratory rate or depth.

    (3) Etiology and pathogenesis. The disease is caused by the ascarid *Parascaris equorum* in the course of its development as an intestinal parasite of foals. When foals are infected with *P. equorum* eggs through ingestion, the larvae penetrate the gut wall and undergo a hepatic–tracheal migration. The larvae arrive by a hematogenous route and then migrate up the airways and return to the intestine to mature. Their presence in the airways stimulates mucus production. Signs are usually transient.

    (4) Diagnostic plan and laboratory tests. As in lungworm infections, a transtracheal aspirate or bronchoalveolar lavage may show eosinophils present in the cytology. However, as the clinical signs are usually mild and the clinical course transient, such diagnostic procedures are seldom performed.

    (5) Differential diagnoses. This infection must be differentiated from other causes of coughing in foals, particularly the far more prevalent viral respiratory infections.

    (6) Therapeutic plan. Most of the commonly used anthelmintics for horses are effective against adult *P. equorum,* with ivermectin also being effective against the larval stages.

2. Bovine parasitic pneumonia

  a. Patient profile and history. This disease occurs most commonly in dairy calves that are younger than 1 year of age in the summer and fall of the first season at pasture. Clinical disease may also occur in adult cattle that have minimal prior exposure to the parasite and have recently moved onto heavily contaminated pasture.

  b. Clinical findings

    (1) Acute form. In acute cases, severe verminous pneumonia occurs. Acute cases **progress quickly,** and death from progressive respiratory failure can occur in 3–14 days. This form of the disease occurs in calves 1–2 weeks after being moved to heavily contaminated pasture, and many calves are affected simultaneously.

        (a) There is a sudden onset of **rapid shallow breathing** with a marked abdominal component. Accompanying this is a frequent **deep cough** and a **fever** that may reach 41°C.

        (b) On **auscultation,** all portions of the lung are affected with increased bronchial tones and fine crackles. The animals can remain reasonably bright and active and attempt to eat, although severe respiratory distress may prevent eating.

    (2) Subacute form. The more common form of the disease is a subacute verminous pneumonia, which has a prolonged clinical course of 3–4 weeks.

        (a) In these cases, the onset is also sudden, with an **increased respiratory rate**

(60–70 beats/minute), frequent paroxysms of coughing, and, in severe cases, an expiratory grunt. The body temperature, however, is normal or only slightly elevated. There may also be evidence of recent **diarrhea.**

(b) On **auscultation** of the lungs, there are crackles and wheezes bilaterally and some areas of ventral dullness on chest percussion, suggesting pulmonary consolidation.

(c) Affected animals **lose weight rapidly,** and although the mortality rate is much lower than in the acute form, surviving calves have severely damaged lungs that result in labored breathing for several months. In addition, these calves are predisposed to secondary bacterial pneumonia or a proliferative pneumonia of possible allergic origin.

c. **Etiology and pathogenesis**

(1) **Etiology.** Both forms of the disease are consistent with bronchopneumonia caused by the pulmonary reaction to the invasion of the larvae of *Dictyocaulus viviparus.*

(a) The **acute form** is likely the result of massive invasion of larvae.

(b) Moderate infestations lead to the **subacute form,** with light infestations resulting in few clinical signs.

(2) **Pathogenesis**

(a) **Transmission.** Pastures are contaminated with the infective third-stage larvae. These larvae develop in feces at pasture, and although they are inactive, the larvae are spread by:

(i) Diarrhea

(ii) Rain

(iii) A high concentration of animals

(iv) Earthworms

(v) The propelling of larvae in the explosive discharge (up to 3 m spread) of the fungus *Pilobolus*

(b) **Route of infection**

(i) The infective larvae are ingested by the susceptible animal and migrate from the intestinal tract, via the lymphatics and venous circulation, to the alveoli (1–7 days).

(ii) After a prepatent phase of 7–25 days, larvae mature in the bronchi and trachea and release eggs, which are coughed up, swallowed, and passed in the feces as larvae (having hatched in the intestine). Larvae are resistant to freezing and can survive the winter on pasture, particularly in cool, moist areas where herbage is long.

(iii) The adult worms survive in the bronchi for approximately 7 weeks, by which time immunity develops, and there is self-cure because most worms die or are discharged.

(c) The **pathology** found is that of **lung lobe consolidation** and an eosinophilic and macrophage response to aspirated eggs and new larvae. Parasitic infection and the subsequent inflammation predisposes the lung to secondary bacterial infection. Therefore, parasitic and secondary bacterial pneumonia may subsequently be difficult to differentiate.

(d) There is also a **reinfection syndrome** in which adults with immunity are exposed to massive numbers of infective larvae. These cattle can develop respiratory disease solely because of their immune reaction, with lymphoid proliferation around dead larvae, no adult worms at necropsy, and no eggs released during the course of the illness.

d. **Diagnostic plan and laboratory tests**

(1) **Clinical suspicion.** When clinically apparent, parasitic pneumonia may be difficult to differentiate from bacterial or viral pneumonia. However:

(a) Failure to respond to standard treatment for these conditions and disease occurring at pasture in the summer or fall support a diagnosis of verminous pneumonia.

(b) A **useful clinical feature** of verminous pneumonia is that the associated cough is relatively soft and paroxysmal rather than the harsh, dry cough of viral pneumonia.

(2) **Necropsy.** In areas of outbreaks, deaths are also frequent enough to allow post-mortem diagnosis, with the adult worms readily observed in the airways by the naked eye.

(3) **Laboratory studies**

(a) A **transtracheal aspirate** or **bronchoalveolar lavage** shows greatly increased numbers of eosinophils and possibly ova or larvae in the sample.

(b) **Fecal sedimentation** of affected animals should be examined by the **Baerman technique** for the presence of lungworm larvae.

e. **Therapeutic plan**

(1) Most modern, **broad-spectrum anthelmintics** [e.g., albendazole at 7.5 mg/kg orally, levamisole (13.6%) at 8 mg/kg subcutaneously, fenbendazole at 5 mg/kg orally] are active against all stages of *D. viviparus.* **Ivermectin** (0.2 mg/kg subcutaneously) is particularly effective against the immature and mature stages, even at one-fourth of the recommended dose. With the full recommended dose, residual protection is provided for up to 28 days.

(2) The topical formulations of both levamisole and ivermectin are also effective. However, killing the parasite does not resolve the damage already present in the lungs.

f. **Prevention**

(1) **Management strategies.** Much of the prevention rests on pasture management, such as preventing overcrowding and avoiding continuous use of the same pasture for young stock. Wet, swampy pastures allow maximal larval development and, therefore, should be used for grazing only the adult (immune) animals.

(2) **Deworming.** After winter housing, yearlings should be dewormed before release onto pasture so that they do not begin a new cycle of pasture contamination.

(3) **Vaccination.** In Europe, a vaccine is available that consists of irradiated larvae that cannot mature. This vaccine is administered orally to calves before they are turned out to pasture. This primes the immune response in advance of any exposure to natural infection.

3. **Ovine and caprine parasitic pneumonia**

a. **Etiology.** Lungworms that affect sheep and goats include *Dictyocaulus filaria, Protostrongylus rufescens,* and *Müellerius capillaris.* Each organism is capable of causing varying degrees of verminous pneumonia, but the former two appear to be of greater clinical significance.

(1) *D. filaria* is usually found in the posterodorsal region of the diaphragmatic lobes and may lead to secondary pneumonia and pleuritis. Although it is primarily a parasite of sheep, it is highly pathogenic to young goats.

(2) *P. rufescens* invades small bronchioles and may lead to secondary pneumonia and pleuritis.

(3) *M. capillaris* infections in adult sheep usually result in nodular or diffuse lesions in the subpleural parenchyma and have been considered to be of minimal significance. However, recent reports suggest that this parasite may cause widespread interstitial pneumonia in goats, with affected animals gradually losing condition.

b. **Clinical findings**

(1) *D. filaria* infection produces a cough that results from bronchial irritation, along with moderate dyspnea and loss of condition. Extreme dyspnea occurs if most airways become plugged with debris.

(2) *P. rufescens* infestations cause clinical signs similar to those of *D. filaria,* with only the kids and lambs showing serious clinical involvement. In contrast to the direct life cycle of *D. filaria, P. rufescens* is indirect, requiring a land snail for the second stage of larval development. Because of this, massive infestations are unlikely to occur.

(3) Infection with *M. capillaris* is relatively innocuous clinically but may constitute a limiting factor in the production of choice lambs.

    c. Diagnostic plan and laboratory tests. The main method of diagnosis is Baerman examination of the feces for the larvae of each lungworm parasite.

    d. Therapeutic plan

       (1) Most of the **broad-spectrum anthelmintics** such as albendazole (3.8 mg/kg), fenbendazole (5 mg/kg), ivermectin (0.2 mg/kg), or levamisole (8 mg/kg), are effective against *D. filaria*. Few of these drugs have been tested against *P. rufescens,* but they are likely effective.

       (2) *M. capillaris* is more difficult to treat, with anthelmintics usually only effective against the adult forms. Efficacy against all forms of the parasite requires treatment with products such as fenbendazole or albendazole in the feed for 2 weeks.

    e. Prevention. Preventing parasitic pneumonia by pasture rotation is difficult. Larvae of *D. filaria* can withstand long periods of freezing. Snails, which are the intermediate hosts of *P. rufescens* and *M. capillaris,* are particularly prevalent in poorly drained pastures. Fencing of wet areas of pastures may be beneficial.

4. Parasitic pneumonia in swine

    a. Patient profile and etiology. Parasitic pneumonia occurs in pigs that are raised in management systems that allow access to earthworms and is most prevalent in pigs ages 4–6 months. Lungworms that infest pigs include *Metastrongylus apri* (most common), *M. salmi,* or *M. pudendotectus,* with mixed infections possible.

    b. Clinical findings. Clinical cases show a barking cough that is easily induced by exercise, resulting from the parasitic bronchitis. In severe cases, pneumonia, poor growth, and debilitation can occur, but minimal clinical signs are apparent after experimental disease.

    c. Pathogenesis. The parasite lays eggs in the lungs of the pig. The eggs are then coughed up, swallowed, and passed in the manure. The embryonated eggs or larvae are eaten by earthworms and develop successively to second- and third-stage larvae. Reinfection occurs when the earthworm is eaten by other pigs.

    d. Diagnostic plan. Necropsy is usually the method of diagnosis.

    e. Therapeutic plan. Many of the broad-spectrum anthelmintics are effective, including levamisole (8 mg/kg) in the feed, mebendazole for 2 days successively in the feed (15 mg/kg), or a single injection of ivermectin.

    f. Prevention

       (1) Pigs that run in dirt yards or at pasture should be moved at short intervals to prevent the ingestion of infected earthworms.

       (2) Rooting by pigs can be prevented by providing adequate feed and by applying nose rings.

       (3) Pastures that are known to be contaminated should not be restocked for at least 6 months.

D. Aspiration pneumonia

1. Patient profile and history. Aspiration pneumonia can occur in any species, and the outcome is largely dependent on the nature of the material aspirated. In horses and cows, this disease can occur as a result of misdirection of a stomach tube and subsequent introduction of fluid destined for the intestinal tract. Horses are also at risk for aspiration pneumonia in cases of choke (esophageal obstruction) or secondary to pharyngeal paralysis associated with guttural pouch mycosis. A severe form of aspiration pneumonia can occur in cows with third-stage milk fever, where regurgitation and aspiration of rumen contents can occur.

2. Clinical findings

    a. The **most severe form** of aspiration, as occurs in cattle with rumen content aspiration, is a necrotizing pneumonia that progresses to pleuritis. There is also toxemia with cardiovascular collapse and rapid death. In these cases, breath odors are usually extremely foul, indicative of the necrotic lung tissue.

    b. When much smaller quantities of material are aspirated (e.g., following choke or pharyngeal paralysis in a horse), the signs of pneumonia are **less severe,** with varying degrees of respiratory distress, fever, depression, and cough.

3. **Diagnostic plan and laboratory tests**
   a. A diagnosis is often apparent from the **history,** such as signs of pneumonia closely following recent unsuccessful attempts at oral or gastric medication. Additionally, **food material at the external nostrils** can indicate pharyngeal dysfunction.
   b. If the animal is not in severe respiratory distress, **endoscopic examination** of the trachea can confirm the diagnosis by observing food material in the lower trachea.
   c. **Other diagnostic aids** include **chest radiographs,** which vary greatly in appearance depending on the many circumstances associated with the aspiration. **Transtracheal aspirate cytology** may show plant material, and the **culture** results are often a mixture of gram-positive, gram-negative, and anaerobic bacteria.

4. **Therapeutic plan**
   a. When aspiration has occurred, treatment is used to control infection and inflammation as the lung defenses deal with neutralizing and expelling the foreign material.
      (1) **Broad-spectrum antibiotics** that are effective against anaerobic bacteria are recommended (e.g., combinations of penicillin with an aminoglycoside, or potentiated sulfonamide).
      (2) **NSAIDs,** such as flunixin meglumine, can help reduce lung inflammation, and cardiovascular support with intravenous fluids is indicated where there are signs of toxemia. Pleuritis is often present in severe cases and may require drainage of the pleural fluid (see I E).
   b. Other treatment measures are dependent on the associated cause, such as choke, milk fever, or pharyngeal dysfunction, which should be corrected concurrently if possible.

5. **Prognosis.** The prognosis for recovery from severe aspiration pneumonia is grave. Although less fulminant cases of aspiration pneumonia are often readily responsive to treatment, a successful outcome is more dependent on resolving the underlying disorder (e.g., choke, pharyngeal paralysis or dysfunction).

E. **Pleuritis and pleural effusion**

1. **Introduction**
   a. **Pleural surfaces.** The pleural surfaces of the thorax are composed of the visceral and parietal pleura.
      (1) The **visceral pleura,** which covers the lung surface, lacks specific pain receptors.
      (2) The **parietal pleura,** which lines the chest wall, diaphragm, and mediastinum, contains pain receptors; thus, when the pleural lining is inflamed, it can be a source of significant pain for the animal.
   b. **Mediastinum**
      (1) In **cattle, sheep, goats,** and **pigs,** the mediastinum, which separates the right from left pleural spaces, is **intact.** In species with a complete mediastinum, disease processes (e.g., pneumothorax, pleuritis) may be restricted to one pleural space, with the opposite lung and pleural space unaffected.
      (2) The **horse** has a thin mediastinum that is frequently perforated. The same disease processes in horses can move from affected to unaffected sides of the thorax.
   c. **Pleural fluid.** The visceral and parietal pleura are in close contact with each other. This proximity creates a potential space that is lubricated by a small amount of pleural fluid in which equal amounts are produced and then resorbed. Effusion in large quantities arises mainly when there is increased vascular permeability and reduction of lymphatic drainage, as occurs in inflammation of the pleura.

2. **Patient profile and history.** The history is variable.
   a. In **horses,** this disease often is associated with stressful events, such as recent transport over long distances or a stressful competition following viral respiratory disease.
   b. In **other species** such as cattle, pleuritis can be part of the pneumonia complex of *Pasteurella* infection (see I B 2).

3. Clinical findings
  a. Pain
    (1) Animals with acute pleuritis show chest pain and are sensitive to touch over the thorax.
    (2) Other signs of pain include abduction of the elbows, reluctance to lie down, and a splinted abdomen. In horses, these signs are sometimes misinterpreted as a sign of colic.
  b. Accompanying signs can include the presence of guarded, shallow respiration with a shallow cough and a nasal discharge, which may have a fetid odor. Anorexia, depression, and fever are usually present. Ventral edema in the brisket area, when present, is a hallmark of the effects of the pleural inflammatory process.
  c. In **chronic cases,** the signs may be less obvious, with weight loss, anorexia, depression, or ventral edema being the only significant clinical findings.
    (1) On **auscultation** of the lungs, there is usually an absence of lung sounds ventrally, which is accompanied by widely radiating heart sounds.
    (2) Pleural friction rubs may be detected but are surprisingly not a consistent finding in pleuritis.
    (3) There is **ventral dullness** on percussion of the chest.
  d. In **acute cases** in the horse, ventral dullness is often associated with a horizontal fluid line. Because the disease in cattle is most often a component of diffuse fibrinous pleuropneumonia, no discrete horizontal line is to be expected on chest percussion.

4. Etiology
  a. Equine pleuritis results from the stress of transport, trauma of perforating thoracic wounds, esophageal perforation, or, less commonly, lymphosarcoma or accompanying equine infectious anemia. Solely infectious causes also are sporadically reported and include infections by *Mycoplasma felis* or *Nocardia* species.
  b. Bovine pleuritis is usually secondary to *Pasteurella* pneumonia or traumatic reticuloperitonitis. An infectious cause of bovine pleuritis, contagious bovine pleuropneumonia *(Mycoplasma mycoides* var *mycoides),* caused large losses in the North American cattle population when the continent was being settled, but this has been eradicated from the continent.
  c. Porcine pleuritis. Pigs have pleuritis and pleural effusion as part of actinobacillosis and in polyserositis of Glasser's disease caused by *Hemophilus suis* or *parasuis* infection, which also results in acute arthritis, peritonitis, and pericarditis (see Chapters 8 and 13).

5. Diagnostic plan and laboratory tests
  a. The **clinical signs** of systemic illness, accompanied by chest pain and shallow breathing, are highly suggestive of pleuritis. Thoracic percussion in the acute phase is suggestive of fluid within the chest.
  b. Of the **laboratory tests** available, both hematology and routine biochemistry are nonspecific. A neutrophilia with or without left shift and possibly an anemia of chronic infection may be noted on hematology, and low albumin accompanied by elevations in fibrinogen and globulins are observed on biochemistry.
  c. More definitive tests for diagnosis include radiology, ultrasonography, and thoracocentesis.
    (1) On **chest radiographs,** there is a pleural effusion line and often signs of an accompanying pneumonia, pulmonary abscess, or both. With adult horses and cows, this finding is often restricted in value because the large chest size reduces the diagnostic quality of the radiographs.
    (2) Chest ultrasound is highly sensitive for the detection of pleural fluid and can provide information regarding pleural thickening, loculation of pleural fluid, and the presence of fibrin. Also, hyperechoic echoes in the pleural fluid can suggest the presence of gas bubbles caused by anaerobic bacteria. These findings dictate highly specific therapy and an unfavorable prognosis.
    (3) Thoracocentesis is often key in assisting in diagnosis, therapy, and prognosis.

(a) Fluid recovered varies from a clear yellow transudate in milder cases to cloudy and even purulent fluid in more severe cases.

(i) **Normal pleural fluid** is difficult to obtain by thoracocentesis and has a cell count of less than 10,000/μl white blood cell count (10 $\times$ 10^9/L). Although cell counts can increase greatly in pleuritis, there is a large range in cell counts, and there has been no correlation of pleural fluid cell numbers with survival.

(ii) Fluid with a **foul odor** suggests an anaerobic infection, such as necrotizing pneumonia.

(b) The pleural fluid should be **cultured** for bacteria and should have a Gram stain performed to give an initial guide to treatment. Frequently, there is no growth from this fluid, and a culture and sensitivity from a transtracheal aspirate is then indicated, as many cases of pleuritis have an underlying pulmonary problem or possibly began as pneumonia.

6. **Therapeutic plan.** Chest drainage, appropriate antibiotics, and supportive nursing care are required for horses with pleuritis. The other large animal species seldom receive similar intensive care; thus, this discussion focuses on the horse. Should treatment be required, similar methods can be used for specific treatment of pleuritis in other species.

   a. **Drainage** of pleural fluid is important if the process in the chest is highly purulent.

   (1) **Continuous drainage** can be managed by using indwelling chest drains with a one-way Heimlich valve, but this is a labor-intensive venture and may not be practical, particularly in many stable environments. This method is associated with complications, such as cellulitis and possible pneumothorax.

   (2) Alternatively, **repeated thoracocentesis** can be performed every several days until the pleural inflammation subsides with treatment. In chronic pleuritis, fibrous adhesions often impair complete drainage.

   b. **Antibiotics.** Selection of the appropriate antibiotic for treatment is initially based on Gram-stain results.

   (1) In horses, **sodium penicillin** (20,000 IU/kg intravenously every 6 hours) and **gentamicin** (2.2 mg/kg intravenously every 8 hours) are commonly chosen because this combination is effective against most gram-positive, gram-negative, and non-*Bacillus fragilis* anaerobic bacteria.

   (2) In circumstances in which *B. fragilis* is involved, (penicillinase producers) **metronidazole** should be added to the regimen (25 mg/kg orally every 12 hours).

   (3) Alternatively in horses, **chloramphenicol** (25 mg/kg orally every 6 hours) can be used as a sole treatment. Chloramphenicol should not be used in food-producing animals.

   c. **Supportive care.** Stress should be minimized. Rest and fluids should be provided as required. Pain relief using NSAIDs (e.g., phenylbutazone, flunixin meglumine) may help the animal regain its appetite and increase its comfort.

   d. **Additional treatment**

   (1) **Heparin** (40 IU/kg subcutaneously every 12 hours) may decrease adhesion formation.

   (2) For chronic, one-sided pleuropneumonia, **rib resection** and **thoracotomy** to drain purulent material has been a successful salvage procedure.

7. **Prognosis.** On initial assessment, the prognosis is often poor, particularly for return to performance. Also, pleuritis is very expensive to treat. However, there is a wide range in recovery, from respiratory cripples to apparently complete resolution. The prognosis is guarded in anaerobic and gram-negative infections with accompanying pneumonia, pulmonary abscess, or both. Conversely, some horses with mild pleural effusion appear to have full recovery. Unfortunately, no one laboratory parameter accurately determines the prognosis.

F. **Noninfectious respiratory diseases**

1. **Metastatic pneumonia** (also called **vena cava syndrome**)

   a. **Patient profile and history.** This disease occurs in cattle older than 1 year and can occur in any breed, sex, or class of cattle. The main complaints may include weight loss, respiratory disturbance, or occasionally thoracic pain.

b. Clinical findings

(1) Affected cattle with a **classic presentation** of this syndrome have tachycardia, tachypnea, and expiratory dyspnea with groaning and wheezes over much of the chest. Accompanying these signs are epistaxis, hemoptysis, pale mucous membranes, and hemic murmurs. The combination of **anemia, widespread wheezes,** and **hemoptysis** is generally regarded as pathognomonic for this disease. The affected animal often has a history of weight loss and cough for weeks to months, but in some cases, the signs may be acute.

(2) **Other clinical signs** include fever, thoracic pain on deep palpation of the sternum, hepatomegaly, subcutaneous emphysema, froth at the muzzle, and melena caused by swallowing the blood that is being coughed up.

c. Etiology and pathogenesis

(1) This disease is thought to develop from an **initial rumenitis secondary to lactic acidosis** (see Chapter 3 1 A 2). As a result of the chemical damage to the rumen epithelium, bacteria (e.g., *Fusobacterium necrophorum, Actinobacillus pyogenes*) are able to penetrate the rumen epithelium to be transported to the liver portal drainage system, where they are filtered and cause liver abscesses. If an abscess is located adjacent to the caudal vena cava, it may result in the development of septic emboli within the caval vein. This condition then showers the lungs and causes pulmonary arterial thrombosis and pulmonary abscessation, along with pulmonary hypertension and aneurysm formation.

(2) The eventual **hemoptysis** that is so clinically distinctive is the result of erosion of a pulmonary abscess into an arterial wall, rupture of a pulmonary aneurysm, or both. Other signs, such as anemia, hemic murmur, melena, and widespread wheezes are directly related to the massive lung bleeding.

d. Diagnostic plan and laboratory tests. In patients with the pathognomonic signs, usually no further diagnostic tests are required.

(1) The **CBC** shows anemia and a neutrophilic leukocytosis. **Serum chemistry** may have hyperglobulinemia and liver enzyme changes (elevated aspartate aminotransferase, γ-glutamyl transferase) merely reflective of passive congestion.

(2) **Chest radiography** usually shows only an irregular increase in lung density, but in some cases, there may be more definitive changes, including small discrete densities indicative of embolic infarction and collapse or large spherical densities with cavitating nodules and gas or fluid interfaces.

e. Therapeutic plan

(1) The **case fatality rate** is **usually 100%.** Thus, when the diagnosis is established, treatment is rarely indicated.

(2) In valuable animals, **supportive treatment** can be undertaken, such as **blood transfusion** in the acute stage, along with **furosemide** (0.4–1.1 mg/kg intravenously or intramuscularly twice daily) and **flunixin meglumine** (0.5–1.1 mg/kg intravenously or intramuscularly given one to three times daily) as needed for the dyspnea. For the organisms usually involved, **penicillin** is the drug of choice, with a dose of 22,000 U/kg intramuscularly twice daily for extended periods (weeks to months).

f. Prevention. Because the initiating basis of this disease is rumenitis with subsequent liver abscess formation, measures to reduce the possibility of developing vena cava syndrome include:

(1) Slowing the introduction of high-energy rations to the cattle

(2) Feeding antibiotics during the periods of increase in concentrate feed

2. Chronic obstructive pulmonary disease (COPD)

a. Patient profile and history

(1) This is a **worldwide disease of horses** that are usually more than 5 years of age and is seen more frequently in stabled animals.

(2) Clinical signs associated with COPD (also known as chronic airway disease, heaves, broken wind, emphysema, chronic bronchiolitis, or recurrent airway

obstruction) are usually exacerbated by **poor environmental conditions,** such as poor ventilation, overcrowding, dusty stables, or breathing molds from stored feeds.

b. Clinical findings

   (1) The **main complaint** is a chronic cough and sometimes an associated exercise intolerance. The cough is usually worse when the horse is stabled. Other common signs include bilateral mucopurulent nasal discharge, dyspnea characterized by nostril flaring, an abdominal lift to the expiration, abdominal muscle hypertrophy (heave line), and pumping of the anus on respiration.

   (2) On examination of the **lung fields,** there are often crackles, wheezes, or both on auscultation, and expanded caudal lung borders with hyperresonance on chest percussion.

   (3) Affected horses are **afebrile** and usually maintain an excellent appetite and demeanor, unless the increased effort of breathing is severe enough to interfere with eating. In such circumstances, weight loss may also occur.

c. Etiology and pathogenesis

   (1) Etiology. Proposed instigating factors for horses developing COPD include previous respiratory viral infection, allergies to dust and fungal spores, dietary factors such as ingestion of 3-methylindole, and, in some horses, genetic predisposition.

   (2) Pathogenesis

   (a) Irrespective of the initiating cause, the affected horse develops **excessive pulmonary reactivity** to ill-defined airborne allergens, which, when present in sufficient concentration in the ambient air, induce clinical signs. Conversely, affected horses can be relatively **free of any clinical signs** when not exposed to these allergens and in dust-free settings.

   (b) The **structural changes** seen in the **lungs** of affected horses with these clinical signs vary from chronic bronchiolitis with diffuse epithelial hyperplasia and mucus plugs to acinar overinflation and peribronchiolar fibrosis and cellular infiltration.

d. Diagnostic plan and laboratory tests

   (1) Clinical signs of chronic recurrent cough in an older horse associated with stabling and no systemic sign of illness is usually sufficient for establishing a diagnosis.

   (2) Laboratory studies. The **CBC** is almost invariably normal. **Transtracheal aspirate** or **bronchoalveolar lavage cytology** reveals large numbers of non-degenerative neutrophils, which are present in the lower airways because of immune stimulation rather than bacterial infection.

   (3) Atropine challenge. Horses can be **tested pharmacologically** for the presence of airway spasm by administering atropine (0.022 mg/kg intravenously). Resolution of clinical signs of dyspnea and improvement of lung sounds constitutes a positive response. These results also determine the proportion of the clinical signs caused by reversible bronchospasm, which can be treated with bronchodilator treatment.

   (4) Arterial blood gas determination and pulmonary function testing. A resting arterial oxygen tension (PaO_2) of less than 83 mm Hg and a maximum change in intrapleural pressure with a tidal breath of greater than 6 mm Hg are suggestive.

   (5) Chest radiographs may demonstrate prominent bronchial and interstitial markings but seldom contribute substantially to diagnosis or disease management.

e. Differential diagnoses. The differential diagnoses can include bacterial pneumonia, pulmonary neoplasia, and diffuse restrictive diseases. Radiography and lung biopsy are the primary tools for these differentiations.

f. Therapeutic plan

   (1) Management strategies

   (a) Improvement of air quality in the horse's environment is the most important factor in managing the clinical signs and decreasing the progression of the disease. The horse should spend as much time as possible outside on pasture.

    (b) During any necessary **period of stabling,** the stall should have ample fresh air (e.g., next to a door or window), and the bedding should be as dust free as possible (e.g., peat moss, shredded newspaper). Hay should be thoroughly soaked in water or the feed changed to a complete pelleted ration. Special moist silage for horses is also commercially available and quite effective in minimizing dust from the feed source. Environmental changes must be complete and permanent, otherwise clinical signs will rapidly recur following lapses in dust control.

  (2) **Medications** include bronchodilators for the bronchospasm, expectorants to aid in decreasing the mucus buildup in the airways, and corticosteroids to decrease airway inflammation.

    (a) Commonly available **bronchodilators** include clenbuterol (available in Canada only), aminophylline-theophylline, ephedrine, and antihistamines.

      (i) **Aerosol therapy** is now possible with products such as terbutaline (a β_2 agonist) or ipatromium bromide (parasympatholytic or atropine-like in action), in conjunction with recent production of medicating face masks for horses.

      (ii) Though not a bronchodilator, the mast-cell stabilizer **cromolyn sodium** also can be administered by the aerosol route and is effective if given to horses that have a component of immediate (type I) hypersensitivity to their airway reactivity.

    (b) **Expectorants,** which include iodides, glyceryl guaiacolate, or simple nebulization with saline, are often used as adjunctive treatment but are of lesser benefit alone in resolving clinical signs.

    (c) **Corticosteroids** are reserved usually for horses that are not responsive to the previous treatment. Although their full effects on the lungs remain poorly understood, corticosteroids do reduce airway inflammation and promote airway smooth-muscle relaxation. **Prednisone** can be given for a severe episode at 1 mg/kg orally twice daily with tapering doses by half every sixth or seventh day and discontinued entirely when the environmental challenge is solved. Some horse may benefit from prolonged administration of low levels of corticosteroids (prednisone 0.5 mg/kg orally every 48 hours).

    (d) **Antibacterials** also may be indicated in selected horses that also have signs of airway sepsis on transtracheal aspiration or systemic signs of bacterial pneumonia. In most North American horses with COPD, antibiotics are seldom indicated or necessary.

3. **Hypersensitivity pneumonitis (extrinsic alveolitis, bovine farmers' lung)**

  a. **Patient profile and history.** This disease occurs almost exclusively in housed adult cattle (particularly dairy cattle) that are fed stored roughage feed. Although the disease occurs sporadically, it appears mainly in the fall, winter, and early spring, when cattle are confined.

  b. **Clinical findings**

    (1) The **main complaint** is usually the increasingly progressive respiratory distress and coughing, along with anorexia and decreased milk production in an individual cow.

    (2) On **clinical examination,** the affected animal shows tachypnea, expiratory dyspnea and a dry, nonproductive cough. There may be a thick nasal discharge, and on chest auscultation, there are increased bronchial sounds and cranioventral crackles. Fever may also be present but it is usually transient.

  c. **Etiology and pathogenesis.** The respiratory distress is attributable to a hypersensitivity reaction to thermophylic molds *(Micropolyspora faeni* and *Thermoactinomyces vulgaris)* that contaminate roughage feeds. Antigen exposure in sensitized individuals activates cellular and humoral immune responses. The pulmonary inflammation results from complement activation, histamine release, and polymorphonuclear neutrophil and macrophage recruitment. The resulting pathology is interstitial infiltration by lymphocytes, plasma cells, macrophages, and granuloma formation. Healing results in restrictive fibrosis.

d. Diagnostic plan and laboratory tests

(1) On **transtracheal aspirate,** there are neutrophils and macrophages in the cytology but no bacteria unless there is a secondary bacterial pneumonia. It is the absence of these signs of infection that suggests consideration of this immune-mediated disease.

(2) Suspect cattle can have **serum samples** analyzed for the presence of precipitins to the antigens of *M. faeni* and *T. vulgaris.* Also, the *M. faeni* antigen can be administered intradermally, and a positive reaction may be noted as a local Arthus reaction after 4–6 hours.

e. Therapeutic plan. Antihistamines and corticosteroids may provide some relief for individual animals, but when the respiratory signs are noticed, the pulmonary damage is usually irreversible.

f. Prevention. When the producer recognizes the problem, the only change possible in management (if the cattle must be housed for extended periods) is to minimize antigen exposure by feeding hay outside or by feeding silage.

4. Acute respiratory distress syndrome [ARDS, acute bovine pulmonary emphysema and edema (ABPE), fog fever]

a. Patient profile and history. This severe type of respiratory distress occurs in late summer and fall mainly in adult beef cattle (ages 3–8 years) that have a history of having been moved from poor to lush pasture in the previous 1–2 weeks. Geographically, this disease appears to be most prevalent in the western part of North America.

b. Clinical findings

(1) The **main complaint** is usually an acute onset of severe dyspnea or open-mouth breathing, expiratory grunt, and tachypnea in mature cattle, often with several to many in a herd affected simultaneously. Although the heart rates are usually elevated, fever (suggestive of an infectious cause) is not usually a prominent feature.

(2) The **mucous membranes** can become **cyanotic** as respiratory embarrassment advances, and **subcutaneous emphysema** over the shoulders and thoracic inlet may appear as a consequence of the severe respiratory effort. There may even be some cattle found dead with few premonitory signs.

(3) In **acute cases,** there are usually increased bronchial tones over the ventral aspects of the lungs, but the dorsal portions of the lungs are surprisingly silent, with a relative absence of breath sounds despite the obvious respiratory distress. Nursing calves running with the cows are usually completely unaffected.

c. Etiology and pathogenesis

(1) This disease is an interstitial pneumonia with lung changes of pulmonary edema and interstitial emphysema, which is the result of ruminal transformation of dietary L-tryptophan to more toxic 3-methylindole (3-MI).

(a) A **sudden feed change** to lush pasture or brassica plants (e.g., rape, kale, tops of turnips) results in the overgrowth of ruminal lactobacillus, which produces toxic levels of 3-MI from dietary L-tryptophan. The ruminally produced 3-MI is then absorbed into the circulation and is metabolized by microsomal enzymes in the Clara cells of the lung to pneumotoxic metabolites that injure the alveolar and capillary epithelium.

(b) Consequently, there is **plasma transudation** in the exudative stage. If the animal survives, there is a proliferation of type II pneumocytes, alveolar epithelialization, and irreversible fibrosis. At necropsy, there is subpleural and interstitial emphysema, alveolar edema, epithelial hyperplasia, and hyaline membrane formation.

(2) There are several other causes of ARDS, with the clinical and pathologic pictures being indistinguishable from the mechanism described in I F 4 c (1). These other causes include:

(a) **Pulmonary damage by mixed function oxidase metabolism of other**

       xenobiotics (e.g., 4-ipomeanol, a toxin from sweet potatoes infested with the mold *Fusarium solani*)

     (b) ***Perilla ketona,*** a pneumotoxic principle found in leaves and seeds of purple mint *(Perilla frutescens)*; there may be a mint-like odor to the edema fluid as noted at necropsy

     (c) **Inhalation of toxic gases,** such as the manure gases (H_2S, ammonia, methane) or nitrogen dioxide from silos

  d. **Diagnostic plan.** Diagnosis usually rests on the clinical history and risk factors for the possible causes, coupled with the signs of an acute onset of severe respiratory distress without fever or toxemia.

  e. **Differential diagnoses.** Additional causes of acute respiratory distress in cattle that appear to be similar in clinical appearance to ARDS include acute immune reactions such as systemic anaphylaxis, milk allergy, or massive pulmonary migration of parasites.

  f. **Therapeutic plan.** There is nothing specific that can be done to reverse the lung damage of affected cattle. Therefore, the main treatment goal is to reduce the adverse effects of the cell damage and inflammation as well as pulmonary edema.

    (1) **Flunixin meglumine** at 2.2 mg/kg intravenously every 12 hours (extralabel use) is useful for its anti-inflammatory effects and **furosemide** at 0.4–1 mg/kg intravenously or intramuscularly every 12 hours reduces pulmonary edema.

    (2) Equally important in management of these animals is the **avoidance of stress** or **exercise** in hypoxic animals and removal of affected animals from any offending site, such as new pasture or feed source.

  g. **Prognosis.** The prognosis is grave in severely affected animals, for which slaughter and salvage is often the most preferred option. For ARDS associated with 3-MI, clients should be cautioned that removal from pasture may not stop further clinical cases from developing in the short term.

  h. **Prevention.** In ARDS associated with 3-MI, the herd should have limited access to pastures with pathogenic potential, such as alfalfa, kale, rape, turnips, or rapidly growing lush pasture. Where the problem is common and not readily avoidable by appropriate pasture management, monensin or lasalocid (200 mg/head/day) before and during pasture change can prevent the disease because these products inhibit overgrowth of ruminal lactobacilli that convert the dietary L-tryptophan to 3-MI.

5. Exercise-induced pulmonary hemorrhage (EIPH)

  a. **Patient profile and history.** This disorder occurs in horses that undertake strenuous exercise such as racing. There is no relation of its occurrence to gender or finishing position, but its incidence may increase with age. The main complaint is either epistaxis at exercise or, more commonly, poor athletic performance without an obvious cause.

  b. **Clinical findings.** In addition to epistaxis, clinical findings are likely to include problems related to athletic performance. Owners may report suspected EIPH horses as losing speed near the end of the race, after which they may take longer to "cool out." Affected horses may be observed to swallow more frequently during this cooling-off period.

  c. **Etiology and pathogenesis.** The bleeding occurs in mainly the dorsal portions of the lung and appears to be related to events during strenuous exercise. Various theories have been offered to explain EIPH. Rupture of blood vessels is likely necessary for hemorrhage to occur.

    (1) An **older theory** proposes that pulmonary hypertension and edema are the mechanisms of action. This was the rationale for treating the problems with **furosemide.** Furosemide therapy remains a popular treatment for "bleeders" on the race track, but there is no clinical evidence showing improvement of the lung bleeding. More recently, furosemide has been shown to have bronchodilating effects.

    (2) A **more recent theory** is that EIPH occurs in horses that have subclinical lung disease, causing some degree of bronchiolar obstruction.

      (a) This **obstruction** may be sufficient to prevent the filling of the alveoli distal to them when the respiratory rate is increased.

      (b) Consequently, there is **asynchrony** between the air movement of the obstructed segment and the adjacent lung tissue. Because of the interdependence between different structures in the lung, this asynchrony may result in tearing of the lung parenchyma and resultant hemorrhage. This may be particularly true if there is lung scarring and pleural adhesions, which may result from past infections.

   (3) This problem in race horses is the subject of study by many veterinary scientists because it appears to occur in a high proportion of race horses, and current understanding of the pathogenesis remains limited, which hampers effective treatment.

  d. Diagnostic plan and laboratory tests

   (1) Endoscopic examination of the trachea and collection of lower airway secretions for **cytologic examination** are the main methods of diagnosis. Confirmation of EIPH requires direct observation of blood in the trachea after a period of intense exercise. The former use of epistaxis as a diagnostic clinical sign is far too insensitive because whereas 75% of race horses have endoscopic evidence of hemorrhage in the trachea after the race, only 3% of these horses have blood present at the nostrils.

   (2) Cytology of the lower airway secretions, either from transtracheal aspirates or bronchoalveolar lavage, shows alveolar macrophages packed with hemosiderin and, often, ingested red blood cells (hemosiderophages). An additional benefit of assessing lower airway cytology may be determining other underlying airway diseases that may be a predisposing factor in the genesis of EIPH. There appears to be no other test available for confirming the occurrence of EIPH.

  e. Differential diagnoses. When EIPH is only suspected as a cause of performance problems in race horses, all other possible problems affecting performance, particularly lameness, should be ruled out. The differential diagnoses for epistaxis should include upper airway bleeding, such as guttural pouch mycosis, ethmoid hematomas, and trauma. In any horse with poor athletic performance, musculoskeletal, cardiac, and other respiratory problems must be ruled out before the EIPH is incriminated as the sole cause of the problem.

  f. Therapeutic plan. There are no proven effective treatments for EIPH, partly because of the limited understanding of its pathogenesis. If a subclinical obstructive disease is present, then rest and environmental management are indicated.

   (1) The most commonly used drug for treatment is **furosemide** at 0.3–0.8 mg/kg intravenously or intramuscularly 3 hours before racing, which is allowed in some racing jurisdictions for use in horses with EIPH confirmed by post-race endoscopy.

   (2) Many other medications (although not approved for racing) are also in current use for treatment of this problem, but most lack any sound scientific basis for their use.

II. DISEASES OF THE THORAX

A. Diaphragmatic hernia

  1. Patient profile and history. The type of animal affected with a diaphragmatic hernia varies. Often the history includes a previous trauma, such as dystocia, breeding, or foaling trauma, or severe physical exertion. Specific to cattle, traumatic reticuloperitonitis (TRP) is a main cause of this uncommon problem.

  2. Clinical findings. Depending on the extent of the damage to the diaphragm and the amount of abdominal content herniated, the signs can range from mild colic and dyspnea to acute severe colic with tachypnea and obvious dyspnea.

  a. Gastrointestinal sounds may be heard over the thorax, and **lung sounds** can be reduced or even absent over one side of the chest.

b. If the small intestine becomes strangulated in the hernia, there may be **gastric reflux.** In cattle with herniation associated with TRP, **forestomach stasis** can occur.

3. Diagnostic plan

a. Radiography. When diaphragmatic hernia is suspected, **chest radiography** is usually diagnostic. Findings include loss of the diaphragmatic shadow and multiple fluid lines in the thorax that are associated with intestines in the thoracic cavity.

b. Thoracocentesis generally yields a serosanguinous fluid, but this is in no way definitive for this specific diagnosis.

c. Electrocardiography. Animals with diaphragmatic hernias usually have decreased amplitude of QRS complexes on an electrocardiogram (ECG).

4. Therapeutic plan and prognosis. Surgical closure of the diaphragmatic defect is the treatment of choice. Given the size of the large animal patients, the prognosis for success is only fair to guarded even if surgery is performed.

B. Pneumothorax

1. Patient profile and history. As in diaphragmatic hernia, all types of animals can be affected with pneumothorax. Usually there is some history of chest trauma. Undergoing an invasive technique, such as thoracocentesis or lung biopsy, may also be part of the recent history.

2. Clinical findings

a. The **main clinical sign** with pneumothorax is a variable degree of dyspnea, the degree depending largely on the amount of air in the chest and subsequent lung collapse. If pneumothorax is associated with an open chest wound, this is usually obvious.

b. On **chest auscultation,** there is an absence of lung sounds over the affected side because of collapse of lung parenchyma away from the chest wall. In some cases, the air also is found under the skin over the chest in the form of subcutaneous emphysema.

3. Etiology. Trauma to chest from external means, such as a penetrating wound, can result in pneumothorax. Alternatively, air leakage through the visceral pleura of the lung from lung damage, such as in rib fracture or ruptured emphysematous bulla, can also result in pneumothorax.

4. Diagnostic plan. Chest percussion often demonstrates a drum-like resonance with the presence of pneumothorax. Aspiration of air freely from the chest cavity by thoracocentesis confirms the diagnosis. With mild cases, chest radiographs may be the only diagnostic method, with retraction of the lung margins from the dorsal-most part of the thorax.

5. Therapeutic plan. The main goals in treatment of pneumothorax are to remove a sufficient amount of air from the chest cavity to resolve signs of dyspnea and to treat, if possible, the underlying cause.

a. Any penetrating chest wound needs closure, at which time routine wound prophylaxis of antibiotics and administration of tetanus antitoxin (for horses) can be performed.

b. To evacuate the chest of air, a teat canula can be placed into the pleural space and continuous suction applied. Medical suction devices are available for such purposes, but it is also possible to perform this in an ambulatory setting on dairy farms by using the suction from the milk line.

DIRECTIONS: Each of the numbered items or incomplete statements in this section is followed by answers or by completions of the statement. Select the ONE numbered answer or completion that is BEST in each case.

1. Which one of the following statements regarding *Rhodococcus* pneumonia is true?

(1) The treatment of choice is oral rifampin combined with a macrolide, such as lincomycin.

(2) Foals up to 4 months of age can be acutely infected from this soilborne organism; thus, a foal with clinical *R. equi* should be isolated from other foals to prevent the spread of infection.

(3) In addition to pulmonary abscessation, other sequelae to infection can include uveitis, nonseptic arthritis, ulcerative colitis, and vertebral body abscesses.

(4) This organism is able to live and grow within macrophages because it can prevent the fusion of phagosomes to lysosomes and has an antiphagocytic capsule (M protein) that prevents phagocytosis by granulocytes.

(5) Seroconversion to *R. equi,* in conjunction with signs of pneumonia and a leukocytosis, is the preferred method of diagnosis.

2. Which statement regarding enzootic pneumonia in calves is true?

(1) This disease is associated with bacterial pneumonia [secondary to bovine respiratory syncytial virus (BRSV) or parainfluenza-3 (PI-3) infection] or mycoplasmas, such as *Mycoplasma mycoides.*

(2) Enzootic pneumonia can occur in beef calves between ages 2 months and 5 months that are housed indoors in the fall and winter.

(3) Vaccination against viral agents such as BRSV or PI-3 in the first several weeks of life can help prevent this disease.

(4) Cold weather can precipitate this disease when producers leave housing ventilation open, exposing calves to cold outside air.

(5) The pathology is usually a consolidation of cranial, middle, and accessory lung lobes, with mycoplasmal involvement classically resulting in alveolitis and bronchiectasis.

3. Regarding pasteurellosis in ruminants, which one of the following statements is true?

(1) In sheep and goats, pasteurellosis due to *Pasteurella haemolytica* can occur in two forms: rapidly fatal septicemia with biotype T and pneumonia with biotype A.

(2) In cattle, shipping fever pneumonia due to pasteurellosis usually peaks several days after the stressful event.

(3) Vaccination against pasteurellosis in cattle should include the leukotoxin of *P. haemolytica* because it increases specific immunoglobulin A production in the lungs.

(4) Vaccination against pasteurellosis in cattle should include the respiratory viruses [infectious bovine rhinotracheitis (IBR), parainfluenza-3 (PI-3), bovine respiratory syncytial virus (BRSV)] because prior viral infection that accompanies the stress of handling is usually required for development of this disease.

(5) Pathogenic *P. haemolytica* strains can be part of normal pharyngeal flora in cattle, whereas the strains in sheep and goats spread from subclinical carrier animals.

4. Which one of the following statements regarding lungworms in large animals is true?

(1) The lungworm *Dictyocaulus arnfieldi* causes a patent infection in donkeys and results in a persistent cough in these infected animals.
(2) *Metastrongylus* species can cause lungworm in pigs raised outdoors, and though minimal clinical disease is found in experimental infection, the infection can result in exercise-induced cough and poor growth in field situations.
(3) Reinfection syndrome of *D. viviparus* in mature cattle causes disease because effective immunity is short-lived and has waned.
(4) *D. filaria* and *Protostrongylus rufescens* in sheep cause similar clinical signs, but because *P. rufescens* has a direct life cycle, it can cause more severe disease in adults.
(5) Although it causes a low-grade productive cough in growing kids and lambs, *Müellerius capillaris* can be effectively treated with a single dose of fenbendazole.

5. Which one of the following statements regarding pleural disease of large animals is true?

(1) Clinical signs of shallow breathing and chest pain are caused by the inflammation of pain receptors on the visceral pleural surfaces.
(2) Pleural fluid accumulation is usually readily apparent in both horses and cattle with pleuritis.
(3) Unilateral thoracic disease is possible in ruminants because of the intact mediastinum, but disease can spread bilaterally in horses and pigs because of the finer, often perforated mediastinum.
(4) Normal pleural fluid has a cell count of less than 10,000/μl white blood cells, but it is usually difficult to obtain in the clinically normal large animal.
(5) A foul odor of the pleural fluid in cases of pleuritis is suggestive of *Escherichia coli* growth, warranting inclusion of aminoglycoside treatment.

6. A herd of cattle is moved from sparse, meager pasture to a lush grazing of turnip tops. The adult cows develop severe dyspnea, open-mouthed breathing, and in some, subcutaneous emphysema. Which one of the following statements best applies to this problem?

(1) The new pasture was likely higher in 3-methylindole (3-MI), which caused the direct lung damage by acting on the Clara cells.
(2) The lung damage from preformed toxin results in eventual hyaline membrane formation and irreversible fibrosis.
(3) Pretreatment of this herd with monensin or lasalocid before pasture change can prevent such outbreaks.
(4) Nursing calves are less severely affected, with signs of mild expiratory dyspnea and cough.
(5) Associated with the severe respiratory distress, lung sounds are typically harsh with crackles and wheezes over the entire lung field.

7. A horse shows blood at the nostrils following intense exercise. Which one of the following statements is true?

(1) The blood likely originated from the caudal lung lobes as a result of left heart failure and fluid overload of the lungs.
(2) The medication *furosemide* is allowable for this condition in certain racing jurisdictions.
(3) The blood most likely originated from the ethmoid region or guttural pouch because this is an uncommon clinical finding in race horses.
(4) The bleeding clearly indicates a performance-limiting problem.
(5) Treatment with procoagulants, such as aminocaproic acid or vitamin K_3, is indicated.

8. Which one of the following statements regarding thoracic disease in large animals is true?

(1) Diaphragmatic hernia in horses is most often caused by trauma, such as dystocia, whereas in cattle it has been linked to traumatic reticuloperitonitis.

(2) Signs of diaphragmatic hernia in horses can be mild to moderate colic and dyspnea, whereas cattle have occult herniation because the rumen is too large to herniate into the thorax.

(3) Gastrointestinal sounds (borborygmi) heard over the ventral chest of the horse are highly suggestive of diaphragmatic hernia.

(4) In cattle with pneumothorax, there is a drum-like resonance to percussion over the chest and very harsh lung sound ventrally because of the collapse of the lung.

(5) Sometimes uncovered incidentally, finding decreased amplitude of QRS and high spikes on the T wave of an electrocardiogram (ECG) of a horse are suggestive of diapragmatic hernia.

ANSWERS AND EXPLANATIONS

1. The answer is 3 [I A 2 b (2)]. The presently accepted and specific treatment for *Rhodococcus equi* pneumonia of foals is a combination of rifampin and erythromycin estolate. In horses, the use of oral lincomycin can induce fatal colitis. There is little benefit in isolating foals with *R. equi* pneumonia. Foals are resistant at 5 weeks of age; therefore, clinically affected foals pose little danger to most foals on the premises. The organism can prevent fusion of phagosome to lysosome but does not have an M protein capsule. Seroconversion is not a measure of disease because many foals seroconvert because of exposure to *R. equi* without ever developing *R. equi* pneumonia.

2. The answer is 2 [I A 3 a]. The disease can occur in any group of calves (not only dairy) that are between 2 months and 5 months of age and housed indoors, particularly when exposed to older cattle. Bacterial pneumonia, which is the end result of the enzootic pneumonia complex, may be secondary to infection by *Mycoplasma* species, but *M. mycoides* has not been described as a precursor agent. Prevention of enzootic pneumonia involves changing management practices. Vaccination has not proven beneficial because levels of colostral immunity interfere with the timing of vaccination. Cold outside air does not precipitate the disease. The buildup of noxious gases in poorly ventilated spaces has the negative impact on mucociliary clearance. The pathologic description in the last choice is accurate; however, this is the result of bacterial not mycoplasmal involvement.

3. The answer is 1 [I B 3 a]. Pasteurellosis in sheep and goats may appear as an acute septicemia as well as a primary pneumonia. The clinical signs of shipping fever in cattle may not occur until 2 weeks after the stressful event (most commonly co-mingling cattle). Viruses are not essential precursors for the disease. Vaccination is not known to produce protective levels of immunoglobulin A antibodies. Pathogenic *Pasteurella haemolytica* strains can be part of the normal pharyngeal flora in cattle, sheep, and goats.

4. The answer is 2 [I C 4 a]. *Dictyocaulus arnfieldi* does not cause clinical signs in its natural host, the donkey. Re-infection syndrome of *D. viviparus* is experienced in cattle with immunity (i.e., this is an immune-mediated reaction to re-infestation with massive numbers of infection larvae). *Protostrongylus rufescens* has an indirect life cycle, with the land snail as the intermediate host. *Müellarius capillaris* is difficult to treat, requiring treatment with fenbendazole over a 2-week period.

5. The answer is 4 [I E 5 c (3)]. The visceral pleura lacks pain receptors and is not the site of pain with pleuritis. In swine, the mediastinum is intact similar to ruminants. Pleuritis may not be obvious on clinical examination, particularly in cattle where the pleuritis is often more diffuse and a component of fibrinous pleuropneumonia. A necrotic foul odor to the breath or pleural fluid indicates the possibility of an anaerobic infection, suggesting treatment with metronidazole.

6. The answer is 3 [I F 4 a, b, h]. The clinical description best fits a diagnosis of acute respiratory distress syndrome in the bovine. In this condition, 3-methylindole (3-MI) is not ingested preformed but as dietary L-tryptophan. Clara cells metabolize the ruminally manufactured 3-MI to pneumotoxic metabolites, which injure the alveolar and capillary epithelium. Nursing calves (preruminants) are not affected because the source of L-tryptophan is the pasture. A very important clinical feature of this condition is the absence of breath sounds over the dorsal portions of the lung fields despite the obvious respiratory distress.

7. The answer is 2 [I F 5 b, f]. Blood at the nostrils following intense exercise of a horse is most likely exertion-induced pulmonary hemorrhage (EIPH). The present accepted theory of pathogenesis is that EIPH results from subclinical lung disease. Asynchrony in movement of various groups of alveoli in the dorsal (distal) airways results in the tearing of lung parenchyma and small vessel hemorrhage. This is a common condition in racehorses but has not been identified as performance limiting. Treatment with furosemide has shown the best clinical response.

8. The answer is 1 [II A 1]. Signs of diaphragmatic herniation in horses can be mild to severe colic. However, borborygmi over the ventral chest is not diagnostic of diaphragmatic herniation because the diaphragm is extremely concave (when viewed from the rear) in the horse, and normal abdominal sounds can be transmitted through the chest cavity. Although decreased QRS amplitude may be found in horses with diaphragmatic hernia, the high spike T wave is not a feature. In cattle with pneumothorax, there is a drum-like resonance but a complete absence of lung sounds over the affected chest.

Chapter 8

Cardiovascular Diseases

Margaret Cebra
Christopher Cebra

I. **INTRODUCTION.** An evaluation of the cardiovascular system is an essential part of any physical examination in large animals. Cardiovascular disorders can affect health, performance, production, and quality of life of the animal. Much of our current understanding of cardiac hemodynamics and heart sounds in domestic animals comes from large animal species.

A. **History and signalment.** The following information should be determined when presented with a patient:

1. Age

2. Sex

3. Environment

4. Management

5. Use of the animal

6. Problems with other animals in contact with the affected animal

7. Information on the animal's appetite, attitude, and symptoms

8. The time of onset of the current problem, attempted treatments, disease progression

9. Vaccination and deworming history, previous illnesses

B. **Physical examination.** A complete physical examination of all body systems is a necessary part of any thorough cardiovascular examination. One should note the animal's attitude, body weight, and body condition.

1. In order to determine the functional status of the cardiovascular system, one should examine the mucous membranes for color, moisture, and capillary refill time, and determine the amount of distention of the peripheral veins. The level of filling of the jugular vein and the patency of the vein should be determined. Peripheral arteries should be palpated for pulse quality and rhythm.

2. **Evidence of edema** along the ventral abdomen, sternum (brisket), submandibular area, and over the pectoral muscles should be sought. Edema of the limbs in horses and udder edema in cattle are less reliable signs of heart disease.

3. **Auscultation** is the most important part of the cardiovascular examination.

4. **Cardiovascular sounds** originate when the mechanical activity of the heart results in the sudden acceleration or deceleration of blood, causing the heart, major vessels, and blood to vibrate.
   a. **Types of heart sounds**
      (1) The **first heart sound (S1)** is caused by the initial ejection of blood from the ventricles, the closure of the atrioventricular (AV) valves, and the opening of the semilunar (SL) valves.
      (2) The **second heart sound (S2)** is associated with closure of the SL valves, rapid reversal of blood flow (blood stops moving out of the heart), and opening of the AV valves.
      (3) The **third heart sound (S3)** is associated with the end of the rapid filling of the ventricles with blood.
      (4) The **fourth heart sound (S4)** is associated with atrial contraction. It is closely followed by S1.

TABLE 8-1. Typical Heart Rates in Adult Animals

Species	Typical Heart Rate (beats/min)
Horses	20–40
Cattle	60–80
Sheep and goats	70–90
Pigs	70–90

  b. In the various large animal species, there are differences in the number of heart sounds, the heart rate, and the rhythm.
  (1) In **sheep, goats,** and **pigs,** only S1 and S2 are heard normally.
  (2) In **horses** and **cattle,** all four heart sounds can be heard.
 5. Heart rate. The heart rate in large animals varies depending on the animal's age and species (Table 8-1). Young animals tend to have a faster heart rate than adults. Sinus arrhythmias are common in normal sheep, goats, and young animals, but uncommon in adult cattle.
 6. Cardiac murmurs are prolonged audible vibrations that occur during a normally silent period of the cardiac cycle. The exact mechanism resulting in the production of a heart murmur is unknown. Murmurs are classified according to timing, intensity, radiation, and quality. In some large animal species such as horses, cardiac murmurs and arrhythmias are extremely common. Thus, the interpretation of such findings should be made in the context of history, physical examination findings, and results of ancillary testing.
  a. Pitch or **frequency** is the number of sound vibrations that occur within a unit of time. Heart sounds consist of a wide range of frequency components and are often not pure tones. However, murmurs may contain a fundamental pitch and overtones that produce a musical quality. Murmurs are described as low-, medium-, or high-pitched.
  b. Quality is a subjective term that is determined by the murmur's frequency, amplitude, and duration. A murmur may be described as harsh, blowing, or squeaking. It can also be described as plateau (band-shaped), crescendo–decrescendo (diamond-shaped), decrescendo, crescendo, or continuous.
  c. Intensity (amplitude) is the loudness of the cardiac murmur. Murmurs are quantified by a grading system (Table 8-2). A **thrill** is a fine vibration felt when the hand is placed over the patient's chest near the point of maximal intensity (PMI) of the heart murmur. It is associated with turbulent blood and the vibration is transmitted in the direction of blood flow. Loud heart murmurs (grades III–V or VI) often have a palpable thrill.

TABLE 8-2. Grading Scheme for Cardiac Murmurs in Large Animals

Grade of Murmur	Description of Murmur
Grade I	Barely audible, requires careful auscultation in a localized area of the chest to discern
Grade II	Faint, but clearly audible after listening to the chest for a few seconds
Grade III	Immediately audible over a wide area. A palpable thrill may accompany the murmur.
Grade IV	Very loud murmur. Heard with stethoscope lightly placed on chest wall. A palpable thrill may be present.
Grade V	Loudest audible murmur. Remains audible when the stethoscope is removed from direct contact with the chest wall. A pronounced thrill is always present.

   d. Timing and **duration** refers to whether the murmur occurs during systole, diastole, or is continuous. (Continuous murmurs encompass both systole and diastole.)

      (1) Pansystolic murmurs encompass both S1 and S2.

      (2) Holosystolic murmurs occur between S1 and S2.

      (3) Holodiastolic murmurs are heard between S2 and S3.

      (4) Presystolic murmurs are heard between S4 and S1.

   e. Radiation describes the location of the PMI of the murmur. This information helps determine the location of the underlying cardiac lesion. A murmur's radiation is often the direction of turbulent blood flow. Intense murmurs may radiate widely over the thorax.

C. **Ancillary tests** for evaluating the cardiovascular system include **electrocardiography, echocardiography, cardiac catheterization,** and **radiography.** Successful diagnosis and management of cardiovascular diseases in large animals involves a proficiency with these diagnostic modalities and a familiarity with cardiac disease presentations, pathophysiology, and prevalence in specific large animal species.

  1. Electrocardiography records the electrical impulses that systematically flow through the heart and are responsible for cardiac contraction. The electrocardiogram (ECG) provides information about cardiac structure and function. Information such as the heart rate, rhythm, and conduction times can also be derived from ECG evaluation.

   a. Technique. The **base-apex lead** is most commonly used. The positive lead is attached to the left fifth intercostal space at the PMI of the apex beat and the negative lead is attached to the right jugular furrow at the level of the base of the heart. The ground lead is attached away from the heart, usually on the dorsum. Leads should be attached to minimize interference due to movement of the animal or skin twitching.

   b. Description of ECG. The form and direction of the electrocardiographic waves depend on the position of the heart, the course taken by the spread of electrical excitation throughout the myocardium, the position of the ECG recording leads, and the relative magnitude of the electrical forces during the cardiac cycle.

      (1) Although large animals typically have very large hearts, measurement of the electrical impulses is difficult due to the size and shape of the thorax and the **multidirectionality** of depolarization. Therefore, the ECG can be used to diagnose arrhythmias in large animals, but is not useful in diagnosing disorders of chamber size.

      (2) The multidirectionality of ventricular contraction in large animals is attributable to an extensive Purkinje fiber network that spreads throughout the ventricular myocardium, enabling explosive depolarization of all parts of the ventricle essentially at the same time. In contrast, small animals and people lack this extensive network and therefore, ventricular excitation occurs in three "fronts" or waves.

   c. Indications. Many cardiac disorders can alter the morphology of the ECG recording in a diagnostically useful fashion. ECGs are particularly useful to characterize **cardiac arrhythmias.**

  2. Echocardiography is a safe, noninvasive way to assess chamber sizes, wall valve motion, wall thicknesses, and blood flow and intracardiac hemodynamics.

   a. Types. There are three basic types of echocardiographic studies:

      (1) M-mode echocardiography is useful for evaluating heart wall thickness, chamber diameters, and valve motion.

      (2) Two-dimensional (2D) echocardiography is useful to depict anatomic relationships between cardiac structures and to define their movement relative to one another. 2D echocardiography is used to detect and display wall motion, abnormal communications, and intracardiac masses.

      (3) Doppler echocardiography evaluates blood flow direction, turbulence, and velocity and allows estimation of pressure gradients within the heart and great vessels. **Color-flow Doppler echocardiography** converts the Doppler signals to an arbitrarily chosen color scale that represents the direction, velocity, and turbulence of blood semiquantitatively.

b. Indications. Echocardiography helps identify and quantify the severity of valvular lesions, septal defects, intracardiac masses, cardiomyopathy, chamber hypertrophy, pericardial disease, aortic disease, and congenital heart disease.

3. **Cardiac catheterization.** An intravascular catheter is introduced through a peripheral vessel and passed into the heart.
   a. **Uses.** Cardiac catheterization allows measurement of pressures in the blood vessels and heart chambers, as well as measurement of the oxygen tension, saturation, and content in the cardiac chambers. It also is used to assess cardiac output and vascular resistance. In **contrast angiography,** radiopaque material is injected and visualized using radiography in order to examine cardiovascular structures and blood flow.
   b. **Indications.** Cardiac catheterization, an invasive technique, may be warranted if elevated artery pressures [such as occur with brisket disease, certain valvular abnormalities, shunts, and congestive heart failure (CHF)] are suspected.

4. **Thoracic radiography**
   a. **Use.** Lateral radiographs are useful for detecting large changes in heart size and shape. Pulmonary pathology secondary to heart disease can be imaged.
   b. **Indications.** Radiographic studies may be indicated if chamber or great vessel enlargement (especially dilatation) is suspected as a result of heart failure, valvular lesions, abnormal intracardiac and extracardiac communications (shunts), or some types of pulmonary disorders.

D. **Pathogenesis.** Heart failure occurs when heart disease from any cause becomes severe enough to overwhelm the compensatory mechanisms of the cardiovascular system. Mechanical inadequacy of the heart results in elevated venous and capillary pressures, leading to congestion and edema formation in the tissues, inadequate cardiac output, or both.

1. **Left-sided heart failure** most commonly manifests as pulmonary edema and signs of respiratory compromise (coughing and exertional dyspnea).

2. **Right-sided heart failure** manifests as ascites, tissue edema involving the brisket, submandibular, or ventral areas, liver congestion, prominent jugular distention, jugular pulsation, and weak arterial pulses. Over time, both right- and left-sided heart disease lead to generalized heart failure.

3. **CHF.** Signs of chronic heart failure referable to edema formation (i.e., pulmonary edema in left-sided heart failure, peripheral edema in right-sided heart failure) are called CHF. Because congestion and edema formation are the most common manifestations of chronic heart failure, the term CHF is often used synonymously with heart failure.

II. BLOOD FLOW DISTURBANCES

A. **Congenital cardiac diseases** are abnormalities of cardiac structure or function that are present at birth. Proposed causes include maternal viral infections, use of pharmacologic agents, exposure to toxins, nutritional deficiencies in early pregnancy, and heredity. A variety of cardiovascular anomalies have been described in domestic animals.

1. **Ventricular septal defect (VSD)** is the most common congenital heart defect in horses and cattle.
   a. **Patient profile and history.** VSD is reported in horses, cattle, small ruminants, and swine.
   b. **Clinical findings**
      (1) Animals with **small defects** may be clinically asymptomatic, except for the presence of a **murmur.**
         (a) The **usual murmur** associated with VSD is grade III–IV, band-shaped, and

pansystolic with the PMI in the right third intercostal space at the heart base.

    (b) A **similar murmur** (usually one grade softer), caused by relative pulmonic stenosis, is auscultable at the base of the heart on the left side with the PMI over the pulmonic valve area.

    (c) Aortic insufficiency (i.e., the prolapse of the aortic valve leaflet into the septal defect during diastole due to lack of aortic root support) may cause a **holodiastolic decrescendo murmur** in the left third intercostal space.

  (2) Animals with **large defects** exhibit **stunted growth, lethargy, dyspnea, exercise intolerance,** and **signs of CHF.**

c. Etiology and pathogenesis

  (1) Etiology. Although the exact cause is unknown, possible causes include those listed in II A.

  (2) Pathogenesis. Failure of the interventricular septum (often the membranous portion of the septum) to completely form in utero leads to the shunting of blood from the left ventricle to the right ventricle and right ventricular outflow tract after birth. This shunting increases the blood flow to the pulmonary circulation and increases the venous return to the left atrium and ventricle. Left atrial and ventricular dilatation occurs secondary to this volume overload, and left-sided CHF may occur.

d. Diagnostic plan and laboratory tests. Diagnosis may be determined by several laboratory tests.

  (1) Thoracic radiographs may reveal enlargement of the cardiac silhouette, prominence of the main pulmonary arteries (PA), and increased pulmonary vascular markings.

  (2) Echocardiography. VSDs greater than 2 cm in diameter are visible on echocardiography. Left ventricular volume overload is also evidenced by a dilated left ventricle.

  (3) Cardiac catheterization usually confirms increased oxygen saturation from the right atrium to PAs and increased pressures.

e. Differential diagnoses

  (1) Tetralogy of Fallot and other complex cardiac anomalies that include a VSD have similar auscultation findings. Cyanosis is often present at rest or following exertion with tetralogy.

  (2) Eisenmenger's complex, which occurs when right ventricular pressure is high, causing the shunt accompanying a VSD to be from right-to-left, and is usually accompanied by cyanosis

  (3) Patent ductus arteriosus (PDA) may cause bilateral systolic murmurs, but a continuous murmur is more common.

f. Therapeutic plan. There is **no treatment** for VSD. A palliative measure for correcting the intracardiac blood shunting associated with large VSDs is **PA banding.** This procedure has been used successfully in a small number of calves.

g. Prognosis

  (1) Small to moderate defects. Horses with defects that are smaller than 2.5 cm may have satisfactory athletic performance, whereas horses with moderately large defects may be used for pleasure only.

  (2) Large defects. Horses with very large defects usually become stunted, exercise intolerant, and have a shortened life span.

2. Atrial septal defect (ASD)

a. Patient profile and history

  (1) ASD has been reported in horses, cattle, small ruminants, and swine.

  (2) The defect may occur in conjunction with other cardiac defects.

b. Clinical findings. Complaints may include fatigue, dyspnea on exertion, frequent respiratory tract infections, and symptoms associated with right ventricular failure.

  (1) Small defects in the atrial septum may be clinically inapparent except for the presence of a cardiac **murmur.**

    (a) Under low pressure, blood flows from the left atrium to the right atrium through the ASD, and the murmur results from increased volume being ejected across the pulmonic valve. The murmur is usually a **holosystolic, crescendo–decrescendo ejection murmur** that is heard best over the left heart base.

    (b) An increased blood flow also may produce a **diastolic murmur** over the tricuspid valve.

  (2) Large defects. If the ASD is large, right ventricular and left atrial dilation may occur. Pulmonary hypertension may result from irreparable changes in pulmonary vasculature due to the increased blood volume.

c. Etiology and pathogenesis

  (1) Etiology. The cause of ASD is unknown. Proposed etiologies include those suggested in II A.

  (2) Pathogenesis

    (a) ASD results from the persistence of direct communication between the left and right atria after birth.

      (i) Ostium secundum defect is the most common type of ASD defect. This defect occurs in the midportion of the intra-atrial septum following failure of the septum secundum to form properly. A patent **foramen ovale** is seen most frequently.

      (ii) Sinus venosus type defect is associated with anomalous drainage of one or more pulmonary veins into the right atrium.

    (b) The hemodynamic significance depends on the size of the defect and whether it is accompanied by other cardiac abnormalities. Typically blood moves from the left atrium into the right atrium because resistance is lower in the right heart chambers relative to the left atrium and ventricle. Volume overload of the right side of the heart results, causing right atrial, right ventricular, and PA dilatation.

d. Diagnostic plan and laboratory tests

  (1) Thoracic radiographs reveal increased pulmonary blood flow, producing increased pulmonary vascular markings. Right ventricular enlargement is particularly apparent as reduced retrosternal lung fields in the lateral view. The PA may be enlarged.

  (2) 2D echocardiography may show an enlarged right atrium, right ventricle, and left atrium. The ASD may be visualized if it is larger than 2 cm. **Color-flow Doppler** can demonstrate the shunt across the atrial septum.

  (3) Cardiac catheterization. Diagnosis can be confirmed by the passage of a catheter across the ASD. Oxygen saturation is higher in the right atrium relative to normal.

e. Differential diagnoses

  (1) Functional murmurs disappear with exertion, whereas the holosystolic murmur of ASD does not.

  (2) Pulmonic stenosis. Cyanosis and polycythemia may occur in conjunction with holosystolic murmur.

  (3) VSD often exhibits a bilateral systolic murmur.

  (4) PDA may cause a systolic murmur on both sides of the thorax, but this condition more frequently causes a continuous murmur (see II A 3).

f. Therapeutic plan and prognosis. There is **no treatment** for ASD. The **prognosis** is good if the animal is asymptomatic. In patients with pulmonary hypertension resulting in right ventricular failure, the prognosis is poor.

3. PDA

a. Patient profile. This disorder rarely occurs as a single defect in large animals, but it can occur in all large animal species.

b. Clinical findings

  (1) Complaints may include stunted growth, exercise intolerance, signs of CHF, and cyanosis.

  (2) Clinical signs depend on the length and diameter of the defect, the direction of the shunted blood, and the presence of other cardiac defects.

    (a) The **murmur** is usually continuous and high pitched. It is heard over both sides of the thorax but is loudest on the left side of the thorax over the aortic and pulmonic valve areas. Often there is a **palpable continuous thrill** over the third or fourth intercostal space on the left side. The murmur is referred to as a **machinery murmur** because it alternates intensity.

    (b) Large defects. If the defect is very large, no murmur may be audible.

  c. Etiology and pathogenesis

    (1) Etiology. The reason for this defect is unknown. There is no evidence to suggest that PDA is hereditary in cattle or horses.

    (2) Pathogenesis

      (a) Normally, the ductus arteriosus closes in response to decreased pulmonary vascular resistance and increased systemic vascular resistance, which occurs at birth when breathing begins.

        (i) Normal foals may have a PDA for a few days after birth, but closure should occur by 96 hours.

        (ii) Normal ruminants rarely have a PDA after birth.

      (b) PDA results from persistent patency of the fetal vessel that connects the pulmonary arterial system to the aorta (bypassing the lungs).

        (i) With **normal pulmonary vascular resistance,** blood from the aorta is continuously shunted into the main PA (left-to-right shunt), resulting in excessive pulmonary blood flow and volume overload of the left atrium and left ventricle.

        (ii) If pulmonary vascular resistance increases due to pulmonary vascular disease or pulmonary hypertension, blood may be shunted from the PA into the aorta (right-to-left shunt). This **reversed PDA** results in poorly oxygenated blood entering the systemic circulation, and **differential cyanosis** may result. With differential cyanosis, the cranial parts of the animal are well oxygenated, whereas the caudal parts are not.

  d. Diagnostic plan and laboratory tests

    (1) Thoracic radiographs may reveal an enlarged cardiac silhouette and prominent pulmonary markings. With left-sided heart failure, pulmonary venous congestion, interstitial pulmonary edema, and alveolar edema may be seen.

    (2) Cardiac catheterization. A catheter usually can be passed from the PA into the descending aorta, confirming the presence of a PDA. The right ventricular and PA pressures and the PA oxygen saturation are elevated.

  e. Differential diagnoses

    (1) Complex cardiac defect with PDA as a component

    (2) VSD. If the defect is very large, aortic insufficiency will result, causing a diastolic murmur in addition to the holosystolic murmur heard with a VSD.

    (3) Vegetative endocarditis involving the AV or SL valves should not produce a continuous murmur.

  f. Therapeutic plan

    (1) Surgical repair is possible, but it is rarely economically feasible in large animal species.

    (2) Pharmacologic closure of PDA with inhibitors of prostaglandin synthesis has been reported to be effective in people, but there is a risk of complications and recurrence. There are no reports of the efficacy of these drugs in large animals.

  g. Prognosis. Animals with large defects have a poor prognosis because of the risk of CHF. It is not known whether small defects impair survival because they are often clinically undetectable and undiagnosed.

4. Tetralogy of Fallot

  a. Patient profile and history. This disorder is reported in all large animal species but may be more common in calves than in foals.

  b. Clinical findings

    (1) Clinical signs often develop very early in life.

      (a) Severe hypoxemia and **cyanosis** of the oral and nasal mucosae, tongue mucosa, and vaginal mucosa are present when hemoglobin is reduced by more than 5 g/dl. Tetralogy of Fallot is one of the more common congenital cardiac defects in large animals that causes cyanosis.

    (b) Exercise intolerance is characterized by dyspnea, worsening cyanosis, and collapse.

    (c) Syncope, CHF, and **sudden death** also may occur.

  (2) Murmurs

    (a) A **loud systolic murmur** (grade IV–V) may be transmitted widely over both thoracic walls.

    (b) A **systolic ejection murmur** may be audible at the heart base over the aortic and pulmonic valve areas, whereas a harsh, more **band-shaped holosystolic murmur** may be heard toward the apex of the heart. There may be a **systolic thrill.**

    (c) With right ventricular hypertrophy and rising right ventricular pressure, the function of the tricuspid valve may be impaired and **regurgitation** may result. A systolic heart murmur that is loudest on the right side over the tricuspid valve may be heard.

c. Etiology and pathogenesis

  (1) Etiology. The cause of this complex heart defect is **unknown.** There is no evidence that this disorder is inherited. Proposed etiologies are listed in II A.

  (2) Pathogenesis

    (a) The **abnormal development of the conal septum** in the embryonic heart leads to the narrowing of the right ventricular infundibulum (i.e., **pulmonary stenosis),** an inability of the conal septum to participate in the closure of the interventricular foramen **(VSD),** and an **overriding aorta. Right ventricular hypertrophy** develops as a result of the pulmonary outflow obstruction. **ASD** may be present as well (pentalogy of Fallot).

    (b) The **degree of blood shunting** is controlled by resistance across the stenotic right ventricular outflow tract as compared with resistance across the aortic valve. Blood moves from the right ventricle, through the VSD, into the aorta.

d. Diagnostic plan and laboratory tests. Diagnosis is determined by the imaging and catheterization studies.

  (1) Thoracic radiographs may reveal right ventricular enlargement and decreased pulmonary vasculature. The ascending aorta may be prominent, causing a loss of the cranial waist of the heart.

  (2) Echocardiography may allow the visualization of the four components of the tetralogy. **Color-flow Doppler** can be used to characterize the abnormalities in blood flow and the severity of right ventricular outflow obstruction.

  (3) Cardiac catheterization reveals equal pressure in the right and left ventricles. There is a pressure gradient between the right ventricle and the PA. Oxygen saturation is decreased in the left ventricle and aorta.

  (4) Hematology. Packed cell volume and red blood cell (RBC) counts may be elevated over time due to chronic hypoxemia and blood sludging. In general, polycythemia is uncommon in foals with cyanotic cardiac disease and is usually present in less than 45% of calves.

e. Differential diagnoses

  (1) Respiratory distress syndrome of neonates. Tachypnea, dyspnea, cyanosis, and abnormal lung sounds are present, but there is no heart murmur.

  (2) Central nervous system (CNS) dysfunction, such as neonatal maladjustment syndrome (NMS) and meningitis. Other neurologic signs are present, and there is no heart murmur.

  (3) Heart failure with or without pulmonary edema or respiratory disease. With this disorder, there is improvement in cyanosis after supplementation with intranasal oxygen.

  (4) Reversed PDA (right-to-left shunt) or VSD. These defects may cause differential cyanosis.

  (5) Tricuspid or right ventricular atresia. The murmur of tricuspid insufficiency is holosystolic and is heard best along the right cardiac apex.

(6) **Aortic anomalies.** A diastolic murmur is heard best over the fourth intercostal space on the left side.

f. **Therapeutic plan and prognosis.** There is no treatment for this condition, and the prognosis for long-term survival is poor.

B. Acquired valvular diseases

1. **Introduction.** Disorders of any of the four cardiac valves commonly result in **valve insufficiency.**
   a. **Etiology and pathogenesis.** Acquired valvular disorders result from degenerative changes, infection (bacterial or viral), inflammation, trauma, or unknown causes. With infectious or inflammatory conditions, vegetative lesions form on the cardiac valves, resulting in **vegetative valvular endocarditis.**
   b. **Clinical findings.** Acquired valvular diseases are usually manifested by a **cardiac murmur** associated with valve incompetence. The murmur is heard over the affected valve and radiates in the direction of the regurgitant blood flow.

2. **Left AV valve insufficiency (mitral regurgitation)**
   a. **Patient profile.** This condition is reported in all large animal species and occurs more commonly in horses than cows.
   b. **Clinical findings**
      (1) **Complaints** include intermittent fever, dyspnea, tachycardia, poor return to resting respiratory rate after exercise, coughing, and signs of CHF.
      (2) **Clinical signs associated with CHF** may be present, including dyspnea due to pulmonary congestion and tissue edema.
      (3) The **murmur** is usually grade III or higher. The murmur is holosystolic and is heard best over the mitral valve area (i.e., left side, fifth intercostal space in horses, fourth intercostal space in ruminants). The sound radiates dorsad and somewhat caudad, dorsal to the mitral valve area.
   c. **Etiology and pathogenesis**
      (1) **Etiology. Insufficiency of the mitral valve** is caused by a deformation of the mitral valve cusps, dilation of the ventricles or valve ring, rupture of the chordae tendineae, or papillary muscle dysfunction. Possible causes for these defects are listed in II B 1 a.
      (2) **Pathogenesis**
         (a) When the mitral valve is unable to close completely, blood flows back into the left atrium during systole, causing volume overload and hypertrophy of the left atrium, endocardial damage to the atrial wall (**jet lesions**), and occasionally a full thickness tear in the left atrium.
         (b) The mitral valve leak also initially leads to a decreased amount of blood pushed forward into the aorta.
         (c) Eventually, **left-sided heart failure** ensues.
   d. **Diagnostic plan and laboratory tests**
      (1) **Thoracic radiographs** may show cardiac enlargement, pulmonary venous distention, pulmonary edema, or pulmonary vascular congestion.
      (2) **Echocardiography** may reveal a vegetative lesion on the mitral valve or prolapse of the mitral valve into the left atrium during systole. A normal to increased shortening fraction may be noted in conjunction with the murmur. Left-sided heart enlargement may be apparent. **Color-flow Doppler** may reveal the regurgitant blood during systole.
      (3) **Cardiac catheterization.** A pulmonary capillary wedge tracing usually shows a large v pressure curve. If radiopaque dye is placed in the left ventricle, it will move into the left atrium during systole.
      (4) **Tests to screen for bacterial endocarditis (BE)** [see II B 6 d] should also be performed.
   e. **Differential diagnoses**
      (1) **Primary respiratory disease.** No heart murmur is present with this condition.
      (2) **Neurologic disorders,** such as meningitis, encephalitis, and encephalopathy. Other neurologic signs may be present in the absence of a heart murmur.
      (3) **Dilated cardiomyopathy.** Echocardiography can be used to distinguish

dilated cardiomyopathy from left AV valve insufficiency. With dilated cardio-myopathy, echocardiography reveals right and left ventricular chamber en-largement with a decreased ventricular shortening fraction. Thoracic radio-graphs may also reveal generalized cardiomegaly.

f. **Therapeutic plan.** For patients with vegetative lesions, treatment consists of the long-term administration of antimicrobials (see II B 6 f). The use of diuretics and anticoagulants may provide some symptomatic relief.

g. **Prognosis** depends on the severity of the mitral valve defect and the age of the patient. If the patient develops CHF, the prognosis is poor.

3. **Right AV valve insufficiency (tricuspid regurgitation)**

a. **Patient profile.** This condition occurs in all large animal species, but it is more common in cattle than horses.

(1) In one report, tricuspid regurgitation murmurs occurred in 16.4% of National Hunt racing Thoroughbreds and 3.7% of nonracing Thoroughbreds.

(2) In cattle, the tricuspid valve is the most common site for vegetative valvular endocarditis lesions.

b. **Clinical findings**

(1) **Complaints** may include exercise intolerance, weight loss, intermittent fever, and weakness.

(2) **Physical examination findings** can include a positive jugular venous pulse wave during ventricular systole, syncope, ascites, venous distention, and pul-monary hypertension in addition to the characteristic heart murmur.

(a) **Right-sided holosystolic murmurs** compatible with tricuspid regurgitation are the **most common murmur reported in athletic horses,** although post-mortem lesions involving the tricuspid valve are not always present in those horses.

(b) The **holosystolic murmur** associated with tricuspid regurgitation is heard best over the tricuspid valve area (right cardiac apex). A **precordial thrill** may be palpable.

c. **Etiology and pathogenesis**

(1) **Etiology** [see II B 2 c (1)]. Tricuspid regurgitation in horses occurs frequently **in combination with mitral regurgitation** and is caused by left-sided heart fail-ure and pulmonary hypertension.

(2) **Pathogenesis.** With the inability of the tricuspid valve to close during systole, blood flows back into the right atrium. Chamber dilation and jet lesions (i.e., damage to the endocardium by a stream of regurgitant blood moving with a high velocity through an incompetent valve) on the atrial wall may result, and right-sided heart failure occurs over time.

d. **Diagnostic plan and laboratory tests**

(1) **Thoracic radiographs** reveal right-sided heart enlargement.

(2) **Echocardiography** may reveal a vegetative lesion on the tricuspid valve, valve thickening or shortening, or prolapse of the valve leaflets into the right atrium during systole. A normal to increased shortening fraction may be noted in conjunction with the murmur. Right ventricular volume overload and right atrial enlargement may be apparent. **Color-flow Doppler** may show the regur-gitant blood during systole.

(3) **Cardiac catheterization.** Radiopaque dye placed in the right ventricle will be seen in the right atrium before it appears in the pulmonary vasculature.

(4) **Diagnostic tests to screen for BE** (II B 6 d) should also be performed.

e. **Differential diagnoses**

(1) **VSD.** VSD can be distinguished from tricuspid regurgitation using echocardi-ography.

(2) **Mitral stenosis** and tricuspid regurgitation may occur concurrently.

(3) **Dilated cardiomyopathy** can be distinguished from tricuspid regurgitation using echocardiography.

(4) **Primary respiratory disease** may cause similar clinical findings, including ex-ercise intolerance and coughing, but no heart murmur is present.

f. Therapeutic plan and prognosis are the same as for left AV valve insufficiency (see II B 2 f–g).

4. **Aortic valve insufficiency**
   a. **Patient profile and history.** This disorder can occur in all large animal species, but it is particularly common in older horses.
   b. **Clinical findings**
      (1) **Complaints.** Usually aortic regurgitation is well tolerated and is not associated with exercise intolerance. However, performance may be impaired.
      (2) **Physical examination findings**
         (a) **Murmur**
            (i) **Location.** The murmur associated with aortic regurgitation is **holodiastolic** with the PMI over the aortic valve (fourth intercostal space on the left side in horses, third intercostal space in ruminants) and radiating toward the left cardiac apex.
            (ii) **Characteristics.** The murmur usually begins at the time of S2 and is generally decrescendo in shape. Sometimes the murmur waxes and wanes in intensity, exhibiting one or more peaks during diastole. It may have a honking quality. Occasionally, atrial contraction may interrupt the aortic diastolic murmur or increase the intensity of the murmur.
         (b) In severe cases, **bounding arterial pulses** may be present, indicating diastolic runoff and left ventricular volume overload.
         (c) **Signs of CHF** may develop rapidly (e.g., jugular venous distention, subcutaneous edema, ascites, respiratory distress).
         (d) **Atrial dysrhythmias,** most frequently **atrial fibrillation (AF),** often develop secondary to atrial enlargement.
   c. **Etiology and pathogenesis**
      (1) **Etiology.** Possible causes are enumerated in II B 1 a.
      (2) **Pathogenesis.** With aortic insufficiency, blood flows from the aorta to the left ventricle through the incompetent valve during diastole. The murmur is associated with leakage of blood back into the left ventricle.
         (a) Initially, the left ventricle cannot accommodate the large blood volume, resulting in elevated pressure in the left atrium and pulmonary circulation.
         (b) Over time, the left ventricle undergoes compensatory changes to accommodate the increased blood flow by dilatation and hypertrophy. With chronicity, there is progressive fibrosis of the left ventricle, which consequently leads to myocardial dysfunction.
         (c) The severity of aortic regurgitation depends on the size of the regurgitant aortic orifice, the pressure gradient across the aortic valve during diastole, and the duration of diastole. Common changes associated with the aortic valve include fibrotic bands, especially along the free edge of the aortic valve cusps at the site of valve closure, and vegetative lesions on the valve itself.
   d. **Diagnostic plan and laboratory tests**
      (1) **Thoracic radiographs** reveal left-sided heart enlargement.
      (2) **Echocardiography** may reveal a vegetative lesion on the aortic valve, nodules or fibrotic plaques on the valve resulting in valve thickening or shortening, or the prolapse of the valve leaflets into the left atrium during diastole. Left ventricular volume overload and left atrial enlargement may be apparent. **Color-flow Doppler** may show the regurgitant blood during diastole. Impaired left ventricular function is noted.
      (3) **Diagnostic tests to screen for BE** should also be performed (see II B 6 d).
   e. **Differential diagnoses**
      (1) **Pulmonic regurgitation** can be distinguished from aortic valve insufficiency using echocardiography.
      (2) **Mitral** or **tricuspid valve stenosis.** In these disorders, the murmur is heard best during mid- to late diastole and is often loudest at the end of diastole.

The murmur associated with aortic regurgitation is heard in early diastole and is decrescendo in shape.

(3) Hyperdynamic states (e.g., those induced by fever, anemia, and exercise) can cause a diastolic murmur as increased blood flow moves across the normal AV valves.

f. Therapeutic plan. No treatment is necessary if affected animals are asymptomatic. If there are symptoms, therapy is the same as for AV valve insufficiency (see II B 2 f).

g. Prognosis is good if the animal is asymptomatic. If the disorder is caused by BE or if signs of CHF develop, the prognosis is poor.

5. **Pulmonary valve insufficiency** is the least common valvular disease in young athletic racehorses and horses that are presented for slaughter.
   a. Patient profile. Although uncommon, this disorder can occur in all large animals.
   b. Clinical findings. This condition may develop in horses with pulmonary hypertension and CHF but is rarely detected clinically.
      (1) Complaints may include severe exercise intolerance, intermittent fever, weight loss, anorexia, or signs of CHF.
      (2) The **characteristic murmur** associated with pulmonic regurgitation is a holosystolic murmur that is heard best over the left heart base in the third intercostal space in horses and the second intercostal space in cattle (i.e., the pulmonic valve region). The murmur may radiate along the pulmonic outflow tract.
   c. Etiology and pathogenesis
      (1) Etiology. In large animals, BE and trauma may cause the primary lesions of the pulmonic valve that result in regurgitation. In cattle, high altitudes may also cause pulmonary valve insufficiency.
      (2) Pathogenesis. The insufficiency of the pulmonic valve allows the regurgitation of blood into the right ventricle during diastole. Severe pulmonary hypertension may lead to pulmonic regurgitation.
   d. Diagnostic plan and laboratory tests
      (1) Thoracic radiographs may reveal right-sided heart enlargement, particularly right ventricular. If pulmonary hypertension is present, increased pulmonary vascular markings or pulmonary edema may be evident.
      (2) Echocardiography may show a vegetative lesion on the pulmonic valve or valvular dysfunction. **Color-flow Doppler** may reveal the regurgitant jet of blood during right ventricular systole. Enlargement of the right ventricle may be apparent because of volume overload.
      (3) Diagnostic tests to screen for BE should also be performed (see II B 6 d).
   e. Differential diagnoses include **aortic regurgitation** and the differentials for aortic regurgitation.
   f. Therapeutic plan and prognosis
      (1) Treatment depends on the etiology, onset, duration, and severity of the lesion. Treatment for BE (see II B 6 f) may be appropriate.
      (2) Prognosis. Generally, the prognosis is guarded to poor when there is clinical evidence of valvular incompetence (e.g., tachycardia, exercise intolerance, signs of CHF, evidence of cardiac chamber enlargement).

6. **Bacterial endocarditis (BE)**
   a. Patient profile. Horses, swine, and cattle can be afflicted with BE.
      (1) Horses. In horses, BE is uncommon and males may be overrepresented.
      (2) Swine. BE occurs more commonly in swine than in other large animal species. Swine younger than 1 year are most often affected.
      (3) Cattle. BE is often undiagnosed or misdiagnosed in cattle; adult cattle are most often affected. Many affected cattle have a history of being treated for pneumonia, reticuloperitonitis, or other infectious diseases.
   b. Clinical findings
      (1) Equine and porcine BE. Although swine may have clinical signs similar to those seen in horses, BE is more often a postmortem finding rather than a clinical condition in swine.

(a) **Complaints** are extremely variable but may include cyclic or intermittent fevers, weight loss, lameness, weakness, or anorexia.
(b) **Physical examination findings**
  (i) A **heart murmur**, associated with a vegetative lesion on one or more heart valves, is often present. In horses, the aortic valve is most commonly involved, followed by the mitral valve. Likewise, in swine, the left AV and SL heart valves are most frequently affected.
  (ii) **Signs associated with CHF** often develop. With **left-sided heart failure** (a sequela of aortic valve dysfunction), signs include **persistent cough, pulmonary edema, syncope,** and **exercise intolerance.**
  (iii) **Signs of other common sequelae** (e.g., **thromboembolism, nonseptic arthritis, embolic showers**) may also be seen. Embolic showers can lead to infarction or metastatic infection at distant organ sites (e.g., the myocardium, lungs, kidney, brain, retina, vertebral vasculature, or synovial membranes).
(2) **Bovine BE**
  (a) **Complaints** may include shifting limb lameness, anorexia, weight loss, cough, diarrhea, and decreased milk production.
  (b) **Physical examination findings**
    (i) A **heart murmur** is often detectable. Vegetative lesions most often involve the tricuspid valve.
    (ii) **Signs of right-sided heart failure** (e.g., tachycardia, jugular and mammary vein distention, jugular pulsation, ventral and submandibular edema) are also associated with tricuspid valve insufficiency.
    (iii) **Other signs** include fever (constant or intermittent), tachypnea, dyspnea, pale mucous membranes, and scleral injection.
c. **Etiology and pathogenesis**
  (1) **Etiology.** Theoretically, any bacteria that gains access to the blood can colonize the heart valves and endocardium, resulting in BE.
    (a) In **horses,** *Streptococcus equi* subspecies *zooepidemicus* and *Actinobacillus equi* are the most common causes.
    (b) In **swine,** *Streptococcus* species and *Erysipelothrix rhusiopathiae* are the most common causes.
    (c) In **cattle,** common causative agents include *Actinomyces pyogenes* and *Streptococcus* species.
  (2) **Pathogenesis**
    (a) **Acute BE.** The only predisposing factor necessary for the development of acute BE is infection with an organism that has the ability to bind to the heart valve endothelium directly. The most common organism capable of causing acute BE in all domestic animals is *Staphylococcus aureus.*
    (b) **Chronic (subacute) BE.** The presence of four factors is necessary for the development of chronic BE: endocardial damage, the formation of a platelet–fibrin thrombus on the damaged endothelium, bacteremia, and a high agglutinating antibody titer toward the infecting organism.
d. **Diagnostic plan and laboratory tests**
  (1) **Blood culture.** Bacteriologic culturing of blood samples should be obtained during febrile episodes before antibiotic administration. Some veterinarians recommend that three blood samples be collected from different sites during a 2-hour period at least 24 hours after the last dose of antibiotics (if administered empirically) or before antibiotic therapy has been initiated.
  (2) **Echocardiography** (M-mode and 2D) may show evidence of a vegetative lesion on the heart valves. The lesion must be at least 2–3 mm in diameter in order to be seen. This test may be less sensitive but more specific than a blood culture.
e. **Differential diagnoses**
  (1) In animals with signs of **left-sided heart failure,** differential diagnoses include respiratory disease and other diseases causing pulmonary edema (e.g., diseases associated with hypoproteinemia).

(2) In cattle with signs of **right-sided heart failure,** the following conditions must be ruled out:

   (a) Septic pericarditis, often a sequela of traumatic reticuloperitonitis

   (b) Cor pulmonale, an effect of lung dysfunction on the heart

   (c) Cardiac lymphosarcoma, an uncommon sequela of bovine leukemia virus (BLV) infection

f. Therapeutic plan. Treatment decisions must take into account the economic value of the animal, the cost of treatment, the owner's emotional attachment to the animal, and the prognosis.

   (1) Antibiotic therapy must be **aggressive** and lasts for weeks to months. **Bactericidal antibiotics** are chosen on the basis of sensitivity patterns and the ability of the drug to penetrate tissue. After completion of therapy, **follow-up blood cultures** should be performed at least once during the next 60 days. If the cultures are positive, antibiotics must be administered again.

   (2) Treatment of specific organ dysfunction may be required. The use of anticoagulants to prevent emboli has not been thoroughly investigated in horses.

g. Prognosis

   (1) Horses. Survival rates in horses with BE have not been reported, but the prognosis appears to be grave.

   (2) Swine. Mortality surveys of sows indicated BE to be the cause of death in 6.4%–8.6% of cases.

   (3) Cattle. Prognosis is poor to grave.

C. Jugular thrombophlebitis (JT). Thrombosis is the formation of a clot that obstructs blood flow.

1. Patient profile. JT can occur in any large animal species. Most affected animals have a history of recent jugular venipuncture or catheter placement. JT occurs most commonly in horses treated for acute toxic enteritis or colitis.

2. Clinical findings include a **noticeable enlargement or mass** associated with the jugular vein. The mass may be warm, red, or painful. Sometimes the jugular has a rope or cord-like appearance. Edema and venous congestion of the area drained by the affected vein may also occur, leading to swelling of the head. Pyrexia, inappetence, and depression may be present.

3. Etiology and pathogenesis

a. Etiology. The **specific causes** of JT are **unknown. Possible causes** of JT include trauma (intimal damage), venous stasis, and catheterization.

   (1) Iatrogenic factors may predispose an animal to JT by causing intimal damage subsequent to placement of a jugular catheter. These factors include the length of time the indwelling catheter has been in place; the site and technique of venipuncture; the composition, contamination, and pH of infusates; the thrombogenicity of catheter material, and the diameter and length of the catheter.

   (2) Hypercoagulable states may lead to JT without intimal damage. These states include dehydration, endotoxemia, anemia, hypotension, stress, or venous stasis.

b. Pathogenesis. Irritation of the intimal lining of the jugular vein, stasis of blood, and/or the existence of a hypercoagulable state trigger the clotting cascade and lead to the development of thrombosis. Blood flow is occluded because of the restricted lumen size. **Secondary thrombosis** can result from perivascular inflammation caused by cellulitis, lymphangitis, or other sources of bacterial invasion around the blood vessels. In severe cases, septicemia leading to endocarditis or pneumonia may occur.

4. Diagnostic plan and laboratory tests

a. Ultrasound may reveal cavitating lesions involving the jugular vein. An echodense thrombus with an anechoic area in the center and restricted blood flow may be seen.

b. Cultures. A needle aspirate of blood and fibrin can be obtained for culture. An ultrasound can be used to identify fluid pockets and guide the placement of the needle into them to obtain an aspirate. The aspirate should be submitted for bacteriologic cultures. The tip of the catheter also can be used for obtaining bacteriologic cultures.

5. **Therapeutic plan**
   a. **Definitive treatment** consists of **removal of the catheter** if present. Subsequently, the affected vein should not be used for any purpose. Surgical removal or drainage of the affected vein should be considered in animals that are unresponsive to medical treatment or those with complications (e.g., bacteremia, toxemia).
   b. **Supportive care**
      (1) **Local treatment** consists of a hot pack, hydrotherapy, and, in horses, the topical application of **dimethylsulfoxide (DMSO)** or other antiphlogistic salves to reduce local inflammation and increase the blood supply.
      (2) **Broad-spectrum systemic antibiotics** are indicated, particularly if cultures are positive. Antibiotic selection should be made on the basis of the bacteriologic culture and a susceptibility study.

6. **Prognosis** depends on the severity and duration of the problem. Recannulation of the vein can occur over time.

7. **Prevention** includes:
   a. Using catheters made out of material with low thrombogenicity (e.g., polyvinyl chloride)
   b. Placing the jugular catheter high enough in the neck so that the tip is not near the entrance of the anterior vena cava
   c. Minimizing trauma to the vein during catheter placement
   d. Maintaining strict asepsis during placement
   e. Using sterile, particulate-free solutions
   f. Securing the catheter by suturing it to the skin and covering the site with a sterile antiseptic dressing
   g. Removing or changing the catheter every 48–72 hours

D. **Aortoiliac thrombosis**

1. **Patient profile and history**
   a. **Patient profile.** Although this condition can occur in any large animal species, it is uncommon in all large animal species. In horses, there may be a predisposition for males and certain family lines.
   b. **History**
      (1) In **horses,** a history of systemic infections (e.g., *Streptococcus equi*, influenza virus), parasites (e.g., *Strongylus vulgaris*), larval migration, back trauma, or racing-associated blood flow turbulence may predispose the animal to aortoiliac thrombosis.
      (2) In **cattle,** a history of severe necrotizing colitis and valvular endocarditis may predispose the animal to this disorder.

2. **Clinical findings**
   a. **Neuromuscular signs** include rear limb weakness, paralysis, and exercise-induced weakness or lameness. Trembling and muscle fasciculations and the reluctance to bear weight on the affected limb may be seen. The affected limb is often cooler and drier than the other limbs. Over time, muscle atrophy over the hind quarters occurs.
   b. **Vascular signs.** Rectal palpation of the abdominal aorta and its branches (the cranial mesenteric, internal, external, and circumflex iliac arteries) may reveal variations in the amplitude of the pulse and asymmetry. The amplitude of the pulse in the great metatarsal and digital arteries is reduced, and saphenous vein refill time is prolonged, particularly after exercise.
   c. **Pain** or **anxiety** (manifested as elevated heart and respiratory rates and profuse sweating) may be associated with an acute ischemic event. Occasionally, horses show signs of colic.

3. **Etiology and pathogenesis**
   a. **Etiology. Trauma** and **infection** may be possible causes. Mechanical factors and blood turbulence can lead to intimal tearing.
   b. **Pathogenesis.** The most commonly proposed pathogenesis is the detachment of an intracardiac thrombus, which then lodges at the aortic–iliac bifurcation. The condition may be induced by moderate to strenuous **exercise.**

4. **Diagnostic plan and laboratory tests.** The thrombus may be visible using 2D ultrasonography if the probe is placed over the terminal aorta per the rectum.

5. **Therapeutic plan**
   a. Treatment consists of **alternate-day aspirin therapy** orally and **controlled** and **continued exercise** (if nonpainful) to maintain or promote the development of collateral circulation. The development of collaterals requires a significant amount of time.
   b. **Surgery** to remove the thrombus is impractical and dangerous.
   c. **Chemotherapeutic agents,** such as streptokinase and tissue plasminogen activator, have not been used in large animals.

6. **Prognosis.** The prognosis is guarded in horses for the return to athletic use. Death may occur in rare cases.

III. CARDIAC DYSRHYTHMIAS

A. Introduction

1. **Definition.** Cardiac arrhythmias or dysrhythmias are abnormalities in the rate, regularity, or site of origin of the cardiac impulse or a disturbance in the conduction of the impulse.

2. **Pacemaker and conductive system.** The specialized pacemaker and conductive system of the heart consists of five components. Any disruption in impulse formation, impulse conduction, or both results in arrhythmias. The components include:
   a. The **sinoatrial node,** where the cardiac impulse is initiated
   b. The **AV node,** where the impulse from the atrium is delayed before passing into the ventricle
   c. The **bundle of His,** which conducts the impulse from the AV node into the bundle branches
   d. The **right and left bundle branches,** which conduct the impulse into the ventricles
   e. The **Purkinje network,** which distributes the impulse to all parts of the ventricle

3. **Classification of arrhythmias**
   a. Arrhythmias can be classified in several different ways. Most arrhythmias fit into one of three categories:
      (1) Autonomic source
      (2) Cardiac source
      (3) Extracardiac source
   b. Regardless of the specific pathologic cause, arrhythmias result from critical alterations in the electrical activity of the myocardial cell.
      (1) **Physiologic arrhythmias.** In horses, most arrhythmias are physiologic and are abolished with exercise and excitement. Examples of physiologic arrhythmias include **first- and second-degree AV blocks** and **sinus bradycardia.**
      (2) **Pathologic arrhythmias** cause poor performance and exercise intolerance. Examples of these arrhythmias include **supraventricular arrhythmias** (such as supraventricular premature complexes and tachycardia, AF, and advanced second- and third-degree AV blocks).
      (3) **Ventricular arrhythmias** are frequently pathologic and include **ventricular tachycardia** and **ventricular premature depolarizations.**

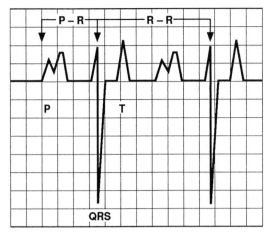

FIGURE 8-1. Enlarged sketch of a normal base-apex electrocardiogram (ECG) from a horse. The P wave, QRS complex, T wave, P-R interval, and R-R interval are indicated. Notice the notched ("M"-shaped) P wave and the absence of a Q wave. Paper speed = 25 mm/sec. Box width = 1 mm.

4. **Incidence.** It has been estimated that cardiac arrhythmias without any other signs of heart disease may occur in greater than 25% of horses. When accompanied by other cardiac problems, an arrhythmia may occur in as many as 40% of horses.

5. **Diagnosis.** Evaluation of the ECG involves identifying electrical events that cause characteristic ECG patterns, identifying abnormal patterns, and measuring the rate of occurrence of each pattern. The normal morphology of the patterns varies, depending on the animal and the placement of the ECG leads.
   a. **Waves and complexes.** The most basic patterns seen on the ECG tracings are the P wave, the QRS complex, and the T wave (Figure 8-1). Normally, a single P wave is followed within 200–550 milliseconds by a single QRS complex, which is followed within 300–600 milliseconds by a single T wave. These complexes occur closer together in animals with tachycardia and in neonates with high heart rates.
      (1) The **P wave** is associated with **atrial contraction** and is usually a single, short deflection of the ECG. The deflection is usually positive (above the baseline) when using the base-apex lead. Because of the size of the atria in large animals, especially in horses, the P wave may have an "M" shape because the two atria may contract at slightly different times.
      (2) The **QRS complex** represents the various waves of **depolarization across the ventricles.**
         (a) The Q refers to a negative deflection of the ECG before the first positive deflection and is often absent in large animals.
         (b) The R refers to the first positive deflection (subsequent positive deflections are referred to as R', R", and so on).
         (c) The S (or S', S", and so on) refers to negative deflections after a positive deflection. Hence, a QRS complex may have one Q deflection and multiple R and S deflections.
      (3) The **T wave** represents **ventricular repolarization.** It may be positive or negative and may vary in appearance between successive heart beats.
   b. **Intervals** commonly measured are the interval between the beginning of a P wave and the subsequent QRS complex (**P-R interval**) and the interval between R deflections of successive QRS complexes (**R-R interval**).
   c. **Interpretation.** On a normal ECG, the P wave and QRS complex recur at regular intervals, and have the same appearance each time. Unless two different wave or complex shapes are present on the same lead tracing, it is often difficult to determine that a P wave or QRS complex is abnormal, even if it has an unusual appearance.

(1) P waves with different shapes often suggest that multiple pacemakers are present **(ectopic atrial pacemaker).**

(2) QRS complexes. The occurrence of QRS complexes with different shapes establishes the presence of an **ectopic ventricular pacemaker,** because all supraventricular impulses conduct through the same system and lead to the same QRS appearance. Abnormal QRS complexes frequently are wider than usual, have bizarre appearances, and occur independent of a preceding P wave.

(3) Intervals. The P-R intervals and the R-R intervals should be compared at different areas on the tracing.

  (a) The **P-R interval** represents the delay in conduction between the atria and ventricles, and can be lengthened by high vagal tone, drugs that slow conduction (i.e., tranquilizers, anesthetics), or pathology.

  (b) The **R-R interval** represents the **heart rate.** The occurrence of one or more P waves or QRS complexes before the time predicted by the R-R interval may represent a **premature contraction** or **paroxysmal tachycardia.** Absence of an anticipated beat may represent a **dropped beat.** An abnormal QRS complex that occurs after a prolonged R-R interval is termed an **escape beat.**

(4) Calculating the heart rate. Assuming a standard ECG paper speed of 25 mm/sec, the heart rate (beats/min) = (1500 mm/min)/(number of mm between beats).

B. | **Bradyarrhythmias**

1. First- and second-degree AV block (incomplete block)

  a. Patient profile. These conditions are more common in horses and cattle than in small ruminants or swine.

  b. Clinical findings. Cardiac auscultation reveals a slow heart rate, an irregular rhythm, and regular S4 that are not associated with S1 or S2.

  (1) First-degree AV block does not cause clinical signs and is unlikely to produce any significant alterations in cardiac function at slow heart rates. Auscultation of animals with first-degree AV block may reveal a separation of S1 and S2 or no abnormalities.

  (2) Second-degree AV block. The jugular pulse may gradually creep up the neck until the beat is conducted. An arterial pulse deficit is palpated. On auscultation, an absence of S1, S2, and S3 is noticed when the block occurs.

  c. Etiology. Bradyarrhythmias, such as first- and second-degree AV block, occur because of impaired impulse conduction. The **specific cause** of first- and second-degree AV block is unknown, but it is speculated to be a waxing and waning of vagal tone. The large cardiac mass in horses and cattle may predispose.

  (1) Possible causes of first-degree AV block include cardiac glycosides, quinidine, or procainamide administration, or the presence of hyperkalemia or hypokalemia. Horses may develop the condition in the presence of systemic illness, such as strangles.

  (2) Possible causes for second-degree AV block include infection, xylazine or digitalis administration, electrolyte imbalances, or AV nodal disease. Although AV block can occur in young horses after viral or bacterial infections, only approximately 20% of adult horses with second-degree AV block have an associated infectious disease.

  d. Diagnostic plan and laboratory tests

  (1) First-degree AV block is characterized by a normal heart rate, normal P-QRS-T complexes and a prolonged P-R interval (greater than 0.44 seconds in the horse).

  (2) Second-degree AV block. Two types can be distinguished by ECG: **Mobitz type I (Wenckebach)** and **Mobitz type II.**

  (a) Mobitz type I is characterized by a P-R interval that is gradually pro-

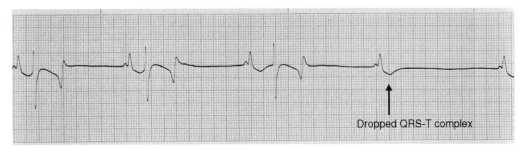

Dropped QRS-T complex

FIGURE 8-2. Base-apex lead-II ECG from a horse with second-degree AV block, Mobitz type I (Wenckebach). Paper speed, 25 mm/sec; 10 mm = 1 mV.

longed until the QRS-T complex is dropped (Figure 8-2). Mobitz type I is the most common type in horses.

- **(b) Mobitz type II** is characterized by a P-R interval that is unchanged, and the blocked beat is unheralded. In both types, the first post-block beat is characterized by a decreased P-R interval, a decreased T-wave amplitude, and a reduction in the negative deflection of the T wave. Sinus arrhythmia frequently accompanies second-degree AV block in horses.

  e. Therapeutic plan and prognosis
  - **(1)** No treatment is required for either AV block. Both of these blocks disappear with exercise.
  - **(2)** Prognosis is excellent, provided there is no underlying cardiac disease.

2. **Advanced second- and third-degree AV block (complete heart block).** A **second-degree AV block** is considered advanced if it persists with exercise and the heart rate does not increase appropriately in response to exercise, excitement, or atropine. A **third-degree AV block** is characterized by a complete block or isolation of the ventricles from the atria.

   a. Patient profile. These bradyarrhythmias are uncommon in large animals and are associated with severe exercise intolerance and syncope.

   b. Clinical findings
   - **(1) Clinical signs.** Horses with advanced second- and third-degree AV block may show no clinical signs at rest, but they exhibit profound exercise intolerance and lethargy with exercise. Animals with third-degree AV block commonly faint (e.g., animals with **Adams-Stokes syndrome**).
   - **(2) Physical examination findings**
     - **(a) Advanced second-degree AV block.** Cardiac auscultation reveals an absence of S1, S2, and S3 when the block occurs.
     - **(b) Third-degree AV block**
       - **(i)** The **pulse rate** in horses with this condition is slow (usually 10–20 beats/min), and the **pulse quality** is poor. The heart rate does not increase appropriately in response to exercise, excitement, or atropine.
       - **(ii)** The **heart rhythm** is frequently regular, but the **intensity** of S1 is variable. The animal often has **high central venous pressure.**

   c. Etiology and pathogenesis
   - **(1) Advanced second-degree AV block.** Underlying cardiac disease is usually present with this block. Chronic inflammatory changes in the AV node and bundle of His have been reported as the causative lesions.
   - **(2) Third-degree AV block.** In this block, the ventricles establish their own rate, which is usually slow (15–20 beats/min). As a result, cardiac output is reduced. The sinoatrial node attempts to compensate and thus, the atrial rate is quite high (94–150 beats/min).

   d. Diagnostic plan and laboratory tests
   - **(1) Advanced second-degree AV block.** Frequently, P waves are not followed by a QRS-T complex. The P-R interval is consistently greater than 0.6 seconds.
   - **(2) Third-degree AV block.** P waves are not associated with QRS-T complexes

and a slower junctional or ventricular escape rhythm is present. The junctional escape rhythm appears as a normal QRS-T complex with a slower rate (20–30 beats/min). A ventricular escape rhythm appears as a QRS-T complex of abnormal morphologic character with a rate of only 10–20 beats/min, which may be uniform or multiform. The P-P interval is regular (Figure 8-3).

e. **Therapeutic plan**

(1) **Cardiac pacemaker.** The definitive treatment of third-degree AV block is the implantation of a cardiac pacemaker, which has been done successfully in a horse.

(2) **Stall rest** and treatment with **corticosteroids** may be beneficial if active inflammation is thought to be present. The administration of **dexamethasone** to horses with third-degree AV block may result in temporary improvement in third-degree heart block.

3. **Sinus arrhythmia, sinoatrial block, and sinus arrest**

a. **Patient profile.** Sinus arrhythmia is not commonly seen in adult cattle, but it is a frequent occurrence in horses, sheep, and goats. This condition also commonly occurs in young large animals. Sinoatrial block is much less common in horses than incomplete AV block.

b. **Clinical findings**

(1) **Sinus arrhythmia** is characterized by a slow to normal heart rate. There is a cyclic variation in the heart rate that may or may not be associated with the respiratory rate. The heart rate is usually faster during inspiration and slower during expiration. The arrhythmia usually disappears with exercise.

(2) **Sinoatrial block** and **sinus arrest** sound similar to sinus arrhythmia on auscultation.

(3) **Fainting** may occur in patients with persistent sinus arrest unless an ectopic pacemaker in the AV junction or in a lower focus takes control of cardiac rhythm. This arrhythmia has not been well documented in horses but has been suspected in some fainting horses with severe atrial myocardial disease.

c. **Etiology and pathogenesis**

(1) **Sinus arrhythmia** is thought to be caused by increased vagal tone. In cattle, this condition may be attributable to acid–base and electrolyte abnormalities as well.

(2) **Sinoatrial block** occurs when an impulse is initiated in the sinoatrial node but is not conducted to the rest of the heart. This block occurs as an apparently normal phenomenon caused by elevated vagal tone at rest.

(3) **Intermittent sinus arrest** is thought to be caused by a reflex increase in vagal tone on inspiration, which leads to an exaggerated sinus arrhythmia. Ocular or carotid sinus pressure may also produce sinus arrest. Other pathologic conditions of the atria, such as dilation and fibrosis, and drug toxicity (e.g., quinidine, digoxin, or propranolol) can cause sinus arrest.

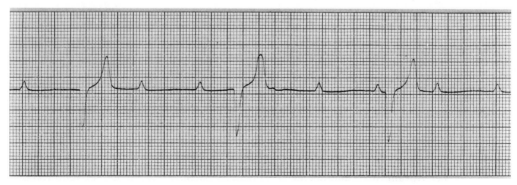

FIGURE 8-3. ECG recorded from a horse with third-degree AV block. Paper speed, 25 mm/sec; 10 mm = 1 mV.

    d. Diagnostic plan and laboratory tests

       (1) Sinus arrhythmia. The P-P intervals differ by more than 10%.

       (2) Sinoatrial block is usually diagnosed when a sinus arrhythmia is present in which the P-P interval is at least twice the sinus interval of preceding or subsequent beats. Often, the condition is diagnosed by inference. A type of sinoatrial block has been described in which the P-P intervals become progressively shorter until there is a long pause, and the P-P interval following the dropped beat is prolonged.

       (3) Sinoatrial block cannot be distinguished from **sinus arrest** when no impulse is initiated from the sinoatrial node, and both atria and ventricles fail to contract.

    e. Therapeutic plan

       (1) Sinus arrhythmia requires no treatment.

       (2) Asymptomatic sinoatrial block does not require therapy and usually disappears after exercise or excitement.

       (3) Symptomatic sinoatrial block or **sinus arrest** may be treated by the administration of **atropine** or **isoproterenol** to elevate the sinus rate. If drug toxicity is suspected, the drug should be discontinued.

C. Tachyarrhythmias

  1. Supraventricular tachyarrhythmias

    a. Atrial premature depolarizations (supraventricular premature complexes) and atrial tachycardia

       (1) Patient profile. Both of these conditions can occur in all large animal species but are uncommon even in association with cardiac disease. Supraventricular premature complexes occur more frequently than ventricular premature complexes.

       (2) Clinical findings

         (a) Affected animals may exhibit **no clinical abnormalities** or **impaired performance** and **exercise intolerance.** The frequency of the premature depolarizations may increase during or after exercise. Other horses may have normal sinus rhythm at rest and develop premature complexes after exercise.

         (b) The **heart rate** is often rapid, irregularly irregular, and closely resembles AF. With atrial tachycardia, the heart rate is often very rapid (120–220 beats/min).

       (3) Etiology and pathogenesis. Causes of both conditions include increased vagal tone, systemic disease, electrolyte and metabolic disturbances, and myocardial disease. Causes of myocardial disease include viruses, bacteria, ischemia, and toxins. Evidence of an underlying cause of the arrhythmia may not be readily apparent.

         (a) Supraventricular tachycardia results from an ectopic focus within the atrium or at the AV junction and may be paroxysmal or sustained. Not all of the atrial impulses are conducted through the AV node and ventricular pathways; thus, second-degree AV block frequently occurs.

         (b) Atrial tachycardia occurs in horses with ventricular pre-excitation (e.g., **Wolff-Parkinson-White syndrome**). This condition also has been noted during quinidine sulfate therapy for AF and may result from digitalis toxicity or hypokalemia. It may be paroxysmal or continuous.

       (4) Diagnostic plan and laboratory tests. An ECG obtained **during exercise** may be necessary to determine the clinical relevance of the arrhythmia or to elicit the arrhythmia.

         (a) Supraventricular (or atrial) premature depolarizations. The ECG reveals a premature P wave, often of abnormal morphologic character, which is followed by a normal QRS-T complex. The premature P wave may be buried in the QRS-T complex and, thus, may be difficult to detect. Occasionally, the premature P wave is not followed by a QRS-T complex,

TABLE 8-3. Digoxin Treatment Protocol for Horses and Cattle with Congestive Heart Failure (CHF)

Digoxin Dose	Horse	Cow
Priming dose	12–14 μg/kg intravenously 34 (elixir)–70 (tabs) μg/kg orally	22 μg/kg intravenously
Maintenance dose	6–7 μg/kg/24 hr intravenously	Infusion of 0.86 μg/kg/hr intravenously
	17 (elixir)–35 (tabs) μg/kg/24 hr orally	11 μg/kg intravenously every 8 hours

particularly if the impulse occurred early in diastole and arrives at the AV node before the tissue has completely depolarized.

   (b) Atrial tachycardia. The conformation of P waves is different from those seen during normal sinus rhythm. Because not all atrial impulses are conducted through the AV node and ventricular pathways, second-degree AV block may be present, making the diagnosis of the arrhythmia from the ECG difficult. Paroxysmal bursts of tachycardia are four or more premature beats, starting and ending abruptly and lasting less than 30 seconds. The R-R interval is usually regular.

  (5) Therapeutic plan
   (a) Identification and **removal** of the primary cause is important in the treatment of both arrhythmias.
   (b) Stall rest for 1–2 months with frequent monitoring of heart rate and rhythm is recommended in horses.
   (c) Digoxin (Table 8-3). If supraventricular tachycardia is sustained and results in CHF, treatment with digoxin may help slow the ventricular response to the atrial impulse. **Application of pressure** to the eye or carotid sinus before and after digitalization may help decrease the heart rate.
   (d) Quinidine sulfate may be effective because it suppresses the ectopic foci and prolongs the refractory period of the atrial musculature.
   (e) Treatment with corticosteroids has been suggested but is controversial and of questionable efficacy.
  (6) Prognosis depends on the underlying problem and the ability to correct the arrhythmia.
 b. AF in horses
  (1) Patient profile. AF occurs in most horse breeds, but the condition appears to be particularly common in young male Standardbreds and draft horses. This apparent breed and sex predilection is probably a reflection of the equine population in areas where studies were conducted. Reports of AF in ponies, yearlings, and foals are rare. AF is the most common arrhythmia affecting equine athletes.
  (2) Clinical findings
   (a) Clinical signs are variable.
    (i) Broodmares and **horses doing light work** are generally asymptomatic, and AF is an incidental finding.
    (ii) Performance horses with AF usually are exercise intolerant and may exhibit exercise-induced pulmonary hemorrhage (EIPH), dyspnea, myositis, ataxia, or collapse after exercise.
    (iii) Horses with moderate to severe left or right AV valvular regurgitation may have signs of CHF, in addition to AF.
    (iv) Horses presenting with colic occasionally have concurrent AF, but generally AF is not associated with gastrointestinal disease in horses.
   (b) Cardiovascular examination is abnormal in affected horses.
    (i) Characteristic findings. An irregularly irregular cardiac rhythm, vari-

able intensity heart sounds, and the absence of S4 are characteristic findings on cardiac auscultation.

   (ii) The **resting heart rate** is usually normal, but heart rates may range from less than 20 to more than 60 beats/min. Heart rates that are more than 60 beats/min generally indicate underlying heart disease and CHF, whereas extremely slow rates suggest an underlying conduction disorder.

   (iii) **Pulse pressures** in affected horses may vary from beat to beat.

   (iv) **Systolic heart murmurs,** consistent with mitral or tricuspid insufficiency, are common.

(3) Etiology and pathogenesis. AF is thought to be initiated by an atrial premature depolarization and sustained by a reentry mechanism. Variation in the ability of adjacent areas of atrial myocardium to be depolarized by an aberrant impulse **(inhomogeneous refractoriness)** is required for reentry to occur.

   (a) AF in the absence of underlying cardiac pathology. The large atrial mass and high vagal tone of normal horses are **predisposing factors** for the development of AF.

   (i) A **large atrial myocardial mass** promotes reentry because it increases the likelihood that an aberrant impulse will encounter a nonrefractory myocardium.

   (ii) **High vagal tone** shortens the effective refractory period and increases inhomogeneous refractoriness, thereby further promoting reentry.

   (b) AF in the presence of underlying cardiac disease

   (i) **Focal myocardial diseases** (e.g., myocarditis) can cause physical heterogeneity of atrial myocardial fibers and may allow AF to persist.

   (ii) **Acquired** or **congenital cardiac diseases** that result in atrial enlargement promote the reentry of aberrant impulses and maintain AF. Moderate to severe left AV valvular insufficiency causes atrial enlargement and has been documented in 10%–84% of horses with AF.

   (c) AF and potassium depletion. Decreased atrial myocardial cell potassium content may contribute to the development of AF. Potassium loss in sweat and the use of potassium-depleting drugs (e.g., furosemide) cause potassium depletion in horses.

   (d) Paroxysmal AF, an arrhythmia that occurs during maximal exercise and resolves within 24 hours, has been associated with transient poor performance in horses.

   (i) **Rapid pacing of the atria** during exercise can cause paroxysmal AF.

   (ii) Paroxysmal AF occurs occasionally in horses with **gastrointestinal disorders** and in horses under **general anesthesia.**

   (iii) **Potassium depletion** may also be cause of paroxysmal AF.

(4) Diagnostic plan and laboratory tests

   (a) ECG findings

   (i) An **irregular R-R interval with the absence of P waves and coarse baseline f waves** is diagnostic of AF (Figure 8-4).

   (ii) Some variation in **QRS and T morphology** may be noted.

   (iii) Occasionally, horses will have **ectopic ventricular depolarizations,** which appear as bizarre-shaped or widened QRS complexes.

   (b) Echocardiographic findings. Echocardiography should be performed to detect underlying cardiac disease, such as atrial enlargement or severe valvular regurgitation in horses with auscultable murmurs.

   (c) Clinical pathology

   (i) **Urinalysis.** Urinary fractional excretion of potassium can be measured to assess the whole-body potassium status.

   (ii) **Cardiac isoenzyme activities** can be determined if an underlying myocarditis is suspected.

(5) Therapeutic plan

   (a) Quinidine, a negative ionotrope and positive chronotrope, is the **drug of**

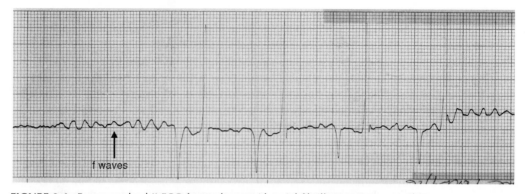

FIGURE 8-4. Base-apex lead-II ECG from a horse with atrial fibrillation. Paper speed 25 mm/sec; 10 mm = 1 mV. Notice the absence of P waves and the presence of flutter waves with irregular rhythm; heart rate = 30 beats/min; 10 mm = 1 mV.

choice for treatment of AF in horses. It prolongs the effective refractory period of the atrial myocardium, thereby suppressing reentry.

(i) **Side effects**

- Quinidine has **anticholinergic properties** that promote AV nodal conductivity and cause tachycardia. This drug should not be used alone in horses with tachycardia (i.e., horses with a heart rate greater than 60 beats/min) or CHF. Concurrent digoxin therapy is required to support the failing heart of such patients.

- Quinidine has *α*-adrenoreceptor blocking properties, which can cause vasodilation and hypotension in treated patients.

(ii) **Administration.** There are **several protocols** for quinidine administration in horses, including intravenous and oral regimens with or without digitalization (Table 8-4). **Oral dosing** requires **nasogastric intubation** because direct oral administration causes oral ulceration.

(iii) **Pharmacokinetics**

- Quinidine concentration peaks ± 2 hours after oral administration.

- Quinidine is 80% protein-bound in plasma and undergoes hepatic metabolism and urinary excretion. In horses, the drug's half-life is ± 6 hours.

- **Therapeutic index.** Quinidine has a narrow therapeutic index. **Therapeutic plasma concentrations** range from 2 to 4 μg/ml. Signs of **toxicosis** occur at plasma concentrations of more than 5 μg/ml. Ideally, quinidine concentrations in plasma should be monitored during therapy, and treatment intervals should be adjusted to maintain concentrations in the therapeutic range.

(iv) **Drug monitoring for quinidine toxicosis.** Because drug monitoring is impractical in many instances, horses undergoing treatment are closely monitored for ECG changes or clinical signs that may indicate quinidine toxicosis. For **horses undergoing intravenous quinidine treatment,** continuous ECG monitoring is preferred and is essential. **Horses that are administered quinidine orally** should have an ECG performed every 2 hours (i.e., immediately before the next treatment and at the peak plasma concentration). Signs indicating quinidine toxicity and the appropriate actions are described in Table 8-5.

(b) **Treatment of CHF**

(i) **Diuretics.** The main treatment includes diuretics (e.g., furosemide), vasodilators, and positive inotropic agents (e.g., digoxin; see Table 8-3).

TABLE 8-4. Quinidine Treatment Protocols for Horses with Atrial Fibrillation (AF)

Description	Protocol	Indications
Quinidine gluconate IV	With continuous ECG monitoring, administer 1.0–1.5 mg/kg quinidine gluconate IV over 1 minute and repeat every 5–10 minutes until sinus rhythm is restored. Stop treatment when (1) a total dose of 11 mg/kg has been administered; (2) the QRS complex duration increases to >25% over baseline; or (3) tachycardia (>90 beats/min) and/or other clinical signs of toxicity are observed.	Horses with AF of <1 week's duration and no evidence of underlying cardiac disease are candidates for this regimen.
Quinidine sulfate PO (standard protocol)	Administer 22 mg/kg quinidine sulfate via nasogastric tube every 2 hours until sinus rhythm is restored. Stop treatment when (1) 6 treatments of 22 mg/kg each (a total dose of 132 mg/kg) have been given; (2) the QRS complex increases to >25% of baseline; or (3) tachycardia (>90 beats/min) and/or other signs of quinidine toxicity are observed. This procedure can be repeated for 3 consecutive days.	Horses with AF of ≤4 months' duration and no evidence of underlying cardiac disease are candidates for this regimen.
Quinidine sulfate PO (modified protocol)	This protocol is similar to the standard protocol. If sinus rhythm is not restored after 4–6 treatments of 22 mg/kg each, treatment intervals are increased to once every 6 hours to maintain steady-state plasma concentrations. These treatments every 6 hours are usually continued for 2 days.	Horses with AF of long duration, or with significant underlying cardiac disease but no evidence of CHF, are candidates for this regimen.
Quinidine sulfate PO followed by digoxin PO	If conversion with the modified protocol has not occurred by day 2, oral digoxin at 0.01 mg/kg every 12 hours should be added to the treatment regimen.	Horses with AF of long duration, or with significant underlying cardiac disease with or without CHF, are candidates for this protocol.

CHF = congestive heart failure; ECG = electrocardiogram; IV = intravenously; PO = orally.

        (ii) Exercise restriction and **dietary sodium reduction** are important.
        (iii) Intravenous fluid support is necessary for the correction of dehydration and electrolyte and acid–base imbalances.
    (6) Prognosis
        (a) In the absence of underlying cardiac disease, AF is treated successfully in 90% of cases. Clinical findings that indicate a good prognosis include:
           (i) Duration of exercise intolerance less than 4 months
           (ii) Intensity of cardiac murmur less than grade III
           (iii) Resting heart rate less than 60 beats/min
           (iv) No evidence of CHF
        (b) Several factors have been associated with the lack of conversion, recurrence of the arrhythmia, or signs of quinidine toxicity. These include:
           (i) A prolonged (i.e., greater than 4-month) history of poor performance
           (ii) Intensity of cardiac murmur greater than grade III
           (iii) Resting heart rate greater than 60 beats/min
           (iv) Signs of CHF

c. AF in cattle
  (1) Patient profile. AF is diagnosed most often in mature, hospitalized dairy cattle. The fact that AF is diagnosed more frequently in dairy cattle than beef cattle reflects the prevalence of dairy cattle in hospital populations where studies were conducted, not necessarily a breed predisposition.
  (2) Clinical findings
    (a) Extracardiac signs
      (i) Cattle with AF generally have evidence of **gastrointestinal disease** (e.g., abomasal displacements, indigestion, diarrhea). AF has also been associated with **foot rot** and **pneumonia** in cattle.
      (ii) Anorexia and **decreased milk production** are common in cows with AF and are likely secondary to underlying gastrointestinal problems.
    (b) Cardiovascular signs
      (i) Heart rate. Affected cows have an **irregular heart rhythm** with no underlying regularity. Heart sounds vary in intensity, and S4 is absent. Heart rates may be slow, normal, or fast; tachycardia in cattle usually is associated with serious underlying gastrointestinal disease.
      (ii) Arterial pulses vary in intensity, but actual pulse deficits are rare.
      (iii) Heart murmurs and **signs of CHF** are extremely rare in cattle with AF.
  (3) Etiology and pathogenesis. The pathogenesis of AF in cattle is the same as in the horse. Predisposing factors include:
    (a) Gastrointestinal diseases, such as displaced abomasum, vagal indigestion, or diarrhea
    (b) Myocardial or **cardiac diseases,** such as myocarditis, BE, cardiomyopathy, or traumatic reticulopericarditis
    (c) Vagal nerve irritation (such as may occur with severe respiratory disease)
    (d) Organic brain disease (e.g., thiamine-responsive encephalopathy), which can cause sympathetic or parasympathetic stimulation
    (e) Electrolyte disturbances, such as hyper- or hypocalcemia or acid–base imbalances, such as metabolic alkalosis

TABLE 8-5. Quinidine Toxicity in Horses

Finding	Action
Cardiac signs	
Prolongation of the QRS complex to >25% of the pretreatment value	Stop treatment.
Sustained increase in ventricular rate of >100 beats/min	Add digoxin (0.002 mg/kg IV; 0.01 mg/kg PO) to slow the ventricular rate.
Severe atrial tachycardia (rare)	Stop treatment.
	Administer isotonic sodium bicarbonate (1 mmol/kg) to increase protein binding of quinidine.
	Administer digoxin (0.002 mg/kg) to slow the ventricular rate.
	Rapidly infuse isotonic fluid to expand plasma volume.
	Administer a pressor agent [e.g., phenylephrine (10 mg in 500 ml of 0.9% saline as a fast drip)]
Extracardiac signs	
Depression, paraphimosis, colic, diarrhea, laminitis, upper airway edema, ataxia, convulsions, and urticaria	Stop treatment and address individual problems. If colic is mild, quinidine therapy can be continued. Flunixin meglumine may be used to control abdominal discomfort.

IV = intravenously; PO = orally.

(f) Other inflammatory or **infectious conditions,** such as foot rot causing pain-mediated vagal disturbance

(4) Diagnostic plan and laboratory tests

   (a) An **ECG tracing** is required for definitive diagnosis of AF. ECG changes in cattle are similar to those described for horses [see III C 1 b (4) (a)].

   (b) Echocardiography should be performed if underlying cardiac disease is suspected. However, in most cases, this test is not necessary.

   (c) Serum analysis

      (i) A **serum biochemical profile** and **blood gas analysis** should be performed to detect electrolyte and blood gas abnormalities. Electrolyte and blood gas disturbances, which are common in cattle with AF, are attributable **to underlying gastrointestinal disease.** Multiple electrolyte derangements in the same individual and high vagal tone associated with gastrointestinal disease may be important in establishing AF in cattle.

      (ii) Metabolic alkalosis is the most consistent finding. **Hypokalemia, hypochloremia,** and **hypocalcemia** also may be present.

(5) Therapeutic plan

   (a) Treatment of the primary gastrointestinal problem and the correction of electrolyte balance in cattle with AF often result in spontaneous conversion to normal sinus rhythm, usually within 5 days.

   (b) Quinidine therapy

      (i) Indications. Quinidine therapy is indicated for cattle that do not convert spontaneously within 5 days, cattle with chronic gastrointestinal problems (e.g., vagal indigestion), and cattle with low cardiac output secondary to AF (e.g., those with poor peripheral perfusion, weak arterial pulses, pulse deficits).

      (ii) Administration. Quinidine sulfate (48 mg/kg suspended in 4 L of isotonic saline or lactated Ringer's solution) is administered at a rate of 1 L/hr while intravenous fluids are administered simultaneously in the opposite jugular vein. The ECG should be monitored frequently during the infusion and the infusion discontinued as soon as conversion occurs. Therapy should be discontinued after the 4-L infusion, even if the cow still has AF.

      (iii) Monitoring and side effects. Cattle should be closely monitored during the infusion. Diarrhea and depression are common side effects, and the infusion can be continued despite their occurrence. The infusion rate should be slowed if the ventricular rate is more than 100 beats/min or if the QRS complex is visibly prolonged.

   (c) Digoxin is used before quinidine therapy in cattle with heart rates greater than 100 beats/min (see Table 8-3).

(6) Prognosis

   (a) The prognosis for cattle with AF is good if spontaneous conversion occurs after the correction of the primary problem. Unless underlying heart disease is present, few cattle revert to AF.

   (b) In rare cases, cattle do not respond to quinidine therapy. These unresponsive animals generally have progressive cardiac disease and are poor producers.

2. Ventricular tachyarrhythmias. Generally, **ventricular arrhythmias** are less common than **atrial arrhythmias** in large animals and are more indicative of cardiac disease.

  a. Ventricular premature depolarizations and tachycardia

    (1) Patient profile. Intermittent or **persistent ventricular tachycardia** is very uncommon in large animals.

    (2) Clinical findings. Common clinical signs include fever, exercise intolerance, weight loss, anorexia, and lethargy.

      (a) Ventricular premature contractions may be detected by auscultation and palpation of the pulse.

       (i) Heart rate. The beats occur earlier than expected and are usually followed by a pause.

       (ii) Heart sounds. A loud diastolic summation sound with a S2 of variable intensity may be heard. The peripheral pulse and S2 may even be absent during the premature beats. After a normal beat, only S1 and S2 are heard immediately. This sound differs from a normal S3, which can be heard in some horses, because it is usually louder and more prolonged.

    (b) Ventricular tachycardia generally is defined as four or more sustained ventricular depolarizations occurring at a rapid rate. With this disorder, the heart rate is rapid and regular. Periods of tachycardia may vary by starting and stopping suddenly, lasting for four or more beats, or persisting for hours or weeks.

  (3) Etiology

    (a) Causes in horses include septicemia or toxemia, severe digestive disturbances, and primary cardiovascular disease characterized by myocardial damage.

    (b) Predisposing factors. Various drugs (e.g., inhalant anesthetics), toxins, and electrolyte disturbances increase myocardial irritability and may exacerbate premature ventricular beats, which are thought to be caused by interference with the conduction of impulses originating from the same focus. Hypoxia, anemia, uremia, acidosis, sepsis, hypokalemia, and exhausting exercise are predisposing factors.

  (4) Diagnostic plan and laboratory tests

    (a) ECG

       (i) Ventricular premature contractions are characterized by the presence of wide, bizarre-shaped QRS complexes that appear earlier than expected and are not preceded by a true premature P wave. The T wave is usually oriented in the opposite direction to the QRS complex. A normal P wave occurs at its expected time but may not be evident if it is buried within the QRS-T complex of the premature systole. The interval between the end of the previous T wave and the beginning of the premature QRS-T complex is usually constant. Two or more different shapes of QRS complexes and different R-R intervals suggest that several different ectopic foci are inducing the contractions. **Ventricular fusion beats** may be apparent. These beats occur if the ventricular ectopic pacemaker initiates an impulse after the impulse from the normal pacemaker has already entered ventricular tissue. As a result, the ventricle is excited from two sources, and a QRS-T complex is created with an appearance intermediate between that of the premature systole and the dominant beat.

       (ii) Ventricular tachycardia produces a series of QRS-T complexes that are bizarre in contour. Sometimes P waves occur independently at a slower rate than the ventricular complexes. Ventricular fusion beats may be present. **Bidirectional ventricular tachycardia** is characterized by alternate QRS complexes that occur in opposite directions.

    (b) Echocardiography may be useful to look for myocardial, endocardial, or valvular damage to the heart. It may be normal.

  (5) Therapeutic plan. Therapy for both arrhythmias should be initiated immediately and should be directed toward the underlying condition, which may be CHF, neoplasia, pericarditis, myocarditis, or secondary problems (e.g., hypoxia, uremia).

    (a) The **correction of acid–base** and **electrolyte disturbances** should be attempted. **Rest, nonsteroidal anti-inflammatory drugs (NSAIDs),** and **systemic antimicrobials** are often indicated.

    (b) Digitalis. The use of digitalis for ventricular premature systole and ventricular tachycardia may eliminate the ventricular ectopic contraction. This agent can be used if the patient has CHF.

    (c) Lidocaine hydrochloride (0.5–1.0 mg/kg intravenously) may be helpful for arresting ventricular premature beats in situations other than cardiac failure. However, lidocaine may cause twitching and convulsions in unanesthetized horses.

    (d) Quinidine sulfate can be used to treat both of these arrhythmias.

        (i) Doses are 20 mg/kg orally every 6 hours until conversion or 6 mg/kg intravenously at a rate of 0.5 mg/kg/hr.

        (ii) Side effects. This drug can result in hypotension and reduced myocardial contractility.

    (e) Magnesium sulfate supplementation has been used successfully in the treatment of ventricular tachycardia in horses.

  (6) Prognosis is guarded. Ventricular tachycardia is particularly dangerous because it may convert to ventricular fibrillation and cause death.

b. Ventricular fibrillation is frequently the immediate cause of death in moribund animals. Transient ventricular fibrillation is not known to occur in large animals.

  (1) Clinical findings. Ventricular fibrillation is so **rapidly fatal** that it is rarely detected clinically except in animals under anesthesia. Few if any clinical signs occur before death. **Cardiac auscultation** may reveal a complete, sudden cessation of heart sounds. A pulse is absent, and there is a precipitous drop in blood pressure.

  (2) Etiology and pathogenesis

    (a) Etiology. Causes are the same as those for ventricular premature beats and ventricular tachycardia [see III C 2 a (3) (a)]. Ischemic damage to the heart is usually the underlying cause of this arrhythmia.

    (b) Pathogenesis. Coordinated contraction of the ventricles ceases with this arrhythmia, and continuous chaotic activity replaces regular systole and diastole.

  (3) Diagnostic plan and laboratory tests. ECG reveals bizarre, irregular oscillations without normal QRS-T complexes.

  (4) Therapeutic plan. No treatment is currently available.

    (a) Electrical defibrillation of adult large animals, such as horses and cattle, has not been successful with available equipment.

    (b) Some work in humans and primates has shown dietary enrichment with **fish oil-derived omega-3 polyunsaturated fatty acids** (to suppress ventricular fibrillation) to be beneficial.

IV. PERICARDIAL DISEASE

A. **Introduction.** Pericardial diseases are rare in veterinary species.

  1. Etiology. There are several reported causes for pericardial disease in large animals, which can be grouped as **congenital** and **acquired.** Acquired pericarditis is more common. Causes include bacterial and viral infections, neoplasia, and trauma. Idiopathic pericarditis is also widely reported.

  2. Pathogenesis

    a. Pericardial disease causes diastolic cardiac dysfunction with minimal alterations in systolic function. Elevated intrapericardial pressure inhibits diastolic cardiac filling, resulting in a reduction in preload for a given venous filling pressure. As a result of the reduction in preload, there is decreased cardiac output if there are no compensatory changes in heart rate, cardiac contractility, and vascular resistance.

    b. Pericardial effusion and **constrictive pericarditis** are the two major pathologic consequences of pericarditis. As the pericardium accumulates fluid or the wall of the pericardial sac becomes thickened, the stretching limit of the pericardial sac is exceeded, and pressure in the pericardial cavity begins to rise. **Cardiac tamponade** occurs when pericardial pressure exceeds the cardiac filling pressures, causing diastolic filling to be impaired.

B. **Pericarditis in cattle**

1. **Patient profile.** Pericarditis is uncommon in cattle, but when it occurs, it usually affects adult cattle and typically lasts 1 week or more. Traumatic pericarditis occurs in less than 10% of cattle with traumatic reticuloperitonitis. This pericarditis often occurs in adult cattle during late gestation or early postpartum.

2. **Clinical findings**
   a. **Complaints** may include weakness, anorexia, weight loss, and depression.
   b. **Physical examination findings**
      (1) Hyperpnea, prominent scleral vessels, fever, and signs of right-sided CHF (e.g., distended jugular and mammary veins; jugular pulsations; mandibular, brisket, and ventral edema; weak peripheral pulses) are usually present.
      (2) **Auscultation** of the thorax often reveals tachycardia and muffled heart sounds, with fluid auscultable in the region of the heart. Lung sounds may be absent in the ventral thorax.
      (3) **Rumen motility** is generally decreased. Signs of cranial abdominal pain are usually present, as well as a reluctance to move.

3. **Etiology**
   a. **Trauma** is a common cause of pericarditis in cattle. Trauma may be induced by external wounds, the penetration of ingested foreign objects, the hematogenous spread of infection (e.g., septicemia), or the extension of infection from other sites, such as the lung, heart, or pleura.
   b. **Other causes.** Pericarditis may also result from vegetative endocarditis that affects one or more cardiac valves, CHF, congenital heart defects, toxins, or neoplasia (particularly lymphosarcoma).

4. **Diagnostic plan and laboratory tests**
   a. **Thoracic radiographs** of the thorax and cranial abdomen in the standing cow may reveal a gas–fluid interface within the pericardial sac. The heart may assume a large, globoid silhouette. Sometimes a linear metallic foreign body can be visualized in the cranial reticulum, the caudal thorax, or both.
   b. **Echocardiography** is the most sensitive, specific, and noninvasive diagnostic test. As little as 15–20 ml of pericardial effusion can be seen using M-mode echocardiography. An **"echo-free space"** is evident between the myocardium and pericardium. The pericardial sac may appear thickened, and poor cardiac contractility is noted frequently.
      (1) **Other cardiac anomalies,** such as vegetative valvular lesions or tumors, may be seen on 2D echocardiograms.
      (2) Evidence of **cardiac tamponade,** such as right ventricular collapse during diastole and right atrial collapse, are common findings with large effusions.
   c. **Pericardiocentesis** can be therapeutic as well as diagnostic. Cytologic, bacteriologic, and viral culturing of pericardial effusion may be done.
      (1) **Technique.** Echocardiography is used to guide needle or catheter placement. Usually the procedure is done from the left fifth intercostal space 2.5–10 cm dorsal to the olecranon.
      (2) **Risks.** The risks associated with this procedure include laceration of the heart, coronary arteries, or lungs, and the development of ventricular arrhythmias. Care must be taken to avoid contaminating the thorax with septic effusion from the pericardium.
   d. **Electrocardiography.** An ECG may reveal decreased amplitude of QRS complexes, **electrical alternans** (i.e., altered configuration of the P, QRS, or T complexes), and ST segment elevation or slurring. Some arrhythmias may be present, particularly sinus tachycardia.
   e. **Cardiac catheterization** demonstrates an elevation in central venous or right atrial pressure, and the atrial and ventricular pressure curve may appear abnormal. Right atrial, right ventricular, and PA end-diastolic pressures may equilibrate.

5. **Therapeutic plan and prognosis**
   a. **Surgery.** Reducing the intrapericardial pressure is the primary goal of treatment.

This can be accomplished by **pericardiotomy** (surgically opening the pericardial sac) or **subtotal pericardiectomy** (partially removing the pericardial sac) to facilitate fluid drainage. Other methods of fluid drainage include surgical **marsupialization** (attaching the pericardial sac to the skin wound) or placement of an **indwelling surgical drain.** At the time of surgery, any foreign body in the thorax can be removed and abscesses can be drained or removed.

  b. **Administration of systemic antimicrobials and analgesics** may be helpful, as well as **lavage of the pericardium.** Fluid support, diuretics, and inotropic agents, such as dopamine or digoxin, may be necessary.

C. **Pericarditis in horses**

  1. **Patient profile.** Pericardial disease, in general, is uncommon in horses. It is seen most often in adult horses, although any age can be affected.

  2. **Clinical findings**
     a. **Clinical signs** may include fever, jugular distention, poor peripheral pulses, tachycardia, tachypnea or dyspnea, ventral abdominal distention, depression, mild abdominal pain, syncope, and weakness. Other signs of right-sided heart failure may be present.
     b. **Auscultation** of the thoracic cavity often reveals muffled heart sounds, pericardial friction rubs, and suspected pleural effusion. Lung sounds may be dull or absent ventrally, whereas heart sounds may radiate over a wider area.

  3. **Etiology.** There are **two major forms of acquired pericardial disease** seen in horses: effusive and nonseptic, and exudative, fibrinous, and often septic.
     a. **Idiopathic pericarditis,** characterized by an aseptic inflammatory exudate, occurs in horses.
     b. **Bacteria.** In several small case series in horses, **fibrinous pericarditis** was attributed to *Actinobacillus equuli.* This organism is a common inhabitant of the tonsils and fecal contents of normal adult horses and may gain access to the heart hematogenously. **Streptococcal infections** and *Actinomyces pyogenes* have been associated with individual cases of equine pericarditis.
     c. **Neoplasia.** A **pericardial mesothelioma** also has been associated with individual cases of equine pericarditis.
     d. **Viruses,** such as equine viral arteritis (EVA), equine herpes virus, equine infectious anemia (EIA), and equine influenza, have been suspected but unproven as causes.
     e. **Trauma** from external wounds

  4. **Diagnostic plan and laboratory tests**
     a. The same methods are used in horses as in cattle, although radiography is less sensitive in horses (see IV B 4).
     b. **Laboratory abnormalities** include anemia, leukocytosis, high fibrinogen and creatinine concentrations, hyponatremia, and hyperkalemia.
     c. **Ancillary diagnostic tests.** The central venous pressure values exceed 45 cm of water.

  5. **Differential diagnoses**
     a. **Pleuritis and pneumonia**
     b. **Circumscribed space-occupying lesions** in the thorax, such as mediastinal or pulmonary abscess, lymphosarcoma, or invading gastric squamous cell carcinoma
     c. **Spontaneous tears in the atria or rupture of the ascending aorta**
     d. **Gunshot wounds**

  6. **Therapeutic plan.** Treatment is similar to that in cattle and should be directed at the primary cause (see IV B 5). **Parenteral corticosteroids** and **NSAIDs** may help control idiopathic or nonseptic pericarditis.

  7. **Prognosis. Relapse** and the **deterioration** of the condition can follow short-term improvements. Resolution is unlikely if the adhesive and exudative changes in the thorax are advanced.

   a. Because of poor response to treatment, the prognosis for **septic pericarditis** is usually guarded to poor.
   b. The prognosis may be fair for **idiopathic** or **nonseptic pericarditis.**

D. **Pericarditis in swine** is similar to that in horses and cattle (see IV B, C).

   1. Patient profile. Young pigs may be affected.

   2. Etiology. Causes include *Streptococcus* species, *Hemophilus parasuis* (Glasser's disease), and *Mycoplasma* species.

   3. Diagnostic plan. The diagnosis of pericarditis is often based on postmortem findings rather than radiographs, echocardiography, or ECG monitoring.

   4. Prognosis is guarded to poor. Death is usually attributable to septicemia.

V. MYOCARDIAL DISEASES

A. **Introduction**

   1. Definitions
      a. Myocarditis is inflammation of the myocardial wall caused by bacterial, viral, or parasitic organisms or thromboembolic disease caused by these organisms. Myocarditis also can occur following bacteremia, septicemia, pericarditis, or endocarditis, regardless of the cause.
      b. Cardiomyopathy is a subacute or chronic disease of the ventricular myocardium that occurs in the absence of valvular disease, congenital malformations of the heart or vessels, or pulmonary disease. In large animals, only dilated cardiomyopathy is important clinically. **Dilated cardiomyopathy** is associated with ventricular dilation, increased ventricular mass, and decreased systolic function.

   2. Patient profile and epidemiology
      a. Patient profile. These diseases have been reported sporadically in all large animal species.
      b. Epidemiology
         (1) Myocarditis. The **prevalence** of acute myocarditis is difficult to estimate because the disease often goes undiagnosed, is mild, or is masked by disease involving another organ system. Also, it is difficult to assess the clinical significance of postmortem evidence of myocardial inflammation and fibrosis. Morbidity due to myocarditis is probably underestimated because it is rarely the cause of death and is associated with infectious conditions that manifest themselves in other ways without specific cardiovascular signs.
         (2) Inherited cardiomyopathy in cattle has an **incidence** in inbred populations of 3%–5%. These cattle may be linked genetically by the presence of the red gene in Holstein-Friesian cattle. There does not appear to be a sex predilection for this inherited cardiomyopathy.

   3. Clinical findings. Some clinical signs are referable to other organ system involvement, including the respiratory system, reproductive tract, gastrointestinal tract, nervous system, or musculoskeletal system. Frequently, animals (particularly pigs) die suddenly with few or no premonitory signs.
      a. Complaints include depression, weakness, anorexia, intermittent or chronic fever, weight loss, or reproductive failure.
      b. Physical examination findings include tachycardia with a gallop rhythm, dyspnea, and other respiratory signs.
      c. Subcutaneous edema of the brisket, ventral thorax, submandibular area, and occasionally the limbs may be noted. **Thoracic auscultation** may reveal cardiac arrhythmias, murmurs (often either tricuspid insufficiency or a pulmonic valve ejection murmur), or weak or muffled heart sounds.

   4. Etiology and pathogenesis

a. **Etiology**
  (1) **Myocarditis.** The causes of myocarditis vary depending on the species.
    (a) **Cattle**
      (i) **Bacterial causes** include *Hemophilus somnus,* clostridial diseases (e.g., *Clostridium chauvoei*), *Staphylococcus aureus,* and *Mycobacterium* species. ***Borrelia burgdorferi,*** a spirochete, also may be a cause of myocarditis in ruminants.
      (ii) **Viral causes** include the picornavirus that causes foot-and-mouth disease.
      (iii) **Parasitic causes** in ruminants include toxoplasmosis, *Neospora caninum,* sarcocystis, and cysticercosis infection.
    (b) **Swine.** *Staphylococcus aureus, Streptococcus suis,* and viruses (e.g., the picornavirus that causes foot-and-mouth disease and the encephalomyocarditis virus) can cause myocarditis in pigs.
    (c) **Horses**
      (i) **Bacterial causes** include *Clostridium chauvoei, Streptococcus equi* or *zooepidemicus, Mycobacterium* species, and *Staphylococcus aureus.* ***Borrelia burgdorferi,*** a spirochete, also may be a cause of myocarditis in horses.
      (ii) **Viral causes** include EIA, EVA, equine influenza, and the reovirus that causes African horse sickness.
      (iii) **Parasitic causes** include strongylosis and onchocerciasis.
  (2) **Cardiomyopathy.** There are several conditions that have been associated with cardiomyopathy, ranging from myocarditis to inherited conditions.
    (a) Cardiomyopathy has been associated with the **ingestion of several different chemicals and plants,** including ionophores such as monensin and lasalocid, salinomycin, gossypol, *Cassia occidentalis,* and *Phalasis* species.
    (b) **Mineral** or **vitamin deficiencies** or **excesses** have been implicated, including vitamin E and selenium deficiency and primary and secondary copper deficiencies.
    (c) Neoplastic infiltration of the heart by **lymphosarcoma** or **fibrosarcoma** may also cause cardiomyopathy.
b. **Pathogenesis.** The pathophysiologic changes associated with myocardial disease depend on the specific nature and extent of the disease. Most infectious etiologies cause septicemia and hematogenous spread to the myocardium. **Myocardial damage** results from either vascular occlusion or direct bacterial, viral, or parasitic action on the myocardium. The end result of myocarditis and cardiomyopathy is reduced myocardial performance (reduced cardiac output).

5. **Diagnostic plan and laboratory tests**
  a. **Clinical pathology.** Myocardial tissue can be evaluated by **histology** and **bacteriologic culture.**
    (1) **Myocardial enzymes.** In animals with acute myocarditis, myocardial enzyme levels, including **aspartate aminotransferase (AST), creatine phosphokinase (CK),** and **lactate dehydrogenase (LDH),** are elevated. The sensitivity and specificity of these tests have not been determined for large animals.
    (2) **Analysis of pericardial or pleural fluids** reveals a transudate with low protein concentration and predominantly mononuclear cells.
    (3) **Tests for specific diseases** may include serology or viral isolation from white blood cells for bovine leukosis infection, tests for nutritional deficiencies and toxicities, and serum or liver copper concentrations. In horses, serologic testing for influenza, EVA, EIA, and herpesvirus may be helpful.
  b. **Echocardiography** may show increased ventricular chamber size, decreased thickness of the interventricular septum and left ventricular free wall, and decreased myocardial function. In animals with **dilated cardiomyopathy,** usually there are increased end-systolic and end-diastolic dimensions of the left and right ventricles, increased left atrial size, and an increased dimension ratio from the left atrium to the aortic root. Mitral valve insufficiency and decreased myocardial function may

be visualized by poor wall motion, which suggests poor contractility. A mass on the right atrium may be seen with BLV-induced lymphoma.

    c. Cardiac catheterization may reveal elevated intracardiac pressures (right atrium, right ventricle, PA, pulmonary capillary wedge, and left ventricular end diastolic) in animals with dilated cardiomyopathy.

6. Differential diagnoses include:
    a. Other cardiac diseases, such as BE or pericarditis, cardiac neoplasia
    b. Septicemia or **toxemia**
    c. Chronic pneumonia (all large animals) or **high-altitude disease** (cattle)

7. Therapeutic plan
    a. Management of myocarditis in all species includes the treatment of the underlying cause (if known) and control of cardiac complications, including dysrhythmias, CHF, or shock.
        (1) Corticosteroids may be of value in cases of severe toxemia, complicated dysrhythmias, or intractable heart failure.
        (2) Rest. Performance animals should be rested until signs of systemic illness have resolved and ECG changes have returned to normal.
    b. Therapeutic management of cardiomyopathy consists of the use of positive inotropes (e.g., digoxin), diuretics, vasodilators, rest, and the drainage of pleural, pericardial, or abdominal fluid.
    c. Supportive care, including intravenous fluids for the correction of fluid, electrolyte, and acid–base imbalances, NSAIDs, and control of cardiac dysrhythmias are important for successful resolution of myocarditis and cardiomyopathy.

8. Prognosis
    a. The prognosis for **myocarditis** is good if there are no signs of heart failure and if cardiac dysrhythmias are managed successfully. The prognosis is guarded to poor if signs of CHF are present.
    b. The prognosis is poor for animals with **dilated cardiomyopathy** and **BLV-induced lymphoma.** Cattle with **inherited cardiomyopathy** may die by 6 months of age, whereas other animals may be asymptomatic until 2–4 years of age.

9. Prevention and control consist of maintaining good vaccination and parasite control programs. Animals with deficiencies or toxicities should receive adequate concentrations of vitamin E, copper, and selenium in their diets.

B. **Gossypol-induced cardiotoxicosis. A significant number of cases** of gossypol toxicosis have been reported in ruminants in the last few years. This may be due to changes in the methods for extracting oil from cottonseed, increases in the amount of concentrates fed to animals, and the amount of creep feed offered to young ruminants.

1. Patient profile and history
    a. Patient profile. Young ruminants (e.g., kids, calves, lambs) and monogastrics (e.g., swine) are more susceptible to toxicosis than adult ruminants. The highest death losses have been reported in bottle-fed calves who are fed starter rations that use cottonseed meal as their protein source.
    b. History. A history of cottonseed in the diet for several weeks to months is necessary for presumptive diagnosis. Often, more than one animal is affected.

2. Clinical findings
    a. Clinical signs may include sudden death, labored breathing, anorexia, stiffness, depression, and occasionally hemoglobinuria. Reproductive problems may be seen in adult ruminants, including sterility in bulls and decreased conception rates in cows. Chronically affected cattle may have decreased heat tolerance, hemoglobinuria, abomasitis, and anorexia.
    b. Postmortem findings may reveal pulmonary congestion, excessive abdominal, pericardial, and pleural fluid, generalized cardiomyopathy, and chronic passive congestion of the liver (i.e., nutmeg liver).

3. Etiology and pathogenesis
    a. Etiology. Free gossypol, a yellow pigment that is most concentrated in the seed of

the cotton plant, is the source of toxicity. Gossypol gives the plant its resistance to insects.

    (1) **Rations** containing either **cottonseed meal** or **whole cottonseed** have been associated with gossypol toxicosis.

    (2) Toxicity is influenced by the method of cottonseed processing, dietary concentrations of iron, calcium, and protein, and the presence of other toxic terpenoids and chemicals found in cottonseed. Rations must be fed for a minimum of 1–3 months to cause toxicity.

  b. **Pathogenesis**

    (1) The **actual mechanism of toxicosis** is not known. However, gossypol forms Schiff's base-type derivatives with some amino acids, making them unavailable for protein synthesis, and forms protein–gossypol complexes. Gossypol affects some enzymatic reactions, such as the ability of cells to respond to oxidative stress.

    (2) Gossypol is primarily a **cardiotoxin,** causing gradual destruction of the cardiac musculature. It may interfere with cardiac conduction. **Adult ruminants** are able to **detoxify** gossypol by binding it to soluble proteins in the rumen and forming stable complexes.

4. **Diagnostic plan and laboratory tests**

  a. **History** and **suggestive postmortem and clinical findings** are important for diagnosis.

  b. **Feed and tissue analysis** for free gossypol concentrations help in diagnosis. Levels of 400 ppm or less free gossypol have been known to cause death in young calves and lambs, whereas older calves and lambs may require levels of 800–1200 ppm.

  c. **Other tests** include those listed in V A 5.

5. **Therapeutic plan and prognosis.** There is **no treatment** currently available.

  a. **Supportive care** may be helpful (see V A 7 a–c).

  b. **Diet.** Gossypol should be removed from the diet. Deaths attributable to toxicity may persist up to 2 weeks after the feed is removed. The ability of animals to recover depends on the severity of the heart damage. Most **gossypol-induced sterility** is reversible when the feed is removed.

6. **Prevention** consists of testing feed for free gossypol concentration or avoiding feeding cottonseed meal to animals under 4 months of age. It is possible to dilute the cottonseed by mixing it with other protein sources.

C. **Ionophore-induced cardiomyopathy**

1. **Patient profile.** This disorder affects horses, cattle, and pigs, with horses being the most susceptible.

2. **Clinical findings**

  a. **Clinical signs** include anorexia, stiffness, depression, weakness (especially involving the hind quarters), sweating, ataxia, colic, and recumbency. Congested mucous membranes, polyuria progressing to anuria, hematuria, hemoglobinuria, and progressive respiratory distress may be seen. Sublethal doses of ionophores may result in myocardial fibrosis. **Signs occur** within 12 hours of ingestion, and **death** may occur 24–36 hours after ingestion.

    (1) **Horses** often show poor performance, ill-thrift, and subsequent signs of CHF. **Chronic exposure in horses** may result in profound exercise intolerance.

    (2) **Cattle** and **sheep** may show diarrhea.

    (3) **Pigs** may exhibit hypermetria, knuckling, and a reluctance to move.

  b. **Postmortem findings** include focal or extensive areas of cardiac muscle pallor and epicardial and endocardial hemorrhages, pulmonary congestion and serous effusions compatible with CHF, fibrosis of skeletal muscles, and passive congestion of the liver. Heart lesions in pigs are often confined to the atria.

3. **Etiology and pathogenesis**

  a. **Etiology**

(1) Toxicoses may result from **ingestion** by sensitive species of **ionophore-containing feeds** prepared for other species. **Mixing errors** may result in toxicosis.

(2) The **toxicity of some ionophores** is increased by various antibiotics (e.g., tiamulin, oleandomycin, chloramphenicol, erythromycin, sulfonamides) administered concurrently.

b. Pathogenesis

(1) **Ionophores form lipid-soluble complexes** with cations to facilitate transport of the cations across lipid membranes.

(a) The **monovalent ionophores** are **monensin, salinomycin,** and **narasin.** They bind sodium and potassium ions, respectively.

(b) **Lasalocid** is a **divalent ionophore** that binds divalent cations such as calcium and magnesium ions.

(2) **Affected muscles**

(a) **Horses.** The cardiac muscle is most commonly affected in horses.

(b) **Ruminants.** Cardiac and skeletal muscles are more equally affected in ruminants.

4. Diagnostic plan and laboratory tests

a. Serum biochemical findings may include elevated enzyme concentrations such as CK, AST, and alkaline phosphatase, and slight elevations in the concentration of unconjugated bilirubin.

b. Hematology. Erythrocyte fragility is increased.

c. Feed sample analysis (ideally performed on several pounds of feed) may reveal ionophore content. Serum, contents of the gastrointestinal tract, and tissues can also be analyzed, but this analysis is not reliable.

d. History, clinical and laboratory findings, and **postmortem results** may suggest the diagnosis.

e. Other tests include those listed in V A 5.

5. Therapeutic plan

a. Antidotes for ionophores are not available. **Mineral oil** or **activated charcoal** may decrease further absorption.

b. Supportive care includes the administration of intravenous fluids to correct electrolyte imbalances, dehydration and shock, diuretics, and stall rest.

6. Prognosis for return to athletic performance is guarded in horses with chronic exposure due to myocardial fibrosis.

7. Prevention of ingestion is the best approach to management.

D. **Nutritional cardiac myodegeneration (white muscle disease, mulberry heart disease)**

1. Patient profile. This disease most commonly affects **neonates** in the first week of life, although it can occur in older animals. In pigs, this disease frequently occurs during the postweaning period (3 weeks to 4 months) and involves rapidly growing pigs.

2. Clinical findings may include dyspnea, cardiac murmurs and arrhythmias, and hemoglobinuria. Affected animals may be weak and exercise intolerant. Death may be immediate as a result of fatal arrhythmias or may occur within a few hours due to exhaustion and circulatory collapse. Other noncardiac signs may include poor reproductive performance (e.g., retained fetal membranes, decreased fertility), ill-thrift, and skeletal muscle weakness or stiffness.

3. Etiology and pathogenesis

a. Etiology

(1) **Selenium deficiency.** Certain regions of **North America** are inherently low in selenium. Acid soils, soils originating from volcanic rock, high-sulfur soils, or soils treated with sulfur-containing fertilizers are often deficient in selenium. Forages grown during seasons with heavy rainfall also may be low in selenium.

(2) **Vitamin E deficiency** occurs when animals are fed poor quality hay, straw, or root crops. Stored grain loses its vitamin E content over time.

b. Pathogenesis. Dietary selenium, sulfur-containing amino acids, and vitamin E act synergistically to protect tissues from oxidative damage.

4. **Diagnostic plan**
   a. **Clinical pathology**
      (1) **Plasma CK** and **serum AST levels** often are elevated. The magnitude of increase in these enzymes is directly proportional to the extent of muscle damage. Specific myocardial enzymes [see V A 5 a (1)] may also be elevated.
      (2) **Selenium and vitamin deficiencies.** Whole blood, liver, or serum **selenium** and plasma, liver, or muscle concentrations of **vitamin E** or **α-tocopherol** (a vitamin E-containing compound) should be determined.
      (3) **Biopsy.** Tissue samples taken by antemortem or postmortem biopsy can be analyzed for concentrations of **glutathione peroxidase** (a selenium-containing enzyme). This enzyme can also be detected in RBCs or platelets.
      (4) **Complete blood cell count (CBC).** Anemia may be seen on a CBC, particularly in swine. Electrolyte and acid–base imbalances may be present, including hyponatremia, hyperkalemia, and metabolic acidosis.
   b. **Echocardiography.** Cardiac lesions can be evaluated by echocardiography (see V A 5 b).
   c. **Soil, forage,** and **grain concentrations of selenium** should be determined.
   d. **Muscle biopsy.** Light microscopic changes suggestive of muscle degeneration and acute necrosis include hyaline degeneration, fragmentation, and lysis of muscle cells. There may be evidence of calcification of necrotic muscle (mineralization).

5. **Therapeutic plan and prognosis**
   a. **Therapy** consists of parenteral administration of vitamin E or selenium (see also V A 7).
   b. **Prognosis.** Animals showing signs of cardiac dysfunction have a poor prognosis. Most animals die within 24 hours.

6. **Prevention** is aimed at proper supplementation of the dam with vitamin E and selenium either by a salt mix or by total ration supplementation. During late gestation, dams may be given parenteral vitamin E and selenium. In addition, neonates may be given a dose at birth.

STUDY QUESTIONS

DIRECTIONS: Each of the numbered items or incomplete statements in this section is followed by answers or by completions of the statement. Select the ONE numbered answer or completion that is BEST in each case.

1. Which grouping correctly describes the heart lesions associated with a tetralogy of Fallot?

(1) Ventricular septal defect (VSD), right ventricular hypertrophy, overriding aorta, pulmonic stenosis
(2) Atrial septal defect (ASD), VSD, left ventricular hypertrophy, overriding aorta
(3) Patent ductus arteriosus (PDA), VSD, right ventricular hypertrophy, pulmonic stenosis
(4) Tricuspid valve atresia, ASD, VSD, overriding aorta
(5) Pulmonary vascular truncation, VSD, right ventricular hypertrophy, overriding aorta

2. When is quinidine sulfate most effective for converting atrial fibrillation (AF) to normal sinus rhythm in horses?

(1) When the resting heart rate is less than 60 beats/min, the duration of AF is 6–10 months, and there are no heart murmurs
(2) When the duration of AF is 1 year, the horse shows signs of congestive heart failure (CHF), the resting heart rate is 80 beats/min, and there are no heart murmurs
(3) When there are no signs of CHF, the resting heart rate is 80 beats/min, the heart murmur is less than grade III, and the duration of AF is more than 6 months
(4) When the duration of AF is less than 4 months, the heart murmur is grade IV, the resting heart rate is 60 beats/min, and there are signs of mild CHF
(5) When the duration of AF is less than 4 months, the murmur is less than grade III, the resting heart rate is less than or equal to 60 beats/min, and there are no signs of CHF

3. An adult dairy cow develops an irregularly irregular heart rhythm with a rate of 90 beats/min. On physical examination, the veterinarian identifies a left displaced abomasum (LDA). What is the most likely type of arrhythmia and the best treatment?

(1) Second-degree atrioventricular (AV) block, no treatment is necessary
(2) Ventricular tachycardia, treated with intravenous lidocaine or digoxin
(3) Sinus arrhythmia, treated by running the cow around the pen to see if the arrhythmia resolves; if it does, no other treatment is required
(4) Atrial fibrillation (AF), treated by correcting the LDA and seeing if the arrhythmia resolves in a couple of days
(5) No arrhythmia is present; cows normally have an irregularly irregular heart rhythm

4. A feedlot in western Canada had several steers that died suddenly with no premonitory signs, often following an episode of pneumonia or meningoencephalitis in the individual or penmates. Postmortem revealed multifocal myocardial infarcts and necrosis and fibrosis with no obvious pulmonary pathology. What is the most likely etiology?

(1) Bovine leukemia virus (BLV)-associated lymphoma involving the right atrium
(2) *Haemophilus somnus* myocarditis
(3) Monensin toxicosis
(4) An aberrant form of infectious bovine rhinotracheitis (IBR) viral infection
(5) Shipping fever disease complex involving the *Pasteurella* species

5. A 26-year-old Standardbred mare is examined by a veterinarian before a routine vaccination. The veterinarian hears a grade III, holodiastolic musical murmur on the left side of the chest that radiates toward the apex of the heart. What is the most likely diagnosis and treatment?

(1) Mitral valve stenosis, no treatment
(2) Bacterial endocarditis (BE) with a vegetative lesion on the mitral valve, long-term antibiotics
(3) Pulmonic insufficiency, no treatment
(4) Aortic insufficiency, no treatment
(5) Ventricular septal defect (VSD), no treatment

6. What is the most common type of incomplete second-degree AV block in fit racehorses and how it is characterized electrocardiographically?

(1) Mobitz type II is characterized by a P-Q interval that is unchanged, and the dropped beat (no QRS-T) is unheralded.
(2) Mobitz type I (Wenckebach) is characterized by a P-R interval that gradually prolongs until the beat (QRS-T) is dropped.
(3) Mobitz type I is characterized by a P-Q interval that is unchanged, and the dropped beat (no QRS-T) is unheralded.
(4) Mobitz type II is characterized by a P-R interval that gradually prolongs until the beat (QRS-T) is dropped.
(5) Mobitz type III (AV dissociation) is characterized by P waves that are completely independent of QRS-T complexes.

7. Several rapidly growing pigs, which were approximately 2 months old, die suddenly. Postmortem examination reveals pericardial effusion, pulmonary and hepatic congestion, and pale discoloration of the grossly enlarged heart. The pigs were fed a diet of soybeans, high-moisture corn, and cereal grain. What is the most likely diagnosis?

(1) Cardiomyopathy caused by vitamin E or selenium deficiency (mulberry heart disease)
(2) Bacterial endocarditis (BE) caused by *Erysipelothrix rhusiopathiae*
(3) Myocarditis caused by the *Sarcocystis* species
(4) Congenital heart defect such as tetralogy of Fallot
(5) Atherosclerosis due to a high-fat diet

8. Heart sounds are generated by the:

(1) impact of valve leaflets coming together.
(2) snapping open of valve cusps.
(3) mechanical activity of the heart resulting in sudden acceleration and deceleration of blood.
(4) turbulent blood moving through incompetent valves.
(5) contraction and relaxation of the cardiac muscle.

DIRECTIONS: Each of the numbered items or incomplete statements in this section is negatively phrased, as indicated by a capitalized word such as NOT, LEAST, or EXCEPT. Select the ONE numbered answer or completion that is BEST in each case.

9. Which one of the following clinical signs is LEAST likely to be seen in cattle with bacterial endocarditis (BE)?

(1) Lameness
(2) Tachycardia
(3) Heart murmur
(4) Fever
(5) Abdominal pain

10. Which one of the following is NOT commonly important in the pathophysiology of pericardial disease?

(1) Diastolic cardiac dysfunction
(2) Elevated intrapericardial pressure, causing a reduction in preload
(3) Systolic cardiac dysfunction
(4) Decreased cardiac output, assuming heart rate, cardiac contractility, and vascular resistance are unchanged
(5) Increased sympathetic tone

11. Which congenital heart defect does NOT cause cyanosis and hypoxemia?

(1) Reverse patent ductus arteriosus (PDA; right-to-left shunt)
(2) Pentalogy of Fallot
(3) Ventricular septal defect (VSD) with pulmonary hypertension (right-to-left shunt)
(4) Tetralogy of Fallot
(5) Foramen ovale

12. Which one of the following diagnostic test results could NOT be used to support a diagnosis of white muscle disease?

(1) Elevated aspartate aminotransferase (AST), creatine phosphokinase (CK), and lactate dehydrogenase (LDH) in serum
(2) Elevated red blood cell (RBC) glutathione peroxidase activity
(3) Urinalysis revealing myoglobinuria
(4) Low selenium concentration in blood
(5) Skeletal or intercostal muscle biopsy revealing hyaline degeneration and lysis

---

DIRECTIONS: Each set of matching questions in this section consists of a list of four to twenty-six numbered options (some of which may be in figures) followed by several numbered items. For each numbered item, select the ONE numbered option that is most closely associated with it. To avoid spending too much time on matching sets with large numbers of options, it is generally advisable to begin each set by reading the list of options. Then, for each item in the set, try to generate the correct answer and locate it in the option list, rather than evaluating each option individually. Each numbered option may be selected once, more than once, or not at all.

Questions 13–15

Match each valvular defect with the appropriate cardiac auscultation finding.

(1) Mitral regurgitation
(2) Tricuspid regurgitation
(3) Pulmonic regurgitation
(4) Aortic regurgitation

13. Holosystolic murmur with point of maximal intensity (PMI) over the left fifth intercostal space

14. Holosystolic murmur with PMI over the left heart base

15. Holodiastolic decrescendo murmur with PMI over the left fourth intercostal space

ANSWERS AND EXPLANATIONS

1. The answer is 1 [II A 4]. Tetralogy of Fallot is a cyanotic heart defect that impairs ventricular emptying. This disorder results from an abnormal dextrad (to the right) development of the great vessels. The four components are a ventricular septal defect (VSD), overriding of the interventricular septum by the aorta (overriding aorta), pulmonic stenosis, and right ventricular hypertrophy. If an atrial septal defect is also present, a pentalogy of Fallot exists.

2. The answer is 5 [III C 1 b (5)]. Quinidine sulfate is the drug of choice for conversion of horses with atrial fibrillation (AF) to sinus rhythm and is most successful when the duration of AF is short (less than 4 months), murmurs auscultated are less than grade III–V, the resting heart rate is less than or equal to 60 beats/min, and there are no signs of congestive heart failure (CHF).

3. The answer is 4 [III C 1 c (2), (5)]. Atrial fibrillation (AF) is the most commonly observed arrhythmia in cattle and can be functional or organic in nature. Functional AF develops without apparent cardiac disease and usually is secondary to other clinical problems, such as gastrointestinal disturbances with associated electrolyte disturbances (LDA in this case). AF will frequently convert to normal sinus rhythm without specific treatment. Correction of the LDA will probably result in return to normal sinus rhythm in a few days. Sinus arrhythmia associated with respiration does not normally develop in cattle. The heart rate is usually slow to normal. There may be cyclic variation in heart rate. Ventricular tachycardia suggests underlying cardiac disease. Auscultation usually reveals a rapid but regular heart rate.

4. The answer is 2 [V A 4 a]. *Haemophilus somnus* produces a syndrome consisting of sudden death with few or no premonitory signs, often following an episode of pneumonia or meningoencephalitis. Necropsy of affected animals often reveals multifocal myocardial infarcts, necrosis, and fibrosis typical of embolic disease. *H. somnus,* which is often isolated from these lesions, is an opportunistic pathogen that has a predilection for the bo-

vine female reproductive tract. The septicemic form, which includes myocardial disease, has been increasing in frequency in western Canada since 1987. Lymphoma involving the right atrium occurs infrequently and usually in older animals. Postmortem findings include a mass on the right auricle or within the right atrium, pericardial effusion, and cardiac dilation. Infectious bovine rhinotracheitis (IBR) is not known to cause myocarditis or cardiomyopathy. Pasteurellosis can cause bacteremia and septicemia with resultant cardiac disease, but it usually manifests as a vegetative lesion on one or more cardiac valves, rather than as myocarditis. Pneumonia is also usually present clinically and at postmortem.

5. The answer is 4 [II B 4]. Degenerative changes involving the aortic valve are common in older horses. The murmur associated with aortic regurgitation is holodiastolic, with the point of maximal intensity (PMI) over the aortic valve and radiating toward the left cardiac apex. Aortic regurgitation is usually well tolerated and is not associated with exercise intolerance. Usually, no treatment is necessary. Atrioventricular valve stenosis is rare in horses. Vegetative lesions on the mitral or tricuspid valve may be large enough to cause narrowing of the valve orifice. The associated murmur is a decrescendo diastolic murmur after S2 and is heard best on the left side of the chest over the mitral valve. Bacterial endocarditis (BE) involving the mitral valve usually results in fever, weakness, anorexia, weight loss, or lameness in addition to the characteristic systolic heart murmur. Pulmonic insufficiency is uncommon in horses. The murmur associated with it is holosystolic with PMI over the pulmonic valve. Usually, horses show other signs of heart disease, such as jugular venous distention and severe exercise intolerance. A congenital heart defect, such as a ventricular septal defect (VSD), produces a holosystolic murmur heard on both sides of the chest.

6. The answer is 2 [III B 2]. Type I Mobitz (Wenckebach) is the most common incomplete atrioventricular (AV) block in horses. It is characterized by progressive lengthening of the P-R interval for several beats until one P wave, representing atrial excitation, occurs

211

without a subsequent ventricular excitation (QRS-T). The post-block P-R interval is shorter.

7. The answer is 1 [V D]. Mulberry heart disease occurs in rapidly growing pigs, particularly during the postweaning period (3 weeks to 4 months). The pigs are usually fed diets deficient in both selenium and vitamin E. Diets may contain a high concentration of unsaturated fatty acids. Diets commonly associated with the condition include mixtures of soybean, high-moisture corn, and cereal grains grown on soils with low levels of selenium. Without selenium, vitamin E, or both, there is widespread tissue lipoperoxidation leading to hyaline degeneration and calcification of muscle fibers such as myocardial fibers. Myocardial muscle is replaced by fibrosis, leading to pale discoloration and firmness. Bacterial endocarditis (BE) usually involves the left AV valve in pigs. Left heart enlargement and vegetative lesions on the AV valves are seen at postmortem. *Sarcocystis* species cause focal myocarditis, not generalized cardiac discoloration and enlargement. A severe congenital heart defect usually causes clinical signs from birth that progressively worsen with age. Evidence of the cardiac defect would be apparent at postmortem.

8. The answer is 3 [I B 4]. Cardiac sounds originate when the mechanical activity of the heart results in sudden acceleration and deceleration of columns of blood, causing the heart, major vessels, and blood to vibrate as a whole.

9. The answer is 5 [II B 6 b (2)]. The most frequently occurring clinical signs associated with bacterial endocarditis (BE) in cattle include tachycardia, weight loss, lameness, heart murmur, and fever. Colic or abdominal pain is uncommon.

10. The answer is 3 [IV A]. Pericardial disease causes diastolic cardiac dysfunction with minimal if any alterations in systolic function. Elevated intrapericardial pressure inhibits diastolic cardiac filling, causing a reduction in preload for any given venous filling pressure. Reduction in preload results in decreased cardiac output, assuming the heart rate, cardiac contractility, and vascular resistance are unchanged. The body responds to the decreased cardiac output by increasing sympathetic tone and stimulating the renin-angiotensin-aldosterone system. The elevated sympathetic tone causes elevations in the heart rate and augmentation of cardiac contractility.

11. The answer is 5 [II A 2 c]. Three congenital heart defects result in hypoxemia and cyanosis. They include tetralogy and pentalogy of Fallot, right-to-left shunting patent ductus arteriosus (PDA), and right-to-left shunting ventricular septal defect (VSD). These defects result in the shunting of blood away from the lungs where oxygenation occurs. Chronic hypoxia may lead to progressive secondary polycythemia and sludging of the blood. A patent foramen ovale (atrial septal defect) usually results in the shunting of blood from the left atrium into the right atrium. This, in turn, results in increased blood volume through the pulmonary circulation. Therefore, hypoxemia is not a common clinical feature.

12. The answer is 2 [V D 4]. Nutritional muscular dystrophy (white muscle disease) may result in elevated muscle enzyme levels [creatine phosphokinase (CK), lactate dehydrogenase (LDH), aspartate aminotransferase (AST)], low selenium in serum, low glutathione peroxidase activity in blood, and evidence of muscle degeneration on a biopsy. All of these tests are used in conjunction with clinical signs and evidence of low or marginal vitamin E or selenium concentrations in the diet.

13–15. The answers are: 13-1 [II B 2 b], **14-3** [II B 5 b], **15-4** [II B 4 b]. Mitral regurgitation produces a holosystolic murmur that is heard best on the left side with the point of maximal intensity (PMI) in the fifth intercostal space.

Pulmonic regurgitation produces a holosystolic murmur that is heard best over the left heart base.

Aortic regurgitation produces a decrescendo diastolic murmur that is heard best on the left side of the chest in the fourth intercostal space. The murmur often radiates over a wide area.

Chapter 9

Metabolic Disorders

Timothy H. Ogilvie

I. METABOLIC DISORDERS OF RUMINANTS

A. Parturient paresis (hypocalcemia, milk fever)

1. **Patient profile and history**

   a. Parturient paresis is most commonly seen in **dairy cattle** and may affect 5%–10% of all adult dairy cows. This disease is less common in beef cattle, sheep, and goats. There is a breed susceptibility, with Jerseys and Guernseys having a higher incidence of disease than other dairy breeds.

   b. Usually, there is a **distribution of cases** around parturition, with 75% of clinical cases occurring within 24 hours of calving, 12% occurring 24–48 hours after calving, and 6% occurring at calving. Hypocalcemia at calving often is associated with dystocia. A subset (7%) also occurs before or unassociated with calving. These forms of the disease are associated with calcium loss but are not caused by an onset of lactation.

   c. There is an **age susceptibility** to the disease in that it parallels milk production, and it is rare in heifers. There is an individual susceptibility and the tendency for the condition to reoccur in susceptible cows.

2. **Clinical findings**

   a. **Cattle.** This condition is divided into three stages:

      (1) **Stage I.** The signs consist of mild excitement and tetany without recumbency. Anorexia is also a consistent finding. These signs may go unobserved because stage I rapidly progresses to stage II (1-hour progression).

      (2) **Stage II**

         (a) There is **depression, paralysis,** and **recumbency.** The head is characteristically turned into the flank or rested on the ground in an extended position. Fine muscle tremors may be evident, and the cow may make threatening motions with the head (e.g., head shaking, open-mouth bellowing).

         (b) **Examination** reveals tachycardia with decreased heart sounds, cool extremities, and a low rectal temperature (35.5°C–37.8°C). Gastrointestinal atony (e.g., mild bloat, constipation), loss of anal reflex, and a slow pupillary light reflex are evident. The clinical signs at this stage may be associated with uterine prolapse. Stage II may last from 1 to 12 hours.

      (3) **Stage III.** Cattle with stage III milk fever exhibit further weakness and progressive loss of consciousness. Bloat may be life threatening because of lateral recumbency and gastrointestinal tract (GIT) atony. There is a danger of aspiration pneumonia, the heart sounds become inaudible, and a pulse may be undetectable. This stage may progress to death in 3–4 hours.

   b. **Sheep** are more likely to develop milk fever in late gestation. Ewes usually exhibit flaccid paralysis; however, tetany or muscle tremors may be evident. Recumbency is less common than with cattle.

   c. **Goats.** Milk fever may occur prepartum, as in sheep, or postpartum, as in high-producing dairy animals. The clinical signs are similar to those in sheep.

3. **Etiology and pathogenesis**

   a. **Hypocalcemia.** When **calcium outflow** is sudden and severe (i.e., lactation in cows, multiple fetuses in sheep), calcium homeostasis mechanisms may fail. Mature cows have increased lactation demands for calcium and older cows have decreased ability to mobilize calcium from the GIT. GIT stasis at parturition (or at other times) also interferes with calcium uptake. **Paralysis** occurs because of inadequate calcium availability at the neuromuscular junction. Calcium is necessary for the release of acetylcholine. Also, low calcium levels impair muscular contractility by hindering calcium-dependent actin and myosin interactions. Neuromuscular dysfunction may be variable (tetany or flaccid paralysis) with mildly decreased calcium concentrations or in nonbovine species (i.e., sheep, goats, horses). Retained placentae are common sequelae to milk fevers.

b. **Hypophosphatemia.** Simultaneous with calcium loss, phosphorus may be lost in milk or not absorbed (decreased intake or decreased mobilization from bone), causing the hypophosphatemia that is seen. Hypophosphatemia may result in enhanced flaccid paralysis and continued recumbency even after low serum calcium levels have been corrected.

c. **Hypermagnesemia** is seen occasionally and also enhances flaccidity. Increased levels of magnesium impair acetylcholine release. The cause for hypermagnesemia is unknown.

4. **Diagnostic plan.** The field diagnosis is based on clinical signs, history, and response to therapy. At the time of treatment, serum should be drawn and held for calcium analysis.

5. **Laboratory tests**
   a. **Total serum calcium determination** is the standard test for all ruminants. Although ionized calcium is the active form, it is difficult to measure in most laboratories and usually closely parallels total calcium concentrations. Total calcium less than 1.9 mmol/L may result in clinical signs, with stage I disease usually characterized by a serum calcium level of 1.4–2.0 mmol/L. Most animals become recumbent before a level of 1.25 mmol/L is reached (the typical range of stage II milk fever is 0.9–1.6 mmol/L). With stage III disease, levels may reach 0.5 mmol/L before the animal dies.
   b. **Serum magnesium and phosphorus determination**
      (1) In dairy cattle with **parturient paresis,** hypermagnesemia (1.5–2 mmol/L) and hypophosphatemia (0.5–1 mmol/L) may be seen.
      (2) In the less common presentation of **nonparturient paresis** (i.e., calcium loss not associated with calving), hyperphosphatemia and hypomagnesemia may occur.

6. **Differential diagnoses** include other causes of recumbency: trauma, peripheral nerve paralysis, calving injuries, or septicemias and toxemias (e.g., acute coliform mastitis).

7. **Therapeutic plan.** Owners may be taught how to diagnose and treat parturient paresis on their own.
   a. **Cattle.** The disease should be treated as an emergency, particularly if the animal is in stage III. Prolonged recumbency results in complications (e.g., bloat, uterine prolapse, muscle necrosis, aspiration pneumonia). Animals do not recover spontaneously. Individuals respond best in early stages and with early treatment. Between 5% and 15% of cows do not respond to initial treatment and remain recumbent for various lengths of time. **Persistent hypophosphatemia** may be an underlying cause for failure to respond.
      (1) **Relieve bloat.** Roll the cow into sternal recumbency before treatment to relieve any bloat.
      (2) **Administer calcium.** Intravenous and subcutaneous calcium solutions each contain between 8 g and 10 g of calcium and are advocated in tandem to lessen the chance of relapse. One 500-ml bottle is sufficient for treatment, but calcium continues to be lost in the milk and is not being absorbed because of GIT atony and increased calcitonin release.
         (a) Administer 500 ml of **23% calcium gluconate** intravenously (calcium borogluconate and glucose, phosphorus, magnesium, and potassium are often found in commercial preparations). Intravenous injections must be given slowly (over 20 minutes) and the heart monitored for signs of irregularity. The heart rate should slow dramatically and become stronger over the period of calcium administration. Other responses to therapy include eructation, urination, defecation, muscle twitching, and an improvement in demeanor. Within 30 minutes of treatment, 60% of animals with uncomplicated milk fever will stand.

      (b) **Subcutaneous calcium.** A subcutaneous calcium preparation without glucose (one 500-ml bottle) is administered as well. For stage I conditions, subcutaneous administration alone may be sufficient. Also, subcutaneous administration without intravenous calcium treatment should be considered in cases complicated by toxemia and shock due to cardiovascular compromise.

   (3) **Follow-up**

      (a) **Full restoration** of calcium homeostasis does not occur for 2–3 days. The owner should request a revisit if there has been no response to therapy within 12 hours of treatment. Retreatment may be warranted up to two more treatments.

      (b) If the animal is **unresponsive** to therapy shortly after administration, prop her up in sternal recumbency, and provide secure footing in case the cow attempts to rise. Provide shelter and easy access to feed and water if recumbency is prolonged.

      (c) **Good nursing care** (i.e., deep bedding, rolling from side to side 4–5 times per day) may be necessary to prevent muscle damage. Mechanical hip-lifting devices may encourage the cow to stand but should be used with great care and discretion to avoid muscle damage. More efficacious lifters include harnesses and inflatable mattresses.

      (d) Consider only **partial milking** for 1–2 milkings post treatment, unless there is concurrent mastitis. **Relapses** of clinical hypocalcemia may occur, and decreasing the milk drain of calcium is thought to lessen the likelihood of relapse.

  b. Sheep and goats. Calcium gluconate should be administered at 50–100 ml of a 23% solution intravenously. Consider cesarian sections for sheep if near term. Sheep developing hypocalcemia in late gestation often relapse.

8. Prevention

  a. Dry cow diets, which are low in calcium content (i.e., nonlegume roughage), are preventive. Diets high in anions (chloride ions and sulfur compounds) compared to cations (sodium and potassium ions) tend to prevent hypocalcemia.

  b. Vitamin D_3 preparations administered prepartum may prevent or ameliorate the clinical signs, but the timing of administration is critical.

  c. Other preventives include culling cattle prone to the condition, keeping cattle on feed at the time of parturition (i.e., reduce episodes of indigestion), and administering oral calcium in the form of calcium gel at calving.

B. Downer cow syndrome

1. Patient profile and history. Cows that remain recumbent 24 hours after initially going down are classified as downer cows. The condition may or may not be related to milk fever, but the vast majority of cases are periparturient and related to parturient paresis.

2. Clinical findings. The animal does not appear to be systemically ill but either is unable to rise or refuses to rise. The cow may have been treated with calcium for parturient paresis. She may pull herself around her enclosure, which accounts for the term **"creeper cow."**

3. Etiology and pathogenesis. Causes of recumbency include parturient paresis, calving paralysis (obturator or sciatic paralysis), pelvic fracture, coxofemoral luxation, lymphosarcoma, and malnutrition. Any large animal that is recumbent is vulnerable to muscle damage. Compressive effects are evident within 6–12 hours on a hard surface. This damage is almost exclusively confined to muscles of the pelvic limbs.

4. Diagnostic plan. Eliminate any obvious causes of recumbency via a general physical examination, and perform a rectal and manual examination of the pelvis. The clinical examination may be aided by the use of a hip lifter or slings. However, the downer animal is often labeled as such by the elimination or exclusion of obvious causes of the condition.

5. **Laboratory tests.** Muscle leakage enzyme (creatine kinase) values rise to moderately high levels but fall to more normal levels after 6 days of recumbency. This may help to differentiate recumbency from other causes from a primary muscular disorder. Serum levels of calcium and phosphorus may be low if the primary disorder is caused by hypocalcemia.

6. **Therapeutic plan**
   a. **Underlying conditions should be treated,** if possible.
   b. **Supplementation** with phosphorus may be efficacious.
   c. **Lifting devices,** such as hip lifters, are useful but only for short periods (e.g., examination, milking). The cow must not be allowed to hang unattended for long periods of time. Abdominal slings are useful but must be well designed. Air bags seem most humane but cause respiratory embarrassment and cows may roll off. Water stalls or pools hold the best theoretical promise but are impractical in field situations.
   d. **Nursing care** is necessary for all down animals and includes rolling, providing deep bedding, cleaning wet skin, feeding, milking, watering, and other supportive measures.
   e. **Analgesics** (e.g., aspirin, phenylbutazone, flunixin meglumine) may be indicated to relieve muscle pain.

7. **Prognosis.** The prognosis for each case depends on the primary disorder and any secondary complications. Any prognosis is extremely difficult to offer if the animal is a true downer without evidence of another or primary disorder.

8. **Prevention**
   a. To prevent **calving injuries** leading to recumbency, provide calving pens for animals rather than calving in stanchions, make sure heifers are large enough at the time of parturition, and provide breeding advice on sire size.
   b. Prevent **parturient paresis** as described in I A 8. Treat recumbent animals vigorously.
   c. Provide **resilient matting** or **deep bedding** in stanchion or comfort stalls.

C. | **Postparturient hemoglobinuria**

1. **Patient profile and history.** Postparturient hemoglobinuria is a disease of mature, high-producing dairy cattle. It is of relatively low incidence, sporadic, and seen in cows 2–4 weeks post calving. It is most commonly seen on particular farms in association with certain diets.

2. **Clinical findings**
   a. There is a precipitous **drop in milk yield** with sudden weakness (e.g., staggering) and anorexia. The urine is reddish-brown to black (hemoglobinuria), and there are signs of anemia (e.g., pale mucous membranes, tachycardia, an increased cardiac impulse). Jaundice develops terminally (3–5 days) with weakness, recumbency, and death.
   b. **Signs of phosphorus deficiency** may be evident in the herd, for example pica, infertility, and poor growth of calves with musculoskeletal disorders (osteodystrophy).

3. **Etiology and pathogenesis**
   a. This condition is associated with **hypophosphatemia** because of low dietary phosphorus intake. It is seen in nonsupplemented cattle grazing on phosphorus-deficient soils. Lactation drain exacerbates phosphorus loss. There may be an association with low total body copper and selenium in individual animals.
   b. It is felt that ingested **hemolytic agents,** such as cruciferous plants (kale and other brassicas), cause erythrolysis, particularly in cases of increased red blood cell fragility. Red blood cells are more fragile with mineral deficiencies (e.g., phosphorus, copper, selenium). The best documented mineral deficiency is chronic phosphorus deficiency.

4. **Diagnostic plan.** The field diagnosis is based on clinical findings. The clinician must differentiate other causes of red urine.

5. Laboratory tests
a. **Serum phosphorus.** Low serum phosphorus levels are found in lactating, unaffected animals (0.65–1.0 mmol/L). Clinically affected cattle have very low serum phosphorus values (less than 0.5 mmol/L).
b. **Complete blood cell count (CBC) and hematocrit.** Cattle are anemic as evidenced by the low total red blood cell count and hemoglobin.
c. **Urinalysis.** There is hemoglobinuria.
d. **Serum copper levels** may be low.

6. Therapeutic plan
a. A **blood transfusion** (5–10 L/cow) must be administered to save the affected animal.
b. **Isotonic fluid therapy** is necessary to provide diuresis and renal support.
c. **Phosphorus** should be given intravenously at a dose of 60 g of sodium acid phosphate in 300 ml of distilled water with a similar amount subcutaneously. The subcutaneous treatment should be repeated once per day for the next 3 days coupled with the same daily dose orally.
d. **Dietary supplementation** with bone meal at 120 g twice daily or some other source of phosphorus is recommended for 5 days post treatment.

7. Prognosis.
The prognosis for any anemic recumbent animal is poor. Kidney failure may occur within 3–5 days, and if an animal survives, a long convalescence may be necessary.

8. Prevention.
Phosphorus, copper, and/or selenium supplementation for the herd is warranted.

D. Clinical bovine ketosis (acetonemia)

1. Patient profile and history
a. **Primary ketosis** is a metabolic disorder that occurs in **lactating dairy cows** 1–6 weeks after calving (usually 3–4 weeks into lactation). It may be seen in high-producing, heavily fed dairy cows indoors, and is rarely seen in cattle on pasture.
b. **Secondary ketosis** may occur as a complication of another disease that usually occurs early in the postpartum period (e.g., metritis, left displacement of the abomasum).

2. Clinical findings
a. **Primary ketosis.** Cows exhibit a gradual decrease in appetite and milk yield for 3–4 days. There is moderate weight loss and depression. Cows are selectively anorexic, preferring hay to grain or silage. Feces are characteristically firm and dry ("bull-like"). When appetite is lost, weight loss may be rapid. A ketone smell may be detectable on the cow's breath. Spontaneous recovery may occur when milk production and caloric intake are stabilized.
b. **Nervous ketosis** is a type of primary ketosis where nervous signs predominate. The cow may appear delirious, walking in circles and head pressing with compulsive licking and chewing movements, hyperesthesia, bellowing, apparent blindness, and a depraved appetite.
c. **Secondary ketosis.** Clinical signs are similar to those of primary ketosis but not as dramatic. The condition is accompanied by another clinical problem (e.g., metritis, left abomasal displacement). Signs may occur earlier in lactation than with primary ketosis (i.e., usually within 1–2 weeks of calving).

3. Etiology and pathogenesis
a. **Primary ketosis.** Subclinical bovine ketosis may be normal in high-producing dairy cattle where there is often a negative energy balance early in lactation. High milk production causes energy (glucose) drain, and the need for energy may exceed capacity for intake. Likewise, the need for energy may exceed that provided for in the ration. A defect in digestion or metabolism may result in inadequate amounts of glucose available at the cellular level.
   (1) **Hypoglycemia** results in an increased requirement for gluconeogenesis in the liver (glucose from amino acids and glycerol). This pathway for glucose pro-

duction normally supplies a high percentage of glucose via the tricarboxylic acid (TCA) cycle. Interference with this pathway (e.g., lack of oxaloacetate) converts ketogenic volatile fatty acids to ketone bodies (acetoacetic and β-hydroxybutyric acid). Depletion of hepatic glycogen occurs and hepatic stores of triglycerides and ketone bodies increase.

(2) **Ketogenic diets** are thought to be low in precursors of propionic acid, which is converted directly to oxaloacetate and glucose. Ketogenic diets (e.g., silages) have high levels of butyric and acetic acid. High-protein diets also may be ketogenic in nature.

b. **Secondary ketosis** is thought to follow the same pathophysiologic sequence as primary ketosis; however, a causative or developmental factor is involved (e.g., a clinical disease). The clinical disease results in a decreased appetite, which, in the presence of the loss of lactose due to lactation, causes the ketotic syndrome to develop.

4. **Diagnostic plan.** The field diagnosis is based on history, clinical findings, cowside tests, and response to therapy. Laboratory tests confirm the diagnosis.

5. **Laboratory tests**
   a. With **primary ketosis,** blood glucose is depressed and blood, urinary, and milk ketones are elevated. A CBC reveals lymphocytosis, neutropenia, and eosinophilia. Cowside tests (i.e., dipstick evaluation) will detect urine and milk ketones.
   b. **Secondary ketosis.** Laboratory changes are similar to those of primary ketosis, but they are less dramatic.

6. **Differential diagnoses** include indigestion, traumatic reticuloperitonitis, abomasal displacements, and metritis. Central nervous system (CNS) diseases also should be considered when presented with a case of suspected nervous ketosis.

7. **Therapeutic plan**
   a. **Routine therapy** is the administration of 500 ml of **50% dextrose solution** intravenously. Relapses are common and follow-up includes the oral administration of propylene glycol (225 g twice daily for 2 days followed by 110 g once daily for 2 more days).
   b. **Corticosteroids** (10 mg dexamethasone intramuscularly given once) may be considered for their effect on repartitioning glucose and depressing milk production. Anabolic steroids (60–120 mg of trenbolone acetate) are also efficacious in treatment. Be aware that this is an off label use in most countries.
   c. **Vitamin B$_{12}$** and **cobalt** may be administered, as may **nicotinic acid,** in the feed.

8. **Prevention**
   a. For **herd problems,** regularly check for ketonuria during the second to sixth weeks of lactation. Reduce the silage component of ration if practical. Sodium propionate or propylene glycol may be fed preventively, although this may be expensive.
   b. Cows should be in **good condition at calving** (not thin or overly fat). Dry off cows in good condition. Gradually increase the grain ration near the end of the dry period, and continue to increase feed after calving relative to milk production.
   c. The most important recommendations center on **nutrition** and **dry cow management.** Dividing the herd into separate feeding groups according to metabolic needs and production indices is necessary. Milking cows should receive good quality feed (16%–18% protein). Cows should receive adequate exercise during any stabling periods.

E. **Subclinical bovine ketosis**

1. **Patient profile and history.** Many high-producing dairy cattle in early lactation are subclinically ketotic. Affected animals are usually housed cattle. Subclinical ketosis can occur at a prevalence rate of 10%–30% in certain herds.

2. **Clinical findings.** Cows suffer from lower than expected milk production and gradual weight loss. There may be an infertility problem (e.g., metritis, ovarian dysfunction).

3. **Etiology and pathogenesis.** Causes are similar to those of clinical ketosis. Cows in negative energy balance with high glucose loss in milk (high milk production) and insufficient capacity for consumption or improper nutrition will be subclinically ketotic. Hepatic stores of glycogen decrease, and triglycerides and ketone bodies increase.

4. **Diagnostic plan.** Consider subclinical ketosis when there is a mild ketonuria, slight fall in milk production, and weight loss in an individual or across the herd. Clinical diseases causing secondary ketosis should be ruled out.

5. **Laboratory tests** confirm ketonuria and hypoglycemia.

6. **Therapeutic plan.** Recommendations are the same as for clinical ketosis (see I D 7).

F. **Pregnancy toxemia of sheep**

1. **Patient profile and history.** Risk factors for ewes developing the condition include late pregnancy, obesity, and carrying multiple (or single large) fetuses. This condition affects intensively raised sheep (i.e., not range sheep) and may be associated with sudden feed changes or inclement weather conditions. This may occur as a flock problem with several animals affected over several weeks.

2. **Clinical findings**
   a. **Neurologic signs** are similar to the signs of nervous ketosis in cattle. There is blindness and changes in demeanor. Animals may head press and circle or stand with a "star-gazing" appearance. Tremors and convulsions may occur interspersed by periods of depression, incoordination, and ataxia.
   b. **Other signs.** Ewes may be constipated and exhibit bruxism and a ketone smell to the breath. Terminally, ewes become recumbent and comatose, resulting in death in 4–7 days. Dystocia may be evident if ewes are in the process of lambing. Death of the ewe may be caused by toxemia resulting from death and decomposition of the fetuses.

3. **Etiology and pathogenesis**
   a. A period of **anorexia** or **starvation** (possibly resulting from feed change) for 1–2 days is the precipitating cause and may have been preceded by a gradual fall in the plane of nutrition during pregnancy. This disorder is not one of undernourished animals, but more often those in good flesh (over fit) with a recent decrease in consumption.
   b. The anorexia and starvation results in a **hypoglycemia** and **hyperketonemia** similar to bovine ketosis. The decrease in consumption is paralleled by a high-glucose drain from a single large fetus or multiple fetuses. The clinical picture is believed to be produced by a hypoglycemic encephalopathy. A terminal uremia may develop and exacerbate the condition.

4. **Diagnostic plan.** The diagnosis is made on the basis of clinical findings and history. Laboratory examination confirms the diagnosis. Collect urine by holding off the nares for a brief period, collecting a free-flow urine sample, and examining for ketone bodies.

5. **Laboratory tests** reveal hypoglycemia, ketonuria, eosinophilia, lymphocytosis, and neutropenia. Plasma cortisol levels are increased.

6. **Differential diagnoses** include hypocalcemia and CNS diseases (e.g., lead poisoning, polio, rabies).

7. **Therapeutic plan**
   a. A **cesarian section** is necessary immediately. Response to therapy without a cesarian is poor, and even with surgery, response is variable to poor.
   b. Clinically affected animals should be treated with **intravenous glucose solutions** and **oral propylene glycol. Corticosteroids** may be administered for their gluconeogenic effects.
   c. **Follow-up.** For recovering animals, force feed a highly palatable, readily digestible ration.

8. Prevention

    a. The rest of the flock should be examined daily for early clinical signs. Animals suspected of developing pregnancy toxemia should be treated orally with propylene glycol. Carbohydrate intake should be increased by providing supplemental feeding.

    b. A rising plane of nutrition should be ensured during the last 2 months of gestation. This may mean restricting feed intake in early gestation to avoid overly fat ewes at parturition. Avoid sudden feed changes during gestation and provide shelter and extra feed during cold and wet periods. Exercise is recommended for confined flocks.

G. **Fat cow syndrome**

1. Patient profile and history. This is a disease of overconditioned beef and dairy cattle. It may be an individual cow disease or a herd problem. There is a history of heavy feeding or a sudden decrease in nutrition in overly fat animals. The disease is sporadic but carries a high mortality rate.

    a. Dairy cows. Fat cow syndrome occurs in the immediate postpartum period, often concurrent with common postpartum diseases (e.g., metritis, retained placenta, displaced abomasum). There may be a history of a prolonged lactation or a dry period.

    b. Beef cows. The condition is most common in late gestation.

2. Clinical findings

    a. Individual

        (1) If an individual cow is affected, it is usually in an intensively managed situation, as with dairy cows. The animal is noticeably fat. The reason for examination may be for a usually responsive postpartum condition that is refractory to therapy. Anorexia and depression are pronounced. Ketosis is commonly severe, and response to therapy is poor and protracted.

        (2) If the cow continues to deteriorate despite therapy, CNS signs of cortical stimulation develop. Eventually, the animal becomes moribund.

    b. Herd

        (1) In **dairy cows,** there may be a high prevalence of unresponsive postpartum diseases (e.g., milk fever, ketosis, retained placenta, metritis). Failure of cows to become pregnant is a common complaint.

        (2) With **beef cattle** in late gestation, the signs may be similar to pregnancy toxemia of sheep. Cattle appear nervous, excitable, and uncoordinated. Feces are firm and scant. Signs progress to recumbency, coma, and death.

3. Etiology and pathogenesis

    a. Overfeeding results in deposition of fat in body stores. Conditions occurring in late gestation (e.g., negative energy balance, hypoglycemia, high concentrations of lipolytic hormones, other poorly understood factors) stimulate mobilization of body fat. This results in increased uptake of fatty acids (FAs) by the liver.

    b. Fatty acids are a normal finding in all postpartum dairy cows as milk production outstrips digestive capacity. Usually, these FAs are esterified to triglycerides in the liver. Under normal circumstances, triglycerides are packaged into lipoproteins and transported to tissues for a source of energy or to the mammary gland for milk fat synthesis. Ruminant fat cow syndrome seems to occur when serum FAs are increased and triglycerides accumulate in the liver, while hepatic lipoprotein production does not increase or is reduced. It is suggested that fat begins to accumulate in the liver in late gestation, is dynamic, and precedes the development of postpartum disease.

    c. Accumulation of fat in the liver disturbs hepatic architecture and function, resulting in hypoglycemia and ketosis. There is also concurrent leukopenia, which may be related to the increased incidence of postpartum diseases seen with the condition.

4. Diagnostic plan

    a. Individual. Liver biopsy is the most reliable indicator of the condition; however, interpretation is difficult. Clinical pathology results are unreliable. Basing the diagnosis on clinical findings, history, and unresponsiveness to therapy often results in a diagnosis by default. This method is prone to error but is the diagnostic plan followed by clinicians.

    b. Herd. On a herd basis, overly fat cows with gestational ketosis and an increase in postpartum diseases leads to a presumptive diagnosis.

5. Laboratory tests

    a. Urinalysis. Urine ketone bodies may range from low to high.

    b. Serum liver enzyme studies. There may be a mild increase in aspartate aminotransferase (AST); however, this is nondiagnostic. Other liver enzymes may be elevated, but the relationship to disease is not invariable.

    c. CBC. There may be leukopenia, neutropenia, and lymphopenia.

    d. A **liver biopsy** is the most reliable and best correlated ancillary test. Fat content may be estimated by the specific gravity (SG) of the sample. Specimens for pathology often are available when there is a herd problem.

6. Therapeutic plan

    a. Standard therapy. Treat concurrent or clinical disease. Promote feed intake with palatable feeds, good quality hay, rumen transfaunation, and the provision of substrate for rumen microbes. Administer intravenous dextrose and oral propylene glycol.

    b. Other therapies that may be attempted in the individual include choline chloride at 25 g every 4 hours subcutaneously or orally, protamine-zinc insulin (200 IU intramuscularly every other day), oral niacin, and glucocorticoids (as in ketosis). Steroids should be used with caution in cases of animals with inflammatory disease.

7. Prognosis and prevention. The prognosis is poor for clinically affected animals. Prevention should center on avoiding obesity in cows. Monitoring body condition scores is helpful in this regard as is separation of cows into feeding groups based on performance and stage of gestation. Exercise is beneficial. Supplement the ration with oral niacin or nicotinic acid (6–12 g/animal/day) for 1–2 weeks prepartum and for 90–100 days postpartum.

H. **Primary protein and energy malnutrition (starvation, emaciation).** This condition may be caused by a **primary lack of feed** or **secondary to parasitism or a disease process** that causes anorexia, an increase in metabolic rate, or both. This chapter considers primary protein and energy malnutrition relating to insufficient feed or improper nutrients.

1. Patient profile and history. Feed insufficiency most often occurs in pregnant or growing animals, and may be the result of poor husbandry or mismanagement. Poor-quality feed in either the roughage or grain component may cause malnutrition. It is often a herd or flock problem.

2. Clinical findings

    a. Individual

        (1) Affected animals may appear normal to the owner one day and recumbent the next. This is a common finding despite the chronic nature of the disease. Loss of body condition may be appreciated by palpation over the ribs and the spinous processes of the vertebrae. Loss of fat and muscle mass will be felt.

        (2) Animals present with an alert mental status despite recumbency. There is hypothermia with a normal to avid appetite. The GIT is usually hypomotile, and in ruminants, the rumen is firm. Diarrhea may be present terminally. Pregnancy usually continues, to the detriment of the dam.

    b. Herd

        (1) In **cattle,** there is **delayed sexual maturity** and **infertility** on a herd basis and signs of poor performance and emaciation. Beef cows that carry fetuses to term have low calf birth weights, decreased milk production, increased calf mortality, and decreased calf weaning weights. Dystocias may increase because of the small size of dams.

        (2) In **sheep,** clinical signs are similar to those in cattle with the added finding of decreased numbers of multiple births.

      (3) In **goats,** the social order may result in malnutrition in submissive animals.

      (4) Malnutrition adversely affects the **immune system,** therefore, the prevalence of diseases may increase. Terminally, there is hypoglycemia and bradycardia.

  3. Etiology and pathogenesis. Insufficient feed may be associated with environmental factors (e.g., heavy snow cover, poor growing season, inclement weather).

    a. With general underfeeding, energy is usually the limiting factor but does not often occur independent of **protein deficiency.** Because of the composition of livestock rations, pure protein deficiency is less common in animals than in people. It can occur with home-mixed feeds where attention is not paid to protein and energy compositions.

    b. With limited nutrients, **animal maintenance requirements** (including growth of the fetus) receive priority. Requirements for growth, production, and fertility will not be met. Body stores of protein and energy are mobilized in the following order:

      (1) Glycogen—from limited stores

      (2) Lipid—as nonesterified FAs from body fat. (Incomplete oxidation of the FAs occurs, but glucose demand is moderate so that ketosis does not occur.)

      (3) Protein—as the major source for glucose to satisfy energy needs. (Catabolism is initiated by decreased insulin and increased corticosteroid secretion.)

    c. In **advanced cases of starvation,** rumen microbes become depleted (because of lack of substrate), as do digestive enzymes. This, coupled with hypoproteinemia and bowel edema, helps explain the rapid deterioration observed in these cases, the prolonged response to therapy, and the diarrhea that may occur. When adequate diets are offered to the animal with malnutrition, diarrhea is often an early response.

  4. Diagnostic plan. The diagnosis is based on history and clinical and subjective findings. It is necessary to rule out other conditions and primary diseases that may be interfering with intake or utilization of feedstuffs. Necropsy findings are diagnostic (serous atrophy of fat).

  5. Laboratory tests are often not reliable and are of little value in the individual animal. Hypoglycemia is a common finding but is not diagnostic.

  6. Therapeutic plan. Treatment of the recumbent animal is often **unrewarding.**

    a. For animals not recumbent and with a good appetite, offer high-quality forages with gradual introduction to concentrate feeding. Force feeding may be helpful combined with transfaunation of microbes. Induction of parturition or cesarian section to relieve fetal demands for energy may be necessary.

    b. Supportive care for recumbent animals should be introduced (e.g., rolling, deep bedding, easy access to food and water). Therapy may be very expensive if total parenteral nutrition is employed.

  7. Prevention. Discuss with the owner the provision of supplemental feeding for the herd or flock. High-quality roughage and natural protein supplements (e.g., soybean meal) should be provided. Good management practices, such as the provision of shelters, attention to animals (body condition scoring), adequate feeder space, group feeding, feed testing, and understanding cold weather needs, are essential.

I. **Hypomagnesemic tetany**

  1. Patient profile and history. The manifestations and epidemiology of hypomagnesemia are variable. All types are usually seen sporadically in individual animals. This condition is seen in:

    a. Mature dairy cattle in early lactation and often on pasture (also called **lactation tetany, grass staggers, grass tetany)**

    b. Calves (age 2–4 months) fed exclusively whole milk or other diets low in magnesium

    c. Cattle or **sheep** grazing on young green cereal crops (also called wheat pasture poisoning)

    d. Beef cattle on poor pasture, during changeable, inclement weather (cold, rain, and wind)

2. **Clinical findings**
   a. **Lactation tetany**
      (1) **Acute form.** Animals may be found dead or with signs of a sudden onset of excitement, hyperesthesia, and frenzy. Cows fall into lateral recumbency in a rigid tetanic spasm, undergoing clonic/tonic convulsions with muscle fasciculations, opisthotonos, nystagmus, chewing movements, and snapping of the eyelids. These short, intense episodes are interspersed with quiet periods but may be precipitated again by noise or physical stimulation. There are very loud heart sounds. Vital signs are elevated, and the mortality rate is high because death often ensues before treatment can be administered.
      (2) **Subacute form**
         (a) There is a more **gradual onset** of signs for 2–3 days with anorexia, hyperesthesia, and some signs of cortical stimulation. Muscle fasciculations, an unsteady gait, trismus, spasmodic, pulsatile urination, and defecation are observed. Milk yield is decreased.
         (b) **Spontaneous recovery** may occur, or there may be progression to advanced clinical signs if the animal's condition is exacerbated by a precipitating event (e.g., physical stimulation). This condition is milder than the acute form, and treatment is often successful.
   b. **Hypomagnesemic tetany of calves**
      (1) **Early signs** are exaggerated movements, hyperesthesia, and a hyper alert attitude. There is opisthotonos, ataxia, and jerky limb movements. A backward carriage of the ears is a characteristic finding.
      (2) **Signs progress** to muscle fasciculations, spasticity, and convulsions. Tetany is not a finding of this condition, despite the name; however, the jaws are clenched tightly during clonic/tonic convulsions. Respirations cease during convulsions, and involuntary urination and defecation occurs. The heart rate is rapid, and heart sounds are very loud. Older calves often die, whereas younger calves may recover for short periods of time. Diarrhea may be a finding.
   c. **Hypomagnesemic tetanies of beef calves, sheep, or cattle grazing cereal pastures.** This condition has clinical signs similar to those of lactation tetany in dairy cattle.

3. **Etiology and pathogenesis**
   a. **Etiology.** Hypomagnesemia occurs with **low dietary intake** (because there are no readily mobilized magnesium reserves in the body), **excessive magnesium loss** (lactation, urinary loss), or both. Young calves absorb dietary magnesium very well, but this ability declines rapidly with age.
      (1) **Low dietary intake** may occur with poor pasture, cereal pasture, milk diet, or lush-growing forage (grasses). Lush pasture growth may occur in the spring, particularly with heavy potassium or nitrogen fertilization. High potassium content of plants may compete with magnesium absorption.
      (2) **Excessive magnesium loss.** Lactation is the main source of excessive magnesium loss, but magnesium is also lost through urine.
   b. **Pathogenesis. Hypomagnesemia** causes the clinical signs and may be precipitated by a sudden period of starvation (e.g., as with inclement weather). Hypocalcemia may be contributory and precede the development of clinical signs in chronically hypomagnesemic animals. Tetanic convulsions may result from CNS stimulation because of low magnesium levels in the cerebrospinal fluid (CSF).

4. **Diagnostic plan.** Diagnosis is based on clinical signs, response to therapy, serum magnesium levels (individual and herdmates), and serum calcium results.

5. **Laboratory tests**
   a. **Serum magnesium levels** are depressed (less than 0.2–0.4 mmol/L; normal is 0.8–1.3 mmol/L). However, serum levels may be variable or higher during episodes of muscular contractions (tetany) because of the release of intracellular magnesium. Magnesium levels in herdmates should be measured and may be low (0.4–0.8 mmol/L).
   b. **Serum calcium levels** are often reduced (1.25–2 mmol/L).

   c. **Urinary magnesium levels** are below normal (less than 0.4 mmol/L).
   d. **Pathology findings** include low magnesium levels in the vitreous humor of the eye if specimens are collected within 48 hours and the animal has been kept cool. CSF magnesium levels (less than 0.5 mmol/L) are diagnostic if collected within 12 hours.

6. **Differential diagnoses** include CNS diseases (e.g., lead poisoning, rabies, nervous ketosis, polio in calves, tetanus, hypovitaminosis A).

7. **Therapeutic plan**
   a. Handle animals quietly before treatment. **Tranquilization** may be necessary.
   b. Treat animals with **calcium** and **magnesium salts.** A recommended treatment is 500 ml of a commercial calcium and magnesium preparation (50 ml for sheep and calves) administered slowly intravenously. This should be followed by 200 ml of 50% solution of magnesium sulfate (20 ml in preruminants or small ruminants) subcutaneously to maintain serum levels.
   c. Follow initial treatment with **oral magnesium supplementation** at the rate of 60 g magnesium oxide/day for 7 days for cows or 1–3 g/day for 6 weeks for calves and small ruminants.

8. **Prevention**
   a. Counsel owners regarding ways to provide increased levels of dietary magnesium (e.g., feeding of magnesium supplements to affected individuals and herdmates, spraying pastures with magnesium sulfate or other magnesium preparations, fertilizing pastures with magnesium products, spraying magnesium on hay). Conversion of pastures from grasses to legumes also increases forage levels of magnesium.
   b. To limit environmental and managemental risk factors for this condition, consider the provision of shelter, adequate nutrition, and supplementing calf diets with legume hay and grain.

II. METABOLIC DISORDERS OF HORSES

A. Hypocalcemic tetany of mares (lactation tetany, eclampsia, transit tetany)

1. **Patient profile and history.** There are two classic presentations of this condition:
   a. **Lactation tetany,** which is seen in heavy milking draft horses at approximately 10 days post foaling or 1–2 days post weaning
   b. **Transit tetany,** which is described in lactating or nonlactating animals transported long distances

2. **Clinical findings.** In both presentations, severely affected animals exhibit tetany and incoordination. Horses are apprehensive and sweating with dilated nostrils, tachypnea, and synchronous diaphragmatic flutter (SDF). Muscular fibrillations and a rapid, irregular pulse are observed. Affected horses are unable to eat, drink, or swallow, and it may not be possible to pass a nasogastric tube. Clinical signs advance to recumbency with tetanic convulsions.

3. **Etiology and pathogenesis**
   a. **Hypocalcemia** is thought to be responsible for the clinical signs, although either hypomagnesemia or hypermagnesemia may be seen in some cases. Hypocalcemia may be produced by heavy lactation, transport, hard physical work, or no apparent cause.
   b. **SDFs** are thought to be the result of diaphragmatic contractions synchronous with the heart beat and caused by changes in the excitation potential of the phrenic nerve because of electrolyte imbalances.

4. **Diagnostic plan and laboratory tests.** The diagnosis is made on the basis of clinical and subjective findings and confirmed by serum calcium levels. There is hypocal-

cemia (1–1.5 mmol/L). Serum magnesium values are variable, but hypomagnesemia may be seen with transit tetany (0.4 mmol/L).

5. **Differential diagnoses** include tetanus, laminitis, enteritis, and colic.

6. **Therapeutic plan.** Calcium solutions are administered intravenously (commercial preparations contain 8 g of calcium per 500 ml). Responses to therapy are gradual, lessening the signs of tetany and the voiding of large volumes of urine. The response is usually good in individual animals.

7. **Prevention.** Oral calcium supplementation or increasing dietary availability of calcium may be considered in heavily lactating mares.

B. **Hyperkalemic periodic paralysis (HYPP)**

1. **Patient profile and history.** HYPP is a genetic disease of Quarter horses, Appaloosas, American point horses, and Quarter horse crosses. Gene frequency is highest in one pedigree of these breeds (i.e., affected horses are all descendants of a single Quarter-horse sire). Animals most frequently observed with the condition are well-muscled males age 2–3 years. The history and observed findings may indicate periods of prolonged recumbency or cutaneous abrasions.

2. **Clinical findings**
   a. Clinical attacks may be triggered by chilling, transportation, exhibitions at shows, and other stressors. In heterozygotes, the most common and earliest clinical sign is **muscle fasciculations,** followed by muscle spasms of the face, jaws, and legs. Weakness and recumbency follow. Death may ensue due to respiratory or cardiac failure, but this is rare. Recovery may take several minutes to several hours. Animals are normal between episodes.
   b. Many horses have **increased respiratory rates** during attacks and may show stridor if laryngeal or pharyngeal muscles are affected. Marked and persistent dyspnea may occur in homozygous foals. There are reports of HYPP attacks following anesthesia.

3. **Etiology and pathogenesis.** HYPP is similar to the human condition and has been transmitted as an autosomal dominant trait that is most likely from a single sire. The disorder is produced by failure of ion transport across the skeletal muscle cell membrane due to an abnormality in the sodium channel. In horses, this has been localized to a point mutation that changes an amino acid (e.g., phenylalanine, leucine) in the α-subunit of the sodium channel protein.
   a. **Defective sodium channels** remain open after membrane depolarization, allowing excessive inward sodium movement and heightened membrane depolarization. Simultaneously, normal sodium channels may be inactivated, preventing normal action potentials from developing. This creates muscular weakness.
   b. **Hyperkalemia** may be secondary to increased release of potassium as potassium channels open to depolarize the muscle membranes. Hyperkalemia also may occur if potassium is less able to enter the myocytes, resulting in serum accumulation.

4. **Diagnostic plan and laboratory tests**
   a. The condition may be diagnosed subjectively by clinical findings and objectively by elevated **serum potassium levels.** Serum potassium is usually elevated to between 6 mmol/L and 8 mmol/L during attacks. These elevations only persist for 1–2 hours. Serum should be separated from clotted samples as soon as possible to prevent red blood cell leakage of potassium into the serum.
   b. Definitive diagnosis is based on a **gene probe for HYPP-type sodium channel DNA.** The test is based on analysis of whole blood and is available commercially.
   c. A **potassium chloride challenge test** also has been used to diagnose the condition; however, this test is difficult to interpret and may be fatal in some horses. Potassium is administered orally at 0.1 g KCl per kg, and both clinical signs and blood potassium levels are monitored. If the horse shows signs of muscle fasciculations and hyperkalemia, the test is discontinued. If results are negative, the test

may be repeated up to four more times, increasing the administered potassium by 0.025 g KCl per kg every challenge up to a total potassium dose of 0.2 g/kg in adults or 0.15 g/kg in foals or weanlings.

   d. Electromyography of suspect horses is practiced for immediate diagnostics and is quite reliable (90% reliability).

  5. Differential diagnoses for presenting clinical signs include colic, trauma, and exertional rhabdomyolysis.

  6. Therapeutic plan

   a. Emergency treatment consists of the intravenous administration of **5% dextrose** (2 ml to 6 ml/kg) together with **sodium bicarbonate** (1 mmol/kg to 2 mmol/kg) or **23% calcium gluconate** (0.2 ml/kg). Dextrose and bicarbonate will move potassium back into cells. Calcium counteracts the effects of hyperkalemia.

   b. Long-term therapy involves removing high-potassium feeds from the diet (e.g., protein supplements, bran, sweet feeds) and feeding a diet low in potassium (e.g., whole grains, grass hay). **Medical therapy** may be used, including acetazolamide (a potassium-wasting diuretic) at 2 to 3 mg/kg orally, 2 or 3 times a day. The dose may be decreased over time until the lowest effective dose is established.

  7. Prevention. There is no cure for HYPP, which is a genetic disease and is inherited as an autosomal dominant trait. HYPP has been diagnosed more frequently during the last few years most likely because the carriers of the condition have been used heavily as sires. Because of the characteristics these carriers have (e.g., well-proportioned, heavily muscled appearance), the disease probably has been unknowingly propagated. Owners should be counseled about parentage identification and DNA gene probe testing. HYPP-positive horses should be removed from breeding use.

C. **Hyperlipidemia (hyperlipemia)** is discussed in Chapter 5 II A 4.

III. **METABOLIC DISORDERS OF NEONATES. Neonatal hypoglycemia** may occur in all neonates but is most common in newborn and weak lambs or piglets. This condition is seen in calves with diarrhea and may be a common cause for crushing deaths, which occur when sows crush piglets against the sides of farrowing crates. Crushing deaths are often accidental, but the incidence increases in piglets with hypoglycemia who are too weak to move out of the sow's way.

A. **Clinical findings.** Animals are shivering, dull, and anorexic. Affected animals have subnormal rectal temperatures, bradycardia, and soft heart sounds. Terminally, convulsions are followed by coma and death.

B. **Etiology and pathogenesis**

  1. In **neonatal pigs,** liver glycogen is rapidly depleted (within 12–24 hours) to maintain blood glucose. Therefore, because the neonate has little carcass fat and poor insulating capacity, the piglet is totally dependant on ingested milk as an energy source. Milk availability may be limited if there is disease in the sow (e.g., mastitis-metritis-agalactia), large litters and competition, sow hysteria, or diseases in the piglet (e.g., transmissible gastroenteritis). In piglets, the critical period lasts until 1 week of age, after which lack of intake only produces weight loss, not hypoglycemia.

  2. In **lambs,** twinning, mismothering, and hypothermia all produce clinical hypoglycemia.

  3. In **calves,** the predisposing factors are hypothermia, diarrhea, and improper or insufficient nutrition. The condition may occur in older calves receiving milk or milk replacer with little or no supplemental feed.

C. **Diagnostic plan and laboratory tests.** The diagnosis is based on clinical signs, subjective assessment, and response to therapy. A laboratory finding of hypoglycemia is confirmatory. Blood glucose findings below 2.2 mmol/L are diagnostic.

D. **Differential diagnoses** include diseases of the CNS. Gastrointestinal disease may be a concurrent and causative condition.

E. **Therapeutic plan**

1. **Piglets.** Treat with 15 ml of 20% dextrose every 6 hours. It may be necessary to provide a foster dam or an artificial diet. Correct the environmental temperature.

2. **Lambs.** Administer 10 ml/kg of 20% dextrose intraperitoneally. Rewarm via warm water baths.

3. **Calves.** Treat with 200 ml of 5% dextrose/50 kg administered rapidly intravenously. Follow with 240 ml/50 kg/hr, and recheck glucose in 1 hour.

F. **Prevention**

1. Provide a **warm environment** for all neonates. Cross-foster offspring from multiple births or with poor milking or mothering dams. Treat concurrent disease in dams or offspring. Provide early colostrum to preruminants (force feed if necessary). Good observation is important.

2. Do not withhold milk too long from diarrheic calves (maximum 48 hours), and **feed small portions** frequently. Increase nutrition for calves during cold weather (12%–14% body weight).

STUDY QUESTIONS

DIRECTIONS: Each of the numbered items or incomplete statements in this section is followed by answers or by completions of the statement. Select the ONE numbered answer or completion that is BEST in each case.

1. Which statement regarding parturient paresis (milk fever) of cattle is correct?

(1) It is caused by calving injuries.
(2) It is relatively rare in heifers.
(3) It produces a fever in stage III presentations.
(4) It causes the heart to sound loud and pounding.
(5) It is associated with diarrhea.

2. Which one of the following findings is consistent with parturient paresis in cattle?

(1) Hypomagnesemia is often a laboratory finding.
(2) Mortality is high despite treatment.
(3) Paralysis occurs because of high calcium concentration at neuromuscular junctions.
(4) Serum phosphorus may be below normal limits.
(5) There is a positive response to anti-inflammatory drugs.

3. The term "downer cow" refers to:

(1) animals remaining recumbent for 24 hours after initially being unable to rise.
(2) milk fever.
(3) cows that have hypophosphatemia.
(4) cows that are recumbent and ill due to systemic disease.
(5) low milk production at the peak period of lactation.

4. Which one of the following statements regarding postparturient hemoglobinuria is correct?

(1) It is a primary renal disorder.
(2) It results from increased red blood cell fragility.
(3) It is secondary to liver disease.
(4) It is usually widespread within a herd.
(5) There is a favorable prognosis in clinically affected animals.

5. Which statement regarding primary bovine ketosis is correct?

(1) It results from insufficient dietary protein.
(2) It is signaled by a rapid decline in milk yield.
(3) It may be seen in beef cattle with diets low in acetic acid.
(4) It is mainly a disease of pregnant heifers.
(5) It may be seen in high producing dairy cattle with insufficient energy intake.

6. Pregnancy toxemia of sheep is best described as:

(1) a condition of range sheep grazing lush spring pastures.
(2) a metabolic disease resulting from kidney failure.
(3) a condition of heavily pregnant ewes carrying multiple fetuses.
(4) responsive to vitamin D and glucose therapy.
(5) resulting from hypocalcemia and hypophosphatemia.

7. Fat cow syndrome in beef cattle and pregnancy toxemia in sheep are similar in that:

(1) animals may present with nervous signs.
(2) the conditions are contagious.
(3) the diseases occur in early gestation.
(4) treatment carries a favorable prognosis.
(5) prevention centers around vaccination programs.

8. Lactation tetany of mares is caused by:

(1) clostridial mastitis.
(2) trauma from foaling.
(3) metritis.
(4) hypophosphatemia.
(5) hypocalcemia.

9. Which one of the following statements regarding hyperkalemic periodic paralysis (HYPP) is correct? HYPP is:

(1) diagnosed by a gene probe for HYPP-type sodium channel DNA.
(2) an autosomal recessive condition of standard breeds in standard-bred crosses.
(3) treated with oral sodium chloride until the animal outgrows the condition.
(4) seen only in animals younger than 2 years of age.
(5) a disease of poor, unthrifty animals on high phosphorus (bran) diets.

10. Hyperlipidemia in mares is best described as:

(1) a result of a high-fat diet.
(2) a disease of fat mares that often develops in late pregnancy.
(3) a common, nonpathologic occurrence.
(4) a disease that occurs spontaneously at the time of heaviest lactation.
(5) secondary to vascular disease.

ANSWERS AND EXPLANATIONS

1. The answer is 2 [I A 3]. Parturient paresis in cattle is caused primarily by hypocalcemia due to calcium losses in milk. Therefore, it is relatively rare in heifers whose lactation demands are not as high as those of older, high-producing cows.

2. The answer is 4 [I A 2 a, 5 b]. Although the primary cause of parturient paresis is hypocalcemia, serum phosphorus levels are often concurrently below normal. Hypermagnesemia also may occur but not hypomagnesemia. Paralysis is caused by low calcium availability at the neuromuscular junction necessary for the release of the neurotransmitter acetylcholine. Treatment is often successful with intravenous and subcutaneous administration of commercially available calcium.

3. The answer is 1 [I B 1]. "Downer cows" may have had milk fever and have not responded fully to calcium therapy by rising, but they are usually no longer hypocalcemic or hypophosphatemic. These animals also may suffer from musculoskeletal problems but are not systemically ill.

4. The answer is 2 [I C 3]. Postparturient hemoglobinuria results from low serum phosphorus levels, which cause increased erythrocyte fragility. This hypophosphatemia may be the result of low intake coupled with lactation losses. Intravascular erythrolysis causes hemoglobinuria and may result in secondary renal damage. Although the hypophosphatemia may be seen on a herd level, it is a condition of individual animals at the peak of lactation. The prognosis is poor to guarded in clinically affected cows.

5. The answer is 5 [I D 3]. Primary bovine ketosis is a hypoglycemia and ketonemia resulting from high glucose losses through lactation combined with insufficient intake or availability. It presents clinically as a gradual decrease in appetite and milk production. Diets known to be precursors for this condition are those high in butyric or acetic acids.

6. The answer is 3 [I F 1]. Pregnancy toxemia of ewes usually occurs in intensively managed sheep carrying multiple fetuses. These are usually over-conditioned animals that may have suddenly faced a declining level of energy in the ration. Terminally, there is renal failure due to shock and dehydration caused by the primary disease. The condition is poorly responsive to any treatment, but the treatment of choice is immediate cesarian section with concurrent glucose therapy.

7. The answer is 1 [I F 2 a, G 2 b (2)]. Fat cow syndrome affects overly fat cows. As in sheep with pregnancy toxemia, beef cattle in late gestation may be affected by fat cow syndrome. This is a noncontagious disease of overly fat animals with an unfavorable prognosis. Prevention of both conditions centers around avoidance of overly fat animals in late gestation and eliminating the possibility of periods of anorexia or starvation.

8. The answer is 5 [II A 3 a]. Lactation tetany of mares is caused by hypocalcemia. This disorder is different than hypocalcemia in dairy cows because cows present with recumbency and flaccid paralysis. The other choices do not cause lactation tetany.

9. The answer is 1 [II B 4]. There is a molecular genetic test to identify the gene mutation. The condition is seen mainly in Quarter horses and is treated in clinical situations with bicarbonate and glucose administered intravenously to drive potassium intracellularly. It is a condition of well-muscled animals, and there is no age predilection. Animals have this condition for life but can often be maintained on low-potassium diets.

10. The answer is 2 [II C]. Fat mares in late pregnancy are most prone to hyperlipidemia. It often occurs in over-conditioned animals at times of decreased feed intake. It is uncommon in occurrence and secondary to stress or disease. It produces a vascular thrombosis and hepatic and renal failure.

Chapter 10

Endocrine Disorders

Timothy H. Ogilvie

I. INTRODUCTION

A. **Patient profile and history.** Endocrine diseases are recognized infrequently in large domestic animals (when compared with the incidence in their smaller, companion animal counterparts). A good history and physical examination is important in the diagnosis of endocrine problems. Endocrine disease should be considered whenever there are complaints of abnormal hair growth, water intake, or sweating.

B. **Clinical findings.** Endocrine dysfunction should be considered when the major problem is poor performance and after other conditions involving the musculoskeletal, respiratory, and cardiac systems have been ruled out.

C. **Diagnostic plan and laboratory tests.** A routine complete blood cell count (CBC) and biochemical profile may be important to eliminate the involvement of other systems. Conversely, abnormal findings may lead the clinician to suspect pituitary or adrenal abnormalities. Specific hormone levels are helpful in some diseases. Cortisol findings are not valuable because of the large normal ranges in some domestic animals (e.g., horses). Endocrine function tests have been used in horses but rarely in ruminants.

II. DIABETES MELLITUS

A. **Patient profile and history.** This disease is rare in large domestic animals. When the disease does occur, the main complaints include polyuria, polydipsia, polyphagia, weight loss, and a strange sweet odor to the urine.

B. **Clinical findings.** The affected animal may be thin with polyuria and polydipsia. Vital signs are normal.

C. **Etiology and pathogenesis**

1. **Etiology**
   a. Diabetes mellitus in the horse has been reported to be the result of a **pituitary tumor** and secondary to equine **Cushing's disease.** Therefore, this condition is not a true diabetes mellitus. Diabetes mellitus correctly refers to only those cases of hyperglycemia resulting from pancreatic islet β-cell deficiency, leading to a decrease or absence of insulin secretion.
   b. **Pancreatic inflammation** and destruction have been reported in both horses and cows as a cause of diabetes. Strongyle migration or localization of *Corynebacterium* species and *Streptococcus equi* have been implicated as causative organisms in horses.

2. **Pathogenesis**
   a. The specific stimulus for the release of **insulin** from β-cells is glucose. Insulin stimulates anabolic reactions, such as the synthesis of protein from amino acids, nucleic acid from mononucleotides, polysaccharides from monosaccharides, and lipids from fatty acids. Thus, a decrease in insulin results in disordered carbohydrate, protein, and lipid metabolism characterized by hyperglycemia and glucosuria.

    b. Counter insulin substances (growth hormone, epinephrine, glucagon and corti-sol) may contribute to the hyperglycemia by interfering with the action of insulin at the cellular level.

D. **Diagnostic plan and laboratory tests.** The clinical index of suspicion is raised by abnormal clinical chemistry findings on blood and urine. The diagnosis is confirmed by responses to insulin and glucose tolerance testing. An animal may have normal results on an insulin tolerance test and abnormal results on a glucose tolerance test.

    1. Laboratory studies. In the few reported cases, there has been **hyperglycemia** (10–20 mmol/L), **glucosuria,** and **ketonuria.**

    2. Necropsy results. In cows, pancreatic adenocarcinoma and infection related to the destruction of the pancreas may be evident at necropsy.

E. **Differential diagnoses**

    1. Polyuria and polydipsia. Chronic renal failure may be ruled out by normal blood urea nitrogen (BUN) and creatinine. Urine-specific gravity is usually normal. Cushing's disease must be considered.

    2. Hyperglycemia and glucosuria. Hyperglycemia of diabetes mellitus is usually greater than that associated with Cushing's disease. Additionally, hyperglycemia secondary to a pituitary tumor is generally insulin resistant, whereas hyperglycemia associated with diabetes mellitus is usually insulin responsive.

F. **Therapeutic plan and prognosis.** Treatment is rarely attempted. To maintain relatively normal blood sugar levels in the horse, 0.5–1 unit of protamine zinc insulin/kg twice daily, intramuscularly or subcutaneously has been used. The prognosis is grave because even with treatment, the long-term client compliance and patient response is poor.

III. DISEASES OF THE PITUITARY GLAND

A. **Equine Cushing's disease**

    1. Patient profile. This condition is most common in aged horses (older than 12 years).

    2. Clinical findings
        a. Vital signs are normal.
        b. Clinical signs. Owners complain of a shaggy hair coat even in summer, gradual weight loss, polydipsia, and polyuria.
            (1) Hirsutism may obscure signs of weight loss.
            (2) Polydipsia. The horse may appear **"sway backed"** or **"potbellied"** and may consume as much as **80 liters of water per day** (normal consumption is 20–30 L/day).
            (3) Chronic infections and **abscess development** are common occurrences with this condition in horses. A common site is around the eyes and masseter muscles. **Laminitis** also is a common secondary finding and may be the presenting problem.
            (4) Neurologic signs may result from compression of the brain stem by a pituitary tumor.

    3. Etiology and pathogenesis
        a. Etiology. The etiology of Cushing's disease in the horse is generally a tumor of the pituitary gland in the pars intermedia region. It has been stated that 75% of horses more than age 12 years have a pituitary adenoma at necropsy, but the majority of these do not exhibit clinical signs.
        b. Pathogenesis. Melanocyte-stimulating hormone (MSH), adrenocorticotropic hormone (ACTH), β-endorphins, and corticotropin-like intermediate lobe peptide are produced by the pars intermedia. These substances often are increased in

horses with Cushing's disease. Increases in these substances probably result from an increase in a precursor molecule. The hypersecretion is insensitive to glucocorticoid negative feedback, which results in adrenal hyperplasia and increased cortisol levels. The elevated cortisol levels or possibly a lack of normal daily secretory rhythm results in hyperglycemia, polyuria, polydipsia, poor wound healing, and loss of muscle tone.

    (1) **Polyuria** may be caused by an increase in the glomerular filtration rate (GFR) brought about by cortisol secretion. Cortisol may block either antidiuretic hormone (ADH) release or its action on the kidney. Secondly, an osmotic diuresis may occur because of glucosuria. Finally, compression of the posterior pituitary, hypothalamus, or both may cause lack of ADH release and result in polyuria.

    (2) **Polydypsia** is secondary to polyuria and necessary to maintain hydration.

    (3) **Sweating (hyperhidrosis)** occurs because of hypothalamic dysfunction or may be in response to the long hair coat.

    (4) **Muscle wasting** and **weight loss** results from deranged carbohydrate metabolism caused by increased cortisol secretion and peripheral insulin resistance. The result is protein catabolism and gluconeogenesis.

    (5) **Infections, laminitis,** and **poor wound healing** result from elevated cortisol levels.

    (6) **Hirsutism** may be the result of androgens of adrenal origin.

4. Diagnostic plan and laboratory tests

  a. Diagnosis relies heavily on laboratory tests. The total white blood cell count will be normal. There is usually an absolute or relative neutrophilia, lymphopenia, and eosinopenia (stress leukogram). Hyperglycemia is evident with blood glucose more than 6 mmol/L. Urinalysis reveals a glucosuria and ketonuria.

  b. Plasma cortisol is high or normal. Interpretation of the findings must take into account the normal daily rhythm for cortisol secretion. In general, evening levels are usually two-thirds of morning values.

  c. ACTH response test is exaggerated because of adrenal cortical hypertrophy. Basal levels of ACTH may be elevated in these cases and used as a diagnostic indication of disease.

  d. Dexamethasone suppression test (DST). Endogenous cortisol is not suppressed by exogenous corticosteroid administration in affected horses because of autonomous secretion of ACTH by the pars intermedia tumor. This is the most reliable test.

5. Differential diagnoses

  a. Chronic debilitation. Chronic weight loss and debilitation in an older horse may be caused by poor management and nutrition. A thorough examination of the mouth should be performed to eliminate dental or oral cavity problems. A fecal flotation should be performed to rule out parasitism. Any chronic systemic disease can result in debilitation (e.g., pulmonary or abdominal abscess, neoplasia, chronic renal/hepatic disease).

  b. Polyuria and polydipsia. Chronic renal failure can be ruled out with BUN, creatinine, and urinalysis findings.

  c. Hyperglycemia and glucosuria. Diabetes mellitus caused by pancreatic islet β-cell deficiency is extremely rare in the horse. There are only a few published reports of diabetes mellitus that are truly diabetes mellitus; the other cases of diabetes mellitus have always been associated with a pituitary tumor and are resistant to insulin treatment.

6. Therapeutic plan

  a. Cyproheptadine has been used with some success in horses with Cushing's disease. This drug has anticholinergic, antihistaminic, and antiserotonin activity and is thought to compete with serotonin for receptor sites. This may prevent serotonin-regulated ACTH release. The initial dose of 0.6 mg/kg orally once a day in the morning is increased to 1.2 mg/kg over several weeks. Improvement, if seen at all, usually occurs between 6 and 8 weeks. This drug may cause tranquilization, which, if severe, will force discontinuation of the medication.

   b. A few reports of the use of **O,P′-DDD (Permax)** in pituitary adenomas have been published. These treatments were not successful, and the drug is expensive.
   c. **Pergolide,** an ergot alkaloid, is being investigated in the treatment of pituitary adenomas. It is a dopaminergic agonist that causes intense vasoconstriction and vascular endothelial damage. This drug may be used at low dose levels (0.75 mg/day) until clinical signs improve and the DST returns to 25% of pretreatment values. Then the horse may be maintained at 0.25 mg/day. Alternatively, a higher dose (2.5–3.5 mg/horse/day) with a gradual decrease over time is advocated by some veterinarians.
   d. **Bromocriptine,** also a dopaminergic agonist, has been used experimentally but is extremely expensive.

7. Prevention. Even without treatment, the animal may live for several years. Special care must be taken to minimize infections and laminitis and to provide a high plane of nutrition.

B. | **Diabetes insipidus**

1. Patient profile and history. A few cases of diabetes insipidus have been reported in horses and food-producing animals. In these cases, the chief complaint has been the occurrence of polyuria and polydipsia in the animal.

2. Clinical findings. Because of a lack of cases, no set clinical signs are known. Polyuria and polydipsia are always present.

3. Etiology and pathogenesis
   a. Diabetes insipidus is characterized by **polyuria** and **polydipsia** in the absence of renal disease or glucosuria. The inability to concentrate urine may be because of a lack of synthesis or release of ADH or a blockage of ADH action on the renal tubules. ADH increases the levels of cyclic adenosine monophosphate (cAMP) in the renal tubule cells, leading to increased tubule cell permeability.
   b. This diabetes can be **congenital** or **acquired,** complete or partial. In humans, diabetes insipidus can result from pituitary adenomas, metastatic neoplasia, postpartum pituitary necrosis, and disseminated intravascular coagulation. In horses, a familial syndrome of diabetes insipidus has been described in sibling colts.
   c. If the animal responds to vasopressin, then a lack of ADH production from the hypothalamus or a lack of release from the neurohypophysis is the cause. Brain lesions that may result in this condition could be abscessation neoplasia or vascular disturbances.

4. Diagnostic plan and laboratory tests. The diagnosis is made based on the clinical findings and the following laboratory tests:
   a. **CBCs** and **chemistry profiles** are usually normal in these cases.
   b. **Urinalysis** is normal except for a low specific gravity [i.e., 1.002 and low osmolality (less than 300 mOsm/L)]. Serum osmolality is often increased (more than 300 mOsm/L).
   c. **Vasopressin response test.** Following the administration of vasopressin USP (100 units is given intramuscularly), the animal should begin to concentrate urine within 1 hour and should achieve peak concentration 4 hours post injection.
   d. **Water deprivation test.** Animals with diabetes insipidus are not able to concentrate urine in the face of dehydration.

5. Differential diagnoses
   a. **Renal disease** is ruled out by a normal BUN and creatinine.
   b. **Psychogenic polydipsia** and **polyuria** are eliminated on the basis of the water deprivation test. Animals with psychogenic drinking are able to concentrate urine if they become dehydrated unless medullary washout has occurred.
   c. **Nephrogenic diabetes insipidus** is not present if the animal responds to vasopressin.
   d. A **tumor** of the pars intermedia presents with polyuria and polydipsia in association with hyperglycemia and glucosuria.
   e. **Partial** or **complete** diabetes insipidus is differentiated by ADH assays and response to chlorpropamide.

6. **Therapeutic plan.** Therapy is seldom attempted in large animals. One case in a cow resolved spontaneously in a few months. The owner should be instructed to ensure an adequate supply of water for the animal at all times.
   a. In cases of **partial diabetes insipidus,** chlorpropamide, a hypoglycemic agent, can be used. This drug acts to increase intracellular cAMP, thereby accentuating the effects of ADH on renal tubule cells. This agent is ineffective in cases of complete diabetes insipidus.
   b. **Pitressin tannate** in oil is the ADH analogue most commonly used in veterinary medicine. This preparation is given intramuscularly and is often painful. Hypersensitivity and resistance can develop. The antidiuretic effect is often variable.
   c. **Desmopressin,** a newer ADH analogue, is used in humans, dogs, and cats. It has not been tried in large animals to date. This agent acts by binding to ADH receptors in the renal tubules, increasing cAMP and, thus, water permeability. The dosage is titrated to effect, and this drug is available for intranasal and parenteral use.

IV. DISEASES OF THE ADRENAL GLAND

A. **Equine pheochromocytoma.** Pheochromocytomas are tumors resulting from the **chromaffin cells** of the adrenal medulla. These tumors may be functional or nonfunctional, malignant or benign. Most of these tumors are unilateral, although bilateral tumors can be found.

1. **Patient profile and history.** Pheochromocytoma has been reported mainly in horses. In most of the cases, the condition occurred in older animals (older than 12 years). There is no specific breed or sex prevalence.

2. **Clinical findings.** Vital signs may be increased, heart sounds may be loud on auscultation, and a bounding jugular pulse may be noted. The animal may appear anxious or overexcited. Hyperhidrosis and muscle tremors are prevalent signs. Pupils are dilated but responsive. Polyuria and polydipsia may be present.

3. **Etiology and pathogenesis**
   a. The **neoplasm** is usually benign and grows slowly, with local destruction of tissue being the only effect of the tumor. On rare occasions, the tumor may **metastasize** to related lymph nodes, liver, lung, and bone. Vascular penetration and invasion of the vena cava and aorta may sometimes occur.
   b. **Functional tumors** may cause an increase in norepinephrine and epinephrine secretion. The high epinephrine concentrations cause hyperglycemia and sweating. Gluconeogenic effects of the catecholamines, catecholamine-induced suppression of insulin secretion, and catecholamine-induced increase in plasma glucagon cause hyperglycemia. Excessive sweating can result in polydipsia. In humans, increased levels of norepinephrine cause hypertension. It is unknown if this occurs in animals.
   c. **Compromised renal function** may result occasionally and is believed to occur because of norepinephrine-mediated vasoconstriction, reducing renal blood flow. In humans, death usually results from cardiovascular collapse, presumed to be caused by muscular hypoxia secondary to vasoconstriction.

4. **Diagnostic plan and laboratory tests**
   a. A detailed physical examination should be performed, and a CBC and chemistry profile should be obtained. Hyperglycemia and glucosuria are the most likely laboratory findings.
   b. **Catecholamine assays** of blood and urine are used in humans. Catecholamines are extremely unstable and samples must be processed within minutes or the results are of no value.

5. **Differential diagnoses**
   a. **Pituitary adenomas** should be considered when the age of the animal and clinical picture fits the disease profile.
   b. **Other conditions** to be ruled out include causes of hyperglycemia, such as diabetes mellitus and equine Cushing's disease. Plasma cortisol levels, an ACTH response test, and a dexamethasone suppression test may help differentiate disorders.
   c. **Pancreatic α-cell tumors** are rare but do increase the secretion of glucagon and cause increased glyconeogenesis.

6. **Therapeutic plan and prognosis.** Treatment usually is not attempted in large animals because a diagnosis is not usually made antemortem. In humans, α-blockers, such as phentolamine and phenoxybenzamine hydrochloride, have been used to control blood pressure. Propranolol (a β-blocker) is used if an arrhythmia is present. Both blockers are effective in decreasing sweating and hypermetabolism. The preferred treatment in humans is a tyrosine analogue (α-methyl tyrosine), which inhibits the rate-limiting step in catecholamine production. The prognosis is grave in all cases.

B. **Equine adrenal insufficiency**

1. **Patient profile and history.** Race horses that have received glucocorticoid or anabolic steroid injections are possible candidates for this condition. Poor condition, poor performance, hirsutism, and lethargy are the complaints. Mares may exhibit anestrus.

2. **Etiology and pathogenesis**
   a. It has been found that only 2 mg of dexamethasone can suppress cortisol secretion for 24 hours in the horse. This implies that small glucocorticoid doses given once or twice a day in the form of anabolic steroid preparations or intra-articular injections may induce adrenal insufficiency. The incidence of Addison's disease (equine adrenal insufficiency) in the horse is unknown, but iatrogenic adrenal insufficiency should be considered in the diagnostic workup of poor performance horses.
   b. **Mares** who have received anabolic steroids while racing appear to go through a "let-down" period when they are retired from the track. It may be 6 months before they begin to put on weight. Reproduction cycles may be interrupted.
   c. In research studies in which horses have been **bilaterally adrenalectomized,** the cause of death is severe hypoglycemia or severe electrolyte disturbances.

3. **Diagnostic plan and laboratory tests**
   a. Diagnosis relies on laboratory findings. Studies that have created bilaterally adrenalectomized horses have shown an increase in the packed cell volume (PCV), increased serum potassium levels, and decreased serum sodium, chloride, and glucose levels. Serum cortisol levels are low, and horses fail to respond to ACTH stimulation.
   b. Normal or depressed serum sodium concentration with a concurrent high-percentage creatinine clearance ratio of sodium in urine indicates salt wasting or hypoaldosteronism (Figure 10-1). Normal levels in the horse are 0.02%–1%.

4. **Differential diagnoses**
   a. Chronic weight loss caused by gastrointestinal involvement
   b. Chronic infection causing lethargy
   c. Lameness that may contribute to poor performance
   d. Cardiovascular disease
   e. Electrolyte disturbances

$$\frac{\text{Urinary Na}}{\text{Serum Na}} \times \frac{\text{Serum Cr}}{\text{Urinary Cr}} \times 100 = \%\text{CrNa}$$

FIGURE 10-1. Calculation of the creatinine clearance ratio of sodium (% *CrNa*). *Cr* = creatinine; *Na* = sodium.

5. **Therapeutic plan and prevention**
   a. **Rest** and **reduction of stress** usually helps mares adjust. If the results of an ACTH stimulation test are still abnormal after 3 months, glucocorticoid supplementation may be necessary.
   b. If **glucocorticoid therapy** is needed in the horse, then alternate-day therapy would reduce the incidence of iatrogenic adrenal suppression. If daily administration of steroids is needed, then the animal should be weaned off the drug gradually. This should be accomplished over 4–6 weeks by cutting the dose in half every fifth day until the last week, when alternate-day therapy is used.

V. DISEASES OF THE THYROID GLAND

A. Equine hypothyroidism

1. **Patient profile and history.** Hypothyroidism occurs rarely, but when it does occur, the disorder is seen most frequently in racehorses, obese mares, and foals. Racehorses present with poor performance, erratic appetite, decreased endurance, dullness, and stiffness of gait. Hypothyroid obese mares often have a history of recurrent laminitis and erratic reproductive function. Foals may be weak, stillborn, or have contracted tendons and tarsal bone collapse.

2. **Clinical findings**
   a. **Foals.** If hypothyroidism begins early in fetal development, the neonate fails to establish normal respiration at birth. Onset in late pregnancy produces a foal that is lethargic and unable to stand and suckle. In studies on surgically created thyroidectomized (THD) foals, the animals are stunted and may die in 1–2 months.
   b. **Adults.** Similarly, THD adults are lethargic, slow moving, have lower rectal temperatures than normal, and an intolerance to cold. They have scaly haircoats, delayed closure of epiphyseal plates, decreased libido, and edema of the distal limbs. This condition is not life threatening and the signs can be reversed with thyroid supplementation.
   c. **Race horses.** Hypothyroidism has been suggested in racing thoroughbred and standardbred horses that present with signs similar to "tying-up" syndrome (see Chapter 13 I B 2 a). These animals do not perform well, are stiff, and may exhibit the percussion dimple of pseudomyotonia.

3. **Normal physiology**
   a. **Iodine** absorbed from the gastrointestinal tract is combined with **tyrosine** in the thyroid gland to form **monoiodotyrosine (MIT)** and then **diiodotyrosine (DIT).**
   b. **Thyroxine (T_4)** is formed by coupling two DIT molecules, and **3,5,3' triiodothyronine (T_3)** is formed by the coupling of one MIT and one DIT molecule. T_3 and T_4 are stored in the follicular colloid in the thyroid gland and are released in response to TSH from the pituitary gland. It is currently thought that when T_4 enters a cell, it is converted to the biologically active T_3. The concentration of T_3 and T_4 are regulated by the negative feedback mechanism on the pituitary.
   c. **Thyroid hormones** affect most body tissues by acting on cells at the level of the nucleus, mitochondria, or plasma membranes. These hormones affect cellular metabolism through amino acid transport and oxygen consumption, both of which impact cellular growth, differentiation, proliferation, and maturation.
   d. **Diurnal variations** in T_4 and T_3 levels occur in horses. T_4 peaks in the late afternoon, with lowest levels in early morning. T_3 peaks in the morning, with lowest levels occurring around midnight. These variations need to be kept in mind when only a single sample is tested. Thyroid hormone levels also decrease with age; foals have twice the T_4 values of adults.

4. **Etiology and pathogenesis**
   a. **Primary hypothyroidism** may be caused by an idiopathic autoimmune disease.

   b. Secondary hypothyroidism may be caused by a lack of thyroid-stimulating hormone (TSH) or TSH-releasing factor from the pituitary or an impaired transport of TSH. This condition may be seen in conjunction with pituitary adenomas of the pars intermedia.

5. **Diagnostic plan and laboratory tests.** Laboratory tests include a CBC, serum biochemistry, T_4 levels, TSH response test, and perhaps a thyroid biopsy. The diet should be evaluated to identify any agents known to affect the thyroid's iodine uptake (e.g., kelp).
   a. **CBC and serum biochemistry.** Abnormal laboratory findings include a normocytic, normochromic anemia. The PCV is in the mid 20s. Serum phosphorus may be decreased and probably relates to decreased feed intake.
   b. **T_4 levels.** Serum T_4 level is low (0.5 μg%; normal is 1–3 μg%). Because radioimmunoassay measures only bound T_4, drugs that compete for protein-binding sites (e.g., phenylbutazone, anabolic steroids) artificially lower T_4 values. Free T_4 levels are not affected by these drugs, and a horse may be euthyroid despite a low T_4 value.
   c. **TSH response test.** TSH (5 IU) is administered intramuscularly, and T_3 and T_4 levels are measured at 1–4 hours post treatment. A normal response would be a twofold increase in T_3 and T_4. An increase less than twofold is considered indicative of primary hypothyroidism.

6. **Differential diagnoses**
   a. In **foals,** consider metabolic bone disease, septic arthritis, contracted tendons caused by lameness, and osteochondritis dessicans.
   b. In **racehorses,** rule out rhabdomyolysis, lameness, polymyositis, or systemic disease.
   c. **Pituitary adenomas** must also be ruled out (see III A).

7. **Therapeutic plan and prognosis.** Sodium levothyroxine (10 mg) is administered orally in 70 ml of corn syrup daily. Measure T_3 or T_4 levels every 1–2 weeks, and adjust dosage as needed. The prognosis is good, but lifetime supplementation may be needed.

B. **Goiter (iodine deficiency)**

1. **Patient profile and history.** This condition is seen in newborn animals of all species and is worldwide in distribution.

2. **Clinical findings.** The major clinical findings are neonatal death with alopecia and visibly enlarged thyroid glands in surviving animals.

3. **Etiology and pathogenesis**
   a. **Primary iodine deficiency.** Iodine-deficient soils are common worldwide because of leaching of soils not replenished by the iodine found naturally in oceans.
   b. **Diets** rich in brassicas and other goitrogenic plants likely produce a thiocyanate in the rumen of ruminants, which may restrict the uptake of iodine by the thyroid. Iodine deficiency results in decreased T_4 production and stimulation of TSH secretion, resulting in hyperplasia of the thyroid gland. Clinical signs are the result of hypothyroidism. Iodine is an essential component for normal fetal development.

4. **Diagnostic plan and laboratory tests.** The diagnosis is made based on clinical findings, necropsy, and laboratory results. Diagnostic strategies include measuring iodine levels in the blood and milk of the herd or flock and obtaining serum T_4 levels.

5. **Therapeutic plan.** Surviving animals should receive iodine supplements. Overdosing can cause toxicity.

6. **Prevention.** Supplement diets with iodine as a salt or mineral mixture.

C. **Equine hyperthyroidism** is a rare condition but may be considered if presented with a high-strung, unmanageable animal.

D. Bovine ultimobranchial (thyroid C-cell) tumor

1. **Patient profile and history.** This condition is seen in older animals (age 6–20 years), usually bulls.

2. **Clinical findings.** There is slight palpable enlargement of the thyroid gland region caused by extensive multiple nodular enlargements along the ventral aspect of the neck. There is severe vertebral osteosclerosis with ankylosing spondylosis deformans and degenerative osteoarthrosis, resulting in clinical lameness in these bulls.

3. **Etiology and pathogenesis.** There is a possible association with long-term ingestion of a high-calcium diet. The chronic stimulation of the C-cells and ultimobranchial derivatives by high levels of calcium absorbed from the digestive tract may be related to the pathophysiology of the neoplasms. Cows do not develop proliferative lesions during similar dietary conditions because of the high physiologic requirement for calcium during lactation.

4. **Diagnostic plan and laboratory tests. Fine needle aspiration** of any masses should be performed. Radiographs should be taken of the thorax and spinal column. Serum calcitonin levels should be measured. **Calcitonin levels** may or may not be increased, and **serum electrolyte levels** are within normal range.

5. **Differential diagnoses.** C-cell adenomas grow slowly. C-cell carcinomas are larger and cause observable enlargements in the anterior neck region of older bulls and frequently metastasize to the anterior cervical lymph nodes and lungs.

6. **Therapeutic plan.** There is no known treatment.

7. **Prevention.** Avoid feeding high-calcium diets to bulls.

E. Equine thyroid tumors

1. **Patient profile and history.** The reported cases have been in horses older than age 8 years. The presenting complaint is swelling in the region of the larynx.

2. **Clinical findings.** There is a palpable mass in the area caudal to the larynx. The animal may be inclined to gulp excessively. Exercise intolerance may be a finding.

3. **Normal physiology.** The thyroid gland in the horse consists of a pair of **encapsulated lobes** that are symmetrically situated on either side of the trachea caudal to the larynx. They measure approximately 2.5 cm $\times$ 5 cm and are frequently palpable in the normal horse.

4. **Etiology and pathogenesis**
   a. **Thyroid adenomas** are common in older horses, but they are usually a postmortem finding.
   b. **Thyroid carcinomas** and **C-cell tumors** have been reported in the horse, but they are uncommon.

5. **Diagnostic plan and laboratory tests.** Fine needle aspiration of the mass, a T_4 test, and a TSH response test should be performed. Serum T_4 and TSH levels are variable. Endoscopy may be useful to rule out an upper airway problem. Thyroid scintigraphy may indicate abnormal uptake.

6. **Therapeutic plan and prognosis.** Surgical removal of carcinomas and C-cell tumors is necessary. Prognosis is good if no metastasis has occurred.

VI. DISEASES OF THE PARATHYROID GLAND

A. Primary hyperparathyroidism

1. **Patient profile and history.** This condition is seen in older horses (older than 15 years) but is rare.

2. **Clinical findings.** There may be lethargy, but there have been too few cases reported to generalize.

3. **Etiology and pathogenesis**
   a. **Etiology.** Primary hyperparathyroidism may be the result of **parathyroid adenoma, parathyroid hyperplasia,** or **carcinoma.** Few cases of parathyroid adenoma have been reported. This may be because the two pairs, or sometimes more than two pairs, of parathyroid glands are widely separated in the horse and are often difficult to identify.
   b. **Pathogenesis.** Primary hyperparathyroidism should always be considered in horses with **hypercalcemia,** particularly if it occurs in the absence of renal failure or neoplasia. When calcium levels increase dramatically, mineralization of soft tissues may occur, leading to renal and myocardial calcification and subsequent renal failure and arrhythmias. Death may follow.

4. **Diagnostic plan.** Serum and urine calcium, phosphorus, and parathyroid hormone (PTH) levels and the percentage creatinine clearance of phosphorus should be obtained.

5. **Laboratory tests.** The CBC is normal, but hypercalcemia and hypophosphatemia are evident. BUN and creatinine levels are usually normal. Urinalysis is normal, but there is an increased fractional urinary excretion of phosphorus (normal is 0%–0.5%).

6. **Therapeutic plan and prognosis.** Therapy rarely has been attempted or reported. Steroid therapy (prednisone) may be rational. Steroids act to decrease calcium absorption from the gastrointestinal tract, decrease release of calcium from bone, and increase urinary excretion of calcium. The prognosis is guarded to grave.

B. **Nutritional secondary hyperparathyroidism (NSH), osteodystrophia fibrosa, big head disease, bran disease, Miller's disease**

1. **Patient profile and history.** Although any age and breed may be affected, young animals are more prone to the condition.

2. **Clinical findings.** There is a transitory shifting leg lameness, generalized joint tenderness, and a stilted gait. Teeth may be loose, and later in the disease a bilateral firm enlargement of the facial bones above and anterior to the facial crests may be noted (**big head disease**).

3. **Etiology and pathogenesis**
   a. NSH occurs because of a compensatory increase in **PTH secretion** as a result of excessive phosphorus intake in the presence of normal or low serum calcium levels.
      (1) **Hyperphosphatemia** lowers blood calcium levels. Hypocalcemia stimulates PTH secretion, which returns blood calcium levels to normal or near normal.
      (2) Stimulation of PTH causes cellular hypertrophy and hyperplasia of the parathyroid glands.
         (a) PTH is involved in the fine **regulation of blood calcium** in mammals. Its direct effects are on bone, causing osteoclastic resorption, and on the kidney, causing calcium retention and phosphorus excretion. PTH also increases calcium absorption in the intestine.
         (b) Fibrous connective tissue is deposited when an excess amount of bone is removed, hence the name osteodystrophia fibrosa.
   b. The ingestion of excessive amounts of **oxalates** also may cause NSH. Oxalates decrease calcium absorption from the gut by forming insoluble complexes, which results in progressive hypocalcemia and PTH stimulation.

4. **Diagnostic plan and laboratory tests.** For a definitive diagnosis, serum and urine calcium and phosphate levels, percentage creatinine phosphate clearance, and serum alkaline phosphatase levels must be obtained. The calcium to phosphorus ratio in the ration also should be evaluated.

$$\frac{\text{Urinary PO}_4^-}{\text{Plasma PO}_4^-} \times \frac{\text{Plasma Cr}}{\text{Urinary Cr}} \times 100 = \%\text{CrPO}_4^-$$

FIGURE 10-2. Calculation of the creatinine clearance ratio of phosphate (%*CrPO*$_4^-$). *Cr* = creatinine; PO$_4^-$ = phosphate.

    a. Hypocalcemia and **hyperphosphatemia** occur very early, but values are often normal later in the course of the condition. Serum alkaline phosphatase (SAP) may be in the high normal range.

    b. Changes in urine phosphates are more consistent. Calcium excretion decreases, whereas phosphate excretion in urine increases. These levels can be measured by the percentage urinary clearance of phosphates (Figure 10-2). Normal percentage creatinine phosphate clearance in horses is 0%–0.5%.

5. Differential diagnoses

    a. Lameness. A thorough lameness examination is necessary to rule out other causes of lameness.

    b. Neoplastic process of the facial bones. A biopsy and radiographs are necessary to rule out other causes of facial bone deformities.

6. Therapeutic plan. Dietary calcium should be increase and phosphorus intake should be decreased. Good alfalfa hay is high in calcium. Limestone (calcium carbonate) supplementation can also increase serum calcium. The clinical signs of lameness should disappear in 1–2 months after dietary correction. Facial swellings may never regress to normal.

C. Pseudohyperparathyroidism (PHT)

1. Patient profile and history. This condition may be seen in older animals with a history of weight loss, polyuria and polydipsia, weakness, and gastrointestinal disturbances.

2. Clinical findings. PHT generally is associated with a neoplastic condition, specifically **gastric adenocarcinoma** and **lymphosarcoma.** Therefore, signs consistent with chronic diseases are evident.

3. Etiology and pathogenesis

    a. The **pathogenesis** of hypercalcemia associated with nonparathyroid tumors is not understood, but it is postulated that these tumors secrete PTH-like substances. Prostaglandins and their metabolites, vitamin D and non-vitamin D steroids, also could participate in bone resorption. The histopathology of the parathyroid glands indicates inactivity, atrophy, or both in response to the hypercalcemia.

    b. There are two mechanisms proposed for the **isosthenuria** that is seen in hypercalcemia.

        (1) Increased calcium in the renal cells interferes with the efficiency of the sodium pump, resulting in decreased sodium in the renal medulla and papilla. This leads to failure of the countercurrent exchange system.

        (2) Locally, increased calcium decreases the permeability of the distal convoluted tubules and collecting ducts to water.

4. Diagnostic plan. Serum calcium levels must be evaluated. Evidence of neoplasia should be sought. Diagnostic workup for neoplasia should include rectal examination, thoracic radiography, abdominocentesis, and gastric endoscopy. PTH levels will probably be normal in horses with PHT.

5. Laboratory tests. Hypercalcemia is the most consistent finding. A low serum phosphorus level may be present. There is an increase in SAP and isosthenuria.

6. Differential diagnoses

    a. Renal disease in horses may present as hypercalcemia, polyuria and polydipsia, and isosthenuria. Concomitant elevation of BUN and creatinine levels will indicate renal disease.

b. Ingestion of **plants with vitamin D activity,** such as *Cestrum diurnum* and *Solanum malacoxylon,* may cause hypercalcemia.

c. **Primary hyperparathyroidism** is rare in the horse.

7. **Therapeutic plan and prognosis.** Treatment is only palliative because of the associated neoplasia. Corticosteroids may be helpful to inhibit the action of PTH and prostaglandins, minimizing the hypercalcemia. Nonsteroidal anti-inflammatory drugs (NSAIDs) also inhibit prostaglandins. Because this disorder is associated with a poor prognosis, euthanasia is often considered.

D. Acute vitamin D₃ toxicosis

1. **Patient profile and history.** There is no age, sex, or breed predisposition with this disease. The client complains that the horse exhibits anorexia, weakness, limb stiffness, and weight loss.

2. **Clinical findings.** Affected horses exhibit depression, anorexia, weakness, and limb stiffness with impaired mobility. There may be polyuria and polydipsia.

3. **Etiology and pathogenesis**
   a. **Etiology.** Causes include accidental excess added to bulk feed, over-supplementation with parenteral vitamin D preparations, or the consumption of plants containing vitamin D-like substances. Two such plants, ***Cestrum diurnum*** and ***Solanum malacoxylon,*** are found in North America.
   b. **Pathogenesis.** Excessive exposure or administration of vitamin D leads to disseminated soft tissue mineralization.
      (1) Vitamin D exerts its effect primarily by increasing calcium and phosphorus absorption in the intestines and may enhance bone resorption. The cardiovascular system appears to be particularly affected.
      (2) Serum calcium levels fluctuate during the course of disease and may remain within normal limits. Therefore, serum calcium is an unreliable indicator of vitamin D toxicosis. Unlike renal disease and hyperparathyroidism, vitamin D toxicosis results in hyperphosphatemia.

4. **Diagnostic plan.** Obtain a thorough history and check serum calcium, phosphorus, and magnesium levels. Request a BUN, creatinine, urinalysis, and urinary clearance of phosphate. Perform a feed analysis if oral exposure is suspected.

5. **Laboratory tests.** There is usually a marked, persistent hyperphosphatemia. Hypercalcemia is a variable finding. BUN and creatinine are normal unless marked kidney mineralization has occurred.

6. **Differential diagnoses**
   a. **Magnesium deficiency** in the horse can present with similar morphologic lesions. Antemortem blood levels of calcium, phosphorus, and magnesium help differentiate the two problems.
   b. **Chronic renal failure, neoplasia,** and **primary hyperparathyroidism** can also cause hypercalcemia in horses and must be ruled out.

7. **Therapeutic plan and prognosis.** Withdraw any contaminated feed, and prevent over-supplementation. Rest and nursing care is the only recommended treatment. The feed supplier should be notified of the problem. The prognosis is poor for horses exhibiting cardiovascular abnormalities. In less severe cases, recovery may take 6 months or longer.

VII. **ANHIDROSIS,** or the inability to sweat, was once thought to result from poor acclimatization of horses native to cooler environments. It is now realized that anhidrosis affects even those horses native to hot, humid climates. Horses undergoing strenuous exercise (e.g., racing, polo, eventing) are affected as well as relatively idle broodmares and "backyard" pleasure horses.

A. **Patient profile and history.** Horses with this condition have a history of exercise intolerance and decreased appetite, and owners frequently notice animals sweat less than expected during periods of extreme heat and exercise.

B. **Clinical findings.** During episodes of exertion, the horse's rectal temperature and respiratory rate often are elevated. There may be no sweating or only patchy sweating. Chronically, there is a loss of body condition.

C. **Etiology and pathogenesis**

1. The **etiology** remains unknown. Cessation of sweating may be complete or partial because some horses maintain some sweating ability over the brisket, perineum, and under the mane. The disorder is most frequently recognized in hot, humid environments and seems to be precipitated by heat stress.

2. **Pathogenesis.** Proposed mechanisms of anhidrosis include the downregulation of sweat gland β_2-receptors in response to higher than normal concentrations of circulating epinephrine secondary to heat stress and also fatigue of sweat gland secretion resulting from prolonged demand. It is interesting to note that horses with anhidrosis do appear to have higher levels of circulating epinephrine than normal horses.

D. **Diagnostic plan.** Diagnosis is aided by the history of inadequate sweat production after appropriate stimulation. An intradermal epinephrine challenge may be applied. A total lack of sweat production at the site of injection is a poor prognostic sign.

E. **Laboratory tests.** There are no laboratory values of diagnostic significance.

F. **Therapeutic plan.** There is no consistent therapy to induce sweating. Oral supplementation of electrolytes is the most common therapy and meets with some success. Iodinated casein supplements have been tried with mixed results. Symptomatic therapy to promote heat dissipation should be employed. These techniques include air and water cooling, shade, and rest.

G. **Prevention.** Moving horses to cooler climates helps.

STUDY QUESTIONS

DIRECTIONS: Each of the numbered items or incomplete statements in this section is followed by answers or by completions of the statement. Select the ONE numbered answer or completion that is BEST in each case.

1. Which statement regarding equine Cushing's disease is correct?

(1) The hyperglycemia associated with equine Cushing's disease is usually insulin responsive.
(2) Surgery is the treatment of choice.
(3) A tumor of the pars distalis of the pituitary gland causes the clinical signs.
(4) A tumor produces excessive glucocorticoid, which decreases in response to a test dose of dexamethasone.
(5) Polyuria, hirsutism, and weight loss are common clinical findings.

2. An equine pituitary adenoma often presents with:

(1) colic and diarrhea.
(2) laminitis and chronic infections.
(3) excessive masculine or feminine behavior.
(4) a loud, pounding heart and renal failure.
(5) bone remodeling and pathologic fractures of long bones.

3. Which statement regarding equine pheochromocytoma is correct? Equine pheochromocytoma:

(1) if functional, causes increased epinephrine and norepinephrine secretion.
(2) is a tumor of the pars intermedia of the pituitary gland.
(3) causes anhidrosis.
(4) is a tumor most often restricted to female thoroughbreds.
(5) is most often treated by surgical removal.

4. Which statement correctly describes equine adrenal insufficiency?

(1) It causes paradoxically high serum cortisol levels.
(2) It has not been reported in mares.
(3) It is seen in horses that have received long-term glucocorticoid therapy.
(4) It can be diagnosed by a dexamethasone suppression test.
(5) It is best prevented by the use of anabolic steroids.

5. Which statement regarding equine hypothyroidism is correct?

(1) It is seen only in racehorses.
(2) It is not a life-threatening condition.
(3) Phenylbutazone administration may artificially increase serum thyroxine (T_4) values.
(4) It may cause horses to exhibit decreased endurance and stiffness.
(5) It is caused by a deficiency of vitamin D.

6. Goiter is best described by which of the following statements? Goiter:

(1) causes hypothyroidism due to iodine deficiency.
(2) is an immune-mediated thyroid disorder.
(3) results in a decrease in thyroid-stimulating hormone (TSH) production.
(4) is a condition restricted to North America.
(5) is of major clinical significance in weak and old animals.

7. Nutritional secondary hyperparathyroidism (NSH) causes which one of the following findings?

(1) Elevated serum phosphorus values
(2) A secondary decrease in parathyroid hormone (PTH) secretion
(3) Renal failure
(4) Lameness and enlargement of facial bones
(5) Decreased calcium absorption from the intestine

8. The hypercalcemia seen in animals with equine pseudohyperparathyroidism (PHT) is related to:

(1) renal disease.
(2) pituitary disease.
(3) the ingestion of certain plants containing high calcium levels.
(4) vitamin C toxicity.
(5) tumors such as gastric adenocarcinoma or lymphosarcoma.

9. Acute vitamin D_3 toxicosis in the horse usually produces which one of the following signs?

(1) Blindness
(2) Marked, persistent hyperphosphatemia
(3) Renal failure
(4) An extremely low serum calcium
(5) Sweating and signs of colic

DIRECTIONS: The numbered item in this section is negatively phrased, as indicated by a capitalized word such as NOT, LEAST, or EXCEPT. Select the ONE numbered answer that is BEST.

---

10. The secretion of which of the following is NOT increased in cases of pituitary adenoma in horses?

(1) Melanocyte-stimulating hormone (MSH)
(2) β-Endorphins
(3) Adrenocorticotropic hormone (ACTH)
(4) Prolactin
(5) Corticotropin-like intermediate lobe peptide

ANSWERS AND EXPLANATIONS

1. The answer is 5 [III A]. The clinical findings of polyuria, hirsutism, and weight loss are associated with equine Cushing's disease. The pituitary tumor causing this disease is confined to the pars intermedia and secretes adrenocorticotropic hormone (ACTH) autonomously, resulting in adrenal gland hypertrophy and excess cortisol secretion. Therefore, the resultant hyperglycemia is not insulin responsive, and the high endogenous cortisol level does not respond to dexamethasone administration. Medical therapy may be attempted, but surgery is not an option.

2. The answer is 2 [III A 2 b]. In horses with pituitary adenoma, the high concentration of circulating endogenous steroids produced in response to excessive adrenocorticotropic hormone (ACTH) secretion from the pituitary tumor results in chronic infections and laminitis. None of the other sets of clinical findings (i.e., colic and diarrhea, excessive masculine or feminine behavior, a loud pounding heart and renal failure, or bone remodeling and pathologic fractures) can be attributed to equine Cushing's disease.

3. The answer is 1 [IV A]. Pheochromocytomas arise from the chromaffin cells of the adrenal medulla, and they will, if functional, secrete epinephrine and norepinephrine. Equine pheochromocytoma does not cause anhidrosis. Therapy is usually not attempted. The tumor is not restricted to female thoroughbreds.

4. The answer is 3 [IV B]. Equine adrenal insufficiency may be seen in a subset of race horses that have received long-term steroid agents to enhance performance. Endogenous cortisol levels are low because of adrenal gland atrophy. Therefore, horses do not respond to adrenocorticotropic hormone (ACTH) stimulation or further dexamethasone suppression.

5. The answer is 4 [V A]. In adult horses, hypothyroidism causes signs of lethargy, poor performance, and stiffness. Although often seen in racehorses, there is no breed or sex predilection. It may also be a disease of the unborn or neonate, in which case it is life threatening. It is diagnosed by measuring thyroxine (T_4) levels, which may be artificially lowered if the horse is receiving phenylbutazone. It may be caused by thyroid or pituitary disease.

6. The answer is 1 [V B 1–3]. Goiter is hypothyroidism due to iodine deficiency. It is seen worldwide and is of major significance in the young. It is not related to thyroid or pituitary disease or dysfunction.

7. The answer is 4 [VI B 2–3]. Nutritional secondary hyperparathyroidism (NSH) results from excessive phosphorus intake concurrent with low or normal calcium intake. The resultant parathyroid hormone (PTH) stimulation causes calcium absorption from the bone, calcium retention by the kidney, and phosphorus excretion. Bone remodeling occurs, causing lameness and enlargement of facial bones. Phosphorus levels may be elevated early in the course of the disease but are very often normal by the time clinical signs are present.

8. The answer is 5 [VI C 3]. Hypercalcemia in horses is often the first indication of a tumor (e.g., gastric adenocarcinoma, lymphosarcoma) and is termed pseudohyperparathyroidism (PHT).

9. The answer is 2 [VI D 2, 5]. Hyperphosphatemia is the most common laboratory finding with vitamin D_3 toxicosis. Blindness, renal failure, extreme hypocalcemia, sweating, and signs of colic do not occur with this condition.

10. The answer is 4 [III A 3 b]. Prolactin secretion is not increased in cases of equine pituitary adenoma. Melanocyte-stimulating hormone (MSH), β-endorphins, adrenocorticotropic hormone (ACTH), and corticotropin-like intermediate lobe peptide are derived from the pars intermedia of the pituitary gland and may be increased with equine Cushing's disease.

Chapter 11

Neurologic Disorders

John Pringle

I. **BRAIN DISORDERS OF THE NEWBORN.** There are many congenital defects of the nervous system of domestic animals. Most defects are lethal and are diagnosed at necropsy. Causes may include genetic or environmental factors. Environmental factors are highly varied and include teratogens, viruses, drugs, trace elements, and physical damage (e.g., rectal palpation of the dam).

A. **Hydranencephaly (normotensive hydrocephalus)** is an absence of cerebral hemispheres in a cranium of normal conformation.

1. **Patient profile.** This condition may be more common than hydrocephalus in large animals (see I B), particularly in calves because hydranencephaly is associated with intrauterine viral infection.

2. **Clinical findings.** Affected animals show signs immediately at birth, with depression and blindness (i.e., dummies) being the key findings. In the viral-associated hydranencephaly of calves, other problems such as cerebellar signs or arthrogryposis may predominate.

3. **Etiology.** In calves, the known causes include intrauterine viral infection by bovine viral diarrhea (BVD) virus, Akabane virus, or bluetongue virus. In some species, a fetal cerebrovascular accident has also been proposed as a cause, but this disease is otherwise poorly understood.

4. **Diagnostic plan and laboratory tests.** An accurate diagnosis in cattle, although challenging, is important for client education and prevention.
   a. **Clinical signs** of blindness and depression from birth are highly suggestive of hydranencephaly. **Arthrogryposis** in calves or lambs is suggestive of intrauterine viral infection as a cause.
   b. **Presuckle serum titers** that are positive to viruses, such as BVD virus in calves or bluetongue in calves or lambs, help confirm a diagnosis of intrauterine viral infection.

5. **Therapeutic plan.** Most affected animals lack vigor at birth and die or are euthanized.

6. **Prevention.** For viral hydranencephaly, vaccination of the dam before breeding can help prevent this problem. However, most cases are sporadic and are unlikely to occur at a high incidence.

B. **Hydrocephalus** (or hypertensive hydrocephalus) is the destruction of tissues within the cranial vault, usually caused by increased hydrostatic pressure in the cerebrospinal fluid (CSF).

1. **Patient profile and history.** Hydrocephalus can affect all animal species as an isolated occurrence, but it is also a rare inherited trait in cattle. Hydrocephalus has been associated with dwarfism in cattle.

2. **Clinical findings.** The animal may be born dead. If the affected animal lives, it is blind and very depressed from birth and usually dies within a few days. Other possible signs include a "domed" cranial enlargement, microphthalmia, and reduced birthweight.

3. **Etiology and pathogenesis**
   a. **Etiology.** This disease is caused by a simple autosomal-recessive trait in cattle (particularly Herefords) or a vitamin A deficiency in cattle.

b. Pathogenesis. Hydrocephalus occurs when there is an accumulation of excessive fluid within the ventricular system.

4. Diagnostic plan
   a. Clinical signs of a domed skull, depression, and blindness from birth suggest hydrocephalus.
   b. Ultrasound examination of the cranial vault through fontanelles in the skull confirms a lack of brain tissue.

5. Therapeutic plan and prevention. Although there is no treatment for the affected animal, genetic planning should be considered if cases are found in purebred Hereford calves.

C. **Cerebellar disease.** Congenital cerebellar diseases can be classified as **neonatal syndromes,** which are present at birth, or **postnatal syndromes,** which may develop weeks to months after birth. Neonatal syndromes are most common.

   1. Patient profile. All species can be affected. Postnatal syndromes have been recognized in Arabian foals, Gotland ponies, Holstein cattle, and Yorkshire pigs.

   2. Clinical findings consist primarily of a **lack of control** of voluntary movement. The neonatal syndromes occur during fetal development and have no progression of signs after birth. Compensation for the deficit may occur over several weeks.
   a. A **key finding** in pure cerebellar disease is **strength without control,** with no paresis or proprioceptive disturbances. **Intention head tremors** are often present and are particularly obvious when the animal moves its head to eat.
   b. Ataxia, hypermetria (or hypometria), and **spasticity** are the major features of gait.
   c. A unilateral or bilateral **lack of menace response** may be present, despite normal vision and normal cranial nerve VII function, because cerebellar processing is required in the normal menace response.

   3. Etiology and pathogenesis
   a. Neonatal syndromes
      (1) Infectious causes are the most common cause of neonatal syndromes.
         (a) Cattle. BVD virus *in utero* infection at 100–170 days' gestation or intrauterine bluetongue virus infection are known to cause cerebellar hypoplasia in cattle.
         (b) Sheep. Border disease virus intrauterine infection at 60–80 days' gestation, as well as bluetongue virus, can result in cerebellar disease in sheep.
         (c) Pigs. Hog cholera virus infection in pigs also causes cerebellar damage.
      (2) Malformation can also lead to neonatal cerebellar disease and has been associated with an autosomal-recessive gene in Hereford cattle.
   b. Postnatal syndromes are classified as **abiotrophies** because they are characterized by lesions of degeneration. Abiotrophies are genetically-induced defects in cerebellar cortical neurons that result in the premature death of these neurons.

   4. Diagnostic plan and laboratory tests. Clinical signs of intention tremors, hypermetria, and spasticity without paresis or decreased sensorium are usually sufficient to suggest cerebellar disease. The time of occurrence (at birth or postnatally) provides further direction regarding cause (e.g., intrauterine or postnatal abiotrophy).
   a. Neonatal syndromes
      (1) Serology. In cases of cerebellar disease at birth, precolostral serology (e.g., BVD in calves) helps establish a viral etiology.
      (2) Postmortem examination
         (a) Intrauterine viral infection. The cerebellum is absent, reduced, or normal in size, with histologic evidence of Purkinje cell loss.
         (b) Malformation. The cerebellum is significantly smaller than normal.
   b. Postnatal syndromes. The cerebellum of the affected animal is of normal size.

   5. Therapeutic plan. There is no treatment for affected animals, but the clinical abnormalities do not usually limit animal survival or growth.

6. Prevention. If a virus is incriminated, the vaccination of dams can prevent future disease.

D. Neonatal maladjustment syndrome [NMS; "Barker foals," hypoxic–ischemic encephalopathy (HIE)]

1. **Patient profile.** This syndrome occurs in foals, most commonly in Thoroughbreds. Foals may be premature or may be from a difficult or prolonged delivery.

2. **Clinical findings.** After an initial period of apparent normality (approximately 24 hours), affected foals lose their affinity for the dam, lose suckling ability, and may wander aimlessly. They may also experience seizures with opisthotonos, appear unaware of their surroundings, and lose their righting reflex.

3. **Etiology and pathogenesis.** The etiology of NMS has not been fully determined. It is felt that hypoxia at parturition or trauma to the central nervous system (CNS) at birth with resulting vascular abnormalities and cerebral hemorrhage may be part of the pathogenesis (see Chapter 18 III A 2). There appears to be poor correlation of clinical signs with severity of brain hemorrhage.

4. **Diagnostic plan and laboratory tests**
   a. **Patient history.** The clinical history of loss of suckle on the first day after initial appearance of a normal foal is suggestive of NMS.
   b. **Laboratory tests.** There are currently no diagnostic tests to detect brain hemorrhage. However, **tests for failure of passive transfer** using zinc sulfate turbidity or a commercially available test (e.g., Cite Test), as well as a **complete blood cell count (CBC)** and **CSF analysis** should be performed to exclude sepsis or meningitis. A **blood glucose level** should rule out hypoglycemia.

5. **Differential diagnoses.** Other causes of loss of suckle can include sepsis and metabolic disturbances. Seizures can occur with hypoglycemia or meningitis.

6. **Therapeutic plan**
   a. Because **sepsis** or **hypoglycemia** can occur concomitantly with NMS, any suggestion of these disorders on laboratory samples is sufficient evidence for treatment with plasma, antibiotics, and/or intravenous glucose.
   b. **NMS.** Seizures should be controlled using **diazepam** or **phenobarbital. Dexamethasone** or **dimethylsulfoxide (DMSO)** can be used in animals with suspected cerebral hypoxia caused by brain hemorrhage. DMSO may be the drug of choice if sepsis is also a possibility.
   c. **Supportive care.** The foal should receive supportive care, including tube feeding, deep soft bedding, and possibly antibiotics and plasma transfusion in the case of failure of passive transfer.

7. **Prognosis.** The prognosis for recovery is guarded if other diseases, such as sepsis, are present. Otherwise, there is a good prognosis (more than 80% recovery rate) with supportive care.

E. Bacterial meningitis (meningoencephalitis)

1. **Patient profile.** Bacterial meningitis is seen in neonates of all species.

2. **Clinical findings** vary depending on the stage of infection.
   a. **Initial clinical signs** include depression and fever. These rapidly progress to signs of hyperirritability (e.g., hyperesthesia, hyperalgesia, opisthotonos, convulsions) and eventually coma.
   b. **Other signs** include muscular rigidity of neck, diarrhea, joint ill (i.e., arthritis), omphalophlebitis, uveitis, or hypopyon.

3. **Etiology and pathogenesis**
   a. **Etiology.** Meningitis in neonates is most often secondary to septicemia. Septicemic strains of *Escherichia coli* are the most common cause, with the exception of *Streptococcus suis* type II, which is the most common cause in piglets.
   b. **Predisposing factors. Failure of passive transfer** of immunoglobulins increases

an animal's susceptibility to septicemia and meningitis. In addition to a lack of colostral transfer, predisposing factors include enteritis, omphalitis, or respiratory infections.

    c. Pathogenesis. Portals of entry for organisms include the pharynx, intestinal tract, and navel. The route of entry to the meninges (leptomeninges) is then hematogenous. Some organisms (e.g., *S. suis* type II in piglets) can infect animals via the cribriform plate.

  4. Diagnostic plan

    a. CSF analysis. A CSF sample (either atlantooccipital or lumbosacral) will show a moderate to high protein content and elevated white blood cell (WBC) count in animals with bacterial meningitis. **Culture** of the CSF is not always positive but should be attempted.

    b. Blood work. A **CBC** often reveals a neutrophilic leukocytosis with or without left shift, but this is not diagnostic for meningitis because other organs may also be involved in the septic process.

    c. Clinical chemistry. A sodium sulfite turbidity test or single radial immunodiffusion (SRID) kit (for calves) often identifies hypogammaglobulinemia, which results from the failure of passive transfer.

  5. Therapeutic plan. When clinical signs are clearly present, therapy is often unrewarding, and the mortality rate is high, despite appropriate treatment.

    a. Early treatment with **broad-spectrum antibiotics** (e.g., synthetic penicillins, aminoglycosides) can be attempted.

    b. Pain relief with **aspirin** (25 mg/kg every 12 hours) or **flunixin meglumine** (2.2 mg/kg intravenously every 12 hours) should be given.

    c. Supportive care includes soft, dry bedding and the administration of nutrition and intravenous fluids during the treatment period.

  6. Prevention. The key to prevention of meningitis in neonates is attention to parturition to ensure adequate colostral intake.

II. BRAIN DISORDERS OF MATURE AND GROWING ANIMALS

A. **Congenital disorders,** such as cerebellar disease (see I C) and Arab foal idiopathic seizures (see II C 4) can manifest in older animals.

B. **Traumatic disorders**

  1. Patient profile and history. There is often a history of head trauma, which is particularly common in young foals that flip over backwards when they are learning to be led.

  2. Clinical findings

    a. Main clinical signs include depression or coma.

    b. Accompanying signs may include **CNS deficits,** such as anisocoria (inequality of pupillary diameter), head tilt, nystagmus, and selected cranial nerve deficits, depending on the site of trauma. If the animal is ambulatory, **ataxia** may also be present.

  3. Pathogenesis. Cranial trauma causes membrane disruption and cellular swelling that proceeds to cerebral edema, with increased intracranial pressure and tissue hypoxia. If a basal fracture occurs, then intracerebral hematoma formation may occur, resulting in focal neurologic signs. These neurologic signs vary depending on the site of the hematoma. However, a localized hematoma may be hard to distinguish because of the more generalized brain disease caused by the intracranial edema.

  4. Diagnostic plan. A key aspect of diagnosis of head trauma is usually the direct observation of the event or the sudden onset of clinical signs in an otherwise normal animal.

a. **Skull radiographs** should be taken to check for fractures, but these may not be diagnostic if the fracture occurs along the epiphyseal lines and is not displaced.
b. **CSF analysis** may reveal **acute frank hemorrhage** into the normally clear colorless fluid. If the trauma is less acute, there may be **yellow discoloration** to the CSF sample (xanthochromia), which is suggestive of blood breakdown products in the fluid. **A CSF sample should not be taken if increased CSF pressure is present** because doing so could result in further brain damage.

5. **Therapeutic plan**
   a. A **patent airway** must be established in comatose patients.
   b. **Cerebral edema reduction**
      (1) Drugs that may reduce cerebral edema include **dexamethasone** (1–2 mg/kg intravenously every 6 hours) or **DMSO** (0.9–1.0 g/kg of 10% solution in 5% dextrose intravenously).
      (2) **Mannitol** (0.25–2 g/kg of 20% solution intravenously), an osmotic diuretic, is also advocated but could cause increased swelling if there is significant vascular leakage in the brain tissue, allowing the mannitol to escape the brain vascular space.
   c. **Seizure control.** If convulsions occur, **diazepam** (25 mg for foals, 100 mg for adults intravenously) reduces the signs of seizures and helps prevent further self-induced trauma.
   d. **Antibiotics** should be administered if there are open fractures on the head.

6. **Prognosis.** With severe head trauma, the prognosis for the return of full function is grave.

C. **Disorders characterized by seizures.** Seizure disorders may occur in all large animals for a variety of reasons. Causes may be idiopathic, metabolic, traumatic, infectious, nutritional, degenerative, neoplastic, or inflammatory. Treatment is directed at resolving the cause of the seizure. In the case of idiopathic seizures, seizure control is the primary focus of treatment.

1. **Polioencephalomalacia (PEM, cerebral cortical necrosis)**
   a. **Patient profile and history**
      (1) **Patient profile.** This disease affects cattle, sheep, and goats. PEM can affect an individual or appear as a herd problem, affecting calves ages 6–12 months and lambs and kids ages 2–6 months. PEM is usually seen in cattle in spring or early summer under feedlot conditions. PEM is less common in adults, and it is more sporadic in small ruminants.
      (2) **History.** Affected animals often have a history of some feed change or access to increased carbohydrates in the feed.
   b. **Clinical findings** are referable to cerebral edema and laminar necrosis.
      (1) **Cortical blindness** (i.e., absent menace with intact palpebral and pupillary light reflex) occurs early in the course of disease.
      (2) **Dorsomedial strabismus** and **nystagmus** are also common findings with PEM.
      (3) **Other neurologic signs** include incoordination, muscle tremors, and depression, which is interspersed with hyperexcitability leading to recumbency, opisthotonos, and paddling with extensor rigidity.
      (4) **Vital signs** can be normal or elevated because of exertion. The rumen usually remains active.
   c. **Etiology and pathogenesis**
      (1) **Etiology.** PEM is the result of **thiamine deficiency.** Thiamine deficiency can result from:
         (a) Decreased thiamine synthesis by rumen microorganisms
         (b) Increased thiamine destruction by thiaminase (found in bracken fern, horsetail)
         (c) Rumen microbial destruction of thiamine by *Bacillus thiaminolyticus* or *Clostridium sporogenes*
         (d) Thiamine antimetabolites (i.e., amprolium)
      (2) **Predisposing factors.** Feeding high concentrate, low-roughage diets has

been linked to PEM, as has high-sulfate dietary or water sources. Major management changes in feeding (particularly with high concentrate diets) may favor the development of thiaminase-producing bacteria in the rumen.

(3) Thiamine is necessary for the production of red blood cell (RBC) transketolase, a major enzyme in the metabolism of glucose via the pentose phosphate pathway. It is postulated that ruminants have increased requirements for glucose via this pathway at the level of the brain.

d. Diagnostic plan and laboratory tests

(1) Response to treatment. Apart from the clinical findings, particularly cortical blindness and a history of feed change or high-carbohydrate feeding, a key method of diagnosis is the response to specific medical treatment (e.g., thiamine).

(2) Assays for metabolic abnormalities. Most routine laboratory findings are not diagnostic, and only in specialized laboratories is it possible to assay for the metabolic abnormalities. These abnormalities include low blood thiamine and decreased erythrocyte transketolase.

(3) CSF analysis. The protein level can be normal to highly elevated, and the cellularity varies from slight to severe mononuclear pleocytosis. The CSF pressure is increased to 200–350 mm of saline (normal pressure is 120–160 mm saline). However, none of these CSF changes are diagnostic for PEM.

(4) Necropsy

(a) If an animal dies, a key finding for a presumptive diagnosis is **autofluorescence** of a freshly cut surface of brain cortex when placed under ultraviolet light.

(b) At necropsy, there is diffuse cerebral edema with compression, yellow discoloration of the dorsal cortical gyri, and laminar necrosis of cerebrocortical grey matter.

e. Differential diagnoses. Diseases that should be ruled out include lead toxicity, pregnancy toxemia in sheep, and nervous ketosis in dairy cattle.

f. Therapeutic plan

(1) Thiamine (10 mg/kg intravenously early in the course of clinical signs), followed by intramuscular or subcutaneous dosing every 6 hours is the drug of choice. A positive response (i.e., the reduced severity of neurologic signs and improved mentation) is seen within 24 hours if the thiamine is administered early in the course of disease.

(2) Corticosteroids, mannitol, or **DMSO** may be indicated for animals with possible cerebral edema.

(3) Tranquilizers. Affected animals that suffer convulsions should be tranquilized to prevent self-induced trauma.

(4) Supportive care. Animals should receive supportive care, including soft, dry bedding while recumbent and parenteral or oral fluid administration.

(5) Diet. When the affected animal shows an interest in eating, it should be given only roughage for several days before being reintroduced to concentrates.

(6) Euthanasia. If no response to treatment is seen within 3 days, euthanasia is warranted because there is likely permanent brain damage.

g. Prevention. Although PEM occurs sporadically, the risk of the disease can be reduced by avoiding sudden feed changes.

2. Lead poisoning

a. Patient profile. Cattle, sheep, and, less commonly, horses can be affected by lead poisoning, with problems more likely to occur in young animals.

b. Clinical findings. Three forms, which are somewhat dose dependent, are described.

(1) Acute form

(a) The acute form most commonly affects young cattle. Affected animals show a **sudden onset** and **short duration** of disease (12–24 hours).

(b) Clinical signs include staggering, muscle tremors, clamping of the jaws, frothing at the mouth, snapping eyelids, rolling eyes, cortical blindness, head pressing, aggressive behavior, and convulsions. Sudden death can also be a finding of the acute phase.

  (2) Subacute form

    (a) The subacute form is found in both cattle and sheep.

    (b) Clinical signs include dullness, anorexia, blindness, circling, abdominal pain, muscle tremor, and constipation followed by diarrhea. Signs of gastroenteritis include ruminal atony (accompanied by constipation in early stages), followed by fetid diarrhea due to abomasitis from lead salts.

  (3) Chronic form

    (a) The chronic form is reported in horses.

    (b) Clinical signs. A degeneration of peripheral nerves usually manifests as paralysis of the recurrent laryngeal nerve and the pharynx. This paralysis may result in recurrent choke, regurgitation of food, and aspiration pneumonia.

c. Etiology and pathogenesis

  (1) Etiology. Lead has been one of the most common forms of toxicity in farm animals.

    (a) Cattle with indiscriminant appetites often ingest toxic quantities in short periods of time. Sources of lead include lead-bearing paints, car batteries, lead shot, and solder or leaded windows.

    (b) The reported source of chronic lead toxicity is the grazing of pastures near highways that have leaded gasoline contamination; however, with the production of all lead-free gasoline, this disorder may soon become less common in North America. Environmental pollution from smelters has also been incriminated.

  (2) Pathogenesis. After lead is ingested and absorbed, it localizes in capillary endothelial cells. The major lesion is vascular, leading to cerebral congestion, edema, and cortical necrosis. Lead also interferes with cell function.

d. Diagnostic plan and laboratory tests

  (1) Clinical signs, including the jaw champing and snapping closed of the eyelids, are highly suggestive of lead toxicity.

  (2) Blood work. A **CBC** may reveal nucleated erythrocytes, but the classic basophilic stippling reported in other species does not occur very frequently in large animals. Whole blood lead levels of 0.35 ppm or greater are considered indicative of lead toxicity in cattle.

  (3) Postmortem examination. Finding lead in renal tissue can confirm the diagnosis.

e. Differential diagnoses. Other neurologic diseases that should be considered include hypovitaminosis A, hypomagnesemic tetany, brain abscesses, poisoning due to arsenic, mercury, or *Claviceps paspali* (ergotism), listeriosis, polioencephalomalacia, and thromboembolic meningoencephalitis. A key clinical sign that helps differentiate lead toxicity from polioencephalomalacia is the finding of an atonic rumen—rumen motility should be normal in polioencephalomalacia.

f. Therapeutic plan

  (1) Removal from access to lead sources may be the only change necessary to halt an outbreak because the slow reversal of signs can occur.

  (2) Therapeutic agents

    (a) Clinically affected individual animals can be treated with **calcium disodium ethylene diamine tetra-acetate** (EDTA) administered by slow intravenous injection as a 6.6% solution (1 ml/0.9 kg daily in two or three divided doses). This drug chelates osseous lead and hastens urinary excretion.

    (b) Magnesium sulfate given orally may aid in precipitating soluble lead salts that remain in the intestine.

    (c) Thiamine is also thought to help by decreasing lead deposition in soft tissue.

  (3) Nursing care is important, particularly to control seizures that may result in self-induced trauma.

g. Prevention. Most cases of lead poisoning result from the careless disposal of lead-containing materials. Proper disposal of these toxic materials aids in prevention.

    h. Economic implications. Carcasses that contain high lead levels may be rejected at slaughter. After lead toxicity in cattle, 6 months may be required for tissue lead levels to drop to background levels.

3. Salt poisoning (water deprivation)

    a. Patient profile. Salt poisoning can occur in all species but has been best studied in swine. Because the main cause is a history of water deprivation, combined with high dietary salt intake (e.g., sodium chloride in the feed or the sole water source), salt poisoning is more likely to occur in confined animals.

    b. Clinical findings

        (1) Affected animals are depressed, may appear blind, wander aimlessly, and exhibit head pressing. They are unresponsive to stimuli and may pivot around a front or hind limb.

        (2) Intermittent convulsive seizures may occur, becoming increasingly frequent until the animal becomes comatose and dies.

        (3) Characteristic signs in pigs include a loss of squeal and "walking-backward" fits.

    c. Etiology and pathogenesis

        (1) Etiology. Water intake can be reduced because of mechanical problems in automatic waterers, frozen water, overcrowding, or refusal to consume medicated water. Drought (resulting in restricted access to fresh water) and high salt intake from water sources contaminated with salt (such as in regions with oil fields) have been associated with this disease in cattle at pasture.

        (2) Pathogenesis

            (a) Increased body sodium levels cause a metabolic blockade and inhibit anaerobic glycolysis at the cellular level, resulting in decreased energy production in the brain and associated depression.

            (b) To compensate for this high sodium level, brain cells begin to produce osmotic products called **"idiogenic osmoles,"** which, over time, change the osmotic gradient to reduce the deleterious influx of the excess sodium ion into brain cells. When water is given to the affected animal in an effort to reduce serum sodium levels (by hemodilution), the osmotic gradient maintained by these idiogenic osmoles causes **cell swelling** and **brain edema,** leading to edema, increased intracranial pressure, and subsequent malacia. **Seizures** and **coma** are resulting signs.

    d. Diagnostic plan and laboratory tests

        (1) Serum and **CSF sodium levels** above 160 mEq/L are suggestive of salt poisoning and water deprivation, with higher levels (170 mEq/L and over) sufficient for a presumptive diagnosis.

        (2) Histopathology. An eosinophilic meningoencephalitis is found on histopathology only in swine; otherwise, microscopic changes are usually nondiagnostic.

    e. Therapeutic plan. When the disease is recognized, the animal should be given small amounts of fresh water per os at frequent intervals. Excessively rapid reduction of sodium levels can result in severe seizures and brain edema. Recovery, if it occurs, may take 4–5 days.

    f. Prognosis. The prognosis for recovery when blood sodium levels are markedly elevated is grave for all affected species.

    g. Prevention. Ensuring unlimited access to fresh water prevents most cases of salt toxicity. For calves, proper dilution of oral electrolyte solutions also helps avoid this disorder.

4. Arab foal idiopathic seizure

    a. Patient profile. This uncommon disease occurs in Arab foals with predominantly Egyptian bloodlines.

    b. Clinical findings. Frequent seizures are preceded by prodromal signs. The seizures may be initiated during attempts to train or discipline foals. Between seizures, affected foals are clinically normal.

  c. Etiology. The cause of Arab foal idiopathic seizure is unknown but, because this disease is seen in a particular bloodline, genetics may play a role. This disease should be considered as a differential diagnosis in Arabian foals that have neurologic signs that may be confused with environmentally-induced problems.

  d. Diagnostic plan and laboratory tests. All laboratory data (e.g., blood, CSF analysis) are within normal limits. A diagnosis is made based on the exclusion of other seizure causes (e.g., trauma, metabolic disturbance) and the appropriate bloodlines of the foal.

  e. Therapeutic plan. The only treatment available is symptomatic. Diazepam is used to control seizures during the clinical episodes. Most animals appear to outgrow the seizures by ages 6–8 months.

D. **Disorders characterized by behavioral and personality changes**

 1. Thromboembolic meningoencephalitis (TEME)

  a. Patient profile. This disease occurs in feedlot cattle of any age but is most common in animals ages 4–12 months, particularly in fall and winter. Signs may begin to appear approximately 4 weeks after arrival to feedlot with several animals affected. The **morbidity rates** in a herd are low (2%), whereas **case fatality rates** are high (90%).

  b. Clinical findings

   (1) Peracute form. Cattle may be found dead.

   (2) Acute form. Early signs include separation from other cattle with depression and apparent blindness. The rectal temperature can be very high, at 41°C–42°C. Anorexia, staggering, recumbency and coma progressing to lateral recumbency, opisthotonos, and partial paralysis of multiple cranial nerves may be present.

    (a) Less severe signs can include polyarthritis, respiratory disease, and occasionally otitis media in affected animals or in penmates.

    (b) Ophthalmologic examination shows retinal hemorrhages (highly suggestive of TEME) in approximately 20% of affected animals.

  c. Etiology and pathogenesis

   (1) Etiology. The cause of TEME is bacteremia due to *Haemophilus somnus. H. somnus* infections can occur in a respiratory, urogenital, or septicemic form. The neurologic signs associated with the TEME are part of the septicemic form of disease.

   (2) Pathogenesis

    (a) Transmission is thought to be via respiratory or urogenital secretions from presumed carrier cattle.

    (b) The pathogenesis of TEME involves a **severe vasculitis,** rather than an embolic phenomenon. It is not known whether the suppurative vasculitis is caused by bacterial attachment to the endothelial cell, leading to destruction of the cell, or whether endotoxin and exotoxin release are responsible for the vasculitis. Animals with TEME may have lesions in the heart, liver, kidney, and joints.

  d. Diagnostic plan. The clinical findings of sudden onset of neurologic signs with high fever, accompanied by respiratory and joint involvement in feedlot cattle, are highly suggestive of this disease.

   (1) CSF analysis. A CSF sample reveals marked pleocytosis with neutrophils predominating, along with high protein levels (i.e., a positive Pandy test).

   (2) Culture of *H. somnus* from CSF, blood, synovial fluid, urine, or a tracheal wash can be attempted, but because of specific growth requirements, this test may be unrewarding.

   (3) Serologic testing for infection can be equally frustrating to interpret because of seroconversion in asymptomatic animals.

   (4) Postmortem examination

    (a) Histopathology of the brain shows a severe vasculitis with neutrophilic infiltrates and occasionally vascular thrombi. **Hemorrhaging retinal vessels,** which reveal the vasculitis, are sometimes considered to be pathognomonic for TEME. Unfortunately, because many affected animals lack these changes, this finding is an insensitive indicator of the disease.

   (b) Multifocal areas of hemorrhagic necrosis are found in the brain and spinal cord.

   (c) There may be a fibrinopurulent meningitis, polyarthritis, laryngitis, tracheitis, retinitis, conjunctivitis, and endometritis.

   e. Differential diagnoses include polioencephalomalacia, lead toxicity, and salt poisoning/water intoxication.

   f. Therapeutic plan. If affected animals are treated before they become recumbent, they can recover within 6–12 hours. The drug of choice is **oxytetracycline** (20 mg/kg intravenously every 24 hours for three days). However, the causative organism is not a highly resistant species and is likely to respond to other antibiotics if chosen.

   g. Prevention. A killed bacterin has been used as a preventative with some success for herd protection. However, given the low morbidity rates associated with this disease, vaccination may not be economically feasible.

2. Nervous coccidiosis

   a. Patient profile. This disease is seen in calves and young cattle, particularly in feedlots. Nervous coccidiosis is almost exclusively a winter disease and occurs mainly in the northwestern United States and western Canada.

   b. Clinical findings

   (1) The **key neurologic findings** are ataxia, muscle tremor, blindness, and hyperexcitability accompanying intermittent or continuous seizures. Seizures may be precipitated by strenuous handling. **Calves** become recumbent with signs of opisthotonos, tonic–clonic movement, medial strabismus, and snapping of the eyelids.

   (2) Affected animals also show **blood flecks in feces** or blood-tinged diarrhea, which is associated with intestinal coccidiosis.

   c. Etiology and pathogenesis. A heat-labile neurotoxin has been identified in the serum of affected calves, but not in the serum of calves with only intestinal coccidiosis. The nature of the toxin is unknown, and the associated mechanism linking nervous coccidiosis to intestinal coccidiosis has not been determined.

   d. Diagnostic plan and laboratory tests. The main method of diagnosis is to **rule out** other possible diseases (see II D 5). A presumptive diagnosis can be made if the location and climate are suggestive of nervous coccidiosis (i.e., cold winter months in western Canada or the northwestern United States).

   (1) Microscopic examination of feces is used to confirm enteric coccidiosis but is not specific for the nervous form.

   (2) Hyperglycemia, hypochloremia, and **low liver copper** and **iron stores** have been found in affected animals.

   e. Differential diagnoses include lead toxicity, PEM, TEME, or salt and water intoxication, for which there are more sensitive and specific diagnostic tests.

   f. Therapeutic plan

   (1) Sulfonamides and **supportive fluid therapy** can be administered to treat intestinal coccidiosis.

   (2) Tranquilizers. Animals with convulsions can be treated by sedation to prevent self-induced trauma.

   (3) Nursing care, including deep bedding and dry shelter, is important.

   (4) Iron or copper salt therapy. It is not known whether iron or copper salt therapy is of any benefit.

   g. Prognosis. Affected calves have a poor prognosis for survival, with a 70%–100% mortality rate expected and death often occurring within 5 days of disease onset. Undoubtedly, part of the mortality may be attributed to the low level of nursing care possible in these management conditions because of the harshness of the climate when the disease is observed.

   h. Prevention. Because little is known about the risk factors involved, there are no known preventative measures.

3. Listeriosis
   a. Patient profile and history
   (1) Patient profile. This disease occurs in all ruminants but is extremely rare in horses. Listeriosis generally affects animals younger than 3 years and is sporadic in cattle, with sheep demonstrating a higher morbidity.
   (2) History. Heavy silage feeding may be a feature of the history, but disease can also occur in animals at pasture.
   b. Clinical findings
   (1) The **neurologic signs** can occur gradually or suddenly, with dullness, head tilt, and circling (hence the name "circling disease" in cattle) as common findings.
   (2) Other signs can include lateral inclination of head and unilateral facial nerve paralysis, dropped jaw, inability to swallow, and pyrexia. Less commonly, *Listeria* species cause septicemia in monogastrics or abortion.
   c. Etiology and pathogenesis
   (1) Etiology. *Listeria monocytogenes* is the causative agent of listeriosis and is commonly found in soil, vegetation, and fecal material.
   (2) Pathogenesis
      (a) Route of infection. The neurologic form and the septicemic form rarely occur together.
         (i) The **neurologic disease** is thought to occur from an ascending infection following a buccal cavity abrasion, with bacteria gaining entry to the brain via the trigeminal nerve.
         (ii) The **septicemic form** of infection is thought to enter the blood via the intestinal tract. Infection may be inapparent with fecal shedding, or septicemia may occur.
      (b) Predisposing factors
         (i) Heavy silage feeding. Because *L. monocytogenes* can live in spoiled silage (with a pH greater than 5.0), heavy silage feeding is a well-recognized predisposing cause.
         (ii) A **sudden weather change** to cold and wet, **overcrowding,** or **unsanitary conditions** may predispose animals to bacterial invasion. These conditions may also favor a buildup of rotting organic debris, such as silage exposed to air.
   d. Diagnostic plan and laboratory tests
   (1) Clinical signs of focal and lateralizing cranial nerve deficits, such as head tilt, circling, inability to swallow, and facial nerve paralysis, along with depression and pyrexia, are highly suggestive of listeriosis.
   (2) CSF analysis. Whereas routine hematology is generally unchanged, a CSF sample has increased protein and leukocytes, typically consisting of small and large mononuclear cells.
   (3) Postmortem examination. The necropsy findings are specific, with **characteristic microabscesses in the pons and medulla.** To culture the organism from the brain, a **"cold enrichment" method** is necessary. Brain suspensions are held at 4°C and cultured weekly.
   e. Therapeutic plan
   (1) Antibiotics. Early treatment with antibiotics such as **tetracycline** (10–20 mg/kg intravenously every 12 hours for 7 days) or **penicillin** (44,000 IU/kg every 12 hours for 7–21 days) is clinically effective. Therapy should be continued for at least 7 days after the resolution of signs.
   (2) Supportive care during clinical disease is also important, with tube-feeding of water and electrolytes to animals that are unable to swallow effectively, and correction of acid–base imbalances that occur with excessive salivary losses.
   f. Prognosis. The prognosis is fair for complete recovery (50%–75%) if the animal is ambulatory and able to swallow.
   g. Prevention
   (1) Management strategies. The only control measures include the isolation of

affected animals and the reduction of silage feeding. In feedlots, constant feeding of low levels of tetracyclines can be considered.

(2) **Human infection.** Because this organism is capable of causing infections in man and is shed in milk and other secretions from cattle, it is particularly important to caution owners of lactating cattle in which the disease has been diagnosed about the risks of consuming unpasteurized milk. Otherwise, infection of man from infected animals is rare.

4. **Brain abscesses**
   a. **Patient profile and history.** Brain abscesses can occur sporadically in mature animals of any species, following a pyogenic disease elsewhere in the body. Affected horses are often younger than 3 years. In cattle, there may be a predilection for the pituitary region, with recent placement of rings in the nose in the history.
   b. **Clinical findings** include an altered mental status, unilateral or bilateral loss of vision, head turn, compulsive circling, a sluggish or ataxic gait, or other focal cranial nerve deficits, depending on the abscess location. These signs also often fluctuate in severity. In **cattle with pituitary abscesses,** a dropped jaw and dysphagia are characteristic findings.
   c. **Etiology and pathogenesis**
      (1) **Etiology**
         (a) In **horses,** *Streptococcus equi* and *Streptococcus zooepidemicus* have been cultured from brain abscesses.
         (b) In **food animals,** *Actinomyces bovis, Mycobacterium bovis, Fusobacterium necrophorum,* and *Actinomyces pyogenes* have been isolated from brain abscesses.
      (2) **Pathogenesis**
         (a) Although *S. equi* and *S. zooepidemicus* are commonly involved with the respiratory tract, infection can result in metastatic abscessation of other organs (e.g., the brain and liver) or mesenteric abscesses.
         (b) Placement of nose rings in bulls has resulted in a higher incidence of brain abscesses in some situations, possibly because of the bacteria gaining ready access to blood flow in the head via wound contamination at the nose ring site.
   d. **Diagnostic plan and laboratory tests.** The diagnosis is often based on clinical signs and neurologic examination.
      (1) **Routine hematology** is unlikely to reflect inflammation unless septic foci are present elsewhere in the body.
      (2) **CSF analysis** often reveals slightly elevated protein levels and the presence of inflammatory cells of a mixed population. However, these changes are not diagnostic for brain abscess.
      (3) **Ancillary diagnostic tests** include cerebral angiography, visual evoked potential recordings, and computed tomography (CT) scans. However, these tests are not accessible at most veterinary facilities.
   e. **Therapeutic plan. Surgical drainage** and **appropriate, prolonged antimicrobial therapy** has been successful in treating brain abscess in horses, but this procedure requires a CT scan for diagnosis and anatomical landmarks for drainage. Antimicrobial therapy alone has not been successful in treating cerebral abscesses in large animals.

5. **Pseudorabies (Aujeszky's disease)**
   a. **Patient profile.** Cases of pseudorabies have been documented in all farm animal species, with the exception of horses. The main carrier animal is the pig. Dogs can also be infected. Although it occurs in some regions of the United States, pseudorabies is exotic to Canada.
   b. **Clinical findings**
      (1) In **ruminants,** signs include intense local pruritus with violent licking or rubbing of the face, limbs, or trunk, accompanied by maniacal behavior (e.g., excitement, circling, vocalization, salivation), ataxia, paralysis, and death within several days. Sudden death can also occur.

(2) In **pigs,** the infection may be asymptomatic in adults or cause abortions. In piglets, a high mortality rate is associated with neurologic signs.

c. Etiology and pathogenesis

(1) Etiology. Pseudorabies is caused by a herpesvirus. Infected swine are the source of infection for other animals.

(2) Pathogenesis. The virus enters abraded skin or the upper respiratory mucosa, and spreads to the CNS through cranial or spinal nerves, causing extensive neuronal damage.

d. Diagnostic plan and laboratory tests

(1) Virus isolation can be used to make a diagnosis in the live pig, but ruminants affected by pseudorabies usually die in 6–48 hours of the onset of clinical signs.

(2) Pathologic findings consist of a nonsuppurative meningoencephalomyelitis.

(3) The **histologic findings** in the CNS include perivascular cuffing and focal necrosis in the gray matter. Intranuclear inclusion bodies may be found in degenerating neurons.

(4) Confirmation of the infection is by virus isolation from postmortem tissue.

e. Differential diagnoses

(1) In **ruminants,** differential diagnoses should include rabies and listeriosis.

(2) In **pigs,** Teschen disease, salt poisoning, hog cholera, streptococcal meningitis, and African swine fever should be considered.

f. Therapeutic plan. There is no effective treatment, but hyperimmune serum given to baby pigs may help during an outbreak in a swine herd.

g. Prevention

(1) Vaccination. The present control method in the United States is through vaccination, but the vaccine's effectiveness has not yet been evaluated.

(2) A **test and removal system** can eliminate the disease from a herd of swine. To prevent exposure to other species, infected and uninfected animals should not be housed together.

6. Rabies. Although rabies is rare in most regions, it is of chief concern because of public health considerations.

a. Patient profile. This disease may occur in all warm-blooded animals. Among large animals, cows are more commonly affected than horses, pigs, sheep, or goats.

b. Clinical findings. The only typical finding in rabies is its atypicalness.

(1) The **mild** or **paralytic form** shows variable signs consistent with progressive ascending paralysis, including knuckling of the hind fetlocks; sagging and swaying of hindquarters; decreased sensation over the hindquarters; paralysis of the tail, anus, and penis; dribbling urine; salivation; recumbency; and eventually death.

(2) The **furious form** occurs if the virus reaches the forebrain and is characterized by tenseness and hypersensitivity to sounds and movement. Affected animals may attack inanimate objects or other animals, bellowing loudly and purposelessly, or they may show sexual excitement.

c. Etiology and pathogenesis

(1) Etiology. Rabies is caused by a rhabdovirus.

(2) Pathogenesis

(a) Transmission. Rabies is transmitted through bite wounds after localizing in the sensory end organs of the olfactory nerve of the infected host carnivore. The **principal reservoirs** in North America are wild carnivores (e.g., skunks, foxes, raccoons), whereas the vampire bat is a key reservoir for the virus in South America. Rabies is also enzootic in insectivorous bats in Western Canada.

(b) Route of infection. The virus spreads from the site of the infection to the CNS via peripheral nerves. The incubation period is 2 weeks to several months, depending on the bite site.

d. Diagnostic plan and laboratory tests. Rabies is extremely difficult to diagnose and should be considered when dealing with any obscure neurologic disease. If rabies is suspected, any diagnostic sampling or animal handing should be performed with caution.

(1) The animal can be treated for any other possible treatable diseases, such as lead toxicosis or metabolic disease, which may also alter behavior.

(2) If rabies is highly suspected, the **regulatory authorities** should be contacted regarding current guidelines for animal handling. Affected animals may be evaluated for a period of 10 days.

(3) **Postmortem examination.** If death ensues, the brain and fresh salivary gland tissue should be submitted to an appropriate laboratory for further diagnostic testing. Half the brain should be fresh and the other half fixed in formalin.

   (a) **Fluorescent antibody testing** and **mouse inoculation studies** are used for confirmation of the diagnosis.

   (b) **Histologic examination** of the brain for Negri bodies is also used but can yield some false-positive results.

   (c) The intracerebral inoculation of weaned mice with brain tissue is highly specific for infection, but this can take at least 3 weeks for confirmation of infection.

  e. **Therapeutic plan.** There is no treatment for animals showing clinical signs. Anti-inflammatory drugs, which may be used concurrently for other diseases, may delay the progression of signs.

  f. **Prevention.** Currently, there are inactivated diploid vaccines that are licensed for all veterinary species. These vaccines appear to be highly protective. In regions where rabies is endemic, horses and other valuable farm animals should be vaccinated.

7. **Equine viral encephalitis**

  a. **Patient profile.** All ages and breeds of horses are susceptible, but the disease is not common in suckling foals younger than 3 months. Equine encephalitis occurs in late spring and summer because of the transmission by insect vectors. However, in the southeastern part of the United States, infection can occur any time of the year.

  b. **Clinical findings**

   (1) The disease may be **subclinical** or may appear in the **septicemic form** with pyrexia, anorexia, and depression. With encephalomyelitis, there is fever, anorexia, and severe depression.

   (2) **Other neurologic changes** may include dementia with blindness, head pressing, ataxia, weakness, and seizures. Severely affected horses can become recumbent and have respiratory arrest.

  c. **Etiology and pathogenesis**

   (1) **Etiology.** The arboviral encephalitides (eastern, western, and Venezuelan) in horses are classified as alphaviruses of the togavirus family.

    (a) **Eastern equine encephalitis (EEE)** is most prevalent in the southeastern United States.

    (b) **Western equine encephalitis (WEE)** is usually restricted to western Canada and the western United States. WEE is less severe than EEE.

    (c) **Venezuelan equine encephalitis (VEE)** occurs outside North America and has far higher morbidity and mortality rates.

   (2) **Pathogenesis**

    (a) **Transmission.** The diseases are transmitted to horses by a mosquito vector.

     (i) **Equine infection.** Horses are considered a "dead-end" host, with infected birds being the reservoir hosts for these viruses.

     (ii) **Human infection.** The equine population acts as a sentinel animal, with equine cases preceding human cases by 2–5 weeks. Human cases tend to be "flu-like," with young and old people susceptible to encephalitis.

    (b) The viruses are neurotropic and cause **direct neuronal necrosis** throughout the entire CNS, particularly in the cerebrum, causing the characteristic severe mental depression.

d. Diagnostic plan and laboratory tests. Diagnosis of EEE and WEE is based on signs, season, locale, and serum titers.

(1) **CSF analysis** reveals increased protein and WBC counts. Neutrophils are present in the acute disease, but mononuclear cells predominate in later stages. A slight xanthochromia may also be present.

(2) **Serologic titers** can be measured by hemagglutination inhibition (HI) or complement fixation (CF). A fourfold rise in titer in samples collected 7–10 days apart or a very high single titer in an unvaccinated animal (1:160 for EEE and 1:40 for WEE) are diagnostic. Additionally, the use of **immunoglobulin M (IgM)-specific enzyme immunoassays** can help in the antemortem diagnosis of EEE.

e. Therapeutic plan. The prognosis is grave for EEE and poor to fair for WEE.

(1) **Supportive and symptomatic care.** If the animal remains ambulatory, it should be given supportive and symptomatic therapy. This includes force feeding and fluid therapy because the depression is often so severe that the animal will leave food in the mouth, although swallowing is not impaired.

(2) **Therapeutic agents.** If depression progresses and pupils become unresponsive to light, cerebral edema may be developing.

(a) **Mannitol** (20%) may be given intravenously at 0.25–0.5 g/kg.

(b) The use of **dexamethasone** is controversial, but in the initial stages, it may be useful at a dose of 0.1–0.25 mg/kg.

(c) **DMSO** (1 g/kg in a 10% solution of 5% dextrose) is probably the drug of choice for treating cerebral edema.

f. Prevention. Vaccination for EEE and WEE is the best preventive method. The animals should receive two injections 3–4 weeks apart 1 month before mosquito season. Semiannual vaccinations may be necessary where mosquito seasons are long. Fortunately, there is no transmission from horse to man, and even the infected horse does not pose a significant risk to other horses.

8. Yellow star thistle or Russian knapweed toxicity

a. Patient profile. This toxicosis is seen in the northwest United States or Australia in late summer or autumn and affects any age, gender, or breed of horse.

b. Clinical findings. Affected horses exhibit an acute onset of rigidity of the mastication muscles. This rigidity results in a characteristic grimacing expression, with the mouth held half open and the lips and nostrils drawn back. Protrusion of the tongue may be present. The difficulty in prehension may progress to a complete inability to eat or drink.

c. Etiology and pathogenesis

(1) **Etiology.** Disease is caused by the ingestion of yellow star thistle *(Centaurea solstitialis)* or Russian knapweed *(Centaurea repens).*

(2) **Pathogenesis.** The plant does not appear to be toxic to ruminants but is thought to contain an antimetabolite that is specifically toxic to horses. Ironically, sheep thrive on a diet consisting solely of these plants.

d. Diagnostic plan and laboratory tests

(1) **Classic clinical signs** and a history of possible exposure to these plants form the basis for diagnosis. There are usually no significant alterations of diagnostic value on laboratory analysis.

(2) **Necropsy.** The major lesion at necropsy is in the brain. It is usually bilateral and consists of areas of necrosis in the globus pallidus and substantial nigra (encephalomalacia).

e. Therapeutic plan and prognosis. There is no cure for this disease, but the animal can be supported via nasogastric tube feeding. However, the prognosis is grave, and the animal usually dies of dehydration or starvation if no nutritional support is given.

f. Prevention. Horses should be kept from pastures that contain these toxic plants, but sheep or cattle can graze these pastures safely.

9. Ammoniated feed toxicity ("bovine bonkers, bovine hysteria")

a. Patient profile. This disease is seen in adult cattle, calves, and sheep that are

given ammoniated feed. Often, a new batch of urea-containing feed has been fed to the animals.
- **b. Clinical findings**
  - **(1) Clinical signs** include acute staggering, recumbency, and even death. Frequent urination and defecation, trembling, sweating, and ear twitching are often observed.
  - **(2) Physical examination.** Bloat, dyspnea muscle tremors, and abdominal pain are found on physical examination. On **neurologic examination,** there is incoordination and blindness, accompanied by hyperexcitability, hyperesthesia, restlessness, colliding with inanimate objects, seizures, and coma.
- **c. Etiology and pathogenesis.** Affected animals have consumed excessive urea in their feed to which their rumen may not be accustomed. Urea is converted to ammonia in the rumen and liver, with alkalosis and ammonia encephalopathy resulting.
- **d. Diagnostic plan and laboratory tests.** An elevated blood and CSF ammonia concentration in the absence of liver disease is diagnostic for urea or ammonia intoxication.
- **e. Therapeutic plan.** Rumen lavage and evacuation is necessary to reduce the ongoing absorption of the urea. Following lavage, acidifying solutions (such as acetic acid) along with cold water should be given orally to help counter the systemic alkalosis.
- **f. Prognosis.** The prognosis is guarded to grave. When clinical signs are obvious, the disease is usually fatal.
- **g. Prevention.** The gradual introduction of feed containing urea should prevent this disease.

10. Hypovitaminosis A
- **a. Patient profile.** This disorder can affect most young growing animals and is also found in adult cattle.
- **b. Clinical findings**
  - **(1) Calves.** Experimental and naturally occurring vitamin A deficiency in calves results in blindness, ill thrift, diarrhea, and pneumonia. The blindness in calves is peripheral, with absent pupillary light reflexes and dilated pupils in severe cases.
  - **(2)** In **adult cattle,** in addition to blindness, there may be convulsions, diarrhea and generalized edema.
  - **(3) Young horses** that are fed vitamin A-deficient diets have shown night blindness, ill thrift, and seizures, but naturally occurring disease in horses is rare.
- **c. Etiology and pathogenesis.** Vitamin A is necessary for **normal bone growth** and **epithelial maintenance.** The pathophysiology appears to be the same in all species, but clinical signs differ according to skull anatomy.
  - **(1) Brain distortion and herniation.** In the CNS, a lack of vitamin A distorts cranial bone development and retards endochondral ossification, resulting in brain distortion and herniation.
  - **(2) Seizures.** Reduced CSF absorption across arachnoid villi leads to increased CSF pressure, which may manifest clinically as seizures.
  - **(3) Blindness** can occur from optic canal restriction, with optic nerve entrapment in the optic foramina.
- **d. Diagnostic plan and laboratory tests.** Serum vitamin A concentrations are usually found to be low (2–15 g/dl).
- **e. Therapeutic plan.** Affected animals should be given vitamin A (440 IU/kg parenterally). There is usually a dramatic response to treatment within 48 hours, with the exception of prominent blindness, which is not likely reversible.
- **f. Prevention.** Current management practices include feeding adequate vitamin A. By merely increasing green feed or hay quality, dietary vitamin A is usually sufficient. Additionally, animals can be given injectable repositol forms of vitamin A.

E. **Disorders accompanied by multiorgan involvement**

1. **Scrapie**
   a. **Patient profile.** This long-recognized disease affects adult sheep between the ages of 2 and 5 years and also goats. Scrapie occurs more readily in some sheep breeds that have genetic predilection for the infection.
   b. **Clinical findings.** The main signs are **cerebellar incoordination** and **pruritus.**
      (1) There are **transient episodes** of nervousness, behavior changes, emaciation, seizures, and recumbency. Eventually death occurs.
      (2) A fine head tremor is often noted. Pruritus is severe, with a characteristic head elevation and nibbling reaction when the skin is scratched.
   c. **Etiology and pathogenesis**
      (1) **Etiology.** The causative organism is a small protein unit (i.e., viroid).
      (2) **Pathogenesis**
         (a) **Transmission.** Scrapie is classified as a "slow virus" infection, with vertical or horizontal transmission and a prolonged incubation period of months to years.
         (b) **Route of infection.** The viroid replicates in lymphoid tissue and invades the central nervous tissue, producing a spongiform encephalomyelopathy with neuronal vacuolation and the degeneration of cerebrospinal, cerebellospinal, and optic nerve tracts.
   d. **Diagnostic plan.** There is no accurate antemortem method to screen for infected animals, and diagnosis is based on postmortem examination of the brain tissue.
   e. **Therapeutic plan and prevention.** There is no treatment, and affected animals should be slaughtered because the disease is invariably fatal. Scrapie has been a reportable disease but was recently removed from this designation in various jurisdictions.

2. **Bovine spongiform encephalopathy (BSE, mad cow disease).** As a consequence of its association with spongiform encephalopathy (Creutzfeldt-Jakob disease) in humans, BSE is currently the cause of a large-scale slaughter of adult cattle in Britain and other European countries. The United States and Canada have imposed strict guidelines for the import of live animals in attempts to ensure that these countries remain free of the disease.
   a. **Patient profile.** This disease affects adult cattle and was first described in Great Britain.
   b. **Clinical findings.** Affected cattle exhibit apprehension, mild incoordination, hyperesthesia that progresses to severe behavioral changes, recumbency, and death.
   c. **Etiology and pathogenesis**
      (1) **Etiology.** BSE is thought to be caused by a "scrapie-like" agent. The causative agent appears to have entered the British cattle population through a change in feed processing, which facilitated the introduction of sheep offal into animal feeds in the early 1980s. This allowed exposure to a "scrapie-like" agent, which, because of the long incubation period, became manifest years later.
      (2) **Pathogenesis.** The infection of the brain tissue by this agent causes a spongiform encephalopathy, but the mechanism is not completely understood.
   d. **Diagnostic plan.** Postmortem microscopic examination of the brain is the only known method to determine the diagnosis.
   e. **Therapeutic plan and prevention.** There is no treatment, and the slaughter of all animals at risk and their offspring has been implemented.

3. **Hepatic encephalopathy** (see also Chapter 5 I B 1 b) occurs in animals with acute or chronic liver failure. Most species and ages can be affected in acute or chronic liver failure, however, affected animals are usually adults. Clinical findings include depression, head pressing, and yawning that may wax and wane, depending on the

time since the last feeding. Hepatic encephalopathy must be differentiated from primary neurologic diseases that may also affect behavior and mental activity.

4. **Leukoencephalomalacia (moldy corn disease)**
   a. **Patient profile and history.** This disease occurs in horses of any breed, sex, or age that have a history of ingestion of moldy corn. Outbreaks can occur.
   b. **Clinical findings.** Affected animals have a sudden onset of dementia, blindness, convulsions, or all of these signs. Sudden death can also occur. Additional **neurologic findings** can include circling, excitability, drowsiness, and ataxia in various combinations and possibly asymmetric findings.
   c. **Etiology and pathogenesis**
      (1) **Etiology.** A toxin, likely fumonisin, produced by *Fusarium moniliform* in moldy corn has been indicated as the causative agent.
      (2) **Pathogenesis.** After ingestion of the toxin, horses develop liquefactive cerebral necrosis and associated brain swelling, which may result in herniation and brain stem compression. Toxic hepatopathy can also develop and may contribute to the clinical signs.
   d. **Diagnostic plan and laboratory tests**
      (1) The **clinical signs, neurologic findings,** and **history** of feeding moldy corn are used as a basis for diagnosis. Finding moldy corn alone does not confirm a diagnosis because up to 80% of corn samples can contain *Fusarium* species.
      (2) **CSF analysis** may be normal or may show a pleocytosis with elevated neutrophils and protein.
   e. **Therapeutic plan.** The only suggested treatment is to **remove horses still at risk from access to the moldy feed** and **give oral cathartics** to those exposed. **Glucocorticoids** or **DMSO** for presumed brain swelling can be given to clinically affected horses.
   f. **Prognosis.** For mildly affected horses, the prognosis for recovery is good, with little or no residual brain damage. Most horses, however, die shortly after the onset of clinical signs.

III. SPINAL CORD DISEASES

A. Equine

1. **Cervical vertebral malformation (CVM; wobbler disease, wobbles, cervical stenotic myelopathy)**
   a. **Patient profile and history**
      (1) **Patient profile.** This disease is found in young horses and usually occurs when the animal is less than 2 years old. There appears to be a sex predilection, with colts being affected more than fillies. Thoroughbreds appear to have the highest incidence.
      (2) **History.** The onset of signs can be sudden and may be related to a traumatic incident, or it may be insidious. Animals are usually in good bodily condition and on a good plane of nutrition.
   b. **Clinical findings.** Clinical signs are referable to **upper motor neuron (UMN) problems** of both the front and hind limbs, suggesting a lesion in the cervical spinal cord.
      (1) **Ataxia.** The animals exhibit varying degrees of ataxia.
         (a) The **hind limbs** are usually more severely affected than the rear, but the signs are usually symmetric from left to right.
         (b) There can be **toe dragging** at the walk and **rear limb circumduction** when the horse is led in a tight circle.
         (c) **Proprioceptive deficits** are exaggerated when the animal is forced to negotiate a hill, turn sharply backward, or step over obstacles.
      (2) **Paresis** may be evident in response to downward pressure over the withers

and loins and when pulling the horse to the side by its tail while at the walk (sway test).

    (3) **Hypermetria** and **spasticity** may also be seen to a lesser degree than the ataxia. When left alone, the animal may assume awkward positions (e.g., legs extended to the side, legs crossed).

  c. Etiology and pathogenesis

    (1) **Etiology.** No specific cause has been identified for CVM. One school of thought favors genetics as a cause, whereas others feel the disease is a result of rapid growth combined with high energy nutrition or nutritional imbalances. Probably both of these factors are involved.

    (2) **Pathogenesis.** Classically, horses suffering from CVM were called "wobblers." A wobbler is a broad term that describes a set of clinical signs that may be caused by several different disease processes. Two forms of CVM have been recognized: a functional (dynamic) stenosis and an absolute (static) stenosis. Both forms occur between the ages of weanling and 3 years, with functional stenosis appearing at a somewhat younger age.

      (a) In **functional stenosis,** spinal cord compression is caused by instability between cervical vertebrae. When the neck is placed in a flexed or hyperextended position, the vertebrae subluxate into the spinal canal.

      (b) In **absolute stenosis,** there is spinal cord compression that is not altered by the positioning of the neck. Osseous changes of the cranial articular processes and medial ingrowth of the articular processes can cause this stenosis.

  d. Diagnostic plan and laboratory tests

    (1) The **neurologic examination** is suggestive of a focal cervical lesion for which **cervical radiographs** should be taken. Remodeling of the caudal vertebrae epiphysis and the articular facets may be seen in functional stenosis.

    (2) A **myelogram** is essential for a positive diagnosis of spinal cord compression, which commonly occurs at C3–4 and C4–5 (for functional stenosis) and at C5–6 and C6–7 (for absolute stenosis).

    (3) **Routine laboratory samples,** such as a CBC and biochemistry panel, are of no diagnostic value for affected horses.

    (4) **CSF analysis,** although useful to rule out other diseases causing similar signs, is usually normal.

  e. Differential diagnoses. Each of the following disorders can be ruled out by its corresponding method of positive diagnosis.

    (1) **Trauma**—myelogram, CSF analysis, history

    (2) **Equine protozoal myelitis**—CSF analysis, asymmetry, lower motor neuron (LMN) involvement

    (3) **Herpes I myelitis**—titer, recovery

    (4) **Equine degenerative myeloencephalopathy**—postmortem examination

    (5) **Cerebrospinal nematodiasis**—CSF analysis

    (6) **Space-occupying lesion (neoplasia, abscess)**—CSF analysis

  f. Therapeutic plan

    (1) **Medical treatment** with anti-inflammatory drugs plus stall rest may arrest the progress of clinical signs for some time, but usually the disease progresses. Additionally, there are ethical questions about treating such cases for which complete recovery is unlikely if the horse is likely to be ridden at high speeds.

    (2) **Surgical treatment** includes **arthrodesis** of the unstable vertebrae in cases of functional stenosis or **laminectomy** to aid in decompression of absolute stenosis. The arthrodesis technique may halt the progress of the ataxia and even allow some return to usefulness.

  g. Prognosis. The prognosis for recovery is guarded to grave. Surgical correction is expensive, and its application to an equine athlete is controversial.

2. Equine degenerative myeloencephalopathy (EDM). First described in 1977, EDM may now account for 25%–50% of ataxic horses seen at referral clinics in North America.

a. **Patient profile.** EDM is an ataxia that affects horses less than 12 months old, with the oldest affected animal about 3 years of age. No breed or sex determination has been noted, and the signs, when observed, can be progressive or stabilize.

b. **Clinical findings**
   (1) Affected horses exhibit **symmetrical ataxia,** with marked proprioceptive deficits when asked to circle or turn. **Paresis** and **spasticity** may also be noted.
   (2) In contrast to CVM, the **front limbs** may have more severe ataxia or paresis than the rear limbs or may be only minimally affected in combination with profound pelvic limb changes, which is not consistent with focal cervical compression.

c. **Etiology and pathogenesis**
   (1) **Etiology.** The etiology of EDM is unknown but is thought to be related to inappropriate vitamin E levels or metabolism in some horses. The roles of hereditary, congenital, toxic, and nutritional factors have not been determined, but the disease resembles heretodegenerative diseases in humans. The disease appears to be associated with increased dependence on hay as the sole diet and with animals that are not allowed much grazing time on fresh forage.
   (2) **Pathogenesis.** The neurohistopathology of EDM indicates a degenerative process throughout the nervous tissue that is more pronounced in the thoracic segments of the spinal cord. There is **diffuse neuraxonal degeneration** of nuclei in the brain. Clinically, the signs are restricted to symmetrical abnormalities in the posture and gait of all four limbs.

d. **Diagnostic plan and laboratory tests**
   (1) **Clinical signs** and **age** may suggest EDM, but there is no antemortem method to differentiate patients from other "wobblers," except by elimination of other causes of ataxia.
   (2) **Cervical radiography** is normal in affected animals.

e. **Differential diagnoses.** The main differential diagnosis is cervical vertebral malformation.

f. **Therapeutic plan.** No curative treatment is available, and signs will plateau. However, high doses of vitamin E have been shown to be effective in preventing the progression of clinical signs and may play a role in prevention in animals at risk.

g. **Prevention.** Supplemental dietary vitamin E (up to 6000 IU/day) can be given to related young horses at risk. Because there may be a genetic factor involved, selective breeding may be advisable.

3. **Equine protozoal myeloencephalitis (EPM)**
   a. **Patient profile and history**
      (1) **Patient profile.** This spinal disease affects horses ages 2–7 years, particularly Standardbreds and Thoroughbreds. EPM has been frequently noted in racing and breeding animals, with males and females equally affected. Serologic evidence suggests widespread exposure to this parasite in the eastern and Midwestern United States, and it is likely that most horses that are seropositive have mounted an immune response and cleared the organism before it reached the CNS.
      (2) **History.** EPM may appear as a mild lameness in the hind limbs that has defied localization.
   b. **Clinical findings.** Signs may occur suddenly or insidiously.
      (1) Clinical signs can be varied, with a history of ataxia, stumbling, falling while being transported, or notable limb weakness. Gait abnormalities may be asymmetric. Mild cases may manifest only as ill-defined hind limb lameness.
      (2) **Muscle atrophy** of isolated muscle groups, most commonly noted in the gluteals, suprascapular, and masseter areas or tongue, have been identified as being highly suggestive of EPM because the disease can result in LMN deficits.

c. Etiology and pathogenesis

(1) Etiology. EPM is associated with a coccidian parasite, *Sarcocystis falcatula.*

(2) Pathogenesis. *S. falcatula* is a parasite that has an obligate two-host life cycle; the definitive host being opossums, and the intermediate host being birds. The disease is sporadic but can occur in several animals in the same locale, and the incidence of disease is said to follow closely the geographic range of opossums.

(a) The parasite encysts in the muscle of birds and when this tissue is eaten by opossums, the organism undergoes sexual reproduction in the intestinal epithelium and is shed as infective oocysts in the feces.

(b) Horses are an aberrant intermediate host for the parasite. Sporocysts are ingested and although tissue cysts do not develop, some of the parasites spread as tachyzoites to the CNS, where they continue to undergo asexual reproduction in neurons and microglial cells. Because cysts do not form, horses cannot transmit *S. falcatula* to other animals.

d. Diagnostic plan and laboratory tests. Diagnosis is based on clinical signs, response to treatment, and recently, analysis of CSF for the presence of antibodies. A CBC and biochemistry panel are invariably of little value.

(1) Clinical signs of an asymmetric ataxia with LMN involvement may aid in a diagnosis, but they may not be present.

(2) Response to treatment. A response to empiric therapy with an antiprotozoal agent [see III A 3 e (1)] aids in differentiating EPM from other spinal cord disorders.

(3) CSF analysis

(a) Presence of antibodies. Recently available serologic tests can provide evidence of exposure to this protozoan parasite. Furthermore, detection of antibodies in the CSF is highly suggestive of intrathecal production of antibodies as a result of nervous tissue infection. However, any blood contamination of the CSF sample can give a false-positive result in a serologically positive horse.

(b) Presence of *S. falcatula* DNA. Testing the CSF for the presence of the parasite's DNA can also be done and provides a highly sensitive test for early EPM infections.

(c) Other findings. Mild xanthochromia, a slight increase in protein level (80–100 mg/dl), and a moderate pleocytosis (10–100 leukocytes/μl, consisting primarily of mononuclear cells) may be noted.

(4) Postmortem findings. Gross necropsy findings may include focal areas of hemorrhage or discoloration in the brain and spinal cord. A multifocal, necrotizing, nonsuppurative myeloencephalitis is seen. Protozoal organisms may be seen in 50% of the cases.

e. Therapeutic plan. Some animals may respond quickly within a few weeks, whereas others may require months of treatment. There may also be no response to therapy.

(1) Antiprotozoal treatment

(a) By extrapolation from the treatment of toxoplasmosis in humans, affected horses have been treated successfully using long-term medication with **trimethoprim-sulfadiazine** (15 mg/kg twice a day), combined with **pyrimethamine** (0.25 mg/kg orally every 24 hours). Both of these drugs impair folic acid metabolism.

(b) When treating with folic acid antagonists, **frequent hemograms** should be evaluated because of a reduction in hematopoiesis. **Folic acid supplementation** (e.g., by adding brewer's yeast to the feed) may be needed if thrombocytopenia or anemia becomes a clinical problem.

(2) Corticosteroids are contraindicated because of their immunosuppressive properties.

f. Prognosis. The prognosis for recovery is fair to good (50%–75%) with appropriate treatment, but depends considerably on the severity and duration of clinical signs when the disease is first identified. A good prognostic indicator is a rapid response to antiprotozoal treatment in the first 2 weeks.

4. Equine herpesvirus 1 (EHV-1) myeloencephalitis
   a. Patient profile and history
      (1) Patient profile. Horses of any age, breed, or sex can be affected.
      (2) History. There may be a recent history of upper respiratory tract infection (see Chapter 6 II A 3 b) or abortion problems on the farm.
   b. Clinical findings
      (1) Ataxia. There is usually an acute onset of weakness and ataxia (in one or all limbs) or even recumbency. Usually the hind limbs are symmetrically affected. These signs may vary in severity from slight involvement to peracute tetraplegia, which quickly stabilizes.
      (2) Fever at 39°C–40.5°C may be present, along with **distal limb edema.**
      (3) Urinary incontinence, bladder distention, and **hypotonia of the anus and tail** may be noted.
      (4) Weakness of the tongue, jaw, or pharynx and **vestibular signs** can also occur, but are less common.
   c. Pathogenesis. EHV-1 myeloencephalitis may be an immune complex disease.
      (1) EHV-1 infection causes abortion and neurologic disease possibly because of its **tropism for endothelium.**
      (2) The myeloencephalitis is primarily a **vasculitis** that affects both the gray and white matter of the brain and spinal cord.
   d. Diagnostic plan and laboratory tests
      (1) CSF analysis. The CSF often has a markedly xanthochromic appearance, with elevated protein levels (100–500 mg/dl), but cell counts are generally within normal limits. These findings are highly suggestive of the vasculitis.
      (2) Serology. Paired serum titers to EHV-1 showing a fourfold rise is good circumstantial evidence of EHV-1 involvement. Preexisting EHV-1 serum-neutralizing titers do not appear protective and may even be required for the neurologic form of the disease.
   e. Differential diagnoses. The differential diagnoses are the same as those for CVM (see III A 1 e).
   f. Therapeutic plan
      (1) Stall rest. Slightly affected animals that remain standing usually recover uneventfully with 2–3 weeks stall rest. **Recumbent animals** are less likely to recover.
      (2) Extensive nursing care is needed to prevent secondary complications of pressure sores, cystitis, and hypostatic lung congestion. Heavy bedding, sterile urinary catheterizations, and frequent rolling of the animal are necessary for success. If practical, slinging may help.
      (3) Corticosteroids. The use of corticosteroids has been suggested by some authors because the process in the CNS is thought to be immune mediated. However, corticosteroid administration is controversial because of the drug's immunosuppressive effects and particularly because EPM may be a possible diagnosis.
   g. Prognosis. For the mildly affected animal, the prognosis for recovery is good.
   h. Prevention. Vaccination against EHV-1 may be beneficial, but the efficacy of vaccination against the neurologic form has not been proven.

5. Cerebrospinal nematodiasis
   a. Patient profile. This disease occurs sporadically, affecting any age, breed, or sex.
   b. Clinical findings. Ataxia, weakness, and head signs vary with migratory sites. Affected horses may be depressed and anorectic.
   c. Etiology and pathogenesis. Several parasites have been found in the CNS in animals with this disease, including *Strongylus vulgaris, Hypoderma* species, *Setaria* species, *Draschia* species, *Micronema* species, and *Parelaphostrongylus* species. Malacic tracts are found along the migratory path. The cause of these aberrant migrations is not known.
   d. Diagnostic plan and laboratory tests. The main method of diagnosis is finding elevated eosinophil counts in the CSF. Other laboratory tests are generally nondiagnostic.

e. **Therapeutic plan**
  (1) **Thiabendazole.** Suggested treatments of a 10-times the normal dose of thiabendazole for 2 consecutive days has been suggested, but this drug is no longer commercially available.
  (2) **Ivermectin** can be given but is unlikely to cross the blood–brain barrier to reach the larvae.
  (3) **Corticosteroids** should be given in conjunction with a larvicide drug to decrease inflammation after killing the parasites (0.1 mg/kg dexamethasone every 12 hours for 2 days).
f. **Prognosis.** As in other spinal cord diseases, the prognosis for recovery is guarded, and the long-term use of the horse for riding should not be expected.

B. **Food animal**

1. **Caprine arthritis-encephalitis (CAE; see also Chapter 13 III D)**
   a. **Patient profile.** This disease affects young goats, usually between the ages of 1 and 4 months, but occasionally is seen in adults. Often, more than one kid is affected over a period of time.
   b. **Clinical findings.** The incidence of subclinical disease is high. Approximately 80% of clinically normal animals are positive on agar gel immunodiffusion (AGID) test for CAE.
      (1) In kids affected with the **neurologic form,** there is ascending paresis and ataxia, usually beginning in one or both hind limbs and progressing to tetraplegia. The animal is bright, alert, and responsive. Spinal reflexes remain intact, which indicates UMN disease. Mild LMN signs (such as hyporeflexia, blindness, head tilt, and facial nerve paralysis) may occur as the disease progresses. The clinical course of the disease can be 7–14 days.
      (2) In **adults,** infection generally results in chronic arthritis. Joint distention and hard udders may be seen in adults belonging to affected herds.
      (3) In the **arthritic form,** there is chronic polyarthritis in adult goats (see Chapter 13).
   c. **Etiology and pathogenesis**
      (1) **Etiology.** This disease is caused by the CAE virus, a retrovirus that is antigenically similar to the Maedi-visna viruses in sheep.
      (2) **Pathogenesis.** Perinatal horizontal spread results from close contact, particularly from colostrum and milk.
   d. **Diagnostic plan and laboratory tests**
      (1) **Serological tests**
         (a) **CSF samples** show a mononuclear pleocytosis with protein elevation.
         (b) **AGID test.** Serum can be tested for presence of antibody to CAE by the AGID test. This is useful for testing exposure in a herd, but is of little diagnostic value for an individual animal.
      (2) **Postmortem findings.** At necropsy, the neural lesions are mainly restricted to the white matter. Marked demyelination, perivascular cuffing with mononuclear cells, and parenchymal infiltration with macrophages are seen on histopathology.
   e. **Therapeutic plan.** There is no effective treatment for the ascending paralysis.
   f. **Prevention.** Control of the disease may be accomplished by separating infected animals from the herd. The CAE virus is passed to the kids through colostrum and milk; therefore, newborn kids should be separated from the dam at birth and fed a safe source of colostrum or pasteurized milk.

2. **Swayback (enzootic ataxia)**
   a. **Patient profile.** This disease occurs in newborn sheep, growing lambs, kids, and possibly piglets.
   b. **Clinical findings.** The course of the disease depends on the age of the animal at presentation.
      (1) **Newborn animals** may be born dead or weak, or they may develop a progressive, ascending paresis and ataxia. Newborns usually die in 3–4 days.
      (2) **Older animals** that are affected may live for 3–4 weeks. LMN signs of

hypotonia, muscle atrophy, and depressed reflexes are present and highly suggestive of the disease. Animals ages 3–12 weeks show progressive ataxia of the pelvic limbs.

(3) **Sheep** exhibit weakness, recumbency, and blindness. Ewes are unthrifty, anemic, and have a poor fleece. Diarrhea, spontaneous fractures, and acute death also may be seen in ewes.

c. **Etiology and pathogenesis**

(1) **Etiology.** Swayback is the result of copper deficiency, which may cause hypomyelinogenesis and porencephaly in utero.

(2) **Pathogenesis**

(a) Swayback develops in lambs, kids, and piglets that are born to dams that either have a copper deficiency or an increase in copper antagonists, such as molybdenum, sulfate, and cadmium.

(b) **Resulting neurologic damage**

(i) **Cavitations** of the **cerebral white matter, chromatolysis,** and **myelin degeneration** in the brain stem and spinal cord may be found on necropsy.

(ii) At the **cellular level,** neuroaxonal defect, myelin degradation, and death of the neuron cell body are found.

d. **Diagnostic plan and laboratory tests**

(1) The **neurologic findings** of ataxia and weakness with LMN changes in lambs, kids, or piglets are highly suggestive of swayback.

(2) **Blood** and **tissue copper levels** confirm the diagnosis. Unaffected herd mates should also be sampled to determine copper levels of the whole farm.

(3) **CSF samples** are normal.

e. **Differential diagnoses** include CAE, listeriosis, and cerebrospinal parelaphostrongylus.

f. **Therapeutic plan.** Copper injections may be followed by some improvement but the neurologic deficits are likely permanent.

g. **Prognosis.** The prognosis for recovery is very poor.

h. **Prevention.** The pregnant animals in the herd should receive injectable copper, or be provided adequate copper in the ration. Orally administered oxidized copper wire or cupric oxide particles, produced for cattle and sheep, may be the most preferred mode of prevention because they provide a sustained supply of blood copper.

3. **Vertebral body abscess**

a. **Patient profile and history**

(1) **Patient profile.** This disorder occurs most commonly in young farm animals, particularly cattle, sheep, goats, and swine, but it can also occur in foals.

(2) **History.** Omphalophlebitis or pneumonia is a common historic or clinical finding. In lambs, these abscesses are commonly associated with the docking of tails.

b. **Clinical findings**

(1) Affected animals may be observed to have **neck** or **back pain** and **ill thrift.** There may be a sudden onset of cervical or back pain, with or without progressive paresis.

(2) If a **pathologic fracture** has occurred, there is **paresis,** with lesion localization to the site of the abscess. At this site, there may also be heat, pain, or swelling, but it can also be nondetectable externally.

c. **Pathogenesis.** Septicemic infection in young animals may localize in vertebral bodies, particularly in the thoracic region in calves. Otherwise, any site on the vertebral column can be involved.

d. **Diagnostic plan and laboratory tests**

(1) **Clinical signs** are suggestive of spinal cord damage.

(2) A **CBC** may also be suggestive of an inflammatory process, with a neutrophilia and increased fibrinogen.

(3) A **CSF sample** can show evidence of compression, with xanthochromia and mild increases of protein and cell content. However, CSF can also be nor-

mal because the septic process is usually external to the dura of the spinal canal.

(4) Radiography and **myelography** may be rewarding when diagnosing young animals.

e. Therapeutic plan. Euthanasia is indicated for all but the most valuable animals. However, high-dose, long-term antibiotic therapy can be attempted for animals of considerable value if the owner wants to continue treatment.

f. Prognosis. Recovery is unlikely when clinical signs are obvious, particularly if there is a pathologic fracture.

 NEUROMUSCULAR DISEASE

A. Tetanus

1. Patient profile and history

a. Patient profile. All farm animals, including horses, swine, cattle, sheep, and goats, can develop tetanus. Horses are most susceptible to the neurotoxin, and cattle are least susceptible.

b. History. Affected animals may have a history of sustaining a penetrating wound in the 3 weeks previous to the onset of clinical signs.

2. Clinical findings

a. Early signs include stiffness, muscle tremors, increased spastic reflex responses to stimuli (e.g., hand clap, head tap), and difficulty chewing, swallowing, or prehending feed.

b. Later signs. As the disease progresses, the animal takes on a sawhorse stance, with elevated ears and tailhead. The animal exhibits "flashing" of the third eyelid, increased jaw tone, and extreme sensitivity to external stimuli, which can induce violent muscle spasms. Cattle can also show mild bloat.

c. Terminally, the animal falls into lateral recumbency, has opisthotonos, and eventually suffers respiratory failure, causing death. These animals die 5–10 days following the appearance of clinical signs.

3. Etiology and pathogenesis

a. Etiology. Tetanus is caused by the toxins of *Clostridium tetani*, a gram-positive facultative to obligate anaerobe.

b. Pathogenesis

(1) Route of infection

(a) Tetanus organisms (i.e., spores) are in the animal's environment and usually enter the body through **penetrating** or **contaminated wounds** (e.g., retained placenta, puncture wounds to the foot in horses, elastrator bands for tail docking or castration).

(b) The **wound site** must have some **tissue trauma** and **lack oxygen** for the spores to grow. Signs can occur any time from 1–3 weeks post injury or occasionally longer.

(c) In **ruminants,** it is postulated that toxin may be produced in the **gastrointestinal tract**.

(2) Neurotoxin migration. *C. tetani* produces a neurotoxin that migrates along nerve fibers and in blood and lymph fluid from its site of production. This neurotoxin acts on four regions of the nervous system: the motor end plate of skeletal muscle, the inhibitory interneurons of the spinal cord, the brain, and the sympathetic nervous system. The inhibitory interneurons predominately involve the antigravity (extensor) muscles; thus, the signs of tetanus reflect the overactivity of these muscles.

4. Diagnostic plan. The diagnosis is made on the clinical signs of hyperesthesia to external stimuli. Demonstrating circulating neurotoxin is not feasible and isolation of the organism from contaminated wounds is difficult.

5. **Differential diagnoses** may include hypocalcemic tetany of mares, hypomagnesemic tetany of cattle and calves, acute laminitis of horses, or PEM of cattle.

6. **Therapeutic plan**
   a. **Tetanus antitoxin (TAT).** Toxin neutralization using TAT is a key part of treatment. Although TAT cannot penetrate nerve fibers or cross the blood–brain barrier, it is administered in an attempt to bind any circulating toxin outside the CSF.
      (1) **Doses** range from 50,000 IU to 300,000 IU given **intramuscularly** or **intravenously** every 12 hours (it must be given within 10 hours of clinical signs).
         (a) In **adult horses,** 50 ml of CSF is withdrawn from the atlanto-occipital (AO) site, and a similar volume of TAT (1000 IU/ml) is injected.
         (b) In a **foal,** 30 ml is used. Also, 150 mg of methyl prednisolone succinate may be administered intrathecally, along with the TAT, to decrease irritation.
      (2) The use of **intrathecal TAT** is controversial. Though some authors report success with intrathecal treatment, others report convulsions and death.
   b. **Cleansing the wound.** Another component of treatment is to prevent further absorption of newly-formed toxin by thorough debridement and cleansing of the wound to allow oxygenation, which ensures a hostile environment for clostridial growth.
   c. **Sedatives.** Uncontrolled muscle spasms and rigidity can be controlled through the use of sedatives (e.g., acetylpromazine, detomidine) or muscle relaxants (e.g., glyceryl guaiacolate).
   d. **Supportive care** involves a heavily bedded, dark stall, minimal manipulation, fluid and electrolyte balance, and bowel and bladder evacuation. Cotton plugs in the ears decrease noise stimuli. A tracheostomy tube should be available for placement if laryngospasm occurs.
   e. **Penicillin.** *C. tetani* is sensitive to penicillin. High doses given intravenously may help.

7. **Prognosis.** The response to treatment in horses and small ruminants is poor but cattle frequently recover. Recovery from clinical tetanus does not confer immunity.

8. **Prevention**
   a. **Vaccination.** A good vaccination program successfully prevents the disease.
   b. **Boosters** with toxoid and antitoxin should be given at times of penetrating wounds.
   c. **Proper care** and **hygiene** for tail docking and castration instruments is necessary.

B. **Botulism**

1. **Patient profile.** Adult cattle, sheep, and horses are periodically affected by botulism, whereas swine appear to be quite resistant. Outbreaks may occur in cattle that are given new batches of oats, rye, or corn silage, or the big grass bale silage. Foals 1–3 months old can also have a form of the disease called **shaker foal syndrome.**

2. **Clinical findings**
   a. In **peracute cases,** there is sudden death with no premonitory signs.
   b. In **acute cases,** there is an abrupt onset of flaccid paralysis or tetraparesis that has no association with systemic illness or trauma.
      (1) A **progressive muscular weakness** and **paralysis** may begin with weakness and ataxia and progress to the inability to rise. Muscle tremors and fasciculation associated with the weakness may be marked. Flaccid paralysis continues until the animal dies of respiratory arrest.
      (2) **Consciousness** and **sensation** are retained until death. Affected animals appear to have normal sensation but depressed reflexes.
      (3) **Urine retention, ileus with constipation,** and **tachycardia** are reported in cattle.
      (4) **Head signs** can include pupillary dilation, tongue paralysis, and dysphagia. Dyspnea and cyanosis may also be noted, which are likely the result of impaired respiratory muscle function.

c. Foals with shaker foal syndrome are vigorous and rapidly growing, usually between 1 and 3 months of age.
  (1) The **main complaint** is that they spend time lying down and walk with a stilted gait. As the disease progresses, the animal can only stand a few minutes at a time before trembling and falling.
  (2) These foals have a **slab-sided appearance** because of the paralysis of the intercostal muscles.
  (3) **Terminally,** inhalation pneumonia may occur.

3. Etiology and pathogenesis
  a. Etiology. Botulism is caused by the effects of one of eight serologically distinct neurotoxins produced by *Clostridium botulinum*. **Two syndromes** are recognized in botulism toxicity: forage poisoning and toxicoinfectious botulism in foals.
    (1) In **forage poisoning,** affected animals have ingested the preformed toxin in spoiled feed (with a pH greater than 4.5) or feed that has been contaminated with carrion. Dried poultry waste, sometimes used as a protein source or bedding for cattle, is another source of the toxin. Outbreaks also happen with new batches of oat, rye, and corn silage and by bale grass silage (anaerobic environment).
    (2) **Toxicoinfectious botulism** of foals is caused by the colonization of *C. botulinum* type B in the gastrointestinal tract with subsequent toxin production within the intestine.
  b. Pathogenesis. The neurotoxin causes muscle paralysis by blocking exocytosis of acetylcholine at the presynaptic membrane of the neuromuscular junction. Thus, only skeletal muscle is affected, resulting in flaccid paralysis. When the toxin has bound to the neuromuscular junction membrane, it must be metabolized before function can be regained.

4. Diagnostic plan
  a. The **clinical signs** of acute onset of flaccid paralysis in the absence of other disease or trauma is highly suggestive of botulism. Decreased tongue tone may be prominent.
  b. Because the toxin is so potent there is usually too little circulating toxin in large animals to be detected by laboratory methods. Samples of the feed ingested should be obtained and submitted to specialized laboratories for detection of the preformed botulinum toxin, where extraction and mouse inoculation can be performed.

5. Therapeutic plan
  a. Supportive care. There is no effective antidote when the toxin has bound to the neuromuscular junction. Therefore, mildly affected animals require supportive care to allow time for toxin metabolism.
    (1) **Nutritional** and **fluid support** can be administered via nasogastric tube, and urinary catheterization may be required.
    (2) **Recumbent animals.** If the animal is recumbent, it should be kept in deep bedding and rolled frequently to prevent muscle ischemia.
  b. Therapeutic agents
    (1) **Mineral oil and sodium sulfate.** Any toxin that may be in the gastrointestinal tract can be eliminated more quickly by administering mineral oil or sodium sulfate.
    (2) **Activated charcoal** may also be given to absorb the toxin within the gastrointestinal tract.
    (3) **Antitoxin administration** may be beneficial to neutralize the circulating toxin that has yet to reach the neuromuscular junction, but these products are extremely expensive.

6. Prognosis. The prognosis for recovery when signs are observed is poor.

7. Prevention
  a. Vaccination against *C. botulinum* type B appears to be effective in areas where foals are affected (e.g., Kentucky).

b. Removal of the source. In forage poisoning, the source of the toxin must be found and eliminated because there is no available vaccine.

C. **Equine motor neuron disease**

1. **Patient profile.** This recently-described disease affects adult horses between ages 2 and 25 years. This disease may be overrepresented in Quarter horses and is more commonly described in the northeastern United States.

2. **Clinical findings** include a marked weight loss, despite a ravenous appetite. This sign is preceded by an acute onset of fine muscle fasciculations, coarse trembling of limb muscles, and a tendency to lie down.

3. **Etiology and pathogenesis**
   a. **Etiology.** Neither toxic nor infectious causes are yet ruled out.
   b. **Pathogenesis.** The clinical signs occur because of neurogenic muscle atrophy, in which there is weakness but no loss of proprioception. There is a widespread degeneration of somatic motor neurons in the ventral horn of the spinal cord. The changes noted are similar to amyotrophic lateral sclerosis (ALS) in humans.

4. **Diagnostic plan and differential diagnoses.** There is no definitive antemortem test; thus, it is important to rule out more treatable diseases, such as rhabdomyolysis, white muscle disease, and botulism.

5. **Therapeutic plan and prevention.** Because little is known of the pathogenesis of this disease, there are no guidelines for successful treatment or prevention.

D. **Periodic spasticity of cattle (barn cramps)**

1. **Patient profile.** This disease affects mature cattle (3–7 years old) of both sexes and all breeds, especially Holstein-Friesian and Guernsey bulls.

2. **Clinical findings**
   a. **Initial findings.** In affected cattle, there are intermittent spastic contractions of the muscles of the back, neck, and legs. Attacks may last for several minutes.
   b. **Progression** of the disease may be accompanied by weight loss, increased recumbency, and prolonged spastic periods.

3. **Etiology and pathogenesis.** The etiology is unknown, but the disease is thought to be inherited as a single autosomal-dominant gene of incomplete penetrance. There is no significant neuromuscular pathologic change.

4. **Diagnostic plan.** Clinical signs are usually sufficiently characteristic to determine the diagnosis.

5. **Differential diagnoses.** Periodic spasticity must be differentiated from spastic paresis, trauma to the CNS, hypomagnesemia, and lameness problems.

6. **Therapeutic plan.** No effective treatment is available, but mephenesin may control severe signs for some weeks.

7. **Prognosis.** Complete recovery never occurs, and the signs are usually progressive.

8. **Prevention.** Because there may be a genetic association to this disease, there can be selection pressure placed against the occurrence of the disease, but this is unlikely to occur.

E. **Stringhalt, lathyrism, and shivering**

1. **Patient profile.** Shivering is a condition described most often in draft horses, whereas any breed of adult horse can be affected by stringhalt or lathyrism.

2. **Clinical findings**
   a. In **stringhalt,** there is an abrupt onset of excessive flexion of the hindlegs that may progressively worsen. This can occur as an outbreak, particularly when related to the ingestion of sweet pea plants (**lathyrism**).
   b. In **shivering,** there are mild muscle tremors to the hind quarters and tail that

occur with movement. Signs are exaggerated when the horse is asked to back up. Some horses are unable or unwilling to back up. It may be impossible to lift the hind legs.

3. **Etiology and pathogenesis.** Many causes have been proposed for these problems, but the underlying feature is likely some alteration of the neuromuscular spindle and gamma efferent fibers to alter the control of muscle tone.

4. **Diagnostic plan and differential diagnoses.** Diagnosis is based on clinical signs, which must be differentiated from upward fixation of the patella.

5. **Therapeutic plan.** There is no treatment, and even muscle relaxants have not been useful in relieving the signs. Horses with stringhalt should be removed from access to any toxic plants.

6. **Prognosis.** The prognosis is unfavorable for shivering, but many cases of horses with sporadic stringhalt slowly improve with time.

V. LOCALIZED PERIPHERAL NERVE DISORDERS

A. Spastic paresis (Elso heel, bovine spastic paralysis)

1. **Patient profile.** This disorder occurs in calves at 6 weeks to 8 months of age. The Holstein breed is more frequently affected, but spastic paresis can be seen in other breeds.

2. **Clinical findings**
   a. **Gait change.** Affected calves walk with straight hind limbs with the angle of the hock close to 180°, but there is no pain associated with this gait change. Usually one hind limb is more severely affected, causing it to be held extended behind the calf at rest, swinging like a pendulum, and bearing little weight.
   b. **As the disease progresses,** there is gluteal atrophy and a raised tail head. The gastrocnemius and Achilles tendon are tense. Involuntary leg jerking may occur, and there is an arched back, flexion of the carpi flex, and weight loss.

3. **Etiology.** The cause is unknown, but certain famous sires (e.g., Elso II, hence the name Elso heel) have been suggested as genetic carriers of this problem. Environmental factors may also contribute.

4. **Diagnostic plan.** Diagnosis is made based on clinical signs and the absence of pain.

5. **Differential diagnoses.** Spastic paresis must be differentiated from gonitis, dorsal luxation of the patella, tarsitis, and fractures.

6. **Therapeutic plan.** Partial or total tibial neurectomy is the treatment of choice and is esthetically pleasing.

7. **Prognosis.** The prognosis for recovery is poor without some intervention.

B. *Sorghum* cystitis and ataxia

1. **Patient profile and history.** This disorder can occur in any age or breed of horse with a history of ingesting sorghum ensilage, fodder, or grain.

2. **Clinical findings.** The main clinical sign is cystitis with urinary incontinence and urine scalding. There may also be ataxia, which becomes exaggerated when the animal is backed up or turned.

3. **Etiology and pathogenesis.** Ingestion of the growing *Sorghum* plant may result in mortality due to the high cyanide or nitrate poisoning. The cause of the cystitis and ataxia is unknown, but white-matter degeneration was observed in the spinal cord.

4. **Diagnostic plan.** Diagnosis is based on the clinical signs of cystitis and urinary incontinence, accompanied by access to *Sorghum*.

5. **Therapeutic plan.** There is no effective treatment.

6. **Prognosis.** When signs are present, the prognosis is grave.

C. **Faciovestibular nerve disease in horses**

1. **Patient profile and history.** All reported cases of this disease have been in mature horses (older than 4 years). Many cases have involved aged horses, and there is usually no history of trauma.

2. **Clinical findings.** There is an acute onset of unilateral paralysis of the facial and vestibular nerves.
   a. The **facial nerve signs** include an ear droop, ptosis, muzzle deviation, or all of these signs. Exposure keratitis of the affected eye may occur.
   b. **Vestibular nerve signs** include head, body tilt, or both; reluctance to move; and ataxia of the limbs (with limbs on the ipsilateral side of the lesion more flexed than the contralateral limbs). Disturbances of balance due to the vestibular changes can be accentuated by blindfolding the animal.
   c. **General signs.** Affected horses are very anxious, and the signs may progress to an inability to stand.

3. **Pathogenesis.** The neurologic signs are attributed to an acute pathologic fracture of the petrous temporal bone. These signs are secondary to a chronic bony proliferation, and fusion is the result of a chronic otitis media. When fusion has occurred, a transfer of forces from tongue movement may be enough to cause a fracture of the petrous temporal bone, which may extend into the cranial vault near the internal acoustic meatus. Damage of cranial nerves VII and VIII occurs here.

4. **Diagnostic plan and laboratory tests**
   a. **Skull radiographs** reveal a thickening of the shaft of the stylohyoid bone, extending to the temporohyoid articulation.
   b. **Endoscopy** of the guttural pouches may also illustrate a thickened stylohyoid bone.

5. **Differential diagnoses** include central vestibular disease caused by abscess or tumor, EPM, trauma, and otitis.

6. **Therapeutic plan.** Prophylactic antibiotic therapy has been suggested but is only of limited success.

7. **Prognosis.** The prognosis for recovery is guarded, but affected horses can compensate visually for vestibular deficits over time.

D. **Radial nerve paralysis**

1. **Patient profile.** All species of any age can incur this nerve damage.

2. **Clinical findings**
   a. In **partial paralysis,** there is an inability to advance the limb, but if the foot is placed, then the animal can support its weight.
   b. In **total paralysis,** there is a "dropped" elbow and an inability to advance the limb. The animal cannot bear weight, and skin sensation over the dorsal and medial aspects of the metacarpus and phalanges is reduced.

3. **Etiology.** Injury to the nerve frequently occurs when heavy animals are restrained in lateral recumbency without adequate padding. The nerve injury may also be caused by a fractured humerus or a severe blow to the lateral aspect of humerus.

4. **Diagnostic plan.** The neurologic examination reveals changes of radial nerve deficits.

5. **Therapeutic plan.** Rest and time may be beneficial for recovery. Following acute radial nerve injury, it is advisable to administer some form of anti-inflammatory agent to decrease local tissue swelling around this nerve.

E. **Suprascapular paralysis (sweeny)**

1. **Patient profile.** Draft horses that pull in harnesses or cows that are crowded through a narrow opening can readily damage the suprascapular nerve.

2. **Clinical findings.** The most prominent changes noted include atrophy of supraspinatus and infraspinatus muscles. The stride may be shortened, but weight bearing is unaffected.

3. **Etiology.** This injury was seen in draft horses that wore heavy collars. Crowding through a doorway may result in trauma to this area.

4. **Diagnostic plan.** The neurologic examination, which reveals selected muscle atrophy, is usually sufficient for diagnosis.

5. **Therapeutic plan.** Apart from the use of anti-inflammatory drugs for trauma, surgical creation of a notch in the scapula has been a suggested treatment, as has the removal of any entrapped tissue.

6. **Prognosis.** The prognosis is guarded, but some acutely affected animals spontaneously recover.

F. **Obturator-sciatic paralysis**

1. **Patient profile.** This is a common calving injury that is seen most often in heifers.

2. **Clinical findings.** Cows and heifers exhibit various degrees of hind limb ataxia, with wide displacement of the hind limbs and frequent kicking of the hindleg. The paralysis is usually bilateral, with uncontrolled abduction of the hind limbs and recumbency, followed by an inability to rise. Provided no other injury is present, there appears to be normal sensation to the hind limbs.

3. **Etiology and pathogenesis.** This paralysis occurs predominately in cattle at parturition as a result of calving trauma. Both the obturator and the L6 branch of the sciatic nerve innervate the adductor muscles of the hind limbs, incurring trauma during calving.

4. **Therapeutic plan.** Tying the hind limbs approximately 1 meter apart prevents excessive abduction and often enables an animal to stand. Muscle massage and rolling the recumbent animal helps decrease decubital ulcer formation.

G. **Cauda equina neuritis (polyneuritis equi)**

1. **Patient profile and history**
   a. **Patient profile.** This relatively uncommon problem occurs in horses and is reported as urinary and fecal incontinence, possibly with colic or rubbing of the tail head. The disease affects adult horses, with no breed or sex predilection. There is a wide age range, although it has not been reported in foals or aged horses.
   b. **History.** A recent vaccination or respiratory illness has been a frequently-mentioned aspect of reported cases.

2. **Clinical findings**
   a. The **initial findings on physical examination** are **urine scald** to the perineum, **obstipation,** and **broken tail head hairs.** On inspection of the **tail region,** there is a ring of **hypersensitivity surrounding an area of analgesia.** A loss of tail tone with paralysis of the bladder, rectum, anal sphincter, and penis or vulva is evident.
   b. A **head tilt** and **facial paralysis** are possible but uncommon.
   c. **Pelvic limb gait abnormalities,** if present, are subtle.

3. **Pathogenesis.** This granulomatous inflammatory disease occurs at the level of the extradural nerve roots and may be an autoimmune disease. Some horses have been found to have circulating antibodies against P_2-myelin protein. Postmortem examination reveals a thickened and fibrotic cauda equina. A similar but less severe reaction may occur at the cranial nerve level.

4. **Diagnostic plan and laboratory tests**
   a. **Clinical signs** of localized hyperesthesia with analgesia around the tail region are typical for cauda equina neuritis.

    b. The **CSF sample** may be normal or may have some protein and cellular increases, but this test cannot confirm the disease.

    c. Biopsy. A caudal epidural biopsy is required for antemortem diagnosis.

5. Differential diagnoses. A thorough rectal examination should be done to rule out a **fractured sacrum,** the most important differential diagnosis for such clinical signs.

6. Therapeutic plan and prognosis

    a. Supportive care. With supportive care of regular bowel and urinary bladder evacuation, affected horses have been maintained for up to 1 year.

    b. Euthanasia. The signs progress, despite glucocorticoid treatment, and necessitate euthanasia.

DIRECTIONS: Each of the numbered items or incomplete statements in this section is followed by answers or by completions of the statement. Select the ONE numbered answer or completion that is BEST in each case.

1. Which one of the following statements regarding listeriosis is true?

(1) It is known as a circling disease when it affects cattle and horses.
(2) Heavy silage feeding is a particular risk factor because the cool acid conditions (i.e., a pH less than 4.5) favor growth.
(3) The changes in the brain are usually multifocal microabscesses, which can cause several cranial nerve deficits as well as depression.
(4) The organism gains entrance to the nervous tissue by intestinal penetration and embolization to cause multifocal brain abscesses.
(5) When signs are evident in cattle, the animals are unlikely to respond to treatment.

2. Regarding pseudorabies or rabies in large animals, which one of the following statements is true?

(1) All farm animals can be affected by both pseudorabies and rabies.
(2) Pigs can carry the pseudorabies virus, with adults showing mild or subclinical signs.
(3) Similar to rabies, pseudorabies is spread primarily by direct bite wounds from infected animals.
(4) Both pseudorabies and rabies are sporadic rare diseases across North America.
(5) Both pseudorabies and rabies are caused by antigenically similar rhabdoviruses.

3. Which one of the following statements regarding some central nervous system (CNS) diseases of the horse is correct?

(1) In arboviral encephalitis, such as eastern or western equine encephalitis (EEE, WEE), the main source of spread is mosquitos that have ingested the viruses from clinically ill horses.
(2) Yellow star thistle can cause rigidity of muscles of mastication in the horse, but signs in cattle are photosensitization.
(3) Equine encephalitis viruses can also affect people; thus, an infected horse should be treated by isolation.
(4) Equine viral encephalitis occurs mainly in summer months in northern climates.
(5) Russian knapweed toxicity in horses can result in starvation because of the induction of paralysis of pharyngeal muscles.

4. Which statement regarding the slow virus diseases in large animals [i.e., scrapie and bovine spongiform encephalopathy (BSE)] is correct?

(1) Both diseases have a long incubation period, with the spread mainly via contaminated animal feeds.
(2) Neither disease occurs in the animal population of North America.
(3) Of the two diseases, BSE is currently of more economic and public health significance.
(4) Both diseases cause a characteristic intense pruritus and emaciation as key clinical abnormalities.

5. Regarding tetanus and botulism in large animals, which one of the following statements is correct?

(1) Horses are highly susceptible to both toxins, with clinical disease occurring in cattle, sheep, and pigs being progressively more common.
(2) For both botulism and tetanus, the administration of specific antitoxin serum can neutralize the toxin at the site of binding.
(3) A horse that recovers from clinical tetanus is subsequently immune to this disease.
(4) Diagnosis of botulism in a cow is usually made by the demonstration of botulinum toxin in the serum.
(5) Botulism in large animals has been associated with feeding newly made silage or big round bale silage, whereas pasture-induced hypomagnesemia could be mistaken for tetanus.

6. When comparing swayback (enzootic ataxia) to caprine arthritis encephalitis (CAE), which one of the following statements is correct?

(1) Swayback occurs in newborn lambs, whereas paresis from CAE is seen only in kid goats.
(2) Swayback exhibits lower motor neuron (LMN) signs with hyporeflexia and depressed reflexes, whereas CAE is mainly seen with upper motor neuron (UMN) signs.
(3) CAE has no cure, but, because swayback is caused by copper deficiency, replacement of copper stores allows affected lambs to return to normal.
(4) Both swayback and CAE are mainly associated with intrauterine processes or infection.

7. Which one of the following statements regarding equine protozoal myeloencephalitis (EPM) is correct?

(1) The causative organism has been identified as *Sarcocystis falcatula*, a parasite whose definitive host is the opossum and whose intermediate hosts are birds.
(2) The parasite only encysts in the central nervous system (CNS) of horses by accident; thus, this parasite only poses a risk if the nervous tissue is eaten by the definitive host.
(3) The presence of antibody to the parasite in the cerebrospinal fluid (CSF) is definitive proof of CNS infection in a seropositive horse.
(4) The drugs of choice are amprolium or spiramycin (another coccidiostat).
(5) Experimentally, the signs of disease first occur when the parasite is undergoing destruction by the immune system within the CNS.

8. Which set of neurologic diseases in large animals warrants isolation of diseased animals to prevent the spread to others in the herd or flock?

(1) Bovine spongiform encephalopathy (BSE), rabies, equine protozoal myeloencephalitis (EPM)
(2) Pseudorabies, listeriosis, nervous coccidiosis, eastern equine encephalitis (EEE)
(3) Caprine arthritis encephalitis (CAE), scrapie, equine herpesvirus-1, EPM
(4) Equine degenerative myelopathy (EDM), thromboembolic meningoencephalitis (TEME), CAE
(5) Pseudorabies, CAE, rabies

9. Which set of neurologic signs and their corresponding etiologies is correct?

(1) In horses that have ingested yellow star thistle or Russian knapweed, there may be an acute onset of flaccidity of the muscles of mastication, resulting in a characteristic grimacing expression of the facial muscles with drooping lips and nostrils.

(2) For leukoencephalomalacia in horses, corn being fed with large amounts of *Fusarium* species is a strong suggestion of the diagnosis in up to 80% of cases.

(3) In hepatic encephalopathy of large animals, affected animals are most commonly neonates because of portosytemic shunts, with signs of depression, head pressing, and yawning that may wax and wane depending on the amount of time since eating.

(4) With vitamin A deficiency, there can be peripheral blindness in calves, with absent pupillary light reflexes and dilated pupils in severe cases. These signs are likely the result of the distortion of bone development involving the optic nerve.

(5) In cauda equina neuritis, initial physical examination findings include urine scald, bladder and tail paralysis, and a central area of hypersensitivity surrounded by a ring of analgesia in the tail region.

10. Which one of the following statements regarding the clostridial diseases in large animals is correct?

(1) Botulism is caused by the effects of one of eight serologically distinct neurotoxins that causes muscle paralysis by blocking acetylcholine at the presynaptic membrane of the neuromuscular junction. Thus, botulism affects only skeletal muscle.

(2) In botulism caused by forage poisoning, affected animals have ingested the preformed toxin in spoiled feed (with a pH less than 4.5) or feed such as new batches of oat, rye, and corn silage or bale grass silage that has had oxygen damage.

(3) The diagnosis of botulism requires the demonstration of a circulating toxin in large animals, and samples of the feed ingested seldom have the toxin identified.

(4) Tetanus is diagnosed based on the clinical signs of hyperesthesia to external stimuli, a demonstrating circulating neurotoxin, and the isolation of the organism from contaminated wounds.

(5) *Clostridium tetani* produces a neurotoxin that migrates along nerve fibers and in blood and lymph fluid from its site of production and acts mainly at the neuromuscular junction to cause muscular spasms.

ANSWERS AND EXPLANATIONS

1. The answer is 3 [II D 3 a–c]. The changes in the brain are usually multifocal microabscesses. Horses are not commonly affected. Decaying organic matter and spoiled silage with a pH more than 5.0 favor growth. The causative organisms enter via abraded buccal mucosa. The prognosis with antibiotic therapy is fair to good in cattle.

2. The answer is 2 [II D 5 a–b; 6 a]. Adult pigs show mild signs when carrying the pseudorabies virus. Not all animals can be affected by both diseases; horses are the exception for pseudorabies. Pseudorabies is spread by contact with abraded skin or through the respiratory tract. Pseudorabies is exotic to Canada, and both rabies and pseudorabies can be more prevalent in certain geographic locales. Pseudorabies is a herpes, which thus can become latent.

3. The answer is 4 [II D 7; 8 b]. Because equine encephalitis is spread by insects, disease occurs in the summer months in northern climates. The reservoirs for arboviral encephalitis are birds, not mosquitos. Yellow star thistle can cause rigidity of muscles of mastication in the horse, but cattle are unaffected. Infected horses do not pose a risk, though people can get this infection. Russian knapweed toxicity can cause horses to starve because of rigid muscles of mastication, not paralysis.

4. The answer is 3 [II E 1 c; 2 a]. Bovine spongiform encephalopathy (BSE) is of more significance because of the large-scale slaughter of mature cattle and the possible link to human dementia. Scrapie is thought to be contracted mainly from vertical or horizontal spread. Scrapie occurs sporadically and is found in sheep flocks. Pruritus is only prominent in scrapie.

5. The answer is 5 [IV A 1; B 1, 3]. Cattle are the least susceptible to tetanus but are highly susceptible to botulism. When bound, the toxin must be metabolized. There is insufficient toxin from clinical tetanus to induce immunity. The amount of circulating botulinum toxin is usually insufficient for detection.

6. The answer is 2 [III B 1 c; 2 a–c]. Swayback also occurs in kids and piglets. The neurologic damage in swayback is most likely permanent and will not be cured by the replacement of copper. CAE is mainly spread by postnatal contact through colostrum or milk.

7. The answer is 1 [III A 3 c]. The causative organism has been identified as *Sarcocystis falcatula*. There appears to be no encysting; thus, there is no infective stage from the horse. Serum contamination of the cerebrospinal fluid sample could give false-positive results. The drugs of choice are pyrimethamine and sulfas. The parasite causes cell neuronal and microglial damage independently, and the immune reaction in the CNS is not vigorous or rapid.

8. The answer is 5 [II D 5, 6 c; III B 1 c]. Pseudorabies, caprine arthritis encephalitis (CAE), and rabies can be spread from infected animals. Bovine spongiform encephalopathy (BSE) is spread in feedstuffs and equine protozoal myelitis (EPM) is not spread from horses. Nervous coccidiosis is sporadic and is only associated with coccidiosis, and equine encephalitis virus is a "dead-end host" in the horse. CAE, scrapie, and equine herpesvirus-1 can theoretically be spread through contact, but EPM is not spread from horses. Equine degenerative myelopathy (EDM) is a noninfectious disease related to vitamin E problems, and thromboembolic meningoencephalitis (TEME) is not thought to be infectious from an infected animal (although it can be carried in other animals).

9. The answer is 4 [II D 10 b–c]. With vitamin A deficiency, there can be peripheral blindness in calves, with absent pupillary light reflexes and dilated pupils in severe cases. Signs include rigid muscles and lips that are drawn back, not drooping features. This mold *(Fusarium)* can be found in up to 80% of samples. Hepatic encephalopathy is uncommon in neonates and is usually seen in adult animals. There is a central area of analgesia surrounded by a ring of hypersensitivity.

10. The answer is 1 [VIII B 3, 4]. Botulism affects only skeletal muscle. Feed is spoiled above pH 4.5, and the toxin needs an anaerobic environment. There is too little circulating toxin for detection, so feed samples are preferred for testing. Culture from the wound is difficult, and it is not readily possible to demonstrate a toxin in circulation because most toxins are bound. The main site of action is at the inhibitory interneurons of the spinal cord. The inhibitory interneurons predominate involve the antigravity (or extensor) muscles, and, thus, the signs of tetanus reflect the overactivity of these muscles.

Chapter 12

Ophthalmologic Disorders

John Pringle

I. DISEASES OF THE CORNEA

A. **Corneal ulceration.** Corneal ulcers are one of the most challenging therapeutic problems in equine medicine but present much less of a problem in food animals. Loss of vision is often disastrous to horses, which often have athletic performance expectations.

1. **Patient profile and history.** Corneal ulceration can occur in any animal regardless of age, breed, or sex. Of the large animals, horses with corneal ulcers are the most challenging to successfully treat. This chapter is directed to the equine, with the understanding that principles of diagnosis and treatment in the other large animal species can be similar.

2. **Clinical findings.** Animals with ulcerated corneas exhibit blepharospasm, epiphora, and often are photophobic. These animals also may appear head shy and reluctant to allow physical examination of the head region.

3. **Etiology and pathogenesis.** Ulcers result from mechanical injury (e.g., entropion in a foal) toxic, infectious, or chemical insults to the cornea, exposure (e.g., moribund septic foals), or decreased tear production. Corneal ulcers can heal without incident or rapidly progress to corneal perforation.

4. **Diagnostic plan.** Early diagnosis is invaluable for optimal success in treating equine corneal ulcers.
   a. **Fluorescein dye staining.** Although some corneal ulcers present with an obviously visible breech in the normally clear uniform surface of the cornea, the eyes of animals with any signs of ocular pain (e.g., blepharospasm, lacrimation) should be stained with fluorescein dye to detect ulceration.
      (1) **Applying the stain** often requires restraint in the form of a twitch or by chemical means.
      (2) If damage to the cornea is only superficial, the site retains fluorescein only minimally, whereas complete loss of the epithelium results in the appearance of a focus of brilliant green at the ulcer site.
   b. **Gram stain and culture and sensitivity testing.** While the animal is restrained, other diagnostic samples can be taken, including a corneal scraping for a Gram stain and a culture and sensitivity evaluation to assist in guiding treatment.
   c. **Staging.** It is also useful in horses to **stage the ulcer** according to size, depth, and involvement of surrounding corneal tissue. This guides both how aggressive the treatment should be and the prognosis.
      (1) **Stage 0** is a healing or static superficial ulceration.
      (2) **Stage 1** is a superficial ulcer of one-third or less of the corneal thickness. The ulcer has distinct, healthy edges.
      (3) **Stage 2** ulcers are large or deep ulcers of more than one-third the corneal thickness with moderate to marked corneal edema. Inflammatory infiltrates and keratomalacia also may be present in animals with stage 2 ulcers.
      (4) In **stage 3** ulcers, corneal perforation is present or imminent.

5. **Therapeutic plan**
   a. **Pharmacologic therapy**
      (1) Although **antibiotics** may not be necessary in the most superficial of corneal ulcers (stage 0), they are usually incorporated in the treatment regimen and are essential in many cases because the site can readily become infected.
         (a) **Broad-spectrum antibiotics** (e.g., the triple antibiotic combination of bacitracin, neomycin, and polymyxin B) or products with **gentamicin** or

chloramphenicol (except in food animals for the latter) can be used every 4–6 hours.

(b) **Antifungal agents.** Corneal ulceration sometimes may be **slow to respond** to treatment or may worsen despite apparently adequate treatment. In such cases, it is important to repeat scrapings and cultures of the ulcer because **mycotic infection** of the site may occur, particularly with the disruption of the balance of normal flora of the eye caused by concurrent treatment with broad-spectrum antibiotics. Most fungi can be readily seen by routine staining techniques. Specific **antifungal drugs** (e.g., miconazole, ketoconazole, natamycin) must then be used for ocular treatment.

(c) **Applying topical treatment.** There may be difficulty applying topical medication because the horse resists treatment or the stage of the ulcer may necessitate treatment on an hourly or every second hour schedule. For these cases, it is preferable to use a **continuous-flow subpalpebral lavage system** so that medication is administered at a site away from the head through the lavage tube. For these systems, it is essential to factor in the volume of medication the tube holds to ensure that an appropriate amount of drug reaches the eye. Additionally, because a lavage system is usually left in place for up to several weeks, strict attention to sterile technique in handling the medication and to sterility of the injection port is essential.

(2) **Atropine** is also a key treatment because of its invaluable cycloplegic and mydriatic effect, which decreases the pain of ciliary spasm and reduces synechia formation when given every 6–12 hours daily.

(3) **Other adjunct treatments** include the installation of collagenase and protease inhibitors, such as acetylcysteine and disodium ethylenediamine tetraacetic acid, to reduce corneal destruction by microorganisms. Serum can also be used topically to provide some of the humoral defenses to this site.

b. In addition to pharmacologic treatment, it is essential to **remove any mechanical causes** that predispose to ulcer formation (e.g., exposure and drying of the eye in an ill foal) or any other mechanical cause of the ulcer (e.g., foreign bodies in the conjunctiva, entropion).

c. **Debridement and surgery.** If **necrotic tissue** is present in the ulcer, debridement of the ulcer edges can be performed using a cotton swab containing dilute povidone-iodine. However, this should not be performed if there is a **desmetocele,** which indicates that corneal perforation is imminent. In this case, surgery is indicated. Support for desmetoceles, or large ulcers, can be managed using a third eyelid flap or a conjunctival flap, the latter being preferred if there is danger of corneal perforation. The conjunctival tissue provides maximum direct support, a direct blood supply, and a source of fibrovascular tissue.

6. **Prognosis.** With early and appropriate treatment, many cases of corneal ulceration can be successfully managed. However, prognosis depends on several factors, including the rapidity of diagnosis and specific treatment, tractability of the animal, owner compliance, and the organisms involved.

B. **Conjunctivitis**

1. **Keratoconjunctivitis**
   a. **Patient profile.** Infected animals show signs of increased lacrimation, blepharospasm, and conjunctival hyperemia.
   b. **Etiology.** There are several causes of the disorder in large animals.
      (1) In **foals,** keratoconjunctivitis can be associated with adenovirus infection.
      (2) In **older horses,** the disorder can be associated with infections such as equine viral arteritis, equine herpesviruses, and with *Moraxella equi.*
      (3) In **sheep** and **goats,** associated infections include *Chlamydia psittaci* in sheep and *Mycoplasma agalactia* in goats.
   c. **Therapeutic plan.** The infectious causes of keratoconjunctivitis are usually transient. Affected animals recover either without treatment or with the use of a short-

term ophthalmic antibiotic ointment. The exception to this is infectious bovine rhinotracheitis (IBK).

2. **Infectious bovine keratoconjunctivitis (IBK)**
   a. **Patient profile and history.** Also known as "pinkeye," this infectious ophthalmia is observed mostly in young animals and peaks in incidence from mid-June to mid-August, coinciding with fly season. Hereford cattle and their crosses are the most susceptible.
   b. **Clinical findings**
      (1) **Initial signs** include serous lacrimation from one or both eyes, photophobia, and blepharospasm. The central part of the cornea usually becomes opaque from edema and cellular infiltrates, after which ulceration of the cornea is common.
      (2) **If untreated,** some cases progress to corneal perforation with resulting painful panophthalmitis, glaucoma, and blindness. However, if corneal neovascularization reaches the ulcer before perforation, corneal healing quickly proceeds, although a permanent corneal scar can remain, appearing as a white or greyish opacity in the central cornea.
   c. **Etiology, risk factors, and pathogenesis**
      (1) **Etiology.** This disease is caused by *Moraxella bovis,* which may exist in the nares of carrier host cattle and can be spread by vectors such as the face fly *Musca autumnalis.* In addition to insect vectors, the organism is transmitted by direct contact, aerosols, and fomites.
      (2) **Risk factors**
         (a) **Development** of the disease is enhanced by ultraviolet radiation damage to the cornea, which lowers the resistance of the cornea to colonization of *M. bovis.* This is probably the reason that cattle with pigmented nicticans and eyelids are more resistant to infection than **nonpigmented cattle.**
         (b) **Other predisposing factors** include **vitamin A deficiency** or **mechanical irritants** to the eye (e.g., high dust or pollen counts, trauma from tall grass on pastures).
      (3) **Pathogenesis.** The organism *M. bovis* has a piliated phase that is necessary for attachment, and the nonpiliated phase is apparently harmless. When the organism has begun growing on the cornea, a bacterial cytotoxin initiates corneal lesions, and deep ulcers follow as a result of the interaction between the host's immune system and the bacterium.
   d. **Diagnostic plan and laboratory tests.** Most cases of IBK are readily diagnosed by the appearance of blepharospasm and tearing associated with developing corneal opacity. Bacterial culture from a swab of the conjunctival sac aids in ruling out other systemic diseases such as infectious bovine rhinotracheitis (IBR) or bovine malignant catarrh (BMC) [see Chapter 6 II B 6 a, f], both of which can cause similar signs, though both eyes are usually equally affected in such cases, and systemic signs are also present.
   e. **Therapeutic plan.** In clinical situations, treatment only occurs when the cornea has already become ulcerated or shows neovascularization. Many cattle, however, heal on their own before corneal ulceration occurs. Therefore, the cost of treatment needs to be weighed by the client against the adverse implications of this disease, which include decreased growth and milk production and disfigurement of cattle resulting in decreased value of feeder calves. Also, the humane aspects of appropriate care for the animals should be considered.
      (1) **Treatment goals** include ridding the eye of *M. bovis,* shortening recovery time, and preventing permanent damage to the eye.
      (2) **Local treatment**
         (a) **Antibiotic.** Therapy is usually effective with most of the commonly used antibiotics, the exceptions being cloxacillin, streptomycin, and tylosin. For convenience of administration, mastitis preparations often are used. Medication is instilled in the conjunctival sac every 8 hours (often less frequently by the client) for several days. Both eyes should be treated at the same time.

(b) Cattle with ulcerated eyes also benefit from the instillation of 1% **atropine ointment** every 8 hours for 2–3 days to decrease the pain of ciliary spasm, but this is seldom incorporated into treatment.

(c) Providing there is corneal neovascularization, a subconjunctival dose of penicillin G (1 ml) with dexamethasone (1 mg) can be highly effective in both treating the infection and hastening clinical recovery. This treatment can be repeated in 3 days if needed, but this should not be used in horses.

(3) Systemic treatment. Other methods of treatment include placing eye patches over the ulcerated eye to protect it from exposure and the systemic administration of **oxytetracycline** (long acting). Systemic penicillin does not appear to be effective because it does not pass readily into lacrimal secretions.

(4) Surgery. For **deep corneal ulcer,** a third eyelid flap may be considered, and where severe ulceration and globe rupture has occurred, enucleation may be necessary.

f. Prevention

(1) Carrier animal reduction. Because *M. bovis* is thought to persist in a herd in the nasal cavities of carrier animals, prevention is possible by reducing the number of carrier animals. Two treatments with long-acting tetracyclines administered intramuscularly 72 hours apart reduces the severity of ocular infection and eliminates most carrier infections. Early aggressive treatment of clinically affected animals is important to reduce the spread of *M. bovis.*

(2) Vaccination. A vaccine that induces secretory antibody (immunoglobulin A) against the pili antigens is available and is reported to lower herd morbidity.

(3) Elimination of insect vectors. Another important component of preventing disease spread is to reduce number of insect vectors, such as the face fly, that can rapidly inoculate many cattle in the herd.

(a) Fly control measures should be initiated early in the season to prevent a buildup of fly populations. Manure should be stored and disposed of in such a manner as to minimize the sites for incubating fly larvae.

(b) Individual animal fly control can be managed with insecticide-containing ear tags or by placing dust bags with insecticide in traffic areas.

C. Ocular trauma

1. Patient profile and history. As in corneal ulcers, the signalment of animals with ocular trauma is highly variable. Blunt, nonpenetrating injuries to the globe are generally less alarming than penetrating or perforating injuries.

2. Clinical findings

a. Signs. Depending on the extent of the damage, signs of trauma vary from mild contusions and abrasions to severe globe perforations or protrusion of the third eyelid. Chemosis, blepharospasm, and epiphora follow as a consequence of the damage.

b. Stages. As in horses with corneal ulcers, the extent of trauma can be staged for purposes of treatment and prognosis.

(1) Stage 0 represents a minor injury with no corneal damage. Although there may be uveitis, there is no hyphema or damage to the posterior chamber.

(2) Stage 1 trauma has minor corneal damage, mild hyphema, and uveitis, but again there is no damage to the posterior chamber.

(3) A **stage 2** injury is more extensive with severe, nonperforating, corneal damage, severe hyphema, and lens luxation or subluxation. Although the injury extends into the posterior chamber, there is neither retinal detachment nor ocular nerve damage.

(4) In **stage 3,** there is perforating ocular injury as well as retinal detachment and optic nerve damage. In these cases, saving the eye is unlikely no matter what the treatment.

3. Diagnostic plan

a. Diagnosis relies mainly on **visual inspection** of the eye along with evaluating all visible structures with a bright light and an ophthalmoscope for lens and retinal appearances.

   b. **Consensual pupillary response** is used for assessing retinal optic nerve involvement. A miotic pupil in the affected eye carries a more favorable prognosis than a dilated pupil (a miotic pupil may still respond to light, whereas a dilated pupil does not).

4. **Therapeutic plan**
   a. **Lacerations.** Large lid lacerations should be sutured to prevent excessive scarring or abnormal lid conformation, and the periorbital tissues should have cold compresses applied for the first 24 hours to reduce swelling.
      (1) **Conjunctival lacerations** and subconjunctival hemorrhage usually heal readily by second intention.
      (2) All **corneal lacerations** and **perforations** should be regarded as stage 2 or stage 3 emergencies. If the anterior chamber has not been entered, treat the eyes with topical antibiotics and cycloplegics as for a corneal ulcer. Healing is usually rapid and suturing not necessary. In more severe lacerations with penetration into the eye, there is a high risk of permanent damage, and these cases are best referred to a specialist.
   b. **Hyphema** is treated with **corticosteroids** and **mydriatics** (see II A 5 a) because there is usually a concurrent iridocyclitis. However, if corneal ulceration has occurred, corticosteroids should not be used, and a nonsteroidal anti-inflammatory drug (NSAID), such as flunixin meglumine, can be administered. Stall confinement limits exercise and exposure to bright light. Topical antibiotics are indicated, and where penetrating wounds are present, systemic antibiotics will be needed. In hyphema that is unexplained or appears excessive in relation to the degree of trauma, clotting disorders should be ruled out.

II. DISEASES OF THE UVEAL TRACT AND OPTIC NERVE

A. **Periodic ophthalmia [equine recurrent uveitis (ERU), moon blindness].** Inflammation within the eye, called uveitis, can result in signs of tearing and blepharospasm without ulceration. Under this general heading of uveitis are **anterior uveitis,** which incorporates iridocyclitis (inflammation of iris and ciliary body); **posterior uveitis,** which involves choroiditis with or without ciliary body involvement, endophthalmitis, or inflammation of the intraocular structures (i.e., uvea, retina, vitreous); and **panophthalmitis,** which includes all the above structures and the sclera.

1. **Patient profile and history.** Uveitis in large animals is most commonly seen in horses. ERU is the leading cause of blindness in horses. Horses with ERU have repeated bouts of ocular pain, which are usually manifested as severe blepharospasm, photophobia, and epiphora. Visual function may be impaired, particularly with ocular damage from repeated episodes.

2. **Clinical findings.** Examination of the eye reveals circumcorneal injection of blood vessels, conjunctival hyperemia, and corneal edema consistent with uveitis. Shining a bright light into the anterior chamber shows an aqueous flare, which is caused by cells or fibrin in the anterior chamber. The pupil is constricted (miotic), and there is often iridal congestion or neovascularization, which causes an apparent color and texture change to the iris.
   a. **Early in the acute stage,** there is slight photophobia and epiphora. The eye will already be hypotonic (decreased intraocular pressure). Other ocular findings can include catarrhal conjunctivitis and vitreal haze.
   b. **After 2–3 days,** hypopyon may be obvious with fibrin in the anterior chamber. A secondary interstitial keratitis (corneal edema) develops as well as conjunctival and circumcorneal congestion, and these precipitate and exudate in anterior chamber. The eye is soft (hypotonic) and very painful to palpation. Photophobia,

miosis, and epiphora continue, and vision is impaired if there is bilateral involvement.

c. **If untreated,** there may be permanent damage caused by cataracts, lens luxation, retinal damage, or phthisis bulbi.

d. **Sequelae.** Resolution of the ocular inflammation also results in the abatement of clinical signs of ocular pain. However, sequelae to repeated bouts of uveitis may be present. These include posterior and/or anterior synechia, corneal opacity, cloudy vitreous, cataracts, pigmented opacities on the anterior lens capsule (from posterior synechiae that have broken loose from the lens), and atrophy or absence of corpora nigra. **Fundoscopic examination** is important because it may detect characteristic retinal lesions of peripapillary alar depigmentation and detachments or "butterfly lesions."

3. **Etiology and pathogenesis**
    a. **Etiology.** There are numerous possible causes of ERU. The **initial stimulus** for ocular inflammation can vary from infectious to immune mediated to traumatic, with infectious causes getting the most attention. However, an etiologic diagnosis is often not possible.
        (1) **Various microbial antigens** have been implicated as the cause of ERU (e.g., leptospirosis, brucellosis, *Streptococcus,* equine influenza, *Toxoplasma, Chlamydia, Mycoplasma*). Infections caused by *Leptospira* species are most commonly associated with ERU.
        (2) **Microfilariae** of the parasite ***Onchocerca cervicalis*** are also a factor in some cases of ERU. The dead or dying microfilaria become immunogenic, whereas the live filaria are often found in the horses with no inflammation.
    b. **Pathogenesis.** When there is a host response to the antigens in the ocular structures, the inflammatory cells (e.g., eosinophils, PMNs, mononuclear cells) and various mediators of inflammation (particularly prostaglandins) alter vascular permeability and participate in ocular inflammation. The disrupted ciliary epithelium and altered vascular permeability allow leakage of protein and fibrin into the eye. This inflammation can be reactivated by the antigens or trauma. Vascular alterations with repeated episodes include endothelial hyperplasia, endothelial hypertrophy, and fibrosis. Glaucoma can occur secondarily to uveitis, but this is uncommon in large animals (see II B).

4. **Diagnostic plan**
    a. A **history** of previous ocular disease or injury is often available, which is sufficient to establish the diagnosis when combined with the typical signs of uveitis in the absence of ulceration.
    b. **Laboratory studies.** Measurements of paired serum titers and aqueous titers to *Leptospira, Toxoplasma,* or *Brucella* species may help, with anterior chamber titers being higher than serum titers. If *Onchocerca* is involved, diagnosis can be aided by a biopsy of the perilimbal conjunctiva, in which microfilaria may be observed or the eosinophils found infiltrating the tissue.

5. **Therapeutic plan.** Early detection and treatment is important to prevent serious ocular sequelae. Specific systemic infections, such as leptospirosis, should be treated, but usually horses with ERU have no evidence of systemic illness.
    a. **Atropine and corticosteroids. Atropine** (administered every 2–4 hours at 0.5%–1% ointment or as a 3% solution) has mydriatic and cycloplegic effects. Relief of the ciliary spasm helps reduce ocular pain. In the absence of corneal ulceration, **corticosteroids** also are indicated to reduce the ocular inflammatory response. Topical treatment with both atropine and corticosteroids can be attempted, but the horse often is in too much pain to allow this; therefore, subconjunctival injections or a subpalpebral lavage system can be used.
    b. **Antiprostaglandins** administered systemically (e.g., flunixin meglumine at 1.1 mg/kg every 24 hours intravenously, intramuscularly, or orally; phenylbutazone at 3–6 mg/kg orally or intravenously every 12 hours; aspirin 25 mg/kg orally every 12 hours) inhibit the release or activity of prostaglandins that are partially responsible for ocular inflammation.
    c. **Microfilaricidal treatment** is indicated if the ERU is associated with onchocerci-

asis (e.g., diethylcarbamazine at 4.4–6.6 mg/kg daily for 21 days; levamisole at 11 mg/kg orally every 24 hours for 7 days; ivermectin at 0.2 mg/kg orally). This treatment is meant to reduce the "load" of antigen and kill microfilariae before they reach the eye. Because it is the dead microfilariae that elicit inflammatory response, anti-inflammatory drugs such as flunixin meglumine should be administered before parasiticide administration. Alternatively, it may be advisable to wait for the acute phase of ERU to subside before initiating parasiticide treatment.

6. **Prevention.** If the diagnosis of ERU is established, the client should be advised of the possibility of recurrence, unsoundness implications in the event of the future sale of affected horses, and the need for early treatment in future episodes to prevent serious sequelae.

B. **Glaucoma** rarely occurs in large animals but can occur secondary to structural changes associated with ERU, uveitis, trauma, or all of these conditions. This disorder may be more common than reported because ocular pressures are seldom examined in these species. If found, management should involve treating the underlying problem, such as in ERU. Chronic glaucoma may require enucleation and placement of an intraocular silicone prosthesis.

III. DISEASES OF THE ADNEXA

A. **Equine periocular sarcoids**

1. **Patient profile.** There is no breed, coat color, or sex predilection, but most affected horses are between the ages of 3 and 5 years.

2. **Clinical findings.** Sarcoids appear on other parts of the horse's skin but can be particularly troublesome as fleshy masses around the adnexa of the eye. They can be verrucous with cauliflowered edges or appear as smooth discrete nodules, or least commonly, a mixture of the two types. These are the most commonly reported tumor of horses.

3. **Etiology and pathogenesis.** The masses are fibroblastic and do not metastasize but are locally destructive with a high probability of recurrence. They appear to be of viral origin, with the viral particle similar or identical to the papilloma virus of cattle.

4. **Diagnostic plan and laboratory tests.** The history and clinical appearance of the masses are often typical. However, a biopsy with histopathologic examination is suggested, as other skin tumors can have a similar appearance. This rules out other types of tumors and habronemiasis.

5. **Differential diagnoses.** The main differential diagnoses for these masses around the eye are squamous cell carcinoma (see III D) and habronemiasis (see Chapter 17).

6. **Therapeutic plan**
   a. **Surgery.** Successful treatment is rare. Surgical excision is only occasionally successful, with up to 50% recurrence rates, often within months. The periocular location of some sarcoids restricts excision because of possible compromise of eyelid function or disfigurement.
   b. **Surgical debulking with adjunct therapy** is another option, but these adjunctive treatments (radiotherapy, cryotherapy, chemotherapy) are also met with limited success.
   c. **Immunotherapy** appears to be the most effective method to treat periocular sarcoids.
      (1) This treatment works by **iatrogenic stimulation** of the immune system for the horse to rid itself of the tumor and generally leaves no disfigurement or altered eyelid function. This form of treatment involves intralesional injection of **bacille Calmette-Guérin** (BCG; attenuated *Mycobacterium bovis*), which stimulates phagocytic activity and induces a delayed-type hypersensitivity

response (cell mediated). The aim is to infiltrate the junction between the tumor and normally appearing tissue with the BCG. BCG is given every 2–3 weeks until the lesion regresses. It takes an average of four injections for cure; one horse was reported to take nine injections.

(2) **Side effects.** Following injection, there is localized swelling, purulent discharge, and ulceration at the site. Because there is a risk of fatal anaphylaxis with repeated injections, pretreatment with flunixin meglumine and/or prednisolone (both 1 mg/kg) may be advised.

B. **Ocular squamous cell carcinoma (SCC)**

1. **Patient profile and history.** This tumor occurs most commonly in older Hereford cattle or crossbreds and peaks at ages 7–8 years. It is uncommon in cattle less than age 3 years. This disorder also occurs in high incidence in horses that are maintained at high altitudes and is most commonly found on the third eyelid.

2. **Clinical findings** include pink, irregularly shaped fleshy masses that occur on the eyelid, third eyelid, cornea, or conjunctiva. They are often ulcerated, particularly if located on the eyelid margin.

3. **Etiology and pathogenesis**
   a. **Etiology. Contributing factors** are both genetic and environmental.
      (1) Predisposition to the disease in Herefords is highly heritable, but ocular SCC is found in other breeds (i.e., Simmentals, Holsteins).
      (2) **Exposure to ultraviolet light** appears to be a major causative factor. Therefore, risk factors include animals living at high altitudes and/or decreased latitudes where there is increased exposure to ultraviolet light. Reflection of light from snow, certain soil types, and irritation of eyes by wind, dust, and flies also are implicated as increasing the risk of ocular SCC development.
      (3) **Previous episodes of IBK** are suspected as contributing to the formation of this tumor in cattle. Fewer than 10% of these masses on the eyes of cattle are carcinomas (malignant).
   b. **Pathogenesis.** The lesions often start as a keratoacanthoma and hyperplastic plaques on the structures of the eye and proceed progressively to papillomas, then to squamous cell carcinomas. At this final stage, there is local invasion with or without metastasis.
   c. **Salvage.** Cattle with extensive squamous cell carcinoma may be condemned for human consumption. The following antemortem and post mortem guidelines are used for determination of the disposal of the carcass.[*]
      (1) "Any animal found on antemortem inspection to be affected and the eye has been destroyed or obscured by neoplastic tissue and which shows extensive infection, suppuration, and necrosis, usually accompanied by foul odor, or any affected animal with cachexia, regardless of extent, shall be condemned.
      (2) Carcasses of animals with the eye or orbital region affected will be condemned if the affection has:
         (a) Involved the osseous structures of the head with extensive infection, suppuration, and necrosis
         (b) Metastasized from the eye or orbital region to any lymph node (including the parotid lymph node), internal organs, muscles, skeleton, or other structure, regardless of the extent of the primary tumor
         (c) Been associated with cachexia or evidence of absorption or secondary changes, regardless of the extent of the tumor
      (3) Carcasses of animals affected to a lesser degree than described may be passed for human food after removal and condemnation of the head, including the tongue, provided the carcass is otherwise normal."

4. **Therapeutic plan.** There are variety of methods to treat these tumors, including surgical excision, cryosurgery, and hyperthermia.

---

[*]Guidelines taken from the Code of Federal Regulations, Title 9, Chapter 3, Parts 309.6, 311.11, and 311.12 (1-1-87 edition).

a. **Surgical excision,** involving removal of the mass or entire eye, can be performed under sedation and local anesthesia. In extensive cases the regional lymph nodes and salivary glands must also be removed. This is moderately successful and often used as a salvage procedure.

b. **Cryosurgery** is highly successful in animals with small (less than 2 cm in diameter) tumors. Freezing the tumor may achieve part of its success by increasing the **tumor cell antigenicity** so that any remaining tumor cells are destroyed by the body's own immunity. **Cryosurgery equipment** is commercially available. The initial cost of purchase is high but warranted if the practice area has a high prevalence of bovine SCC.

   (1) This treatment involves a **double freeze and thaw cycle** using liquid nitrogen. The process requires a rapid freeze to -25°C, unaided thaw to 5°C, and rapid refreeze. Temperature probes in the tissue during the freeze cycle can ensure these criteria are met.

   (2) This method has been reported to result in **complete regression** of 97% of tumors treated that were less than 2 cm diameter; whereas only 73% of those over 2 cm diameter regressed. During this procedure, other ocular structures need to be protected with a water-soluble lubricant and Styrofoam strips (a Styrofoam coffee cup makes a suitable and readily available shield).

c. **Hyperthermia** is also effective, easily performed, and an economic treatment for early forms of ocular SCC or large tumors that are surgically debulked before hyperthermia. The technique involves using a probe that emits a radiofrequency current to create moderate heat. Tissues are heated to 50°C, but the tissue penetration is only 4 mm. For treatment of appropriate sized tumors, this method has an 80% regression rate.

5. **Prevention**

   a. Clients should be advised of the implication of **breed predisposition** in SCC. They are unlikely to decide to change breeds because of SCC, however, and so could try to breed for pigmentation around the eyes.

   b. Far more important in managing this disease is **early recognition** and treatment of lesions when they are still small and circumscribed. These are often best screened for at the time of pregnancy testing or branding.

C. **Entropion**

1. **Patient profile.** This disorder can affect up to 80% of lambs between the ages of 1 week and 3 weeks. It is often bilateral and, if uncorrected, will result in ulceration and corneal vascularization.

2. **Therapeutic plan.** Treatment is to evert the eyelids, either using a simple stitch or staple in the skin of the eyelid or by injection of a bleb (0.5 ml) of antibiotic, usually procaine penicillin, in the lower eyelid. Even the trauma of the suturing process or the injection is often sufficient to evert the eyelid. Entropion also occurs commonly in weak, premature or ill foals secondarily to enophthalmos. It is found as a congenital abnormality in cattle, particularly in Herefords, and requires surgical correction to protect the cornea.

D. **Ectropion,** or eversion of lower lid, can occur from overzealous correction of entropion or, rarely in foals, be a congenital abnormality.

IV. **CONGENITAL OCULAR DISEASE.** Although ocular abnormalities occur in up to 50% of stillborn calves, these disorders are far less common in live calves (2%–3% of births). A common abnormality is microphthalmos, which may be unilateral or bilateral and may have other associated abnormalities (e.g., cataracts). Most cases are sporadic and idiopathic, and although all breeds can be affected, this disorder is more common in Thoroughbreds. However, there is no proof that microphthalmos is an heritable trait, and in cattle, bovine viral diarrhea (BVD) and hypovitaminosis A are possible causes.

Other congenital ocular abnormalities include dermoids, blockage of nasolacrimal ducts, corneal, iris and lens, and retinal abnormalities.

A. **Dermoids** are focal masses that resemble skin affecting eyelid margin, palpebral and bulbar conjunctiva, nictitating membrane, and most commonly the cornea. This disorder can occur on any newborn but is more likely to be found in Herefords. Surgical removal is the treatment.

B. **Congenital blockage** of the nasolacrimal ducts appears as persistent epiphora from birth. Fluorescein dye can be instilled in the eye, and the lack of its subsequent appearance at the external nares establishes the absence of duct patency.

C. **Corneal abnormalities** are rare apart from dermoids but include microcornea, corneal melanosis, corneal opacities, and iridocorneal angle abnormalities.

D. **Iris and ciliary body abnormalities** are usually of little clinical significance.

  1. **Heterochromia** occurs particularly in light-colored horses, Holstein, Simmental, Limousine, and Angus cattle. Albinism is most likely to be seen in Herefords. Aniridia, bilateral absence of the iris, occurs as an autosomal recessive defect in Belgian horses. Structural defects in the iris (coloboma) may be hereditary in albino Herefords.

  2. **Lens changes,** such as cataracts, are a common congenital ocular defect in foals. Both eyes usually are affected, and they are associated with microphthalmia. The precise etiology is unknown, but suggestions include heredity, trauma (pre- or postnatal), poor nutrition, or in utero infections. There seem to be higher numbers of Arabian foals affected, but there is no proof of this being heritable. Progression of lens changes is unlikely, but if the cataracts are severe, they can interfere with vision.

  3. **Retinal problems** occur in horses, resulting in night blindness affecting mainly the Appaloosa but also other breeds to a lesser extent. **Fundic examination** is normal and the diagnosis is based on a history of reduced vision in low light. The disease can be confirmed with an electroretinogram. In cattle, retinal degeneration can be present at birth and has been linked to *in utero* bluetongue infection.

V. OCULAR MANIFESTATIONS OF SYSTEMIC DISEASES

A. **Exophthalmos.** Whether unilateral or bilateral, exophthalmos is a hallmark of orbital disease. Retrobulbar tumors (lymphosarcoma), chronic frontal sinusitis, or carcinomas of nasal cavities or sinuses are the main causes of exophthalmos.

B. **Horner's syndrome.** This syndrome consists of a combination of signs that include ocular changes of slight miosis, ptosis, and a slight enophthalmos. Other signs include ipsilateral facial warmth or sweating and, in cattle, a dry muzzle on the affected side. In older cattle, the cause can be a carcinoma in the nasal cavity, whereas in horses, the most likely cause of the signs is perivascular jugular injection, resulting in irritation to vagosympathetic trunk.

C. **Other manifestations**

  1. **Eyelid abnormalities** can reflect systemic disease, such as facial nerve palsy in listeriosis, which results in an associated ptosis and exposure keratitis. Also, "flashing" of the third eyelid to tactile stimuli is a classic sign in tetanus. With urticaria, there is bilateral edematous swelling of eyelids along with other mucocutaneous-cutaneous junctions.

  2. **Conjunctivitis** is particularly obvious in **IBR** and may be the only or the salient feature in some outbreaks. It is also a component of **equine viral arteritis** and **MCF,** the latter of which also results in corneal edema.

3. **Changes in the uveal tract** as a reflection of systemic disease are common in septicemia, where fibrin or pus (hypopyon) appears in the anterior chamber of one or both eyes. This is particularly common in colostrum-deprived calves.

4. **Blindness** results from a number of systemic diseases. Vitamin A deficiency causes blindness with dilated, nonresponsive pupils. This is caused by pressure on the optic nerve (noted by ophthalmoscope as papilledema) that occurs because of problems in the bony remodeling of optic canal.

5. **Cortical blindness,** blindness in the presence of light-responsive pupils, is a change that is associated mainly with polioencephalomalacia (thiamine responsive disease) but also is found in lead poisoning and in hypoglycemia that occurs in severe ketosis of cattle or in starving, chilled calves.

STUDY QUESTIONS

DIRECTIONS: Each of the numbered items or incomplete statements in this section is followed by answers or by completions of the statement. Select the ONE numbered answer or completion that is BEST in each case.

1. Which one of the following statements regarding infectious bovine keratoconjunctivitis (IBK, "pinkeye") is true?

(1) The causative organism, *Moraxella bovis*, is frequently spread from carrier animals in the herd by mosquitos (*Culicoides* species) or deer flies (*Tabanidae* species).
(2) The causative organism, *Moraxella bovis*, uses pili to attach itself to the cornea and secretes a toxin that causes corneal lesions.
(3) The clinical signs of IBK include tearing, photophobia, and blepharospasm, but there is seldom permanent ocular damage from this disease.
(4) Preventive treatment is with long-acting penicillin to reduce the carrier state.
(5) There are seldom adverse clinical effects, other than the ocular signs, associated with IBK.

2. In regard to periodic ophthalmia of horses ["moon blindness," equine recurrent uveitis (ERU)], which one of the following statements best applies?

(1) The ocular pain and tearing are usually associated with increased intraocular pressure.
(2) A corneal ulcer is more likely if blepharospasm and corneal edema are present.
(3) Infectious organisms (e.g., the microfilaria of *Onchocerca cervicalis*, *Leptospira* species) cause direct tissue damage, leading to ERU.
(4) The treatment of this disease should include a broad-spectrum topical antibiotic and a cycloplegic, but corticosteroids are contraindicated.
(5) Sequelae to repeated bouts of this uveitis can include anterior and posterior synechia, cataracts, cloudy vitreous, and butterfly lesions on the retina.

3. Regarding ocular tumors in large animals, which one of the following statements is correct?

(1) Ocular sarcoids in horses are locally invasive tumors caused by a virus similar to cattle papilloma virus; they are readily treated by cryotherapy.
(2) Ocular squamous cell carcinomas (SCCs) appear almost exclusively in Hereford cattle and their crosses.
(3) Periocular sarcoids appear to occur in young horses, with no breed, coat color or sex predilection, whereas ocular SCCs occur more commonly in older cattle that lack pigmentation around the eyes.
(4) In cattle with an eye destroyed by SCC and an ongoing localized infection, the entire head and neck must be discarded before the carcass can be used for human consumption.
(5) Immunotherapy with intralesional bacille Calmette-Guérin (BCG; attenuated *Mycobacterium bovis*) is the treatment of choice for ocular SCC in cattle.

4. Which one of the following statements regarding ocular problems in large animal neonates is true?

(1) Entropion in Hereford calves and in foals is most likely a congenital abnormality.
(2) Entropion in lambs can affect many in a flock and can be successfully treated by application of a stitch or staple to evert the lower eyelid.
(3) Microphthalmos in calves has been associated with intrauterine bovine viral diarrhea (BVD) infection, and in foals with midgestation equine herpes virus-1 (EHV-1) infection.
(4) Dermoids in calves are most common in Holsteins; cryosurgery is required to prevent regrowth of the masses.

5. Conjunctivitis is a common clinical sign in:

(1) Equine viral arteritis, equine influenza, and equine herpes virus (EHV) infection in horses.
(2) *Moraxella bovis* infection in sheep and cattle.
(3) *Chlamydia psittaci* infection in sheep and *Moraxella equi* infection in horses.
(4) Equine viral arteritis in horses and *Chlamydia psittaci* infection in sheep.
(5) *Mycoplasma agalactia* infection in goats and *Moraxella equi* infection in horses.

6. In a horse with a corneal ulcer that is slow to respond to conventional treatment or suddenly worsens, which one of the following is an appropriate course of action?

(1) Perform a corneal scraping for cytology and culture; mycotic keratitis is a high possibility.
(2) Perform a corneal scraping for cytology and change to a broad-spectrum antibiotic; superinfection by a drug-resistant species of bacteria is likely occurring.
(3) Create a third eyelid flap to facilitate blood supply to the ulcer.
(4) Perform a corneal scraping for culture, and while waiting for the culture increase the frequency of drug administration to every second hour.
(5) Create a third eyelid to deprive the invading organisms of oxygen.

7. A 7-year-old Hereford cow has an ulcerated fleshy mass measuring 5 cm in diameter on the lower eyelid. The cow's eyes appear normal otherwise and she is in good body condition. Her vital signs are normal. What advice can you give the owner regarding treatment and the potential for salvage?

(1) Surgical excision and immunotherapy with bacillus Calmette-Guérin (BCG, attenuated *Mycobacterium bovis*) is advisable; the cow will likely have its head and neck discarded if sent to slaughter.
(2) The eye should be removed surgically and the cow will likely pass for slaughter, with condemnation of the head and tongue.
(3) Surgical excision and cryotherapy is advised because the most likely tumor is only locally invasive and does not spread to lymph nodes.
(4) Immunotherapy with BCG after surgical debulking is the preferred treatment because the cow will be condemned if sent to slaughter at this time.

8. Which one of the following statements regarding entropion in large animal newborns is true?

(1) In most cases, congenital entropion in foals should be surgically corrected because if untreated, corneal ulceration and neovascularization can occur.
(2) Entropion in calves only occurs secondarily to profound dehydration and thus corrective surgery should not be performed.
(3) Overzealous correction of entropion can lead to ectropion.
(4) Treatment is by saline injection into the lower eyelid margin.

ANSWERS AND EXPLANATIONS

1. The answer is 2 [I B 2]. The organism responsible for infectious bovine keratoconjunctivitis (IBK, "pinkeye"), *Moraxella bovis*, has a piliated phase, during which it is able to attach to the cornea, and a nonpiliated phase, during which it is apparently harmless. Once the organism has colonized the cornea, it secretes a bacterial cytotoxin that is responsible for initiating the corneal lesions. Untreated cases of pinkeye may result in corneal perforation and blindness. The ocular signs of this disease are certainly most prominent, but other adverse effects include decreased feed efficiency and milk production. *M. bovis* is spread from carrier cows to susceptible animals via the face fly (*Musca autumnalis*). Systemic penicillin is not an effective preventative treatment because it does not pass into lacrimal secretions in high enough concentrations.

2. The answer is 5 [II A]. Sequelae of periodic ophthalmia ["moon blindness," equine recurrent uveitis (ERU)] include anterior and posterior synechia, cataracts, cloudy vitreous, and butterfly lesions on the retina. Glaucoma (i.e., increased intraocular pressure) is rare in large animals and, in fact, there is most often decreased intraocular pressure in animals with ERU. Corneal ulceration is not a feature of ERU. Infectious organisms (e.g., *Leptospira* species or *Onchocerca cervicalis*) can cause this disease; however, they do not do so by direct invasion. Rather, disease occurs when dead or dying organisms cause antigenic stimulation, leading to inflammation and pain. Treatment of ERU includes corticosteroids (unless a concurrent corneal ulcer is present), nonsteroidal anti-inflammatory drugs (NSAIDs), and mydriatic cytoplegics. Topical antibiotics are of little value because the disease is immune-mediated, not infectious.

3. The answer is 3 [III A–B]. Equine periocular sarcoids are often seen in young horses, with no breed, coat color, or sex predilection, whereas ocular squamous cell carcinomas (SCCs) in cattle are seen most commonly in older cattle that lack pigmentation around the eyes. Although SCCs are over-represented in Hereford cattle, other breeds are also suscepti-

ble, including Holsteins and Simmentals. Ocular sarcoids in horses are difficult to treat and many methods, including radiotherapy, cryotherapy, and chemotherapy, are met with very limited success. An animal with an eye destroyed by SCC and with an ongoing localized infection is unfit for human consumption and must be condemned. Bacille Calmette-Guérin (BCG, attenuated *Mycobacterium bovis*) is the treatment of choice for periocular sarcoids in horses, not SCC in cattle. In cattle with SCC, surgical treatments are the most effective.

4. The answer is 2 [III C]. Entropion, a common congenital condition in lambs, is not so common in foals and calves. In lambs, the majority of the flock can be affected. Treatment entails eyelid eversion, using either a simple stitch or staple. Microphthalmos, while induced by infection with the bovine viral diarrhea (BVD) virus in calves, is regarded as idiopathic or genetic with no association with equine herpes virus-1 (EVH-1) infection in foals. Dermoids are most common in the Hereford breed, not the Holstein breed.

5. The answer is 4 [V C 2]. Conjunctivitis is often a clinical sign of equine viral arteritis in horses and *Chlamydia psittaci* infection in sheep. Equine influenza virus, equine herpes virus, *Moraxella bovis*, *Moraxella equi*, and *Mycoplasma agalactia* infection are not associated with conjunctivitis.

6. The answer is 1 [I A 4 a (1) (b)]. With corneal ulcers that are slow to respond or resistant to treatment, a secondary mycotic keratitis is a distinct and the most likely possibility. Therefore, a corneal scraping for cytology and culture should be performed, and the administration of antifungal drugs may be appropriate pending the results. Any treatment that increases the dose of antibiotic or closes the eye can potentiate fungal growth.

7. The answer is 2 [III B 3 c, 4]. Squamous cell carcinoma (SCC) is the most likely diagnosis. The ocular and periocular involvement is minimal; therefore, in all likelihood, the cow would not be condemned (exclusive of the head and tongue) if sent to slaughter. The treatment of choice in this case is surgical excision of the eye. The description of the case does not indicate spread to other tissues, but the ocular SCC can metastasize to the lymph nodes. Intralesional instillation of bacille Calmette-Guérin (BCG; attenuated *Mycobacterium bovis*) has not proven useful in the treatment of SCC.

8. The answer is 3 [III C]. Overzealous correction of entropion will result in permanent eversion of the lower eyelid (ectropion). Entropion is not recognized as a congenital problem in foals, but is seen as a congenital problem in lambs and Hereford calves. Injection of a bleb of procaine penicillin will serve as satisfactory treatment for entropion, but saline is too rapidly absorbed to be effective.

Chapter 13

Musculoskeletal Disorders

Timothy H. Ogilvie

I. **DISEASES OF THE MUSCLES**

A. **Nutritional myopathy in young animals**

1. **Patient profile and history**
   a. **Affected animals**
      (1) Nutritional myopathy is seen mainly in **young, rapidly growing calves** and **lambs.** This disorder occurs most commonly at 2–4 months of age but can occur in younger or older animals. It often accompanies unaccustomed exercise. Disease may occur in outbreaks with up to **15% morbidity** and a **100% case fatality rate.**
      (2) In **foals,** it usually affects individual animals and is not associated with exercise.
      (3) Myopathy may occur with vitamin E and selenium deficiency in **piglets** but is overshadowed by other major pathologic findings (e.g., mulberry heart disease, hepatosis dietetica).
   b. The condition is most common in **selenium-deficient areas** (e.g., northeast and northwest North America) and in dams that are fed winter diets deficient in vitamin E and selenium. Occurrences may be associated with diets containing unsaturated fats (e.g., fish oils, corn oils).

2. **Clinical findings**
   a. **Calves and lambs**
      (1) **Acute enzootic muscular dystrophy.** Calves and lambs may die suddenly. If the animals survive, they may be found in lateral recumbency. They are seen to be bright, alert, and usually able to swallow. Tachycardia (150–200 beats/minute) is a feature often coupled with an irregular heart beat.
      (2) **Subacute enzootic muscular dystrophy.** The most common presentation of nutritional myopathy is **white muscle disease** in calves and lambs.
         (a) Animals present in sternal recumbency and are bright, alert, and unable to stand. If animals are standing, they are weak, stiff, and trembling.
         (b) On **bilateral palpation, muscles** may be firm and swollen, particularly over the gluteal and shoulder muscles. Calves and lambs are often dyspneic because of intercostal muscle involvement, and a transient fever (41°C) may be present. There is tachycardia, but the heart rhythm is regular.
   b. **Foals.** Myopathy may occur in foals from 1 week to 5 months of age. Clinical expression is recumbency, difficulty in rising, trembling, unsteadiness, failure to suckle, polypnea, and tachycardia. A specific localized presentation occurs where face and neck muscles degenerate. Therefore, foals may appear to have a stiff neck and be unable to nurse.

3. **Etiology and pathogenesis**
   a. **Etiology.** Although their exact relationship is unknown, dietary selenium, sulfur-containing amino acids, and vitamin E work together to protect cells from oxidative damage. Therefore, a deficiency in these agents can cause nutritional myopathy.
   b. **Pathogenesis**
      (1) **Selenium** is an essential component of **glutathione peroxidase (GSH-Px).** GSH-Px detoxifies lipid peroxides by reducing them to nontoxic hydroxy fatty acids. A deficiency of selenium limits the production of GSH-Px and other selenoproteins, thereby allowing a buildup of oxygen (free radicals), which causes cellular destruction.

(2) Vitamin E prevents fatty-acid hydroperoxide formation and protects cellular membranes from lipoperoxidation. High levels of **dietary unsaturated fatty acids** may overwhelm the protective mechanism of vitamin E but are not a prerequisite for disease. Selenium may limit the amount of dietary vitamin E required.

(3) Affected muscles. Presentations may not be distinct and can occur together in the same animal.

    (a) In **young lambs, calves,** and **foals, myocardial** and **diaphragmatic muscles** are most often affected, resulting in a presentation of acute heart failure, respiratory distress, and rapid death.

    (b) Older animals, particularly calves, often present with **skeletal muscle** involvement.

4. Diagnostic plan

    a. Acute cases. The diagnosis for acute enzootic muscular dystrophy is often based on postmortem findings, but laboratory results are diagnostic in the live animal.

    b. Subacute cases. The diagnosis for subacute enzootic muscular dystrophy is based on clinical findings and dramatically increased muscle enzymes and decreased serum selenium and GSH-Px.

5. Laboratory tests

    a. Plasma creatine phosphokinase (CPK) is the most commonly used laboratory measurement. CPK is highly specific for cardiac and skeletal muscle and will show a 10- to 50-fold increase in clinical cases of nutritional myopathy. CPK has a short half-life (2–4 hours) but will indicate muscle damage for up to 3 days.

    b. Elevations of **aspartate aminotransferase (AST)** indicate muscle or liver damage. Levels remain high for 3–10 days at three to ten times the normal values. The magnitude of increase in both CPK and AST is proportional to the amount of muscle damage.

    c. Serum and **whole-blood selenium levels** correspond to whole-body selenium status. Serum levels are the most reliable; however, neither test is available outside of research institutions or major reference laboratories.

    d. Levels of the **enzyme GSH-Px,** which is found in red blood cells (RBCs), parallel the selenium status of the animal because selenium is incorporated into the erythrocyte during erythropoiesis.

    e. Vitamin E status may be measured via α-tocopherol or vitamin E levels in the blood; however, these tests are less reliable as indicators of disease.

    f. Myoglobinuria does not occur. Muscle mass is still limited at this age, and myoglobin content of muscle is low.

6. Differential diagnoses

    a. Acute cases. Differential diagnoses include pneumonia, septicemia, and toxemia.

    b. Subacute cases may appear similar to pneumonia, neurologic disease (e.g., meningitis), trauma, blackleg, or toxicities, as with organophosphates. In lambs, enzootic ataxia and swayback may appear similar.

7. Therapeutic plan

    a. With the **acute myocardial form,** there is generally an unfavorable response to vitamin E and selenium therapy. Animals usually die within hours despite therapy.

    b. For the **subacute form,** a single treatment of the recommended therapeutic dosage of a vitamin E and selenium preparation at 2 ml/45 kg is curative. Animals respond to therapy in 2–5 days.

8. Prevention. Dietary supplementation with vitamin E and selenium is necessary in deficient geographic locations. During a dam's pregnancy, this supplement may be provided in the feed as mineral or salt mixtures. Calves should be treated intramuscularly at birth (and 4–6 weeks later if necessary) with vitamin E and selenium at 1 ml/45 kg.

B. Myopathy in older animals

1. Muscular dystrophy (paralytic myoglobinuria) of cattle

    a. Patient profile and history. This myopathy is seen sporadically in cattle up to 2 years of age. There is a recent history of increased exercise and a patient profile of heavily fed, well-muscled animals.

b. Clinical findings. Affected animals are found in lateral recumbency, with a bright and alert attitude. Skeletal muscles may feel firm, particularly the semimembranosus and semitendinosus muscles. Myoglobin may be present in the urine, which is brown.

c. Etiology and pathogenesis are the same as with young animals (see I A 3).

d. Diagnostic plan and laboratory tests
   (1) The **preliminary diagnosis** is based on clinical findings and history. Other causes of recumbency (e.g., trauma, malnutrition) must be eliminated.
   (2) The diagnosis is **confirmed** through clinical pathology findings. CPK is very high in clinical cases (usually more than 20,000 IU/L). Vitamin E levels are low in herdmates.

e. Therapeutic plan
   (1) This condition is treated with **parenteral solution of vitamin E** and **selenium** at recommended dosages.
   (2) It is important to maintain **deep bedding** while the animal is recumbent to limit pressure necrosis of muscles. Recumbency may be prolonged for days or weeks during convalescence, which clouds the prognosis and limits economic salvage of affected animals.

f. Prevention. Dietary supplementation with vitamin E and selenium is recommended for the herd.

2. Exertional (post-exercise) rhabdomyolysis in horses

a. Patient profile and history
   (1) The **most common presentation** of the condition (also called **equine paralytic myoglobinuria, tying-up syndrome,** and **azoturia**) is in horses after unaccustomed exercise or insufficient training.
   (2) There may be a **familial basis** to the disease in certain breeds (e.g., Quarter horse), but the condition is common among all breeds and is overrepresented in young, female animals.
   (3) The condition may be **chronic** and **recurring** in certain animals.

b. Clinical findings. There is a sudden onset of muscle soreness, which may range from stiffness (a rigid stance) to recumbency, and the animal sweats profusely after exercise. There is swelling and rigidity of various skeletal muscle groups. Myoglobinuria is evident clinically.

c. Etiology and pathogenesis
   (1) Etiology
      (a) Predisposing factors include heavy musculature, irregular exercise, high-grain diet, and a nervous disposition. There is degeneration of muscle cells and muscle bundles associated with **unaccustomed exercise** (e.g., Monday morning disease).
      (b) The condition is not associated with the vitamin E or selenium status of the animal.
   (2) Pathogenesis. Recent studies have indicated that the pathogenesis may be a **glycogen storage disorder** with a possible autosomal-recessive pattern of inheritance. However, there may be multiple causes for the accumulation of glycogen and polysaccharide.

d. Diagnostic plan and differential diagnoses. Clinicians should rely on history, clinical findings, and laboratory results to establish the diagnosis. For chronic or relapsing cases, a muscle biopsy may be useful in differentiating the clinical picture from that of lameness.

e. Laboratory tests. There is an increased CPK level (5000–10,000 IU/L) and myoglobinuria.

f. Therapeutic plan
   (1) Early therapy is essential, including rest, analgesics, and supportive therapy (e.g., bedding, intravenous fluids if necessary to increase excretion and dilute myoglobin).
   (2) Sodium bicarbonate intravenously is warranted in cases with acidemia.

g. Prevention. The only recommended prevention includes training modifications and attention to diet. Overconditioned animals are more prone to exertional rhabdomyolysis. Dantrolene sodium has been used to slow calcium release and decrease muscular contraction.

3. **Ischemic myopathies**
   a. **Patient profile and history.** Large animals in prolonged recumbency on hard surfaces (e.g., horses following anesthesia, downer cows with hypocalcemia or calving injuries) are most prone to this condition.
   b. **Clinical findings.** Hind limbs or areas of pressure during recumbency are affected. Animals appear bright and alert with normal appetite but are unable to rise. Cattle may creep along, pulling themselves forward using their front legs.
   c. **Etiology.** Ischemic myopathy is caused by muscle degeneration resulting from local ischemia. Prolonged muscle compression results in tissue anoxia, cellular damage, inflammation, cell death, and muscle degeneration.
   d. **Diagnostic plan.** The condition is diagnosed by a combination of history, clinical findings, and laboratory results. The clinician must rule out trauma or other causes of recumbency.
   e. **Laboratory tests.** Muscle enzymes are elevated but less so than with nutritional or exertional myopathies. Occasionally, post-anesthetic myopathies can cause great elevations in CPK, where the serum enzyme level may exceed 100,000 IU/L.
   f. **Therapeutic plan**
      (1) Consider the administration of **analgesics,** and institute **supportive care** (e.g., deep bedding, rolling, limited lifting or slinging).
      (2) **Immersion** in a specially designed water tank aids in physiotherapy for down cows. Horses have responded occasionally to the use of an equine swimming pool.
      (3) Correction of any fluid or electrolyte imbalance and administration of **intravenous fluids** to increase excretion of myoglobin are necessary therapies.
   g. **Prognosis** for individual cases is highly variable and must take into account the length of recumbency, muscle mass and size of the individual, flooring and surface characteristics, as well as attention to supportive care.
   h. **Prevention.** Advise the client regarding the primary cause (e.g., hypocalcemia), and institute appropriate preventive measures for the herd.

4. **Porcine stress syndrome [PSS, pale soft exudative (PSE) pork, malignant hyperthermia].** It is thought that these terms are all **synonymous.** The names correspond to the stage of identification.
   a. **Economic implications.** This condition concerns the **meat-packing industry** because the keeping quality and presentation of cuts of pork are affected by the soft, pale, weeping condition of the meat [pale soft exudative (PSE) pork].
   b. **Patient profile and history**
      (1) If the condition is seen in **finishing pigs,** it is characterized by acute death induced by stressors (e.g., transport, fighting, high environmental temperature).
      (2) This disorder may also be seen in **other species** associated with the administration of **anesthetics** or **muscle relaxants.**
   c. **Clinical findings**
      (1) In **pigs,** the most dramatic sign is **acute death,** often after transport. If animals are found alive, they appear stiff or recumbent with tremors and have a high rectal temperature, dyspnea, and skin blanching with areas of erythema.
      (2) In **other animals** with an anesthesia-precipitated event, the signs are similar.
   d. **Etiology and pathogenesis**
      (1) **Etiology.** The condition is caused by an **inherited susceptibility** (single recessive gene) in all breeds of pigs but is most common in Landrace, Pietrain, and Poland China pigs and particularly in pigs selected for heavy muscling and rapid growth.
      (2) **Pathogenesis.** Biochemical events include a rapid onset of anaerobic glycolysis and loss of control of skeletal muscle metabolism. This results in excessive lactate production and the development of heat, which, in conjunction with peripheral vasoconstriction, results in hyperthermia.
   e. **Diagnostic plan and differential diagnoses.** Differential diagnoses are key to pri-

mary diagnosis. The clinical and postmortem findings help rule out other causes of sudden death, such as heatstroke.

f. Laboratory tests. Clinical pathology is of little relevance in acute disease because of the rapidity of disease progression.

g. Therapeutic plan. There is no treatment other than cooling and the immediate relief of stress; however, this therapy is invariably futile in clinical cases.

h. Prevention

(1) Screening

(a) For many years in test stations, the **halothane test** was used to test for expression of the gene causing the condition but was only effective in revealing homozygous carriers. Test matings were then established to identify heterozygotes.

(b) Other screening methods include blood creatine kinase levels, blood typing, meat quality evaluation for PSE pork, and erythrocyte fragility. The most recent test used to identify carriers is the **DNA-based assay** (gene probe) for a C–T mutation at base pair 1843 of the skeletal muscle ryanodine receptor (ryr1). This mutation is highly correlated with PSS.

(2) Control of the condition in a susceptible population includes the **reduction of stressors** (e.g., ventilation, spray cooling, rapid transport). **Tranquillizers** have also been used, including azaperone (40–80 mg). Dantrolene sodium has been used prophylactically. It is hypothesized to slow the release of cellular calcium, thus limiting muscular contraction.

5. Other conditions that can cause myopathy in older animals include:

a. Neurogenic myopathies (Akabane virus)

b. Neoplasia (rhabdomyosarcomas)

c. Congenital myopathies (double muscling)

C. **Myositis of domestic animals.** Myositis is manifested as either an **acute inflammation** with muscle swelling and pain or a **chronic inflammation** manifested by atrophy and joint and limb contracture. Many cases are traumatic in origin, with specific clinical signs and therapies related to the type and location of trauma.

1. Clostridial myositis (clostridial myonecrosis, blackleg, malignant edema)

a. Patient profile and history. Clostridial myositis may follow **intramuscular injections,** which cause tissue necrosis. This has been described most frequently in horses.

(1) Clostridial myonecrosis occurs primarily in cattle, sheep, goats, and wild ruminants. There is no sex or breed predilection. This is most often a disease of prosperous animals older than 3 months in age.

(2) Blackleg

(a) Cattle may develop resistance to ***Clostridium chauvoei*** after 2 years of age. The term *blackleg* most often refers to gangrenous myositis, which is caused by *C. chauvoei.*

(b) In **sheep,** this infection is associated with wounds such as those associated with shearing, docking, and castrations, particularly in unsanitary conditions.

(3) Malignant edema is more likely to be associated with wound infection *(C. septicum, C. novyi* type B, and occasionally *C. sordellii* and *C. chauvoei).* This disease usually affects sheep; however, it can affect other species of all ages.

b. Clinical findings

(1) Blackleg

(a) Cattle. Usually, this disease is characterized by **sudden death.**

(i) Clinical signs may include lameness, depression, anorexia, rumen stasis, reluctance to move, and fever (40°C).

(ii) Muscle swelling resulting from subcutaneous emphysema can be seen or felt on the thigh, rump, loin, or brisket. Crepitation occurs on palpation. Swellings may be warm but progress rapidly to cold. The skin over these areas feels dry, is insensitive to pain, and is discolored (blue, black). The course rapidly progresses to dyspnea, prostration, coma, and death.

    (b) Sheep. The clinical signs are similar to those in cattle.

  (2) Malignant edema presents as a rapidly spreading edema, and sometimes emphysema is seen around the site of a wound. Blood-tinged edema fluid gravitates from the wound to dependent areas through tissue planes. Death is rapid with this disease.

  (3) *C. sordellii* infection produces a highly fatal myositis and can cause death in cattle and horses. The disease course is rapid, and clinical signs often do not develop before death.

 c. Etiology and pathogenesis

  (1) Etiology. Clostridial diseases are infectious but not contagious. *Clostridium* organisms are common inhabitants of the gastrointestinal tract but are mainly found as soilborne organisms. They are a constant threat to livestock, particularly those not in confinement.

  (2) Pathogenesis. These organisms may persist in soil as spores for years and gain access to the animal through injections, wound contamination, or puncture wounds. If introduced as spores (particularly via the gastrointestinal tract), the organisms may sequester in tissue until a suitable anaerobic environment occurs (e.g., trauma, circulatory disturbances). Exotoxins elaborated by the organisms cause further necrosis, which encourages more bacterial growth.

 d. Diagnostic plan

  (1) The disease usually is diagnosed by **postmortem findings;** however, postmortem decomposition is particularly rapid with these diseases, and differentiation of organisms is difficult, particularly with overgrowth of other clostridia.

  (2) Diagnosis is aided by an **accurate history** (e.g., occurrence of disease in the area, no vaccination history) and **tissue smears** from fresh carcasses.

 e. Therapeutic plan. If clinically ill animals are observed, penicillin (44,000 IU/kg twice daily) or broad-spectrum antibiotics are administered for 5–7 days. The mortality rate with these diseases approaches 100%.

 f. Prevention. In clinical cases in a herd, all exposed animals should be treated with a **multivalent clostridial vaccine.** Herd or flock immunization is effective and inexpensive. It should be practiced regularly, particularly in areas known to have outbreaks of clostridial diseases.

2. Other conditions
  a. Eosinophilic myositis
  b. Fibrotic myopathy
  c. Ossifying myopathy
  d. Parasitic myositis

II. DISEASES OF THE BONES AND JOINTS

A. Osteomyelitis

1. Patient profile and history. Osteomyelitis affects all species but is most common in young animals.

2. Clinical findings. Initial presentation includes a soft, sometimes painful lesion over bones or joints. The pain persists and becomes more severe (lameness), resulting in cellulitis, discharge from the sinuses, and pathologic fractures.

3. Etiology. The infection is introduced traumatically or hematogenously.

 a. Specific causes include spinal abscesses from tail docking, tail-biting pigs, and omphalophlebitis or septicemias that result in infectious arthritis, meningitis, and osteomyelitis.

 b. In **foals,** the cause is usually a hematogenous source for suppurative polyarthritis and concurrent osteomyelitis. There is physeal, metaphyseal, and epiphyseal involvement. Septicemia does not have to be clinically apparent. Causative organisms include *Escherichia coli, Actinobacillus equuli, Rhodococcus equi,* and others.

    c. Horses. In adults, open fractures commonly result in osteomyelitis.

    d. In **calves,** the cause may be similar to that in foals. Lesions are usually restricted to physeal or metaphyseal involvement.

    e. Cattle. A common osteomyelitis in cattle is **lumpy jaw** (see II B), which is caused by *Actinomyces bovis.* Traumatic causes are also common because of a variety of organisms, commonly *A. pyogenes.*

4. Diagnostic plan and laboratory tests. Diagnosis is based on clinical findings, radiographic changes, cytology of an aspirate from the lesion, and possibly culture.

    a. Bacterial culture. In the case of concurrent arthritis, consider a **synovial biopsy** for bacterial culture. A synovial biopsy is often more likely to yield a positive culture than the fluid aspirate from a joint.

    b. A **blood culture** should also be performed in septicemic or bacteremic animals.

5. Differential diagnoses should include trauma, arthritis, and osteodystrophy.

6. Therapeutic plan

    a. Medical therapy may arrest clinical progression but is rarely curative. Long-term treatment is necessary with broad-spectrum antibiotics. Anaerobes may be involved, therefore, consider penicillin or metronidazole as an adjunct to other antibiotics (e.g., trimethoprim-sulfas). Intra-articular antibiotics have not proven to be more efficacious than systemic.

    b. Surgery is often the treatment of choice and involves arthrocentesis, surgical drainage, irrigation, and bone curettage or removal. Polysulfated glycosaminoglycan should be used as intra-articular therapy following surgical intervention.

7. Prevention. Proper neonatal management, attention to wounds, and early treatment are essential.

B. | **Actinomycosis (lumpy jaw)**

1. Patient profile and history. Lumpy jaw is most common in cattle, although occasionally it is seen in pigs and horses. This disease is usually sporadic in young adult cattle and can occur in calves. There may be a farm or animal predisposition.

2. Clinical findings

    a. Swelling. Lumpy jaw presents as a **painless, bony swelling,** usually of the mandible and occasionally of the maxilla. The result is disfigurement that leads to improper mastication, which causes a loss of body condition.

    b. Lesion. The lesion is usually most prominent on the lateral aspect of the jaw but may occur on the inside of the mouth. Progression of the lesion is variable. In advanced cases, pus is discharged from various fistulae. The pus is described as "sticky" and "honey-like" and may be granular.

    c. Soft tissue. Involvement of soft tissue may occur, with clinical signs dependent on the area involved (e.g., lower esophagus).

3. Etiology and pathogenesis

    a. Etiology. The causative organism is *Actinomyces bovis.*

    b. Pathogenesis. *A. bovis* is a common inhabitant of the bovine mouth, gaining entrance to subcutaneous tissues through compromised mucosa (trauma). Also, foreign bodies, plants, or infected teeth may aid in the introduction of infection. *A. bovis* also may invade the alveolus via erupting teeth.

4. Diagnostic plan. The diagnosis is based on clinical findings, smears of discharging pus, and granules submitted for microbiologic staining.

5. Therapeutic plan. All that can be hoped for is an arrest in the progression of the lesion. Many of the listed therapies can be carried out simultaneously in order to carry an animal for a short period of time (e.g., to calving).

    a. Iodides are recommended but are less effective with advanced lesions than early in the course of disease. Potassium iodide (6–10 g/day orally for 7–10 days) or

sodium iodide (1 g/12 kg intravenously as a single treatment, may repeat once) are used.
b. **Sulfa drugs** (1 g/kg daily for 4–5 days), **streptomycin** (5 g/day for 3 days intramuscularly), or **isoniazid** (10–20 mg/kg, orally or intramuscularly, for 3–4 weeks) may also be tried.
c. **Surgical debridement** also has been used.

6. **Prevention.** Cleanup of the environment is recommended to remove sharp foreign objects.

C. **Osteodystrophy**

1. **Patient profile and history.** Defective or abnormal formation of bone can occur in all species and is usually most evident in groups of animals (adults or young).

2. **Clinical findings** are usually less marked in adults than in young animals.
   a. **Bone curvature** and **shifting lameness** are the earliest clinical signs (bowing of long bones) and are most common in young, growing animals. Also, there is an enlargement of the distal ends of long bones. Epiphyses may be painful to palpation.
   b. **Unexpected fractures** may occur commonly in mature animals. The rib cage becomes flattened, and the animal appears "slab-sided."
   c. **Other clinical findings** occur with primary deficiencies or imbalances of certain nutrients (e.g., infertility, unthriftiness, teeth abnormalities).

3. **Etiology and pathogenesis**
   a. **Etiology**
      (1) **Nutritional causes**
          (a) **Imbalances** or **deficiencies** of **calcium, phosphorus,** and **vitamin D,** alone or in combination, produce bony abnormalities. Examples include rickets in young animals, osteomalacia in adult ruminants, and osteodystrophia in pigs and horses.
          (b) Other primary nutritional causes include **copper deficiency** (e.g., osteoporosis in lambs, epiphysitis in young cattle) and **inadequate dietary protein,** which leads to osteoporosis. **Hypo-** or **hypervitaminosis A** produces skeletal abnormalities in pigs and cattle.
          (c) **Secondary protein or mineral imbalances.** Chronic parasitism produces skeletal abnormalities resulting from protein deficiency. High levels of aluminum in the ration interfere with calcium and phosphorus metabolism.
      (2) **Chemical agents**
          (a) Chronic **lead poisoning** leads to osteoporosis in lambs and foals.
          (b) Chronic exposure to **fluorine** results in osteoporosis and exostosis.
      (3) **Poisonous plants.** Plants can interfere with mineral balance. For example, oxalate accumulators (e.g., rhubarb, sorrels, wild dock) can cause skeletal disease because of oxalic acid's great affinity for calcium and magnesium in the gastrointestinal tract.
      (4) **Inherited or congenital conditions.** Some known conditions include:
          (a) **Achondroplasia** and **chondrodystrophy** (dwarfism)
          (b) **Osteogenesis imperfecta**
          (c) **Osteopetrosis**
          (d) **Arthrogryposis**
          (e) **Splayleg in piglets**
          (f) **Angular limb deformities**
          (g) **Flexural deformities**
          (h) **Ovine hereditary chondrodysplasia in Suffolk lambs** (spider syndrome)
      (5) **Environmental causes**
          (a) **Indoor housing with hard flooring** has been associated with osteochondrosis, arthrosis, and epiphysitis.
          (b) Vertebral osteochondrosis or spondylitis is a described syndrome of **older bulls in breeding units.**
      (6) **Unknown causes.** Hypertrophic pulmonary osteoarthropathy is a disease of in-

creased bone formation and has been reported in horses, cattle, and sheep. The cause, although unknown, is related to pulmonary lesions, such as tumors or chronic infectious processes.

- **b. Pathogenesis**
    - **(1) Imbalances of calcium, phosphorus, and vitamin D**
        - **(a) Absorption.** Calcium is absorbed from the small intestine according to need. Absorption is influenced by nature of diet, amounts of calcium and phosphorus in the diet, and requirements of the individual. Phosphorus is available in forage and grain diets.
        - **(b) Metabolism** of calcium and phosphorus is under the control of parathyroid hormone and vitamin D. Parathyroid hormone is secreted in response to hypocalcemia and stimulates conversion of 25-dihydroxycholecalciferol to 1,25-dihydroxycholecalciferol (1,25-DHCC). Together, these stimulate bone resorption, and 1,25-DHCC alone stimulates intestinal absorption of calcium. This activity is balanced by calcitonin when serum calcium levels return to normal.
    - **(2) Copper deficiency** causes changes in osteoblastic activity and impairment of collagen formation.
    - **(3) Fluorine toxicosis.** Chronic ingestion of fluorine causes deposition in bones and teeth. Calcium and phosphorus are excreted in the urine in conjunction with fluorine, resulting in osteomalacia, osteoporosis, and exostosis.
- **4. Diagnostic plan.** It may be difficult to define a specific disease entity, deficiency, or imbalance unless there are obvious characteristics of a specific condition (e.g., big head in horses, rickets in sheep). Conditions usually are diagnosed on the basis of history, clinical findings, laboratory results, feed analysis, and necropsy.
- **5. Laboratory tests. Serum calcium** and **phosphorus** are not reliable indicators of primary disturbance or whole-body status. Combinations of feed samples, pathology specimens, blood chemistry, and urine chemistries (fractional excretions of electrolytes) may add to diagnostic evidence. For example, serum copper levels may be combined with a liver biopsy to determine copper reserves in suspected cases of epiphysitis due to copper deficiency.
- **6. Therapeutic plan**
    - **a. Early treatment of animals affected by a dietary imbalance** may yield positive results if lesions are not too far advanced or if the primary disease is treatable. For example, nutritional secondary hyperparathyroidism carries a better prognosis than renal secondary hyperparathyroidism.
    - **b. Specific conditions** may respond to medical therapy. For example, selected cases of fetlock flexural limb deformities in foals often respond to intravenous tetracycline injection combined with splinting, foot trimming, phenylbutazone, and a slow return to exercise. The recommended dosage of intravenous tetracycline is a single 3-gram dose that may be repeated in 24 hours if there has been no response to therapy.
    - **c. Treatment of the group** requires nutritional counseling and dietary management (supplementation or balancing). A balanced diet with adequate protein and good-quality roughage is extremely important in the growing animal. Injectable calcium, phosphorus, and vitamins may be considered.
- **7. Prevention** is based on the specific diagnosis but often centers on nutritional management.

III. LAMENESS

A. Lameness of cattle

1. **Foot rot (pasture foot rot, infectious pododermatitis, interdigital phlegmon, interdigital necrobacillosis).** The disease is sporadic, but up to 25% of cows may be affected per year, making this an important economic disease.

a. Patient profile and history
- **(1)** This is a contagious and relatively common condition that affects mainly **mature dairy cattle** that are on pasture or living in unsanitary housing conditions.
- **(2)** This disease is seen most commonly during **wet periods** and under management conditions that cause abrasions between the claws (e.g., stones, rough ground, sharp objects).

b. Clinical findings
- **(1)** There is the sudden appearance of **obvious foot lameness** almost exclusive to the **hind limb.** The cow's temperature ranges from 39°C to 40°C, with a loss of milk production, loss of condition, or both. The limb bears little weight.
- **(2)** **Heat, pain,** and **swelling** of the coronet and between the claws is obvious. On closer examination, the lesion is seen to be a fissure in the interdigital space. The fissure is moist, red, swollen, and has a characteristic foul odor. If left untreated, this fissure may progress to produce deeper involvement of soft tissues, bones, and joints. In these cases, there is more severe lameness with swelling higher in the leg.

c. Etiology. It is thought that injury or compromise to the skin of the interdigital space (e.g., constant moisture) predisposes the animal to infection by *Fusobacterium necrophorum.* Other bacteria may be involved or may occasionally be isolated (e.g., *Bacteroides melaninogenicus, Dichelobacter nodosus*), but these organisms are not a requirement for disease.

d. Diagnostic plan. The diagnosis is based on history and clinical findings of a moist, red fissure in the interdigital space.

e. Differential diagnoses that are usually ruled out by clinical examination include traumatic lesions, hoof growth abnormalities, laminitis, and stable foot rot.

f. Therapeutic plan. Parenteral antibiotics and local treatment of early lesions often achieve success.
- **(1)** **Procaine penicillin G** (22,000 IU/kg intramuscularly, twice daily for 3–5 days) is often the treatment of choice. Other broad-spectrum antibiotics may be used but are no more successful (remember milk withdrawal). Occasionally, a highly resistant strain of *F. necrophorum* may be encountered, which limits the success of therapy.
  - **(a)** Cows should be kept inside with dry footing until systemic therapy is complete.
  - **(b)** Non-milking cattle may respond to long-acting antibiotics to reduce the number of parenteral injections necessary.
- **(2)** **Local treatment.** The foot should be examined by rope lift, chute restraint, and chemical tranquilization. **Disinfectant creams** or **solutions** (e.g., copper sulfate-5% paste) may be applied following **thorough cleaning** and **debridement.** Bandaging usually is not necessary in uncomplicated cases.
- **(3)** **Surgery.** For deeper involvement of tissues (synovitis, tenosynovitis, arthritis, osteomyelitis), surgical therapy may be necessary.

g. Prevention
- **(1)** Employ **pasture modifications** if possible (e.g., rotate pastures more often, fill mud holes, remove sharp objects).
- **(2)** With **herd involvement,** provide a **foot bath** of a 5%–10% solution of formaldehyde and copper sulfate in an area where cattle must walk (e.g., doorway). Copper sulfate may be used alone. Animals may try to drink the solution, so restrict access. Alternatively, **dry lime** may be used in a walkway box to coat feet and decrease moisture and bacterial proliferation.
- **(3)** With **feedlot cattle,** the feeding of **chlortetracycline** or **ethylene-diamine dihydriodide (EDDI)** has been advocated with some empirical efficacy. However, with dairy animals, both antibiotic and iodide residues are a concern in milk.
- **(4)** **Commercial vaccines** are available but efficacy is yet unproven.

2. Stable foot rot (underrun sole)
- **a. Patient profile and history.** This condition occurs in cattle that are housed for

long periods (i.e., stanchioned cattle). It is associated with poor hygiene, and as in pasture foot rot, hind claws are more commonly affected.

    b. Clinical findings. The animal may be lame and tends to stand with the hind feet placed further behind than usual. Inspection of the plantar surface of the foot reveals necrosis and erosion of the heel and horn at the heel, as well as lateral hoof wall overgrowth over the sole.

    c. Etiology and pathogenesis

      (1) Etiology. Conformationally weak pasterns, overgrown hooves, or lesions caused by chronic laminitis may shift weight bearing to the heel, thus predisposing the animal to the condition. The lesion begins as heel necrosis from which ***Fusobacterium necrophorum*** can be isolated. ***Dichelobacter nodosus*** can also be recovered in some cases.

      (2) Pathogenesis. The heel necrosis and the change in hoof angle and foot placement causes the hoof to overgrow, which in turn traps debris and necrotic material between the hoof wall and sole. The separated sole, impacted debris, and necrosis of the sole cause lameness in advanced cases.

    d. Diagnostic plan. Clinical examination is sufficient for diagnosis.

    e. Therapeutic plan. Remove all abnormal horn via trimming, and restore normal conformation to the foot.

    f. Prevention. Regular foot trimming and nutritional counseling regarding laminitis are two of the primary preventive practices that may limit the incidence of disease. Foot baths and attention to dry-lot hygiene may help control the secondary invaders.

3. Sole ulcer (pododermatitis circumscripta)

    a. Patient profile. This condition most commonly is seen in stabled cattle, with hard flooring and diet being likely risk factors.

    b. Clinical findings

      (1) The **foot lesion** is a circumscribed ulcer on the sole, exposing corium. It is usually of the hind limb on the lateral claw at the heel–sole junction. If an ulcer is not obvious on initial examination, it may be exposed by trimming.

      (2) The **sole** overlying the lesion feels spongy. Granulation tissue may be seen extruding through the sole defect, and severe lameness is often present.

    c. Etiology and pathogenesis. The pathogenesis is still somewhat debatable, and although there may be an anatomical or mechanical predisposition of the lateral claw, a localized ischemia resulting from chronic laminitis may be the underlying cause of the condition.

    d. Diagnostic plan. The diagnosis is made by examination with careful attention to both hind feet.

    e. Therapeutic plan

      (1) Remove undermined sole with trimming, and pare away granulation tissue.

      (2) Medications such as an astringent powder may be considered in combination with a pressure bandage to control granulation tissue.

      (3) The unaffected claw (medial claw) may be **blocked up** to provide relief to the affected claw while the animal walks or stands. Commercial blocks or slippers are available for this purpose.

4. Digital dermatitis (hairy heel warts, strawberry foot rot)

    a. Patient profile and history. This worldwide disease was first described in North America in the early 1980s. It is now common with a high herd prevalence, particularly in dairy herds. **Milking cattle** are most commonly affected.

    b. Clinical findings

      (1) The **early lesion** of the foot is an interdigital roughness and reddening. This progresses to a red, papilloma-like lesion with erect hairs. The lesion usually is confined to the hind feet at the point of the cleft of the heels or up to the dewclaws. Further progression results in continued proliferation with a slimy or velvety appearance and the isolation of secondary bacterial organisms.

      (2) Lameness is not a constant feature, and it is assumed that any pain associated with the disease is sporadic.

    c. Etiology. A spirochete-like bacteria is associated with this disease, although its etiology is unproven. Reproduction of the condition has been unsuccessful. Because topical antibacterial solutions and antibiotics have proven somewhat successful in treating the condition, the bacterial cause has remained the most popular.

   d. **Diagnostic plan.** Diagnosis relies on the clinical findings and is based on observation of the lesion.
   e. **Therapeutic plan.** Because **lameness** is not always associated with the lesion, treatment of only lame cows is the most rational economic decision. Various **topical therapies** are used, including sprays containing **tetracycline** and **lincomycin.** Topical solutions may be paired with bandaging for best results.
   f. **Prevention.** In **herds** where the disease is prevalent, formalin, tetracycline, or lincomycin footbaths or sprays may be used as a preventive. The disease is thought to be transmissible, so practices that limit the introduction of infected cattle into uninfected herds are recommended.

5. **Laminitis (founder, diffuse aseptic pododermatitis)** is a diffuse, aseptic inflammation of the corium.
   a. **Patient profile and history.** Laminitis is a condition usually affecting **young dairy cattle** or **feedlot cattle.** This disease is seen occasionally in **older dairy animals** 2–3 months **after parturition** or **associated with periparturient diseases** (e.g., mastitis, metritis).
   b. **Clinical findings.** This disease is recognized in several forms. Subclinical laminitis is perhaps the most common form, but in the clinical sense, it is recognized as either acute or chronic.
      (1) **Acute laminitis** is seen sporadically in individual animals. Clinical signs of foot disease may be overshadowed by associated diseases.
         (a) There may be severe **lameness, stiffness,** and **pain** in any or all legs and a reluctance to walk. The cow may stand with an arched back, forelegs extended, and hind legs underneath. Recumbency is common.
         (b) There is **swelling** and **tenderness** of the heel bulbs and the coronary band. The sole may become soft, and trimming reveals subsolar hemorrhage and bruising.
      (2) **Chronic laminitis** is more prevalent than recorded. Signs are mild or unobserved (subclinical). Clinical signs occur mainly in the hind feet and consist of wide, flat, long, and misshapen feet. The pasterns and heels tend to drop. Trimming reveals hemorrhage at the white line, beneath the cranial sole, or both.
   c. **Etiology and pathogenesis.** The cause and pathogenesis is uncertain for any of the forms (acute or chronic, clinical or subclinical).
      (1) **Acute laminitis** is associated with an acute systemic disease or carbohydrate overload (ruminal acidosis). Hemodynamic and vascular changes occur, which decrease the blood supply to the laminae likely by the establishment of arteriovenous shunts. Laminar degeneration occurs, and the sensitive laminae of the third phalanx (P_3) separates from the interdigitating laminae of the hoof. Clinical signs and destructive lesions are not as severe as in horses, but pedal rotation may still occur.
      (2) **Chronic laminitis** is likely associated with heavy, interrupted feeding of diets high in grain. Chronic constrictive vascular lesions at the level of the laminae may cause blood stasis in the capillaries. This blood stasis results in stagnant hypoxia, which interferes with the production of keratohyalin and hoof growth.
   d. **Diagnostic plan.** The diagnosis is made based on history, clinical findings, and foot trimming to identify subsolar hemorrhages and to rule out other causes of foot lameness.
   e. **Therapeutic plan**
      (1) For **individual cases,** treat associated diseases, and consider the use of nonsteroidal anti-inflammatory drugs (NSAIDs) if cleared for use in the species of animal under care.
      (2) For **chronic cases,** the only treatment is trimming the affected feet, which is not usually warranted or practical.

f. Prevention
    (1) Affected cattle become more susceptible to chronic misshapen feet, thus requiring **frequent trimming.** Laminitis may predispose to other conditions (e.g., sole ulcer).
    (2) For **chronic laminitis** and **herd** or **feedlot problems,** the owner may have to **reduce feeding,** which affects herd production. A better alternative is to establish bunk management practices, which allow for more frequent feeding of smaller amounts of carbohydrates.

6. Other conditions
  a. Interdigital dermatitis
  b. Verrucose dermatitis
  c. Trauma
  d. Horizontal cracks
  e. Sand cracks

B. **Lameness of horses**

1. Thrush is a moist exudative dermatitis of the central and lateral sulci of the frog.
  a. Patient profile and history. Thrush is most common in adult horses that are kept in confinement under unhygienic conditions.
  b. Clinical findings. Soft, spongy, disintegrated frog horn is observed in advanced cases. This finding is accompanied by a characteristic fetid odor. Clinical cases are characterized by lameness and, if advanced, inflammation of the coronet and discharge of pus from fissures in the coronet and heels may be evident.
  c. Etiology and pathogenesis
    (1) *Fusobacterium necrophorum* is commonly isolated from foot lesions, but the pathogenesis is debatable.
    (2) **Unhygienic conditions, lack of exercise,** and **poor foot care** lead to accumulations of soil and fecal material in the hoof sulci.
    (3) **Lameness** may predispose to the condition by decreasing weight bearing and natural cleaning of the sole or by causing improper hoof growth. Infection is confined to superficial layers but will affect deeper tissue in untreated cases.
  d. Diagnostic plan. Diagnosis is based on clinical findings and the examination of the sole.
  e. Therapeutic plan
    (1) **Loose** and **necrotic material** must be pared away.
    (2) **Antiseptic products** (e.g., iodines, copper sulfate) should be administered daily.
    (3) **Bandaging** may be necessary.
  f. Prevention. Educate the client regarding proper hygiene, foot care, picking out the feet, and trimming. Correct any chronic lameness.

2. Laminitis is a local, inflammatory condition of the foot that is often a manifestation of a systemic disturbance.
  a. Patient profile and history. Equine laminitis occurs most commonly in ponies but can affect all horses and is more common in the spring. Overweight ponies on pasture, mares with retained placenta, and horses with acute systemic diseases are most susceptible to this disease.
  b. Clinical findings
    (1) **Acute laminitis.** Clinical signs may involve all feet, although the front feet are more commonly affected.
      (a) **Lameness** may develop rapidly. The horse shifts its weight onto the hind limbs (under its body), while front limbs are placed out in front. When forced to walk, the horse walks with short strides and places the feet down quickly. Recumbency is common.
      (b) **Affected hoof walls** feel warm, and a bounding digital pulse is felt. Pain is most prominent over the sole, as evidenced by hoof testers.
    (2) **Chronic laminitis.** The chronic form may be seen in individual limbs, particularly in overweight horses.

- **(a) Clinical signs** include recurrent bouts of variable lameness or of chronicity following the acute form.
- **(b)** Classic **hoof wall "rings"** are seen, and a dropped or flattened sole with a long toe develops.

(3) **Clinical description.** Lameness caused by laminitis has been graded according to the following scale:

- **(a) Obel grade 1**
  - **(i)** Foot discomfort without pain
  - **(ii)** A short and stilted gait at the trot
  - **(iii)** No lameness
- **(b) Obel grade 2**
  - **(i)** Some discomfort and lameness as evidenced by a stilted gait at the walk
  - **(ii)** Forefeet lifted without difficulty
- **(c) Obel grade 3**
  - **(i)** Reluctance to move
  - **(ii)** Resistance to lifting forefeet
- **(d) Obel grade 4.** The horse does not move without being forced.

(4) **Other clinical findings** associated with laminitis include a heel-to-toe placement while walking and recumbency. There may be additional clinical signs found with the associated systemic disease.

c. **Etiology and pathogenesis**
(1) **Etiology**
- **(a)** Diseases that produce **systemic disturbances** often result in laminitis. These diseases include **endometritis, salmonellosis,** and **colitis X.**
- **(b) Carbohydrate overload** is also a common cause of the condition.
- **(c) Predisposing factors** include:
  - **(i) Excessive trauma** resulting from concussive forces on hard surfaces (e.g., road founder)
  - **(ii) Excessive weight bearing** forced on a single limb after injury to the contralateral limb

(2) **Pathogenesis**
- **(a)** The condition may be **initiated** by events such as grain engorgement, toxic metritis, and septic shock, which may allow circulating endotoxins to initiate the **peripheral vascular response.** This vascular response (e.g., changes in vascular resistance) deprives the laminar corium of blood supply, resulting in separation of the sensitive laminae at the junction of P_3 and the hoof. In addition to vasoconstriction, there may be platelet aggregation, microthrombosis, perivascular edema, and arteriovenous shunting.
- **(b)** The effect is **most clinically apparent** at the distal aspect of P_3, which angles downward resulting in the characteristic radiographic evidence of **pedal rotation** seen with the disease. Also, **disseminated intravascular coagulation (DIC)** develops just before the lameness due to laminitis occurs, and corticosteroids are capable of inducing laminitis. These findings and the complexity of the disease discourages an overall accepted hypothesis from emerging.

d. **Diagnostic plan and laboratory tests**
(1) The **diagnosis** is often made based on the clinical signs and history.
(2) **Radiology** confirms changes to the angulation of P_3 and shows evidence of gross laminar degeneration. Radiographs should be taken early in the course of the condition and are used to monitor changes to P_3.

e. **Therapeutic plan**
(1) **Acute form.** Laminitis is an emergency. Treat any initiating disease (e.g., mineral oil for carbohydrate overeating, antibiotics for metritis). If **response to therapy** is not evident within 48 hours, a poor prognosis is warranted and therapy should intensify. With no response in 3–4 days, pedal bone rotation will have almost invariably occurred. Penetration of the sole may then follow, with resultant pedal osteitis or abscessation requiring heroic measures or euthanasia.

(a) Agents used for **pain relief** include:
   (i) **Phenylbutazone** 8.8 mg/kg (4.4 mg/kg in ponies and foals), which should be given immediately and continue for 4–5 days in decreasing doses
   (ii) **Flunixin meglumine** (1.1 mg/kg), which may be given as an anti-inflammatory or .25 mg/kg for its postulated anti-endotoxic activity
   (iii) **Aspirin** (10 mg/kg daily)
(b) Treatments used to **restore digital blood flow** include:
   (i) **Acepromazine,** which should be administered for its analgesic and α-adrenergic effects (40 mg every 4–6 hours)
   (ii) **Phenoxybenzamine** as an α-adrenergic antagonist (2 mg/kg every 12 hours)
   (iii) **Isoxsuprine hydrochloride,** which is used at a dose of .6 mg/kg twice daily
   (iv) **Dimethylsulfoxide (DMSO)** for its effects as a free radical scavenger, an anti-inflammatory, analgesic, vasodilator, and inhibitor of platelet aggregation
   (v) **Sodium heparin** at 44–66 IU/kg intravenously every 4 hours to prevent microvascular thrombosis
   (vi) **Nitroglycerine** (2% paste); 15–30 mg applied over each digital vessel daily, for a total dose of 30–60 mg. Alternatively, nitroglycerine patches may be used at the rate of 1 patch every 24 hours.
(c) **Nerve blocks** (posterior digital nerve desensitization) may be used to localize the pain to the feet.
(d) **Trimming** the foot and padding and supporting the sole can be effective and helpful. However, removing shoes during the acute episode may be painful. The use of local nerve blocks may help decrease the pain and resultant release of more vasoactive substances. Lowering the heels will help bring a rotated P_3 in better alignment with the ground but will also increase the tension on the deep digital flex or tendon. Therefore, this is a controversial practice.
(e) **Walking** the horse is controversial. Walking may promote blood flow but may further traumatize the sensitive laminae.
(f) **Dietary modification.** In the case of **carbohydrate engorgement** causing laminitis, feed only grass hay until clinical signs disappear.
(2) **Chronic form.** Chronic laminitis is expensive to treat in terms of labor and cost.
(a) **D-l methionine** has been advocated to restore disulfide bond substrate for maintenance of the hoof wall pedal bone bond. Attention to trimming and shoeing is necessary to provide support and allow for optimal hoof growth and foot conformation.
(b) **Hoof-wall resection** may be necessary to return more appropriate conformation and angle to the hoof wall.
f. Prognosis
(1) **Acute form.** P_3 rotation has been used as a prognostic indicator for return to function. If the rotation is greater than or equal to 11.5 degrees, there is an unfavorable prognosis. If the rotation is 6.8–11.5 degrees, the prognosis is guarded. Less than this, there is favorable prognosis for return to function.
(2) **Chronic form.** The long-term prognosis for return to function is very poor.
g. Prevention
(1) **Acute form.** To prevent the disease, discuss predisposing causes and dietary management. Make clients aware of the recurrent nature of the condition in some instances. Horses that recover should not be put back into work for a minimum of 45 days.
(2) **Chronic form.** To prevent the recurrence of chronic laminitis, maintain good dietary management, reduce weight in overweight horses, and consider the use of support pads.

C. **Infectious foot rot in sheep**
1. Patient profile and history
a. Infectious foot rot is a significant, production-limiting disease of sheep, but it may

also occur in goats. There is a species variability in susceptibility and a variation in incidence associated with climate and environment.

b. The disease occurs most commonly on pasture during **wet springs** or at times of persistent moisture. **Hot, dry conditions** are unfavorable for the spread of disease.

c. Foot rot is more common in areas with **heavy population pressures.** It may occur as outbreaks with up to **75% morbidity.** The disease is of economic importance because of the cost of treatment and loss of production.

2. Clinical findings

a. Early clinical signs include inflammation (moistness and swelling) of the interdigital space, a break at the skin–horn junction, and separation of the soft horn. Lameness is mild at this stage. The clinical condition progresses to severe lameness (non-weight bearing) with a foul odor. The horn becomes loose and sloughs, creating an underrun sole.

b. Virulent foot rot may exhibit systemic signs of fever and anorexia because the lesion extends to deeper tissue (osteomyelitis) with sloughing of the foot.

c. Intermediate foot rot has only moderate clinical signs.

d. Benign foot rot. Because there are various strains and serotypes of the causative organism (*Dichelobacter nodosus*), infection may occur with mild or no clinical signs. This form is called benign foot rot or footscald.

3. Etiology and pathogenesis

a. Etiology

(1) ***Dichelobacter nodosus,*** the causative organism, has varying virulence (proteolytic activity) and produces a variety of clinical signs (virulent, intermediate, benign).

(2) **Predisposing factors**

(a) ***Fusobacterium necrophorum*** causes an initial interdigital dermatitis, which may resolve as the pasture dries up. However, this infection may predispose for invasion by *D. nodosus.*

(b) **Trauma** (e.g., stones, strongyloides parasites) may be a predisposing factor to invasion by *D. nodosus.*

(c) During times of **moisture and warmth,** the bacteria more readily penetrate the skin of the interdigital space.

b. Pathogenesis

(1) **Route of infection.** *D. nodosus* invades horn by producing keratolytic enzymes. Discharges from affected feet serve as a source of infection for other sheep. The condition spreads rapidly.

(2) **Carriers.** *D. nodosus* does not persist on pasture but may do so for years in the feet of **carrier sheep.** Carrier sheep usually are not lame but may have misshapen feet and a pocket of infection beneath the underrun sole. Consequently, the disease may be introduced into a flock by the purchase of an infected animal.

4. Diagnostic plan and laboratory tests. It is important to diagnose the condition accurately because of the expensive and dedicated measures necessary to treat and eliminate the condition.

a. The **preliminary diagnosis** is based on clinical findings.

b. Bacterial cultures confirm the diagnosis but must agree with clinical and epidemiologic findings.

5. Differential diagnoses. Conditions that should be ruled out include foot abscesses, foreign bodies, granulomas, fibromas, trauma, contagious ecthyma, bluetongue, ulcerative dermatosis, strawberry foot rot (dermatophilosis), and laminitis.

6. Therapeutic plan. All forms of the disease respond to therapy, but the condition may be extremely difficult to eradicate. Treatment includes:

a. Trimming to expose necrotic sole

b. Applying local disinfectant (e.g., 5% formalin, 10% $ZnSO_4$, 5% $CuSO_4$)

c. Administering antibiotics (*D. nodosus* is susceptible to many antibiotics, and one treatment with penicillin is often all that is necessary if dry weather intervenes.)

d. Rechecking of feet if wet environment continues

7. **Prevention.** Eradication and control is the long-term goal when the disease has been diagnosed, but this is often difficult to achieve.
   a. **Eradication.** The **objective** is to cull or cure infected animals and return them to clean pastures. When sheep have been removed from contaminated pastures, these pastures can be considered free of *D. nodosus* after 14 days. The disease is best eradicated during the dry season.
   b. **Vaccination** is proving promising.

D. Caprine arthritis-encephalitis (CAE)

1. **Patient profile and history.** This disorder is common in **adult dairy goats** and is prevalent in North America, Europe, and Australia. It is common to have a high prevalence of serological conversion within a herd or population with a much lower expression of clinical signs.

2. **Clinical findings**
   a. **Enlarged carpal joints** (called **big knee)** are seen in goats older than 6 months of age. The onset of this arthritis may be acute or insidious, but lameness usually is not severe.
   b. There is **gradual weight loss** with the development of a **poor hair coat** and swollen joints. Terminally, there is emaciation and recumbency.
   c. **Other clinical findings** may include interstitial pneumonia or mastitis and development of a hard udder. The CAE virus also causes a leukoencephalitis in kids.

3. **Etiology and pathogenesis**
   a. **Etiology.** The etiologic agent is a **retrovirus** (subfamily lentivirus), which has similarities to the virus of **Maedi-visna.**
   b. **Pathogenesis**
      (1) This disease is **transmitted** to kids principally through milk and colostrum, although cross-infection can occur. Between 65% and 81% of the goats in most goat herds are seropositive to the CAE virus (CAEV).
      (2) CAE is a **multisystemic disease** involving synovial-like connective tissue. It is a lymphoproliferative disease caused by continual viral stimulation and the resultant immune response. This disease produces a hyperplastic synovitis.

4. **Diagnostic plan.** The diagnosis is based on history, clinical findings, and laboratory tests.

5. **Laboratory tests**
   a. **Synovial aspiration** yields a brownish red synovial fluid.
   b. **Cytologic evaluation** reveals a mononuclear reaction with high cell counts.
   c. An **agar gel immunodiffusion (AGID) test** and **enzyme-linked immunosorbent assay (ELISA)** on serum are positive.
   d. **Radiologic evidence** suggests soft tissue changes, which progress to proliferative bony changes.

6. **Differential diagnoses.** Clinicians should rule out other infectious causes for arthritis (e.g., *Mycoplasma, Chlamydia, Corynebacteria*).

7. **Therapeutic plan.** There is no known treatment.

8. **Prevention**
   a. **Total eradication** of CAEV from a goat herd is unlikely because vertical transmission does not seem to be the sole mode of spread and seroconversion may be delayed after exposure to the virus.
   b. To **decrease infection pressures** in the herd, identify infected animals through serology, and cull or house separately. **Separate kids at birth** and feed either colostrum from negative dams or pasteurized colostrum/milk. Because antibodies from positive animals are not protective, there is no need to feed colostrum from seropositive animals. Continue regular serological survey of the herd.

Directions: Each of the numbered items or incomplete statements in this section is followed by answers or by completions of the statement. Select the ONE numbered answer or completion that is BEST in each case.

1. Which statement regarding nutritional myopathies is true? They:

(1) do not occur in foals or mature ruminants.
(2) are subclinical in nature only and produce losses due to poor performance.
(3) may be caused by deficiencies of vitamin A.
(4) are most common in animals found in the arid interior of North America.
(5) produce high elevation in serum creatine phosphokinase (CPK) levels.

2. Mature dairy cattle recumbent for prolonged periods of time on a hard surface develop which one of the following disorders?

(1) Ischemic myopathy
(2) Milk fever
(3) Obturator paralysis
(4) Fat cow syndrome
(5) Blackleg

3. Which of the following terms are used interchangeably in swine?

(1) Blackleg, malignant edema, malignant hyperthermia
(2) Malignant hyperthermia, porcine stress syndrome, pale soft exudative pork
(3) Pale soft exudative pork, blackleg, malignant edema
(4) Porcine stress syndrome, malignant hyperthermia, malignant edema
(5) Blackleg, pale soft exudative pork, porcine stress syndrome

4. The best test to establish the carrier state of porcine stress syndrome is:

(1) test mating of suspect boars to suspect sows.
(2) serum ionized calcium concentrations.
(3) a gene probe for a C–T mutation.
(4) analysis of muscle biopsy for fast-twitch fibers.
(5) an adrenocorticotropic hormone (ACTH) stimulation test.

5. Which one of the following descriptions characterizes blackleg in cattle?

(1) Sudden death
(2) Chronic lameness
(3) The presence of a contaminated wound
(4) Overrepresentation in housed dairy cattle
(5) Resistance to herd level immunization

6. In young foals, the most common cause of osteomyelitis is:

(1) trauma inflicted by the mare.
(2) improperly placed vitamin injections.
(3) consuming mastitic milk from the mare.
(4) trauma during the foaling process.
(5) hematogenous spread of infectious organisms.

7. The organism most commonly associated with causing pasture foot rot in cattle is:

(1) *Dichelobacter nodosus.*
(2) *Actinobacillus pyogenes.*
(3) *Bacteroides melaninogenicus.*
(4) *Fusobacterium necrophorum.*
(5) *Staphylococcus intermedius.*

8. Examination of the left rear foot of a mature dairy cow reveals a red, papilloma-like lesion at the point of the heels. Which one of the following disorders is the most likely diagnosis?

(1) Pasture foot rot
(2) Hairy heel warts
(3) Laminitis
(4) Stable foot rot
(5) Benign foot rot

9. Laminitis in young dairy or beef cattle is considered to be associated with:

(1) *Fusobacterium necrophorum.*
(2) *Dichelobacter nodosus.*
(3) rumen acidosis.
(4) conformational defects.
(5) heredity.

10. Which statement best describes thrush in horses?

(1) An exudative dermatitis of the frog
(2) A yeast infection of the mouth
(3) A lymphangitis
(4) Laminitis
(5) Quarter cracks

11. Which one of the following statements regarding laminitis in horses is true?

(1) It seen most commonly in Draft breeds.
(2) The disorder is mainly a subclinical disease.
(3) Radiography best determines the diagnosis.
(4) Frequent walking of affected horses is the best treatment.
(5) It is a local manifestation in the foot of a systemic disturbance.

12. Which statement best describes infectious foot rot of sheep?

(1) It occurs most commonly in hot, dry environments.
(2) The disease is relatively simple to eradicate.
(3) It is the same as contagious ecthyma.
(4) This disease often responds to penicillin therapy.
(5) It causes lameness in carrier sheep.

13. Which one of the following statements regarding caprine arthritis-encephalitis (CAE) is true?

(1) The disease is not seen in North America.
(2) It demonstrates a high prevalence of seroconversion in affected herds.
(3) It is also known as mastitis, metritis, and agalactia syndrome.
(4) The disease produces a severe, sudden, debilitating lameness.
(5) Intra-articular antibiotics are the best treatment.

ANSWERS AND EXPLANATIONS

1. The answer is 5 [I A 1 5]. Creatine phosphokinase (CPK) is released from degenerating muscle cells and reaches very high (diagnostic) levels in the serum. Nutritional myopathies are caused by deficiencies of vitamin E and selenium. These myopathies occur in foals, lambs, calves, piglets, and mature ruminants. Disease is uncommon in the selenium-rich areas of the North American plains. Losses are most commonly caused by clinical disease.

2. The answer is 1 [I B 3 a]. Pressure necrosis and ischemic myopathy occur when large animals are recumbent on hard surfaces for extended periods. Milk fever and obturator paralysis may cause cows to become recumbent but are not the result of recumbency. Fat cow syndrome is a ketotic condition of obese cows, and blackleg is a clostridial myositis unrelated to recumbency.

3. The answer is 2 [I B 4]. These are different manifestations of the same inherited susceptibility for excessive skeletal muscle metabolism in swine. Blackleg and malignant edema are clostridial diseases of ruminants.

4. The answer is 3 [I B 4 g (2)]. Test matings have been replaced by a polymerase chain reaction gene probe and the other choices do not pertain to porcine stress syndrome.

5. The answer is 1 [I C 1 b (1)]. The most common presentation of blackleg in cattle is sudden death of growing beef animals on pasture. Wounds often are not present (as opposed to malignant edema), and immunization is preventive.

6. The answer is 5 [II A 3 b]. Although trauma may cause osteomyelitis, the most common cause is hematogenous spread from an infective process.

7. The answer is 4 [III A 1 c]. *Fusobacterium necrophorum* is a requirement for pasture foot rot (infectious pododermatitis) in cattle. Other organisms (e.g., *Bacteroides melaninogenicus, Dichelobacter nodosus*) may occasionally be

recovered but are not necessary for disease. *Actinobacillus pyogenes* and *Staphylococcus intermedius* do not cause foot rot.

8. The answer is 2 [III A 4 b]. The clinical findings support a diagnosis of hairy heel warts (digital dermatitis).

9. The answer is 3 [III A 5 c (1)]. Interrupted feeding of high-grain diets causes bouts of rumen acidosis. This is thought to initiate the systemic hemodynamic changes that result in laminitis.

10. The answer is 1 [III B 1]. Thrush is a disease of the foot of the horse. It is a moist dermatitis of the frog that emits a sour, foul odor. In advance cases, thrush may cause lameness.

11. The answer is 5 [III B 2]. Diseases such as salmonellosis and endometritis may result in laminitis. Although laminitis may be irreversible in severe cases, early, vigorous therapy is often successful. Laminitis is diagnosed best by clinical findings, although radiology helps to provide prognostic information in more longstanding cases. Walking is controversial as a therapy but should not be considered in severely lame horses. Although often a subclinical disease in cattle, the condition is more often clinical in horses.

12. The answer is 4 [III C 6]. The causative organism, *Dichelobacter nodosus,* causes the most significant clinical signs in affected sheep. The organism is susceptible to penicillin therapy. The disease occurs most commonly on pasture under conditions of moisture. Although straightforward to treat, this disease is difficult to eradicate because the organism is protected in the feet of carrier sheep. These carrier sheep are not lame.

13. The answer is 2 [III D 1]. Caprine arthritis-encephalitis (CAE) is prevalent across North America, Europe, and Australia. It produces a chronic, progressive arthritis, and there is no known treatment.

Chapter 14

Hematopoietic and Hemolymphatic Disorders

Christopher Cebra
Margaret Cebra

I. **ANEMIA.** Although anemia literally means "no blood," medically it refers to a state of inadequate oxygen transport by circulating hemoglobin. Anemia is rarely a primary disease and is usually a secondary problem related to trauma, infection, toxicosis, or another disease process.

A. **Clinical evaluation of anemia**

1. **Clinical findings**
   a. **History.** A complete history of the affected animal should be taken, including:
      (1) Anthelmintic and acaricidal treatments and risk factors for infestation
      (2) Drug treatments or exposure to toxins
      (3) Dietary history (e.g., exposure to toxic plants and minerals)
      (4) Frequency of erythrocyte parasites in the region
      (5) Hemorrhage or other illnesses
   b. **Clinical signs** generally include weakness, lethargy, exercise intolerance, pallor of mucous membranes, and a loss of prominence of retinal or scleral vessels.
      (1) **Chronic anemia.** Poor growth and peripheral and ventral edema may be seen with chronic anemia, particularly if there is concurrent protein loss.
      (2) **Severe anemia.** Exertion can lead to tachycardia and tachypnea with severe anemia. If anemia is accompanied by a decrease in blood volume, tachycardia and poor jugular filling are common.
   c. **Physical examination.** The following should be noted during the physical examination:
      (1) **Degree or presence of pallor**
      (2) **Degree or presence of icterus.** (It must be noted, however, that icterus can develop in the absence of hemolytic anemia—anoretic horses frequently develop icterus due to alterations in bilirubin metabolism, and animals with liver disease also may develop icterus without hemolytic anemia.)
      (3) **Urine discoloration. Red urine** can be caused by hematuria, hemoglobinuria, or myoglobinuria. **Dark urine** can result from these factors, as well as from a high bilirubin or methemoglobin content.
      (4) **Fever.** Often, animals with immune-mediated hemolysis and infectious conditions present with a fever. The absence of fever does not exclude these conditions.
      (5) **Signs of internal or external blood loss** (e.g., epistaxis, melena, hematuria, hematochezia)

2. **Classification of anemia.** Anemia can be classified by mechanism, regenerative response, red cell indices, and morphology.
   a. **Mechanisms.** There are four causes of anemia:
      (1) **Egress of red blood cells (RBCs) from the vasculature (i.e., hemorrhage)** can occur due to internal or external bleeding or parasitic ingestion. Peracute blood loss results in a **loss of intravascular volume** and possibly **hypovolemic shock.**
      (2) **Destruction of RBCs (hemolysis)**
         (a) **Intravascular hemolysis** occurs when damaged erythrocytes are lysed in the blood stream.
            (i) Intravascular hemolysis can occur with some infections and toxins, osmotic damage, or with immunoglobulin M (IgM)-mediated hemolysis.
            (ii) Free hemoglobin is released into the blood, resulting in **hemoglobinemia** and **hemoglobinuria** (red urine).

      (iii) Some hemoglobin is metabolized to **bilirubin,** causing **icterus** and **dark urine.**

      (iv) Free hemoglobin can lead to **secondary renal tubular necrosis.**

  (b) Extravascular hemolysis occurs when damaged erythrocytes are removed by the reticuloendothelial organs.

      (i) Oxidative damage to hemoglobin, membrane changes due to drugs or infectious agents, and antibody binding (IgG) to the erythrocyte membrane are the most common causes of extravascular hemolysis.

      (ii) Hemoglobin is metabolized by the reticuloendothelial cells to bilirubin and is not released into the peripheral blood.

      (iii) Hyperbilirubinemia leads to **jaundice** and **dark urine.**

(3) Impaired production of RBCs can result from the suppression of bone marrow activity or the replacement of hematopoietic stem cells. Examination of bone marrow cells should reveal:

  (a) A lack of hyperplasia of the precursor cells of the erythroid line

  (b) Possibly a lack of megakaryocytes and myeloid precursor cells

(4) Impaired oxygen-carrying capacity of RBCs is extremely rare in large animals, but it is seen in cows with erythropoietic porphyria.

b. Regenerative response. The body's reaction to anemia is to increase erythrocyte production and release by the erythroid stem cells in the marrow. The direct stimulus for increasing erythrocyte production is **erythropoietin,** which is released into the blood by renal tubular cells in response to hypoxemia.

(1) Anemia can be classified as **regenerative** or **nonregenerative,** depending on the effectiveness of the marrow response.

  (a) All anemias are initially nonregenerative, because it takes several days for marrow hyperplasia to occur.

  (b) A strong regenerative response is more common after acute blood loss or in the presence of hemolytic anemia. A regenerative response is less likely when the anemia is caused by impaired production or chronic disease.

(2) Evidence of a regenerative response varies among large animal species.

  (a) Ruminants and pigs can release large numbers of **reticulocytes** (i.e., large, immature erythrocytes) and other immature erythrocytes into the peripheral blood.

      (i) Immature erythrocytes are larger than mature cells, resulting in **anisocytosis** and **macrocytosis,** and contain less hemoglobin per unit volume, resulting in **hypochromasia.**

      (ii) The reticulocytes often contain DNA or RNA remnants, which are visible after staining as **polychromasia (basophilic stippling).**

      (iii) The reticulocyte count adjusted for anemia can be used to test the effectiveness of the regenerative response. The **adjusted reticulocyte count** is calculated and interpreted as shown in Table 14-1.

  (b) All large animal species should develop **hyperplasia of erythroid precursor cells in the bone marrow.** Lack of this reaction is strong evidence of a nonregenerative anemia.

  (c) An **increase in erythrocyte count over time** is the best evidence that regeneration is occurring.

TABLE 14-1. Calculating the Adjusted Reticulocyte Count

$$\frac{\text{Reticulocyte count}}{\text{Total erythrocyte count}} \times \frac{\text{PCV}}{\text{Mean PCV for species}} \times 100$$

A value of **2.0 or greater** indicates a **regenerative response.**
A value of **0.5 or less** indicates a **nonregenerative response.**
A value of **0.5–2.0** indicates an **early** or **impaired response.**

PCV = packed cell volume.

TABLE 14-2. Calculation of Red Cell Indices

$$\text{MCV (fL)} = \frac{\text{PCV} \times 10}{\text{Erythrocyte count (millions)}}$$

$$\text{MCH (pg)} = \frac{\text{Blood hemoglobin concentration (g)} \times 10}{\text{Erythrocyte count (millions)}}$$

$$\text{MCHC (g/dL)} = \frac{\text{Blood hemoglobin concentration (g/dL)} \times 100}{\text{PCV}}$$

MCH = mean corpuscular hemoglobin; MCHC = mean corpuscular hemoglobin concentration; MCV = mean corpuscular volume; PCV = packed cell volume.

c. **Red cell indices.** Calculation of the mean corpuscular volume (MCV), mean corpuscular hemoglobin (MCH), and mean corpuscular hemoglobin concentration (MCHC) aids in the classification of anemia (Table 14-2).
   (1) **MCV.** The MCV of small ruminants is typically half that of cattle or horses. **Normocytic, microcytic,** and **macrocytic** refer to normal, low, and high MCV, respectively.
      (a) **Microcytosis** occurs with **iron deficiency** and some immune-mediated hemolytic anemias.
      (b) **Macrocytosis** occurs with **maturation defects** (e.g., cobalt or vitamin B_{12}/folate deficiency, some systemic diseases) or the release of immature erythrocytes into the peripheral blood, which is a normal regenerative response to anemia (particularly anemia due to acute blood loss or hemolysis).
   (2) **MCH** decreases with most causes of anemia as a result of decreased erythrocyte count. MCH may increase artifactually with intravascular hemolysis because free hemoglobin in the blood is also measured.
   (3) **MCHC. Normochromic, hypochromic,** and **hyperchromic** refer to normal, low, and high MCHC, respectively.
      (a) **Normochromasia** is common with nonregenerative anemia.
      (b) **Hypochromasia** can accompany microcytosis (and low MCH) with iron deficiency or macrocytosis (with a normal to high MCH) with the release of immature erythrocytes into the blood as part of a regenerative response.
      (c) **Hyperchromasia** can occur with intravascular hemolysis due to the measurement of free hemoglobin in the blood.
d. **Morphology.** Microscopic examination of a blood smear can be used to describe the size, shape, and staining characteristics of erythrocytes.
   (1) **Reticulocytosis** occurs when reticulocytes are released into the blood as part of the regenerative response to anemia. Reticulocytosis is seen only in ruminants and pigs, never in horses.
   (2) **Anisocytosis** refers to cells of varying sizes in peripheral blood. **Mild anisocytosis** is common in ruminants, but **marked anisocytosis** (due to macrocytosis and reticulocytosis) is usually a sign of a regenerative response. Anisocytosis may also be seen after a transfusion if the host and donor erythrocytes are different sizes.
   (3) **Basophilic stippling (granulation)** in erythrocytes stained with Romanowsky stain is the result of DNA remnants. This stippling is seen as part of the regenerative response in cattle and with chronic lead toxicosis. **Howell-Jolly bodies** are similar dark-staining nuclear remnants that are normally seen in horse erythrocytes and, thus, are of little value in determining regenerative response.
   (4) **Spherocytosis** refers to small erythrocytes that lack central pallor. Spherocytosis usually results from partial removal of the red cell membrane by reticuloendothelial cells and often accompanies extravascular hemolysis. Spherocytes

are difficult to identify in large animals because of the small size of normal erythrocytes.

(5) Heinz bodies are aggregates of hemoglobin that have undergone oxidative denaturation. Heinz bodies are visible as refractile bodies when stained with Romanowsky stain or as round, darkly staining peripheral bodies within erythrocytes when stained with new methylene blue stain.

(6) Methemoglobin is formed when the **ferrous (2^+) iron** of hemoglobin is oxidized to its **ferric (3^+)** form. A small amount of methemoglobin is present normally and more is formed in some animals with oxidative injury (often in conjunction with Heinz body anemia). Methemoglobinemia and methemoglobinuria cause brown discoloration of the blood and urine, respectively.

(7) Erythrocyte aggregation can result from rouleaux formation or autoagglutination.

  (a) Rouleaux are normal in horses and dissipate when diluted with saline.

  (b) Autoagglutination is seen during inflammatory reactions and when erythrocytes are coated with antibody. Autoagglutinating erythrocytes do not disperse as readily with saline dilution.

3. Diagnostic plan and laboratory tests

  a. Blood work

   (1) Complete blood cell count (CBC) and morphologic examination. Anemia can be quantified by measuring the:

     (a) Packed cell volume (PCV). The PCV, the percentage of blood volume occupied by erythrocytes, can be determined by automated counter or centrifugation. Microcentrifugation may be necessary to adequately pack small ruminant erythrocytes.

     (b) Blood hemoglobin concentration

     (c) Blood erythrocyte count

     (d) Microcytic hypochromic anemia is suggestive of iron deficiency, whereas **macrocytic hypochromic anemia** is suggestive of a regenerative response (seen with acute blood loss or hemolysis). **Normocytic normochromic anemia** is seen before the regenerative response has started (2–4 days) or with nonregenerative anemia.

     (e) Anemia with **hypoproteinemia** is suggestive of acute blood loss, whereas anemia with **hyperproteinemia** is suggestive of an inflammatory reaction.

     (f) Agglutination may be seen. If not, a Coombs' test may be performed to test for antibody binding.

     (g) Erythrocytes should be examined for morphologic abnormalities, regenerative response, or parasites.

     (h) Yellow plasma is seen with hyperbilirubinemia, whereas **pink plasma** is seen with hemoglobinemia. Whole blood may be **dark brown** with severe methemoglobinemia.

   (2) Direct Coombs' test. Specific anti-immunoglobulin and anticomplement antibodies may be mixed with host erythrocytes. If host erythrocytes are coated with these factors, as often occurs with immune-mediated hemolysis, agglutination may occur. The test is usually performed at body temperature (warm agglutination) for IgG and below body temperature (cold agglutination) for IgM. A Coombs' test cannot be performed on blood that autoagglutinates.

   (3) Iron-binding capacity. Serum iron concentration and unbound iron-binding capacity can be measured. Both are low with anemia of chronic disease, whereas unbound iron-binding capacity is high with iron deficiency anemia.

  b. Fecal occult blood test detects the presence of blood peroxidase in feces and, therefore, helps identify gastrointestinal hemorrhage. Dietary factors in ruminants and small subclinical ulcerations affect the diagnostic value of this test. The sensitivity and specificity of this test has not been established for large animals. However, test results can be used to raise or lower clinical suspicion of gastrointestinal bleeding.

  c. Urinalysis

   (1) Urine sediment should be examined for erythrocytes. If hematuria is present, **urinary tract hemorrhage** may be the source of blood loss.

(2) Tests may be performed to differentiate **hemoglobin** from **myoglobin** in red urine. Hemoglobinuria is seen with hematuria or intravascular hemolysis.

(3) A high urine bilirubin concentration may be seen with **hemolysis** or **liver dysfunction** (or fasting in horses).

d. **Bone marrow examination** can be performed in order to examine the stem cell response to anemia. Because horses do not get reticulocytosis, cytologic examination of marrow is the best way to determine if anemia is regenerative. Hyperplasia of stem cell lines, particularly erythroid precursor cells, suggests a regenerative response.

B. **Acute blood loss anemia**

1. **Clinical findings.** Animals with rapid external blood loss may have obvious hemorrhage or ectoparasitism. With internal hemorrhage, the site of hemorrhage may not be obvious.

   a. Signs of anemia include **pale pink to white mucous membranes, disappearance of visible scleral vessels,** and **prolonged capillary refill times.**

   b. Animals with blood loss anemia also often have **tachycardia, weak pulses, poor jugular filling,** and **cold extremities.**

   c. Animals with poor organ perfusion become **weak** and **dull.**

2. **Etiology and pathogenesis**

   a. **Etiology.** Rapid loss of blood from the vascular compartment can occur internally or externally. Blood loss can be caused by the rupture of a large, blood-filled viscus (e.g., vessel, spleen, heart), thrombocytopenia, a clotting factor defect, bloodsucking parasites, or severe ulceration of an epithelial membrane.

   b. **Pathogenesis.** Decreased intravascular volume and hemoglobin content result in low cardiac output and poor tissue perfusion. Severely affected animals develop hypovolemic shock and may die.

3. **Diagnostic plan and laboratory tests**

   a. **Clinical findings** support a diagnosis of blood loss anemia, particularly when external hemorrhage is present.

   b. **Blood work**

      (1) **With peracute blood loss,** blood appears normal and has a normal PCV, total protein, and hemoglobin concentration.

      (2) **With acute, subacute, or chronic blood loss anemia,** blood appears thin and watery and has a low PCV, total protein, and hemoglobin concentration.

      (3) After a few days of blood loss, there should be evidence of a **regenerative response.**

4. **Therapeutic plan.** Treatment is dictated by the degree, rapidity, and severity of blood loss. Efforts should be made to correct the cause of blood loss. Less aggressive intervention is required with gradual blood loss because of the animal's ability to compensate.

   a. **Fresh whole blood** is the best treatment.

   b. **Isotonic** or **hypertonic fluids** should be given intravenously to restore vascular volume in patients with hypovolemic shock.

   c. **Stress** to the animal should be minimized.

C. **Chronic blood loss anemia**

1. **Clinical findings**

   a. Affected animals typically appear **unthrifty,** with **poor body condition** and **hair coats. Pallor of mucous membranes** may be present, but often is not remarkable.

   b. Animals with longstanding concurrent hypoproteinemia often develop **edema** of the ventrum and extremities.

   c. Severely affected animals are **weak** and **lethargic** and may die if stressed.

2. **Etiology.** Chronic blood loss can be caused by all of the causes of acute blood loss (see I B 2). **Parasitism** and **gastrointestinal mucosal ulceration** are the two most common causes in large animals. Because of the animal's ability to maintain circulatory

volume with chronic blood loss, hypovolemic shock is not seen. Clinical signs result from the decreased oxygen-carrying capacity of blood.

3. **Diagnostic plan and laboratory tests**
   a. **Blood work.** Determination of the **PCV** and **hemoglobin concentration** are necessary to diagnose chronic blood loss anemia. The **regenerative response** often is absent or poor, and there is occasionally hypochromasia and microcytosis compatible with **iron deficiency.**
   b. **Identifying the cause** of blood loss through **fecal examination** for endoparasites, **visual inspection** for ectoparasites, and **endoscopic examination** for gastric ulceration may be useful.

4. **Therapeutic plan.** Specific treatment for chronic blood loss anemia usually is not indicated. Iron supplements may be helpful. Efforts should focus on treating the cause of blood loss.

D. **Hemolytic anemia (HA)**

1. **HA of horses**
   a. **Infectious causes of HA**
      (1) **Babesiosis (piroplasmosis)**
         (a) **Clinical findings.** Fever and icterus are common findings with both causative organisms, whereas hemoglobinuria is more common with *Babesia equi* than with *Babesia caballi.* Generalized signs are seen with severe anemia and include weakness, anorexia, and depression. Eyelid swelling and naso-ocular discharges are common with severe disease.
         (b) **Etiology and pathogenesis**
            (i) **Etiology.** This disease is caused by the protozoan parasites *B. caballi* and *B. equi.* Both organisms are predominately found in tropical and subtropical areas but potentially can be found anywhere within the ranges of their host, ticks. Both organisms live within erythrocytes; *B. equi* also has a lymphocytic stage.
            (ii) **Pathogenesis.** *Babesia* species are spread by *Dermacentor, Hyalomma,* and *Rhipicephalus* ticks. Vertical transmission in ticks occurs with *B. caballi* but not with *B. equi.* The parasites cause both intra- and extravascular hemolysis, and most infected horses remain carriers for life.
         (c) **Diagnostic plan and laboratory tests.** Identification of *Babesia* in a blood smear examination from a horse with compatible clinical signs is diagnostic. *B. caballi* are large and pyriform, whereas *B. equi* piroplasms are small and rounded. Multiple organisms can be found inside a single erythrocyte, occasionally forming the "Maltese cross" shape with *B. equi.* Serologic tests are also available.
         (d) **Therapeutic plan. Imidocarb** is the drug of choice to treat equine babesiosis. High doses are needed to treat *B. equi* and to prevent the carrier state with *B. caballi.* High doses (4 mg/kg body weight) have been associated with colic signs and death, particularly in donkeys.
         (e) **Prevention.** There is no vaccine for equine babesiosis. Tick control is essential to prevent the spread of the organisms.
      (2) **Equine infectious anemia (EIA; swamp fever)**
         (a) **Patient profile.** EIA only infects horses and other Equidae, regardless of age, breed, or sex. The disease is found worldwide.
         (b) **Clinical findings.** The clinical and hematologic manifestations vary depending on the virulence of the virus, host resistance factors, and environmental stressors. Ninety percent of acute and subacute episodes occur within the first year of infection. **Recrudescence** of clinical signs may occur in association with corticosteroid administration, stressors (e.g., transport, heavy work), intercurrent disease, or adverse environmental factors. There are **three forms** of clinical disease:
            (i) **Acute form.** Clinical signs include intermittent fever, depression, pe-

techial hemorrhages, progressive weakness, weight loss, anemia, swelling of the legs, brisket and ventral abdomen, or sudden death.

(ii) Subacute to chronic form. Clinical signs include recurrent episodes of fever, depression, anemia, icterus, lymphadenopathy, petechial hemorrhages, edema, and weight loss. Occasionally, there are neurologic alterations. Clinical signs usually occur within the first few months after infection.

(iii) Chronic or inapparent form. There may be few clinical or hematologic signs. Occasionally, carrier animals have periodic fever or weight loss.

(c) Etiology. EIA is caused by a **lentivirus,** which is a nononcogenic retrovirus that infects cells of the immune system.

(d) Pathogenesis. EIA virus is host-specific and is transmitted from animal to animal through body fluids, particularly blood. Infected horses are carriers for life.

(i) Transmission. Contaminated needles, syringes, and **surgical** or **dental instruments** may spread the disease. **Horse flies** and **deer flies** can also transmit infected blood to uninfected horses. The chance of spread of EIA virus via arthropod transmission is dependent on the distance between infected and uninfected horses, the number of vector flies feeding on the horses, the amount of infected blood ingested, and other factors.

(ii) Viral life cycle. The virus multiplies in lymphoid tissues throughout the body within monocyte and macrophage cells. The virus elicits brisk humoral and cellular immune responses. It incorporates into the host genome and is disseminated throughout the body. The virus escapes the host's immunosurveillance by remaining intracellular and by altering its surface glycoproteins to appear unrecognizable to surface neutralizing antibodies.

(iii) Clinical manifestations. Many of the clinical manifestations of EIA infection are thought to be immune-mediated. Hepatitis, lymphadenopathy, and splenomegaly are caused by infiltrates of virus-infected mononuclear cells. Anemia results from the negative effects of the virus on hematopoiesis, viral hemagglutinin-mediated hemolysis and phagocytosis, and relative iron deficiency.

(e) Diagnostic plan and laboratory tests

(i) Clinical pathology. There may be a mild lymphocytosis and monocytosis during acute disease, but changes in the leukogram are inconsistent. Inapparent carriers may have a normal hemogram except for a marginally low erythrocyte count.

(ii) Agar-gel immunodiffusion (AGID, Coggins) test is a highly specific and accurate indication of EIA infection. Test results may be negative in the first 10–14 days of disease. **False-positive tests** may occur in foals born to infected dams because of the absorption of antibodies from the colostrum.

(iii) Competitive enzyme-linked immunosorbent assay (ELISA) is more sensitive but less specific than AGID.

(f) Therapeutic plan. There is no effective treatment for EIA. State and federal regulations require that infected horses be reported. Only seronegative horses can be moved between states and internationally for participation in equestrian events.

(g) Prevention. It is generally recommended (and may be required) to humanely destroy infected horses because even clinically normal chronic carrier horses pose a health risk to other horses. To avoid euthanasia, infected horses must be **separated** by at least 200 yards from healthy horses, and **strict insect control** must be practiced to ensure no transmission of disease. Strict attention to contaminated needles, syringes, or surgical instruments is also necessary.

b. **Immune-mediated causes of HA**
   (1) **Neonatal isoerythrolysis (NI)**
      (a) **Epidemiology.** In Thoroughbreds, NI occurs in approximately 1% of births. In Standardbreds, NI occurs in approximately 2% of births. The prevalence of NI is higher in mule foals (10%) because of the unique donkey erythrocyte antigen, which is present on donkey but not horse erythrocytes. Because mule foals are the product of a donkey sire and a horse dam, NI is possible in all such breedings, particularly if the dam has previously carried a mule foal.
      (b) **Clinical findings.** The severity of clinical signs appears to relate to the amount of colostrum absorbed; therefore, vigorous foals are often the most severely affected.
         (i) Foals are born healthy but develop progressive **lethargy** and **weakness** 24–36 hours postpartum after ingesting colostrum.
         (ii) **Mucous membranes** are initially pale and later become icteric.
         (iii) There may be **hemoglobinuria** and **hemoglobinemia** before death.
         (iv) **Other signs** include rapid, shallow breathing followed by labored breathing, tachycardia, excessive yawning, and seizure-like activity.
      (c) **Etiology and pathogenesis.** Coating of foal RBCs with maternal alloantibodies absorbed from colostrum causes RBC destruction.
         (i) **Blood group antigens.** This condition can occur whenever the sire and foal share a blood group antigen that is not present in the mare. The Aa and Qa blood group antigens, as well as a unique donkey blood group antigen, appear to be strongly immunogenic and are responsible for most cases of NI.
         (ii) **Exposure in the mare.** In order to have antibodies against these blood types in colostrum, the mare's blood must lack the antigen, and the mare must have been previously exposed to this antigen by blood transfusion, exposure to blood from a previous foal (usually sired by the same male) during parturition, or exposure to the foal's blood during gestation due to placental pathology.
         (iii) **Exposure in the foal.** When antibodies are absorbed from the colostrum into the foal's circulation, they attach to the foal's erythrocytes, leading to accelerated erythrocyte removal and destruction by reticuloendothelial cells.
      (d) **Diagnostic plan and laboratory tests**
         (i) **Clinical pathology** reveals anemia, hemoglobinemia, elevated bilirubin (mostly conjugated), and hemoglobinuria. Mule foals may also have thrombocytopenia. The leukogram should be evaluated to help eliminate sepsis as the cause of clinical signs.
         (ii) **Lytic** or **precipitation tests** detect antibodies in the colostrum or the mare's serum against the foal's whole erythrocytes. The **jaundice foal agglutination (JFA) test** is performed by mixing the mare's serum or colostrum with the foal's erythrocytes. Agglutination should occur with NI.
         (iii) **Direct Coombs' test.** This test also detects antibodies in the colostrum or the mare's serum against the foal's whole erythrocytes.
      (e) **Therapeutic plan**
         (i) **Blood transfusion.** If anemia becomes severe (i.e., when the PCV is less than 15% and decreasing over time), a whole blood transfusion should be considered. If the mare is used as the donor, all plasma must be removed by washing the mare's erythrocytes. Almost any horse's blood can be used for mule foals, but donkey blood should not be used. In general, horses that lack the Qa or Aa antigens or antibodies against them are the best donors.
         (ii) **Supportive care** includes intravenous fluids to maintain hydration, promote diuresis of hemoglobin, and correct electrolyte and acid–base imbalances. Efforts should be made to **minimize stress** and **restrict activity** until the foal's condition is stable.

      (iii) Immunosuppressive drugs are not effective against NI because the agglutinating antibody is exogenous.

    (f) Prevention includes:

      (i) Blood typing. Broodmares at risk for the development of NI can be identified by blood-typing. Any mare that is negative for either Aa or Qa antigen is at risk and should preferably only be bred with Aa- or Qa-negative stallions.

      (ii) Serum screening. If blood typing cannot be done before breeding or if a potentially incompatible match cannot be avoided, the mare's serum should be screened for the presence of antierythrocyte antibodies within 30 days of foaling. This is done by mixing the mare's serum with the stallion's erythrocytes and looking for agglutination. This test can be repeated closer to foaling if the results are equivocal. If the blood test is positive, a JFA test should be performed before allowing the foal to nurse. If the JFA test is positive, colostrum from another source should be provided to the foal, or antibodies should be supplied by plasma transfusion from a suitable donor. When the foal can no longer absorb colostral antibody (usually by 48 hours postpartum), the foal can be allowed to nurse from the mare.

(2) Immune-mediated HA

    (a) Clinical findings. Clinical signs, including fever and icterus, resemble those seen with parasitic immune-mediated hemolytic disorders (e.g., Babesiosis).

    (b) Etiology and pathogenesis. Host antibodies and complement may bind to host erythrocyte membranes. This may result in intravascular hemolysis but more commonly leads to erythrocyte phagocytosis or partial phagocytosis by reticuloendothelial cells (extravascular hemolysis). This antibody binding may occur for two reasons: the alteration of the RBC membrane or an overzealous immune response. Changes in the membrane are more common and can result from:

      (i) Intraerythrocyte parasites

      (ii) Chronic bacterial and viral infections

      (iii) Lymphosarcoma

      (iv) Disorders of immune function (e.g., systemic lupus erythematosus, neonatal isoerythrolysis)

      (v) Medications (particularly penicillin)

      (vi) Idiopathic causes

    (c) Diagnostic plan and laboratory tests. Spontaneous autoagglutination or a positive Coombs' test should be used to confirm immune-mediated hemolysis.

    (d) Differential diagnoses. Parasitic diseases and EIA should be ruled out by a blood film examination or serologic tests.

    (e) Therapeutic plan. All prior medications should be discontinued.

      (i) Immunosuppressive drugs. If an acute or chronic infectious condition can be ruled out, an immunosuppressive course of corticosteroids or cyclophosphamide can be initiated. The dosages of these drugs should be gradually reduced, and their administration should be discontinued within 1 month, if possible.

      (ii) If a noninfectious disease state (e.g., lymphosarcoma, systemic lupus erythematosus) is identified, **treatment of the primary disease** may result in the resolution of hemolysis.

      (iii) Infectious diseases should be treated with the appropriate drugs, but classes of drugs that may have precipitated hemolysis should be avoided.

      (iv) A **blood transfusion** is rarely necessary.

c. Toxic causes of HA

  (1) Oxidative injury (red maple leaf, onion, and phenothiazine toxicosis)

    (a) Patient profile. Red maple leaf toxicosis occurs in late summer and fall.

Any horse or pony is susceptible regardless of age, breed, or sex. Horses are less susceptible to onion toxicity than cattle, but they are more susceptible than sheep or goats. All horses are susceptible to phenothiazine toxicosis.

(b) **Clinical findings**
  (i) **Clinical signs.** Polypnea, tachycardia, weakness, depression, anorexia, and cyanosis are common. Death may occur in 4–6 days.
  (ii) **Fever** may be present during the hemolytic episode.
  (iii) A **brownish discoloration of blood** and **urine** may occur with red maple leaf toxicosis.

(c) **Etiology.** Ingestion of onions or wilted, dry red maple leaves or the administration of phenothiazine sedatives or anthelmintics can lead to severe, acute hemolytic anemia.

(d) **Pathogenesis.** Oxidative denaturation of hemoglobin by n-propyl disulfide (an alkaloid) from onions, by an unknown toxin in red maple leaves (*Acer rubrum*), and by phenothiazines results in the production of Heinz bodies within RBCs. Red maple leaf toxicosis also causes methemoglobinemia.
  (i) **Onion toxicity.** The alkaloid n-propyl disulfide depletes the intraerythrocytic enzyme, glucose 6-phosphate dehydrogenase, which maintains glutathione in its reduced state. When glutathione is oxidized, mixed disulfide linkages form between globin chains of hemoglobin and glutathione. These linked molecules precipitate within the cell, forming Heinz bodies.
  (ii) **Phenothiazines** are also strong oxidizing agents.
  (iii) **Red maple leaf toxicosis.** Erythrocytes containing Heinz bodies are removed from the circulation by the reticuloendothelial system (extravascular hemolysis), leading to anemia. With severe oxidative damage, some intravascular hemolysis can occur. There are two patterns of toxicity with red maple leaf toxicosis. The **peracute form** results from massive methemoglobinemia, causing marked tissue anoxia and sudden death. The **hemolytic form** is caused by continuous oxidative stress on RBCs, causing Heinz body anemia with subsequent intra- and extravascular hemolysis.

(e) **Diagnostic plan and laboratory tests**
  (i) **Clinical pathology.** Anemia is present with all three diseases. Spherocytes, Heinz bodies in peripheral blood, and elevated total bilirubin (mostly unconjugated) may also be seen. **High MCHC** and **MCH** values support the diagnosis of intravascular hemolysis. **Urinalysis** may reveal elevated protein and blood and the presence of hemoglobin, bilirubin, and urobilinogen. **Methemoglobinuria, methemoglobinemia,** and **low glutathione levels** should be found with red maple leaf toxicosis but should not be evident with the other two diseases.
  (ii) **Postmortem findings** include generalized icterus, petechiae and ecchymoses on serosal surfaces, and splenic engorgement. There may be a dark brown discoloration to the blood and tissues and changes in liver architecture. **Histopathologic findings** include the presence of hemoglobin, renal tubular casts and mild nephrosis, and extensive erythrophagia by macrophages.

(f) **Differential diagnoses.** Other causes of hemolysis or methemoglobinemia should be eliminated.

(g) **Therapeutic plan**
  (i) **Eliminate red maple leaves** or **onions** from the diet by moving the horse. **Discontinue** the use of **phenothiazines.**
  (ii) **Intravenous isotonic fluids** are useful for diuresis, the correction of dehydration, electrolyte depletions, and acid–base abnormalities.
  (iii) **Whole blood transfusion** may be necessary if the PCV is less than 12% and decreasing over time.
  (iv) **Dexamethasone** may help stabilize erythrocyte membranes and re-

duce the risk of a transfusion reaction. Steroids must be used with caution because they may lead to laminitis.

    (v) Ascorbic acid (125 mg/kg orally initially, followed by 50 mg/kg subcutaneously twice daily) has been used as an antioxidant for the treatment of red maple leaf toxicosis.

(2) Iatrogenic causes of HA. Several medications that are commonly administered to large animals cause hemolysis. Unless large amounts of the medication are administered, hemolysis is rarely clinically significant.

    (a) Hypotonic solutions can cause osmotic lysis of RBCs when administered intravenously.

    (b) Phenothiazine tranquilizers and **anthelmintics** cause oxidative injury to RBCs [see I D 1 c (1)].

    (c) Some concentrated drugs, notably **tetracycline** and **dimethylsulfoxide (DMSO),** cause hemolysis by an undescribed mechanism. To avoid this, these drugs should be diluted (less than 10% solution for DMSO) before intravenous administration.

2. HA of ruminants can also be categorized as intra- or extravascular. Each type leads to the characteristic abnormalities as discussed with horses (see I D 1).

  a. Infectious causes of HA

    (1) Anaplasmosis

      (a) Clinical findings are related to the immune-mediated loss of circulating erythrocyte mass. Calves under 1 year of age show few clinical signs. Severity of clinical disease increases with age, such that cattle older than 3 years often die of peracute disease. All of the following forms can occur in infected sheep and goats, but clinical disease is rare.

        (i) Acute anaplasmosis is common in young adult cattle. Anemia, fever, tachycardia, tachypnea, weakness, depression, and icterus are seen. Blood appears thin, and mucous membranes appear pale.

        (ii) Peracute anaplasmosis is more common in older cattle. Signs are similar to the acute disease, except that death often occurs before icterus develops.

        (iii) Chronic anaplasmosis can follow acute infection and is characterized by ill-thrift and decreased production. The animal becomes a reservoir for the infection of herd mates.

      (b) Etiology. The disease in cattle is caused by *Anaplasma marginale marginale* and *Anaplasma marginale centrale* of the order Rickettsiales. The disease in small ruminants is caused by *Anaplasma ovis.* These organisms are obligate intracellular parasites of erythrocytes.

      (c) Pathogenesis

        (i) Transmission. The organisms are spread by the passage of blood between animals. Chronically infected animals and wild ruminants act as reservoirs. **Argasid** and **ixodid ticks, biting flies,** and **veterinary instruments** are the most common means of transmission. Transmission is seasonal, based on the life cycle of the arthropod vectors. **Experimental transplacental transmission** has been documented.

        (ii) Disease progression. After an incubation period of 2–7 weeks, parasitized erythrocytes begin to be removed by the reticuloendothelial system. Immune-mediated extravascular hemolysis leads to anemia.

      (d) Diagnostic plan and laboratory tests. Because clinical signs are specific to hemolytic anemia but not anaplasmosis, laboratory tests can be used to confirm the diagnosis.

        (i) Blood smears reveal reticulocytosis, polychromasia, Howell-Jolly bodies, and basophilic stippling. *Anaplasma* may be visible on direct smear as refractile bodies or in Giemsa-stained smears as small, round, purple bodies. *A. marginale marginale* are located at the periphery of erythrocytes, whereas *A. marginale centrale* are located toward the center.

        (ii) Serologic tests and DNA probes. Chronically infected animals have fewer visible rickettsia and may be better diagnosed by serologic tests or DNA probes.

- **(e) Therapeutic plan.** The three considerations of treatment include the resolution of acute parasitemia, maintenance of organ perfusion, and prevention of the carrier state.
  - **(i) Oral chlortetracycline** and **parenteral oxytetracycline** are the most commonly used drugs to treat acute or chronic infection. Low concentrations of a tetracycline (usually chlortetracycline) added to the feed or water can be used to reduce morbidity during periods of high transmission in endemic areas. Higher doses or longer treatment courses are required to eliminate infection.
  - **(ii)** Although **fluids** or **blood transfusions** can be used to maintain organ perfusion, these treatments are usually impractical.
  - **(iii)** Efforts should be made to **minimize stress** and **exertion** of severely affected cattle until parasitemia is reduced and circulating erythrocyte mass has been restored.
- **(f) Prevention.** The control of vectors, reduction of parasitemia through the continuous use of antimicrobial drugs, elimination of the carrier state, or vaccination can be used to reduce the losses caused by anaplasmosis.

(2) Babesiosis (piroplasmosis) has been eradicated from North America.
- **(a) Patient profile.** Cattle, goats, sheep, and swine may be affected.
  - **(i)** Cattle of all ages are susceptible to this disease, although calves between the ages of 2 and 9 months appear to be resistant. Offspring of exposed dams are protected against clinical disease by colostral antibody during the neonatal period. Exposed calves develop long-lasting resistance to clinical babesiosis.
  - **(ii)** *Bos indicus* cattle and their calves appear to be more resistant than other cattle.
- **(b) Clinical findings**
  - **(i) Clinical signs. Fever** often is present for several days before other signs appear. **Anemia, depression, tachycardia, icterus,** and **weakness** are common. **Hemoglobinuria** helps distinguish babesiosis from diseases characterized by extravascular hemolysis (e.g., anaplasmosis). **Neurologic signs** (e.g., convulsions, somnolence) are common in the hours before death.
  - **(ii) Necropsy lesions.** With anoxic organ damage, severe disease ensues, and death is common. Necropsy lesions include icterus and dark, swollen internal organs.
- **(c) Etiology.** The disease is caused by protozoan parasites of the species *Babesia*. *Babesia bigemina* and *Babesia bovis* are the main pathogenic species. These organisms are obligate intracellular parasites of erythrocytes.
- **(d) Pathogenesis**
  - **(i) Transmission** between animals is by ticks. *Boophilus* species and *Ixodes ricinus* are the most important tick vectors. Transovarial transmission to the next generation of ticks plays a major role in the transmission to cattle.
  - **(ii)** After an **incubation period** of 2–3 weeks, the number of parasites can increase enough to become clinically relevant. Intraerythrocyte parasitism leads to intravascular hemolysis with hemoglobinemia and hemoglobinuria ("redwater"). Babesia also releases toxins that cause vasodilation, increased vascular permeability, and erythrocyte aggregation. These effects on the vasculature impair circulation, leading to tissue hypoxia and necrosis. Renal damage also results from exposure to hemoglobin.
- **(e) Diagnostic plan and laboratory tests.** Clinical signs and necropsy lesions often are adequate to diagnose babesiosis in an endemic area.
  - **(i) Hemogram evaluation** should reveal anemia with evidence of a regenerative response.
  - **(ii)** The parasites can be seen on **Giemsa-stained smears** and are seen as

single or paired large ovoid or pyriform organisms within erythrocytes. Organisms are more readily seen on smears of peripheral blood (as opposed to jugular blood).

    (iii) Serologic tests are also available.

  (f) Therapeutic plan and prevention. A variety of babesiocides are available for the treatment of clinical disease. These include **imidocarb, diminazene, phenamidine,** and **amicarbalide.** Imidocarb and diminazene can also be used for short-term prophylaxis. Any treatment or prevention protocol should include provisions for tick control.

(3) Eperythrozoonosis. *Eperythrozoon* species, rickettsial parasites, are similar to *Anaplasma* because these organisms stimulate immune-mediated hemolysis. There are two principal species that affect ruminants and a third that affects pigs.

  (a) *Eperythrozoon wenyoni*

    (i) Patient profile. Cows of all ages appear to be susceptible to infection by this organism.

    (ii) Clinical findings. Affected cattle typically have transient fever, lymphadenopathy, depression, and decreased milk production. Swelling of the udder and hind legs is common in dairy cattle. Icterus is uncommon and mild when present.

    (iii) Etiology. Although arthropod vectors are suspected, this has not been proven. Most infections appear to result in minimal clinical disease, but some cattle show clinical signs of inflammation and hemolytic anemia similar to those seen with acute anaplasmosis. Chronic infections and a subclinical carrier state are thought to occur.

    (iv) Diagnostic plan and laboratory tests. Diagnosis is made by identifying the parasite on a peripheral blood smear examination. The organism is small, frequently round (but occurs in a variety of shapes), and found within erythrocytes. The organism may be seen singly, in clumps, or in a ring form. The ring form, together with a relatively large number of free organisms in blood, helps differentiate this disease from anaplasmosis.

    (v) Therapeutic plan. Clinical signs usually resolve spontaneously in 7–10 days, except in immunocompromised or splenectomized cattle. More rapid resolution is seen after the administration of a single dose of a **long-acting oxytetracycline** or a 3-day course of a **short-acting oxytetracycline.**

  (b) *Eperythrozoon ovis*

    (i) Patient profile. All ages of sheep appear to be susceptible to this organism, but clinical disease is most common in young animals.

    (ii) Clinical findings. Fever, depression, weakness, icterus, and hemoglobinuria are seen with severe disease. The more common manifestation is ill-thrift syndrome in lambs. Affected lambs grow poorly, have poor hair coats and pot bellies, and are easily stressed by exertion.

    (iii) Etiology and pathogenesis. Other pathogens have been isolated from sheep with ill-thrift syndrome, so *E. ovis* is only one of several possible etiologic agents. Ticks, keds, and mosquitos are thought to be important vectors. Similar to *E. wenyoni* in cattle, *E. ovis* infection is thought to result in minimal clinical disease in most affected sheep. However, hemolytic anemia and the inflammatory response appear to cause morbidity and mortality in some sheep.

    (iv) Diagnostic plan and laboratory tests. Similar to *E. wenyoni* infection in cattle, the diagnosis is made by identifying round or pleomorphic organisms both within plasma and erythrocytes. Clumps, crosses, and rings are a common finding.

    (v) Therapeutic plan. Oxytetracyclines are probably the best drugs to treat this infection. Other drugs have been used with mixed results. In some cases, treatment failure may result from failure to identify another primary pathogen.

(4) Leptospirosis

(a) Clinical findings and diagnostic plan. Leptospires are slender spirochetes that require special laboratory techniques to stain and detect. Leptospires may be identified in body fluids (usually urine) by dark-field microscopy, immunofluorescence, or DNA hybridization. Single high (greater than or equal to 100:1 dilution) or a fourfold increase in paired samples on the microscopic agglutination tests are considered diagnostic.

(b) Etiology. Clinical disease is caused by serovars of *Leptospira interrogans*. Serovars *hardjo* and *kennewicki* (formerly *pomona*) are responsible for disease in ruminants.

(c) Pathogenesis. A maintenance host (cattle for variant *hardjo*; wild mammals for variant *kennewicki*) infects moist soil and pools of water. The organism may be ingested or penetrate intact skin. Acute disease coincides with the subsequent leptospiremia. Among other pathogenic mechanisms, cold-agglutinating IgM attaches to host erythrocytes, leading to intravascular hemolysis.

(d) Therapeutic plan. Intravenous fluid therapy should be initiated. Patients may require treatment for acute renal failure (see Chapter 15), disseminated intravascular coagulation [DIC; see II B 3 b (5)], or both. Antibiotic therapy includes penicillin initially, followed by dihydrostreptomycin or tetracycline therapy when renal function has returned to normal.

(5) Bacillary hemoglobinuria is very similar to Black's disease (see Chapter 5 III A 3).

(a) Clinical findings. Affected ruminants often are found dead due to peracute disease. Other affected animals are extremely depressed, walk with hunched backs, and are very sensitive to abdominal palpation. Normal bodily functions are reduced or absent. Tachycardia, tachypnea, and fever are common. Animals that survive more than 1 day may have icterus and hemoglobinuria, and icteric tissues are commonly found on postmortem examination.

(b) Etiology and pathogenesis. *Clostridium hemolyticum* is a large, spore-forming, gram-positive anaerobic rod. Spores survive in the environment for a long time, are ingested or inhaled, and are transported to the liver of ruminants. With hepatic injury, commonly due to fluke migration, spores germinate. Mature bacteria produce exotoxins, which cause local necrosis and intravascular hemolysis.

(c) Diagnostic plan and laboratory tests. Postmortem examination, revealing severe hepatic necrosis with infarcts, hemorrhagic exudates, and subcutaneous edema, is strongly suggestive of this disease. The organism may be found by bacteriologic culture or impression smear of liver lesions. Hemoglobinuria should be present.

(d) Therapeutic plan. Treatment is rarely rewarding. If pursued, treatment should consist of large doses of penicillin and supportive care.

(e) Prevention. Vaccination with clostridial toxoids and fluke prevention are both efficacious in preventing this disease.

(6) Yellow lamb disease

(a) Patient profile. This hemolytic disease has only been identified in lambs.

(b) Clinical findings. Affected lambs are depressed, weak, and often in distress. Anemia, icterus, and hemoglobinuria are common.

(c) Etiology and pathogenesis

(i) Etiology. *Clostridium perfringens* type A, the causative agent, is a large, spore-forming, gram-positive anaerobic rod. Spores survive for long periods in the soil, and the organism may inhabit the gut of healthy animals.

(ii) Pathogenesis. The organism proliferates in the gut and releases exotoxins. One of these exotoxins, the α-toxin, causes vasculitis and intravascular hemolysis due to phospholipase activity.

(d) Therapeutic plan. Most affected lambs die within 12 hours of the onset of clinical signs. Treatment with large doses of penicillin and supportive care can be attempted.

(e) **Prevention.** There is no toxoid useful in preventing this disease.

b. **Immune-mediated causes of HA**

(1) **NI**

(a) **Patient profile.** NI does not occur without human intervention in cattle, sheep, or goats. There is no breed or sex predisposition.

(b) **Clinical findings.** Clinical signs usually develop within 24–36 hours postpartum. Sudden loss of appetite and weakness are seen. Death usually occurs within 24 hours. The animal may show anemia, tachycardia, and rapid or shallow breathing, which progresses to labored breathing.

(c) **Etiology.** This immune-mediated RBC destruction in neonates is associated with the ingestion of colostrum containing antibodies to the neonates' erythrocytes.

(d) **Pathogenesis.** Blood transfusion or the administration of whole erythrocyte vaccines (such as those against anaplasmosis and babesiosis) to breeding females may sensitize the dam to certain blood groups, most commonly in the A and F systems. If the blood types of the sire and offspring contain these antigens and the dam has produced alloantibodies against them, an immune-mediated hemolytic crisis may appear in the calf associated with successful passive transfer.

(e) **Diagnostic plan and laboratory tests**

(i) **Clinical pathology** reveals a low PCV, hypoproteinemia, and high (conjugated) bilirubin. In sheep, NI may be more of an extravascular hemolysis.

(ii) A **direct Coombs' test** should be performed.

(f) **Therapeutic plan.** Treatment consists of blood transfusions or intravenous fluids.

(2) **Bovine colostrum fed to sheep**

(a) **Patient profile.** Disease is usually seen in lambs between the ages of 7 and 21 days that are fed bovine colostrum. No sex or breed predisposition has been reported.

(b) **Clinical findings.** Clinical signs include a sudden loss of appetite and weakness, without evidence of icterus or hemoglobinuria. Death may occur in less than 24 hours.

(c) **Etiology.** Immune-mediated destruction of sheep RBCs may occur because of antibodies directed against sheep blood group antigens, which are present in bovine colostrum.

(d) **Pathogenesis.** The presence of antibodies to sheep blood group antigens in bovine colostrum is a common occurrence. These antibodies are called "heterophile antibodies" and result from the production of antibodies to common cross-reactive antigens that are present on the surfaces of bacteria and protozoa. When bovine colostrum is fed to lambs, these antibodies bind to sheep RBCs and lead to extravascular destruction.

(e) **Diagnostic plan and laboratory tests**

(i) A **direct Coombs' test** with anti-sheep immunoglobulin and anti-bovine immunoglobulin may demonstrate immunoglobulin on the surface of RBCs.

(ii) **Direct immunofluorescence** may also demonstrate antibodies.

(iii) **Clinical pathology** reveals anemia, hypoproteinemia, icteric plasma, and hyperbilirubinemia (73% unconjugated). Hemoglobinemia or hemoglobinuria are usually not seen.

(f) **Therapeutic plan.** Whole blood transfusions or intravenous fluids may be necessary.

c. **Toxic causes of HA**

(1) *Brassica* **species plants (e.g., kale, canola)**

(a) **Patient profile.** Cattle appear to be more sensitive to *Brassica* plants than horses or small ruminants.

(b) **Clinical findings.** The severity of clinical signs relates to the duration and dose of feeding the toxin. Because oxidant damage to erythrocytes usually results in extravascular hemolysis, only cows with a concomitant disease, which increases erythrocyte fragility (postparturient hemoglobinuria), should have intravascular hemolysis and hemoglobinuria.

- (i) Most affected animals exhibit **pallor, weakness, decreased milk production, dark urine,** and mild to moderate **icterus.**
- (ii) **Neurologic signs** and **pulmonary emphysema** are seen occasionally in cows fed *Brassica* plants, but the mechanism is unknown.

(c) **Etiology and pathogenesis**
- (i) The **toxin content** of *Brassica* plants increases as these plants mature but is destroyed by heating or ensilage. Feeding these plants worsens the hemolytic crisis seen with postparturient hemoglobinuria [see I D 2 d (2)].
- (ii) *Brassica* plants contain **S-methyl cysteine sulfoxide,** which is metabolized by rumen bacteria to dimethyl disulfide. This toxin decreases the activity of glutathione within erythrocytes, allowing disulfide bonds to form between hemoglobin chains, resulting in Heinz body formation. As erythrocytes containing Heinz bodies are removed by the reticuloendothelial system, anemia develops.

(d) **Diagnostic plan and laboratory tests.** Feeding history, clinical signs, and the identification of Heinz-body anemia are critical to making a diagnosis. Dimethyl disulfide concentration in blood or rumen fluid can be measured using gas chromatography.

(e) **Therapeutic plan.** The removal of animals from the feed and blood transfusions for severely affected animals are the only treatments.

(2) **Onion**
(a) **Patient profile and history.** Cattle appear to be more sensitive to onions than other farm animals. History of exposure to onions is important in establishing a diagnosis.
(b) **Clinical findings.** Affected animals can develop clinical signs within 1 week of being fed an all-onion diet.
(c) **Pathogenesis.** The toxic principle of onions is n-propyl disulfide, which causes Heinz-body anemia by the same mechanism as *Brassica* plants [see I D 2 c (1)]. S-methyl cysteine sulfoxide has also been reported to be found in onions.
(d) **Therapeutic plan.** Treatment is the same as that for *Brassica* toxicosis [see I D 2 c (1) (e)].
(e) **Prevention.** Clinical disease can be prevented by mixing onions with other feedstuffs so that onions compose less than 25% of the dry matter of the ration. However, cattle fed as little as 5% onions have laboratory evidence of HA.

(3) **Copper**
(a) **Clinical findings.** Severely affected animals have icterus, hemoglobinuria, weakness, and thin, watery blood. Vomiting and sudden death may also be observed. If mucous membranes are not severely jaundiced, pallor may be seen.
(b) **Etiology and pathogenesis.** Ingestion or injection of a toxic dose of copper can precipitate an acute episode of intravascular hemolysis. A similar syndrome is seen in animals that are chronically overfed copper. It is thought in this latter circumstance that hepatic saturation or another stress leads to the massive release of liver copper stores into the blood.
(c) **Diagnostic plan and laboratory tests.** Feeding or treatment history and clinical signs are strongly suggestive of this disease. For confirmation, copper concentrations in blood, liver, and feed can be determined.
(d) **Therapeutic plan.** Except for supportive care, most treatments for copper toxicosis are experimental.

(4) **Nitrate and nitrite toxicosis**
(a) **Clinical findings**
- (i) **Acute toxicosis.** Clinical signs of acute nitrite toxicosis begin within

6 hours of ingestion of toxic feedstuffs. Animals display **signs compatible with severe anoxia,** including weakness, depression, cyanosis, and tachycardia. Animals die if 60%–75% of hemoglobin is oxidized to methemoglobin (this usually occurs within 24 hours of ingestion). **Gastrointestinal signs** include salivation, diarrhea, and vomiting.

    (ii) Chronic toxicosis has been blamed for abortion and an increased vitamin A requirement.

(b) Etiology. Cereal crops, *Astragalus* plants, other plants, and deep water wells may accumulate nitrate, particularly in areas where nitrogenous fertilizers are used heavily.

(c) Pathogenesis. Nitrate is reduced to nitrite in the rumen. Heat may also reduce nitrate, so that hay stacked in strong sunlight or heat-prepared feedstuffs may contain nitrites and cause toxicosis in nonruminants. Absorbed nitrite oxidizes hemoglobin to methemoglobin and causes mild vasodilation. These effects result in tissue anoxia and hemolysis. Nitrates also cause gastroenteritis.

(d) Diagnostic plan and laboratory tests

    (i) Clinical findings, history of exposure to nitrate-accumulating plants, and **inspection of blood** for methemoglobinemia are strongly suggestive of the disease.

    (ii) A **diphenylamine test** can be performed on blood, urine, or feed (the inside of the plant stalk or root is best) to detect toxic nitrate levels. Tests on animal tissue must be performed quickly because nitrite is converted to other compounds.

(e) Therapeutic plan. Methylene blue (1% solution) can be given to reduce methemoglobin to hemoglobin. A single treatment (1–2 mg/kg of body weight given intravenously) is usually sufficient in nonruminants, whereas higher doses (up to 20 mg/kg) and repeated dosing (every 8 hours) may be necessary in ruminants that have ingested large quantities of nitrates.

d. Other causes of HA

  (1) Water intoxication

    (a) Clinical findings. This is primarily a neurologic disease. Affected animals show apparent blindness, a staggering gait, dullness, and head pressing. Severely affected animals often have seizures and become comatose. Hemoglobinuria is seen in some cases.

    (b) Etiology. Water intoxication occurs when free access to water is allowed after a period of deprivation. The condition is more severe if the animal has become dehydrated or is fed a high-sodium diet.

    (c) Pathogenesis. With water deprivation, there is a gradual increase in the plasma sodium concentration due to insensitive water loss and an inability to excrete excess ingested salt. There is also a gradual increase in the sodium concentration in the brain and cerebrospinal fluid (CSF), although this occurs slowly because of the relative impermeability of the blood–brain barrier to sodium. When the animal is re-exposed to water, a rapid drop in plasma osmolality can cause osmotic lysis of RBCs and rapid transfer of free water into the brain. These result in intravascular hemolysis and cerebral edema, which lead to hemoglobinuria and neurologic signs, respectively.

    (d) Diagnostic plan and laboratory tests. Information concerning diet and access to water helps confirm a diagnosis of water intoxication. Hemoglobinuria and the detection of a substantially higher CSF sodium concentration are also of diagnostic value. (There is usually a 10 mEq/L difference between the CSF sodium concentration and the plasma sodium concentration.)

    (e) Therapeutic plan

      (i) Treatment of **comatose** and **seizing animals** is rarely successful.

      (ii) In less severely affected animals, the goal is to normalize the plasma and CSF sodium concentrations without causing rapid shifts in water. This can be accomplished through limited access to free water and slow administration of intravenous fluids. Fluids containing sodium concentrations close to that in normal plasma are preferable to 0.45% sodium chloride solutions. Administration of full-strength solutions are less likely to cause pathologic rapid decreases in plasma osmolality.

(2) Postparturient hemoglobinuria

(a) Patient profile. Cattle in the first 6 weeks of lactation are most susceptible. Herd outbreaks can occur, although the disease usually affects single cows.

(b) Clinical findings. Affected cattle have red urine, pale mucous membranes, absent scleral vessels, tachycardia, tachypnea, weakness, and decreased milk production. Clinical signs last several days, and icterus may be seen toward the end of the disease course. Tissue anoxia or renal damage can cause death.

(c) Etiology and pathogenesis

(i) Etiology. The cause of this disorder is unknown and may differ in different parts of the world.

(ii) Pathogenesis. Increased erythrocyte fragility in postpartum dairy cows leads to intravascular hemolysis, anemia, and hemoglobinuria. In **North America,** hypophosphatemia is thought to impair function of the Na^+/K^+ pump, causing erythrocyte lysis. In **New Zealand,** hypocupremia is thought to make erythrocytes more sensitive to the hemolyzing activity of oxidant-containing plants.

(d) Diagnostic plan and laboratory tests. Clinical findings aid in the diagnosis. Laboratory tests can be used to confirm hemoglobinuria and to investigate underlying mineral deficiencies.

(e) Therapeutic plan

(i) Blood transfusion. Severely affected animals should be transfused with fresh whole blood.

(ii) Fluids. If blood is unavailable, **crystalloid fluids** can be used to increase cardiac output and protect the kidneys against the toxic effects of hemoglobin.

(iii) Phosphorus or **copper supplements** can be administered, if indicated, and efforts should be made to avoid feeding oxidant-containing plants.

(3) Inherited congenital porphyria

(a) Clinical findings. Plasma and urine from affected animals are red or reddish brown. Photosensitization of unpigmented skin occurs in cattle exposed to direct sunlight. Teeth and bones may have a pink or brown discoloration and fluoresce red on exposure to ultraviolet (UV) light.

(b) Etiology and pathogenesis. Congenital porphyria appears to be an autosomal recessive defect of cattle. Similar diseases in people are caused by the insufficiency of an enzyme in the pathway of heme synthesis. As a result, hemoglobin synthesis and RBC maturation are impaired, and porphyrins accumulate in body fluids and tissues. Anemia results both from impaired erythrocyte production and hemolysis. Porphyrin pigments are red or brown and act as photosensitizing agents.

(c) Diagnostic plan and laboratory tests. Clinical features are strongly suggestive of this disease.

(i) Histopathologic examination of bones and teeth reveals large amounts of porphyrin pigments. Porphyrin pigments may be identified in urine by **spectroscopic examination.**

(ii) Anemia is usually characterized by **macrocytosis** and **normochromasia** due to impaired erythrocyte production.

(d) Therapeutic plan. Affected cattle should be shielded from direct sunlight. There is no other specific treatment.

3. Eperythrozoonosis of swine

a. Clinical findings. During the acute reaction, affected pigs are febrile and have a rapidly decreasing PCV.

    (1) **Adult pigs** are depressed and inappetent.
    (2) **Lactating sows** may have reduced milk production.
    (3) **Piglets** less than 2 weeks old and **feeder pigs** may have weakness, detectable pallor and icterus, and poor growth.
  b. Etiology and pathogenesis
    (1) **Etiology.** Disease is caused by the rickettsial organism *Eperythrozoon suis,* which is an obligate parasite of RBCs and is thought to be spread by arthropods.
    (2) **Pathogenesis.** Organisms initially multiply rapidly within erythrocytes. The body's immune response leads to the coating of infected RBCs with cold-agglutinating IgM. These cells are removed in reticuloendothelial organs, causing **extravascular hemolysis** and **anemia.**
  c. Diagnostic plan and laboratory tests. Identification of round, dark-staining organisms within RBCs on **Giemsa-stained blood smears** is the most common form of diagnosis. There are also **serologic tests** for eperythrozoonosis.
  d. Therapeutic plan. Spontaneous recovery is common, but infected pigs rarely reach full growth potential, and some may be chronic carriers of the organism.
    (1) **Injections.** Clinical signs usually resolve after a single shot of a **long-acting tetracycline.** A second injection may be necessary in some cases.
    (2) **Tetracycline feed additives** usually are ineffective because of decreased intake, but **water supplements** have proved beneficial. These same protocols may improve performance of chronically infected animals.
  e. Prevention. Arthropod control (i.e., **ivermectin** for mites) should be improved in piggeries with endemic eperythrozoonosis.

E. **Depression anemia.** Reduced bone marrow production is a common cause of mild nonregenerative anemia in large animals. There are several possible causes of reduced production.

1. Nutritional deficiency anemia
  a. Iron deficiency
    (1) **History.** Iron deficiency is most commonly seen with chronic blood loss due to parasitism but is also a common finding in calves on an all-milk diet or neonates (particularly piglets) housed without access to dirt.
    (2) **Pathogenesis.** Iron is necessary for hemoglobin synthesis, and iron deficiency leads to a decrease in hemoglobin production.
    (3) **Diagnostic plan and laboratory tests.** Iron-deficient animals typically exhibit:
      (a) Low iron stores visible in marrow stained with Prussian blue stain
      (b) High serum iron-binding capacity with low serum iron concentrations
      (c) Microcytic hypochromic anemia
    (4) **Therapeutic plan.** Supplemental iron may be given orally (ferrous sulfate) or parenterally (iron dextran or cacodylate), but these treatments have been associated with fatal reactions.
  b. Copper deficiency. Copper is vital for iron transport; thus, copper deficiency anemia resembles iron deficiency anemia. Copper deficiency also may be a factor in some cases of postparturient hemoglobinuria.
    (1) **Etiology.** This deficiency may be primary or secondary to dietary excesses in molybdenum, sulfates, or zinc.
    (2) **Clinical findings.** Copper deficiency causes anemia, ill thrift, dilute hair color, chronic diarrhea, and neurologic disease.
    (3) **Diagnostic plan and laboratory tests.** Copper levels can be measured in serum, liver tissue, or hair.
    (4) **Therapeutic plan.** Supplemental copper may be given orally or parenterally.
  c. Cobalt, folate, and vitamin B$_{12}$ deficiency
    (1) **Clinical findings.** Cobalt or vitamin B$_{12}$ deficiency is associated with ill thrift, weight loss, poor growth, and anemia. Anemia is usually normocytic, normochromic, and probably associated with impaired protein and energy metabolism. Macrocytosis may also be seen.
    (2) **Etiology and pathogenesis**

      (a) Etiology. Inadequate dietary cobalt results in inadequate ruminal vitamin B_{12} production in ruminants. Horses require preformed vitamin B_{12} in their diets.

      (b) Pathogenesis. Vitamin B_{12} is necessary in all large animal species for folate metabolism and is necessary in ruminants for gluconeogenesis from propionate. Deficient folate metabolism leads to impaired erythrocyte maturation.

    (3) Diagnostic plan and laboratory tests. Diagnosis of cobalt deficiency can be established by the measurement of vitamin B_{12} concentrations in serum or liver tissue.

    (4) Therapeutic plan. Supplemental vitamin B_{12} can be given parenterally, or cobalt can be added to the diet.

2. Anemia of chronic disease

  a. Clinical findings. Affected animals have mild normocytic normochromic anemia and low serum iron concentration and binding capacity.

  b. Etiology and pathogenesis. Chronic inflammatory reactions appear to cause mild anemia by altering iron metabolism. Iron is stored in a nonuseful form. Shortened erythrocyte lifespan may also contribute to the anemia.

  c. Diagnostic plan and laboratory tests. Prussian blue staining of marrow reveals adequate iron stores, but much of the iron appears to be unavailable for heme synthesis.

  d. Therapeutic plan. Treatment efforts should be directed toward the primary disease.

3. Anemia secondary to organ dysfunction

  a. Overview. In addition to the effects of chronic disease, dysfunction of specific organs can lead to nonregenerative anemia.

    (1) Gut function is necessary for the absorption of essential nutrients.

    (2) Liver function is necessary for the proper distribution of nutrients.

    (3) Liver and kidney function together are necessary for the adequate production of **erythropoietin,** the major stimulus for erythropoiesis.

  b. Therapeutic plan

    (1) Treatment efforts are usually directed toward the **primary disease.**

    (2) Recombinant erythropoietin therapy may prove to be of some value in treating depression anemia in large animals.

4. Anemia secondary to bone marrow dysfunction or dysplasia

  a. Clinical findings. Because erythrocytes are among the longest-lived blood cells (more than 140 days in most large animals), neutropenia, thrombocytopenia, and their clinical effects (e.g., infection, hemorrhage) may be seen before anemia develops.

  b. Etiology. All normal blood cells are generated through the hyperplastic activity of stem cells in the marrow. Replacement of lost cells may be insufficient if there are too few stem cells, or if the activity of those cells is suppressed.

    (1) The most common cause of loss of stem cell populations is **crowding out through the proliferation of a neoplastic cell line.** In all large animals, the most common neoplasm associated with marrow destruction is lymphoma.

    (2) Suppression of stem cell hyperplasia, **aplastic anemia,** is most commonly an idiosyncratic reaction to a drug or toxin. **Nonsteroidal anti-inflammatory drugs** (NSAIDs; e.g., phenylbutazone), **synthetic estrogens**, and **bracken fern toxicosis** (in cattle) have been associated with aplastic anemia.

  c. Diagnostic plan and laboratory tests

    (1) Blood work. Anemias caused by suppression or replacement of bone marrow are usually normocytic and normochromic, with minimal evidence of a regenerative response.

    (2) Cytologic examination of bone marrow. Because animals affected by these processes frequently have a chronic disease, differentiation between anemia secondary to bone marrow dysfunction or dysplasia and anemia of chronic disease is difficult and best achieved by cytologic evaluation of bone marrow.

      (a) With anemia of chronic disease, the bone marrow contains numerous stem cells and frequently contains large iron stores, although evidence of active hyperplasia and maturation is less than expected.

(b) With anemia caused by crowding out of the marrow, stem cell lines are present in small numbers and another neoplastic cell line is also present.

(c) With suppression of bone marrow, stem cells are present, but evidence of hyperplasia and maturation is minimal.

d. Therapeutic plan

(1) When marrow suppression is suspected to be caused by a drug or toxin, the animal should be removed from the source of that drug or toxin.

(2) If marrow cells have been crowded out by neoplastic cells, chemotherapeutic agents may be administered to treat the neoplastic process.

(3) There are currently no specific therapeutic agents licensed for use in stimulating marrow hyperplasia in large animals. If nonerythroid cell lines [white blood cells (WBCs), platelets] are affected, fresh plasma or whole blood administration and prophylactic antibiotic administration may be beneficial. Treatments used in humans and small animals, including marrow transplants and administration of synthetic hormonal stimuli for marrow activity (colony stimulating factors) are currently impractical for use in large animals, but may be available in the future.

II. HEMOSTATIC DYSFUNCTION

A. Petechial hemorrhages

1. Vasculitis

a. Equine purpura hemorrhagica (EPH)

(1) History. Typically horses with EPH have a history of respiratory infection 2–4 weeks before the onset of clinical signs. Respiratory infections may be caused by *Streptococcus equi, Streptococcus zooepidemicus,* or equine influenza virus.

(2) Clinical findings. This condition is characterized by fever and edema, primarily of the limbs and sometimes the head, ventral abdomen, thorax, and prepuce. Occasionally, horses are depressed. Lymphadenopathy may be found. Sometimes, petechial hemorrhages are seen on mucosae. Wheals may occur and glomerulonephritis has occasionally been reported. **Colic** associated with hemorrhage, edema, and necrosis of the intestinal wall has been reported. Affected horses may be reluctant to move.

(3) Etiology. The cause is unknown, but the disorder may be associated with an allergic reaction to streptococcal or viral antigens.

(4) Pathogenesis. EPH is an immune complex-mediated disease. *S. equi* or other antigens bind to specific antibodies, particularly IgA, leading to immune complex formation. These complexes are deposited in vessel walls, with subsequent complement activation and chemoattractant production. Infiltrating inflammatory cells release proteolytic enzymes that cause vessel-wall necrosis, with subsequent edema, hemorrhage, and infarction of supplied tissues. Death may occur.

(5) Diagnostic plan and laboratory tests

(a) A **history** of recent respiratory tract infection and **clinical signs** lead to a diagnosis. Isolation of a respiratory pathogen from the upper respiratory tract or pharyngeal lymph node is supportive of a diagnosis.

(b) A **skin biopsy** may reveal leukocytoclastic venulitis.

(c) Serum levels. Horses have elevated levels of serum IgA with normal IgG and IgM levels.

(6) Therapeutic plan. Treatment is directed at removing the antigenic stimulus, reducing the immune response, reducing vessel wall inflammation, and providing supportive care.

    (a) Edema can be minimized by **hydrotherapy,** the **application of pressure wraps,** and the **administration of diuretics.**

      (i) NSAIDs may reduce inflammation and provide analgesia.

      (ii) High doses of **dexamethasone** may be required initially.

      (iii) Antimicrobial therapy may reduce the incidence or severity of cellulitis and other septic sequelae.

      (iv) Intravenous fluids may be required to prevent dehydration.

    (b) Isolation. Affected horses should be isolated for 4–5 weeks or until there are three negative nasal swab cultures.

  (7) Prognosis. The prognosis for EPH is fair with early, aggressive therapy and supportive care. Possible complications include skin sloughing, laminitis, cellulitis, pneumonia, and diarrhea.

  (8) Prevention. There is no means of prevention other than avoiding exposure of previously sensitized horses to antigens such as *S. equi.*

b. Equine viral arteritis (EVA)

  (1) Patient profile. The host range of EVA is restricted to equids. The disease is widely distributed in horse populations throughout the world. EVA infection is endemic in Standardbreds, although there does not appear to be any difference in susceptibility to infection between the Standardbred horses and other breeds.

  (2) Clinical findings

    (a) Subclinical infections with EVA are very common, particularly in mares that are bred to carrier stallions. No carrier state has been demonstrated in the mare. Abortion with no other clinical signs can occur between 3 and 10 months' gestation.

    (b) Clinical signs may include pyrexia (up to 41°C) that can last 2–9 days, depression, anorexia, leukopenia, limb edema (particularly of the hind limbs), stiffness of gait, nasal and lacrimal discharges, conjunctivitis, periorbital edema, and ventral edema involving the scrotum, prepuce, or mammary gland.

  (3) Etiology. The causative agent is a non–arthropod-borne group of togaviruses in the genus *Arterivirus.* Only one major serotype of the virus has been recognized.

  (4) Pathogenesis. Exposure to EVA may result in the development of clinical or inapparent infection, depending on the strain of virus involved, size of the virus challenge, the age and physical condition of affected animals, and environmental contamination. Except for the potential of abortion, mortality does not occur following infection with naturally occurring strains of EVA.

    (a) Transmission

      (i) Inhalation of infectious aerosolized particles is the primary means of transmission during outbreaks.

      (ii) Venereal infection of a long-term carrier stallion represents the primary means whereby EVA is maintained in horse populations. Venereal transmission to a susceptible mare can trigger an outbreak of the disease.

      (iii) Rarely, **transplacental transmissions** of EVA can occur when a pregnant mare is exposed to the virus during gestation. If infection occurs during late gestation, the fetus can acquire the infection. Infected foals are aborted after developing rapidly progressive fulminating interstitial pneumonia and a fibrinonecrotic enteritis.

    (b) Viral growth. Initial multiplication of the virus occurs in bronchial macrophages in the lung. Within 48 hours of infection, EVA disseminates to regional lymph nodes, and by the third day, viremia develops.

    (c) Disease progression. Characteristic vascular lesions first appear in the pulmonary blood vessels and later in the small arteries and veins throughout the body. The virus localizes in some epithelial sites, particularly the adrenal gland, seminiferous tubules, thyroid gland, and liver. The virus can persist in the reproductive tract long after it is no longer detectable in most body fluids.

(5) **Diagnostic plan and laboratory tests.** Both clinical and inapparent EVA infections often go undiagnosed due to limitations in available diagnostic capability and because the disease can be readily confused with other clinically similar respiratory diseases of horses.

  (a) **Acute EVA.** Confirmation of a diagnosis of acute EVA is based on viral isolation, corroborative serologic data, or both.

   (i) **Serologic tests.** Acute and convalescent sera samples should be taken 21–28 days apart. A fourfold rise in antibody titers is suggestive of an acute infection.

   (ii) **Viral isolation** can be done on nasopharyngeal swabs or washings, conjunctival swabs, and citrated, ethylenediamine tetraacetic acid (EDTA), or heparinized blood samples. Virus isolation can be attempted from placental and fetal fluids, placenta, lymphoreticular organs, lung, and other tissues.

  (b) **Identifying carrier stallions** can be done by **serologic testing.** Horses testing positive at a serum dilution of 1:4 or greater should be considered potential carriers of the virus. Isolation of the virus can be attempted from a semen sample. The virus is usually found in the sperm-rich fraction of the ejaculate.

(6) **Therapeutic plan**

  (a) There is **no specific treatment** for horses infected with EVA. Spontaneous recovery usually occurs within 4 weeks.

  (b) **Symptomatic therapy,** including rest, diuretics, and NSAIDs, may be helpful to counteract edema and pyrexia.

(7) **Prevention**

  (a) **Vaccination.** A modified-live vaccine appears to be safe and effective for stallions and nonpregnant mares. This vaccine is not recommended for pregnant mares or foals younger than 6 weeks of age.

   (i) Protection after vaccination lasts for at least 1–3 years. However, it does not prevent reinfection and limited replication of the challenge virus.

   (ii) Vaccinated horses cannot be distinguished from infected horses by serologic tests and, therefore, cannot be transported when a negative titer is required.

  (b) **Isolation.** In order to reduce the chances of introducing EVA into a group of susceptible horses, all horses returning from other farms, sales, or racetracks should be isolated for 3–4 weeks. In the event of an outbreak of EVA, the movement of breeding stock should be restricted. Selective vaccination may help curtail the spread of disease.

  (c) **Control programs.** Kentucky and New York are the only states that have formulated preventative and control programs for their respective Thoroughbred breeding industries.

c. **Equine ehrlichiosis**

  (1) **Patient profile.** There appears to be a seasonal incidence of infection, with most cases occurring during the fall, winter, and early spring.

  (2) **Clinical findings.** Clinical signs vary according to the age of the affected horses.

   (a) **In horses younger than 1 year old,** fever may be the only sign.

   (b) **Horses ages 1–3 years** may develop fever, depression, limb edema, and ataxia.

   (c) **Horses older than 3 years** often are most severely affected. Clinical signs include anorexia, depression, severe limb edema, fever, mucosal petechiation, and restricted movement.

  (3) **Etiology and pathogenesis**

   (a) **Etiology.** The causative agent is *Ehrlichia equi,* a rickettsial organism.

   (b) **Pathogenesis**

    (i) The **mode of transmission** is unknown, but, in most cases, affected horses have been exposed to or infested with ticks.

        (ii) After natural infection, the **incubation period** is unknown. Experimentally infected horses develop clinical signs in 1–9 days.

        (iii) *E. equi* organisms live in the cytoplasm of neutrophils and eosinophils and cause a necrotizing vasculitis in many parts of the body.

    (4) Diagnostic plan and laboratory tests

        (a) Giemsa- or **Wright-stained blood smears** demonstrate the characteristic cytoplasmic inclusion bodies in neutrophils or eosinophils.

        (b) Indirect fluorescent antibody testing, using paired serologic samples, can also be used.

    (5) Therapeutic plan. Intravenous administration of **oxytetracycline** can be used. Recovery usually occurs within 10 days with supportive care, including NSAIDs.

    (6) Prognosis is excellent in uncomplicated cases.

2. Thrombocytopenia

  a. Clinical findings. Thrombocytopenia often results in petechial hemorrhages in the mucous membranes. Hematuria, epistaxis, and melena may be seen.

  b. Etiology and pathogenesis. Thrombocytopenia may be the result of platelet consumption, decreased platelet production, or platelet destruction.

    (1) Platelet consumption is most common with septic conditions or DIC.

    (2) Decreased platelet production is most common with aplastic anemia or infiltration of the marrow with neoplastic cells.

    (3) Platelet destruction (in addition to that caused by consumption) usually occurs through an immune-mediated process. Drug treatments (particularly penicillin), lymphosarcoma, and systemic bacterial infections are the most commonly described triggers for immune-mediated thrombocytopenia. In many animals, a source cannot be identified.

  c. Diagnostic plan and laboratory tests

    (1) Platelet counts are usually very low (less than 40,000/μL). Overt hemorrhage may be seen if platelet counts drop below 10,000/μL.

    (2) Total clotting time is prolonged, but activated partial thromboplastin time and prothrombin time should be normal.

    (3) Measurement of antiplatelet antibodies is not currently practical for large animals, so the diagnosis often is based on the response to treatment. Efforts should be made to find an underlying disorder.

  d. Therapeutic plan. All medications should be discontinued. If the action of a particular drug is essential, a different class of drug (anti-inflammatory or antibiotic) should be used, if possible.

    (1) Immunosuppressive drug treatment. When immune-mediated thrombocytopenia has been diagnosed and all identified underlying factors have been removed or treated, a course of an immunosuppressive drug (usually dexamethasone) can be given. A 2- or 3-week course with decreasing dosages is usually sufficient, but platelet counts should be monitored to determine that the disease is in remission before immunosuppressive treatments are discontinued.

    (2) Fresh whole blood or **platelet-rich plasma** can be used to immediately increase platelet counts in animals with severe thrombocytopenia.

B. | Abnormal hemorrhage from large vessels

  1. Overview. This disorder almost always reflects a defect in the coagulation cascade and is, therefore, independent of platelet function. However, platelet dysfunction can be present and may contribute to bleeding tendencies.

    a. Clinical findings. Clotting deficiencies can result in excessive bleeding after trauma or surgery, bleeding into body cavities (e.g., hematoma, hemoperitoneum, hemothorax, hemopericardium, hemarthrosis), or bleeding from epithelial surfaces (e.g., epistaxis, hematuria, melena, hematochezia).

    b. Etiology. Coagulopathies can be inherited or acquired. Acquired coagulopathies can result from toxins, infections, trauma, or neoplasms.

2. **Inherited coagulative disorders**
   a. **Pathogenesis.** All inherited clotting factor deficiencies affect the intrinsic pathway and, therefore, prolong the activated partial thromboplastin time (APTT) but not the prothrombin time (PT).
   b. **Therapeutic plan.** Except for periodic transfusion with fresh plasma, specific treatments are not available.
   c. **Specific conditions**
      (1) **Deficiencies in factors VIII, IX, XI,** and **prekallikrein** have been described in horses.
         (a) **Factor VIII deficiency** (hemophilia A) is sex-linked and recessive.
         (b) Inheritance patterns for the **other deficiencies** are not known.
      (2) **Factor XI deficiency** has been described in Holstein cows and is thought to have an autosomal recessive pattern of inheritance.
      (3) **Factor XI deficiency** causes only slight bleeding tendencies.

3. **Acquired coagulative disorders** are usually related to a lack of production, consumption, or inhibition of clotting factors. Because multiple factors are affected, both the intrinsic and extrinsic pathways are impaired.
   a. **Inhibition of vitamin K-dependent factors**
      (1) **Sweet clover**
         (a) **Patient profile.** Cattle appear to be more sensitive than sheep or horses.
         (b) **Clinical findings.** Clinical signs are caused by internal or external hemorrhage. **External hemorrhage** can lead to anemia, weakness, and hypovolemic shock, whereas **internal hemorrhage** additionally leads to subcutaneous swelling and pain. **Spontaneous hemorrhage** is rare and usually results from a traumatic insult, such as calving or dehorning.
         (c) **Pathogenesis. Coumarol,** which is normally found in sweet clover, can be converted to **dicoumarol** by molds during spoilage. Dicoumarol inhibits the synthesis of the vitamin K-dependent coagulation factors (factors VII, IX, X, and prothrombin), leading to bleeding tendencies. Chronic feeding either of spoiled hay or silage is usually necessary to cause clinical signs, with hay more likely to contain toxic concentrations of dicoumarol than silage.
         (d) **Diagnostic plan and laboratory tests**
            (i) **Evidence of internal** or **external hemorrhage** with **history** of exposure to moldy sweet clover feeds is indicative of dicoumarol toxicosis.
            (ii) **Abnormal tests of clotting function** in animals exposed to the feeds is also supportive. **Determination of prothrombin** time is the most accurate of these clotting function tests.
            (iii) **Feed samples** should be submitted for analysis to determine dicoumarol content. Multiple samples should be analyzed because dicoumarol production may be localized.
         (e) **Therapeutic plan**
            (i) **Transfusion.** Animals with severe anemia or hypovolemic shock should be treated with whole blood, if possible.
            (ii) **Crystalloid fluids** should be administered to animals in shock if blood is not available. Feeding of the affected feedstuffs should be discontinued immediately.
            (iii) **Vitamin K_1** and **K_3** have both been shown to reduce prothrombin times in cattle with dicoumarol toxicosis; Vitamin K_1 appears to be more effective.
         (f) **Prevention.** Efforts should be made to reduce moist aerobic conditions in sweet clover products. Moldy hay and silage should not be fed. If all suspected feed cannot be discarded, it should be fed in combination with other feeds and fed intermittently. Cattle appear to be able to maintain normal coagulation function if they are completely removed from affected feed every second or third week.

(2) Warfarin toxicosis
- **(a) Patient profile.** Pigs appear to be the most susceptible farm animal species because of their small size and eating behavior.
- **(b) Clinical findings.** Overt hemorrhage and rapid death may occur with massive dosages. Chronic exposure to smaller dosages causes a similar syndrome to moldy sweet clover.
- **(c) Pathogenesis.** Warfarin is related to dicoumarol and also induces hypocoagulability by preventing the synthesis of the vitamin K-dependent clotting factors. Warfarin and related compounds are used as rodenticides. Large animal exposure can occur due to accidental ingestion of rodent bait or contaminated feed.
- **(d) Prevention.** The source of the toxin should be determined to prevent subsequent exposure.

b. DIC is a disorder that may be characterized by widespread thrombosis, bleeding tendencies, or both.
- **(1) Clinical findings.** The most notable signs usually are referable to the primary disease that triggers DIC.
  - **(a) Organ thrombosis** may contribute to morbidity and mortality. Clinical signs of thrombosis include weakness, colic, oliguria, and neurologic deficits.
  - **(b) Bleeding tendencies** (coagulopathy) rarely result in overt hemorrhage but may result in mucosal petechiation, melena, retinal hemorrhage, and prolonged bleeding from venipuncture sites.
- **(2) Etiology.** The exact mechanism of DIC has not been described and may vary from case to case. It is generally accepted that a triggering insult leads to diffuse activation of the coagulation cascade. **Triggering insults** include:
  - **(a) Sepsis**
  - **(b) Neoplasia**
  - **(c) Vasculitis**
  - **(d) Ischemia**
- **(3) Pathogenesis.** Diffuse coagulation can lead to thrombosis and ischemic damage to organs. Clotting factors and platelets are consumed in the process, leading to subsequent clotting deficits. With ensuing fibrinolysis, hemorrhage may occur.
- **(4) Diagnostic plan and laboratory tests.** Because DIC can be characterized by either hypercoagulation or hypocoagulation, tests of clotting function may be normal or abnormal. However, the finding of thrombocytopenia and prolonged clotting times is suggestive of DIC, as are findings of low plasma antithrombin III concentrations with concurrent high fibrin degradation product concentrations.
- **(5) Therapeutic plan.** Many treatments have been proposed for DIC, but most have not been evaluated critically. Treatment of the primary disorder is essential.
  - **(a) Intravenous fluids** help maintain organ perfusion and may decrease susceptibility to thrombosis.
  - **(b) Corticosteroids** and **heparin** may be contraindicated because of their unpredictable effects on coagulation. Low doses of **NSAIDs** may be helpful in some cases when endotoxin is thought to be an inciting factor for DIC.
  - **(c)** Treatment is generally unsuccessful if there is evidence of a hypocoagulable state.

c. Suppression. A lack of production of clotting factors is most common with **severe chronic hepatic disease.** Because factor VII has the shortest half-life, deficits in the extrinsic pathway are seen before there is overt hemorrhage. Animals with severe hepatic disease will have reduced blood coagulability, as measured by clotting assays and reduced plasma concentrations of most clotting factors, including fibrinogen. Coagulopathy is only one of many clinical signs seen in animals with severe chronic liver disease (see Chapter 5).

III. LYMPHATIC DISEASES

A. **Lymphoproliferative and myeloproliferative disorders**

1. **Bovine leukosis.** Lymphomas in cattle are characterized by the presence of soft tissue masses consisting of immature lymphocytes within a fibrous stroma. Bovine lymphomas can be subdivided into **sporadic** or **enzootic,** based on the etiology.

   a. **Sporadic lymphoma**
      (1) Overview
         (a) Patient profile. Although small "outbreaks" have been reported, usually only single animals are affected.
         (b) Clinical findings and diagnostic plan. Affected cattle may have serum titers against the **bovine leukemia virus (BLV)** due to transfer of maternal antibody or concurrent infection with the virus, but BLV is not thought to contribute to these diseases.
         (c) Etiology and pathogenesis. No cell type, etiologic agents, or risk factors have been identified.
         (d) Diagnostic plan and laboratory tests. Diagnosis is by histopathologic examination of tissue biopsies.
         (e) Therapeutic plan. Treatment is rarely attempted.
      (2) Specific conditions. There are **three forms** of sporadic lymphoma.
         (a) Juvenile multicentric lymphoma
            (i) Patient profile. This sporadic lymphoma is seen in cattle younger than 2 years old (most commonly between ages 4 and 8 months).
            (ii) Clinical findings. Affected calves develop fatal progressive weight loss, lymphadenopathy, and depression. Many different internal organs can be infiltrated. Half of affected calves develop lymphoid leukemia.
         (b) Thymic lymphoma
            (i) Patient profile. This disease is seen in cattle between ages 6 and 24 months.
            (ii) Clinical findings. Affected calves die after developing presternal swelling, jugular distention, and local edema. Muffling of heart sounds and respiratory distress can be present with intrathoracic tumor growth. Leukemia is present in one-third of affected calves.
         (c) Cutaneous lymphoma
            (i) Patient profile. This lymphoma occurs in cattle between ages 1 and 4 years.
            (ii) Clinical findings. Affected cattle develop multiple dermal or epidermal nodules, which can be covered by normal or hyperkeratotic skin. Cutaneous lesions may regress spontaneously, but most animals die of internal metastatic tumors.

   b. **Enzootic lymphoma**
      (1) Patient profile
         (a) Prevalence of infected cattle in individual herds varies, but in general, **dairy cattle** are more likely to be infected than beef cattle. A variety of domestic and nondomestic ruminants are also reported to be susceptible.
         (b) Approximately 30% of infected cattle develop **persistent lymphocytosis** (i.e., high peripheral blood counts of normal lymphocytes). **Less than 10%** of cattle infected with BLV develop **lymphoma,** and most of these are between ages 4 and 8 years.
      (2) Clinical findings. Persistent lymphocytosis does not appear to predispose those cattle to subsequent tumor development.
         (a) Tissue masses. The most common sites for tissue masses are the lymph nodes, abomasum, heart, uterus, kidney, lumbar spinal cord, and in the retrobulbar space. Multiple sites are usually affected.
         (b) Nonspecific clinical signs include weight loss, decreased milk production, anorexia, and occasionally fever.
         (c) Specific signs relate to the organs affected and can include

lymphadenopathy, signs of heart failure, exophthalmos, reproductive failure, melena, and posterior paresis.

   (d) **Death** usually occurs within 30 days of the onset of clinical signs.

(3) **Etiology and pathogenesis**

   (a) **Etiology.** Bovine enzootic or adult lymphoma is caused by **BLV,** an oncogenic retrovirus.

   (b) **Pathogenesis.** The virus infects and replicates in B cells and appears to be spread by the introduction of infected lymphocytes into a susceptible host. Repeated use of blood-contaminated equipment, including dehorning tools, hypodermic needles, and rectal sleeves, appears to be the major cause of transmission, although the virus can also spread transplacentally and possibly through biting flies and infected semen or milk.

(4) **Diagnostic plan and laboratory tests.** Because enzootic lymphoma is the most common internal neoplasm in cattle, finding a tissue mass in one or more of the above organs is strongly suggestive of this disease.

   (a) **Histopathology** can confirm the diagnosis.

   (b) **Serologic tests,** most commonly the **AGID test,** can be used to confirm BLV infection, but it must be remembered that most infected animals do not develop clinical disease. **False-positive tests** can occur in calves due to colostral antibody, and **false-negative tests** can occur in recently infected cattle and in periparturient cows.

(5) **Differential diagnoses.** Approximately 10% of cattle with lymphoma have lymphoid leukemia, which can be differentiated from persistent lymphocytosis by the presence of immature cells.

(6) **Therapeutic plan.** Treatment is rarely attempted.

(7) **Prevention** of disease through reduced exposure to contaminated body fluids (sanitation of instruments) is vital. Serologic tests can be used to identify infected cattle for removal from the herd.

2. **Equine lymphosarcoma.** There are **four different forms** of equine lymphoma, with each form characterized by the accumulation of abnormal lymphocytes in a different location.

   a. **Classifications and their clinical findings**

      (1) **Multicentric or generalized.** Multiple internal organs and lymph nodes are affected, causing depression, weight loss, and anorexia. This is the most commonly reported form of lymphosarcoma in mature horses, but it can occur in horses of any age.

      (2) **Intestinal.** Masses are most common in the bowel wall and abdominal lymph nodes without peripheral lymphadenopathy. This is the most commonly reported form in juvenile or young adult horses. Affected horses develop generalized ill-thrift due to nutrient malabsorption and protein-losing enteropathy. Anemia and hypoalbuminemia are common.

      (3) **Mediastinal or thymic.** Masses form in the cranial mediastinum and retropharyngeal lymph nodes, causing tachypnea, pleural effusions, and respiratory distress.

      (4) **Cutaneous.** This may be the most common form of equine lymphoma, although it is not frequently reported. Affected horses develop multiple subcutaneous or dermal nodules of varying sizes. Spontaneous enlargement, regression, and regrowth are common. Nonaggressive forms can be present for years without morbidity, whereas aggressive forms lead to lymphadenopathy, internal metastasis, and death.

   b. **Etiology.** There does not appear to be an infectious etiology.

   c. **Diagnostic plan and laboratory tests**

      (1) **Biopsy.** Diagnosis of any form of lymphoma is best made by histopathologic examination of a biopsy sample taken from a mass. Aspirates from masses are not as reliable. Masses can be found by external or rectal palpation or by thoracic radiographic examination.

      (2) **Abnormal lymphocytes** also may be seen occasionally on examination of peripheral blood or thoracic or abdominal fluid.

(3) **Clinical pathology abnormalities** are usually nonspecific and reflect dehydration or organ damage caused by a tumor.

(4) **Hypercalcemia** and **leukemia** are each seen in less than 20% of horses with lymphoma.

d. **Therapeutic plan.** Except for the nonaggressive form of cutaneous lymphoma, most horses die within 30 days of the onset of signs.

(1) **Chemotherapeutic protocols** similar to those used in people and dogs have been used to prolong the life of some horses.

(2) The **nonaggressive cutaneous form** can be treated with **long-term corticosteroids,** but recurrence is common if treatment is discontinued.

3. **Plasma cell myeloma**

a. **Patient profile.** Affected horses can be any age.

b. **Clinical findings.** Most affected animals exhibit some degree of weight loss and anorexia. Some animals have limb edema, bone pain, paresis, lymphadenopathy, and fever.

c. **Etiology and pathogenesis.** No etiologic agent has been identified. The malignant expansion of plasma cells leads to the infiltration of multiple organs, including bones and lymphoreticular organs. The secretion of immunoglobulin by neoplastic plasma cells frequently leads to monoclonal gammopathy.

d. **Diagnostic plan and laboratory tests**

(1) **Protein electrophoresis** to confirm monoclonal gammopathy is the best means of establishing an antemortem diagnosis.

(2) **Radiographic examination** of the bone may reveal multiple focal areas of bony lysis and periosteal reaction.

(3) **Bone marrow** and **mass aspirates** may reveal a homogeneous population of mononuclear tumor cells, some of which have nuclei with a "clock face" pattern. **Normal aspirates** may also be obtained from affected horses. **Immunofluorescent stains** can be used to label intracytoplasmic and surface immunoglobulin on these cells to confirm their identity.

(4) **Clinical pathology abnormalities** include anemia, hypoalbuminemia, and hyperglobulinemia caused by monoclonal gammopathy. Proteinuria and a hypocoagulable state are also common.

e. **Therapeutic plan.** Most horses die within several months of the onset of signs. Chemotherapy can be attempted.

B. **Lymphadenitis** is the enlargement of lymphoid tissue due to inflammation. Lymphadenitis often is suppurative, leading to accumulations of purulent fluid (abscesses), which may be lanced or break open spontaneously for drainage. **Caseous lymphadenitis** is so named because abscesses frequently contain thick pus.

1. **Patient profile.** This disease primarily affects small ruminants.

2. **Clinical findings.** Infected animals usually develop caseous lymphadenitis within a few months of infection.

a. **Goats** usually develop abscesses in the superficial lymph nodes of the head and neck.

b. **Sheep** can develop similar lesions or peripheral abscesses but also commonly develop internal abscesses.

c. **Lesions**

(1) Animals with **external lesions** usually are bright and appetent, but the value of fleece and hide are decreased.

(2) Animals with **internal abscesses** usually are culled because of poor reproductive or production performance and chronic wasting disease.

3. **Etiology and pathogenesis**

a. **Etiology.** The disease is caused by *Corynebacterium pseudotuberculosis,* a short, curved, gram-positive rod.

b. **Pathogenesis.** *C. pseudotuberculosis* is usually introduced into a flock through an infected animal, which contaminates the environment and fomites with discharges from draining lesions. The organism may persist in the environment for up to 6 months. Infection occurs when susceptible animals inhale or ingest the organism or when the organism gains entry through contact with damaged skin. Shearing instruments are particularly important in transmission.

4. **Diagnostic plan and laboratory tests.** Findings of internal or external suppurative lymphadenitis in small ruminants without evidence of another inflammatory focus is strongly suggestive of caseous lymphadenitis.
   a. **Bacteriologic culture.** The diagnosis can be confirmed by bacteriologic culture of pus.
   b. **Serologic tests** have been developed to identify infected animals, but the accuracy of these tests has not been established.

5. **Therapeutic plan**
   a. **Isolation.** Animals with signs of caseous lymphadenitis should be isolated from healthy animals. Animals may be returned to the flock when all of the lesions have healed, but these animals should be observed for recurrence of lesions. Healthy animals should not be allowed to contact equipment or facilities used for infected animals.
   b. **Draining lesions** should be lavaged with dilute antiseptic solutions. **Thin-walled abscesses** may also be lanced to facilitate drainage.
   c. **Antibiotics** are not thought to speed recovery.

6. **Prevention**
   a. **Environmental hygiene.** Facilities and shearing procedures should be checked to minimize skin trauma, and shearing blades should be sanitized between animals in diseased flocks.
   b. **Vaccinations** that appear to reduce severity of infection are available in Canada.
   c. **Serologic tests** and the **removal of infected animals** can be used to eradicate the disease from a flock.

IV. IMMUNE DEFICIENCY SYNDROMES

A. Immune deficiency syndromes of horses

1. **Failure of passive transfer (FPT)** is discussed in Chapter 18 IV.

2. **Combined immune deficiency syndrome (CID)**
   a. **Patient profile.** CID usually affects Arabian foals during the first few months of life as the maternal antibody wanes. As many as 25% of Arabian horses may be CID carriers.
   b. **Clinical findings** are associated with several diseases.
      (1) **Infectious diseases.** Chronic or recurrent pneumonia, enteritis, and sepsis are the most common infectious diseases associated with CID. These diseases can be caused by organisms not normally considered pathogenic.
      (2) Affected animals usually have **persistent lymphopenia** (less than 1000 cells/μL) and **hypoglobulinemia,** but CID also can be seen with other **acute inflammatory conditions.**
   c. **Etiology and pathogenesis.** CID is an autosomal recessive immunodeficiency of Arabian foals. The genetic defect has not been identified; affected animals appear to have a defect in stem cell maturation to both B and T cells.
   d. **Diagnostic plan and laboratory tests.** Because the parents of an affected foal are both carriers of the trait, care must be taken in establishing this diagnosis. Foals with CID have **four characteristic findings:**
      (1) Persistent lymphopenia
      (2) Absence of serum IgM either at birth before drinking colostrum or after 3 weeks of age (when the maternal antibody has been metabolized)
      (3) Absence of germinal centers and perivascular lymphoid sheaths in lymphoid tissue

  (4) Abnormal lymphocyte function assays, including failure to respond to intra-dermal phytohemagglutinin

  e. Therapeutic plan. Symptomatic treatment of infections can be attempted, but most foals with CID die before reaching the age of 6 months.

  f. Prevention. There is no test for CID carriers, except for the production of an affected foal.

3. Transient hypogammaglobulinemia

  a. Patient profile. Foals are most vulnerable in the first 3 months of life.

  b. Clinical findings. Chronic or recurrent infectious disorders are characteristic.

  c. Etiology and pathogenesis. There are few reports of this disorder, and it may often go unrecognized. When this disorder does occur, neonatal immunoglobulin synthesis does not begin early enough to replace metabolized colostral antibody. This immunodeficiency spontaneously resolves as the foal's antibody synthesis increases with time.

  d. Diagnostic plan and laboratory tests. Hypogammaglobulinemia with low concentrations of other classes of immunoglobulins is characteristic. Histopathologic examination of lymphoid tissue and lymphocyte function assays are normal.

  e. Therapeutic plan. Symptomatic treatment of the infections is indicated. Immunoglobulin synthesis increases with time, making foals less susceptible to repeated infections.

4. Agammaglobulinemia

  a. Patient profile. This disease has only been reported in male Thoroughbred and Standardbred foals.

  b. Clinical findings. Chronic and recurrent infections are common.

  c. Etiology. A suspected defect in B-cell maturation leads to an absence of B cells and antibody production. Cell-mediated immunity is normal. That the disease only seems to occur in male Thoroughbred and Standardbred foals suggests x-linked inheritance.

  d. Diagnostic plan and laboratory tests. Although affected horses have normal blood lymphocyte counts, labeling demonstrates a lack of B cells. All classes of immunoglobulin are absent or found in very low concentrations. Tests of T-cell function are normal.

  e. Therapeutic plan. Symptomatic treatment of infections may be attempted. Affected horses may live for several years, whereas most other horses with congenital immunodeficiencies die as foals.

5. Selective IgM deficiency

  a. Patient profile and history. Animals of any age may be affected, but cases often occur in one of three groups of horses:

  (1) Foals that show signs similar to CID and die in the first year of life

  (2) Juveniles that show signs similar to agammaglobulinemia and die before adulthood

  (3) Adult horses, many of which have or develop lymphoproliferative disorders

  b. Clinical findings. Affected horses show signs of poor growth and chronic or remittent infection.

  c. Etiology. The cause of the disease is unknown. Some forms may be hereditary, but this has not been determined.

  d. Diagnostic plan and laboratory tests. Affected horses have persistently low serum IgM concentrations, with normal to high concentrations of other immunoglobulins. In most affected horses, lymphocyte function tests and lymphoid tissue histopathology are normal. Older horses should be examined for lymphosarcoma.

  e. Therapeutic plan. Symptomatic treatment of infection can be attempted, but most affected animals die within 1 year.

B. **Immune deficiency syndromes of ruminants**

1. FPT is discussed in Chapter 18 IV.

2. Bovine leukocyte adhesion deficiency (BLAD)

  a. Clinical findings

    (1) Infections. Affected calves, within the first months of life, develop chronic or recurrent bacterial infections. Oral infections, bronchopneumonia, enteritis, and dermatitis are the most common diseases.

    (2) Clinical signs. Fever, lymphadenopathy, and very high (more than 40,000 cells/μL) peripheral blood neutrophil counts are commonly reported.

    (3) Serum biochemical abnormalities are not specific to BLAD but include hypoalbuminemia, hyperglobulinemia, low serum creatinine, and electrolyte loss with diarrhea.

  b. Etiology and pathogenesis. BLAD is an autosomal recessive immunodeficiency of Holstein calves. A point mutation in the CD18 gene leads to a defect in the Mac-1 surface glycoprotein, a β-2 integrin, causing impaired leukocyte adhesion and migration in homozygotes.

  c. Diagnostic plan and laboratory tests. Young Holstein cattle with the mentioned clinical signs and laboratory abnormalities should be suspected as having BLAD. Additionally, **histopathologic demonstration** of the absence of neutrophilic infiltrates around bacterial foci is supportive. Definitive diagnosis can be made using a **polymerase chain reaction test.** This test identifies both heterozygous carriers and homozygotes.

  d. Therapeutic plan. Most affected calves die within the first year of life. **Antimicrobial drugs** can be used to treat infections temporarily.

  e. Prevention. Bulls used for stud should be tested as potential carriers. Efforts should be made to limit inbreeding.

3. Chédiak-Higashi syndrome

  a. Clinical findings. Affected animals have a dilute coat color and complete or partial ocular albinism. They suffer from chronic or recurrent pulmonary and gastrointestinal infection and typically grow poorly.

  b. Etiology and pathogenesis. Chédiak-Higashi syndrome is an autosomal recessive immunodeficiency of Hereford and Brangus calves. The defect leads to fusion and enlargement of granule-containing cells, including granulocytic leukocytes and melanocytes. This causes impaired immune function and abnormal coat color.

  c. Diagnostic plan and laboratory tests. In addition to characteristic clinical features and abnormal tests of immune function, granulocytic leukocytes and melanocytes typically contain very large granules.

  d. Therapeutic plan. Symptomatic treatment of infections is possible, but most affected animals die within 1 year.

4. Immunodeficiency induced by viral or bacterial infections

  a. Clinical findings. Secondary immunodeficiency includes a broad spectrum of possible disease signs caused by the recrudescence of latent infections, as well as new infections. Clinical signs relate to the site and nature of the infection. Typically, secondary infections are recognized as the abrupt worsening in clinical condition. In some cases, the primary infection may be subclinical.

  b. Etiology. Many infectious conditions cause secondary immunodeficiency by consuming or sequestering leukocytes, suppressing marrow production, or altering leukocyte function. Bovine viral diarrhea virus and sepsis are just two of many possible etiologies.

  c. Diagnostic plan and laboratory tests. Bacteriologic and virologic culture techniques and serologic tests are used to identify both primary and secondary infectious agents.

  d. Therapeutic plan. Treatment should be based on the nature and site of the secondary infection. If possible, the primary infection should also be treated.

DIRECTIONS: Each of the numbered items or incomplete statements in this section is followed by answers or by completions of the statement. Select the ONE numbered answer or completion that is BEST in each case.

1. Which one of the following neoplastic diseases has the best prognosis for long-term survival?

(1) Cutaneous lymphoma in a 1-year-old calf
(2) Multicentric lymphoma in a 6-month-old calf
(3) Thymic lymphoma in a 9-month-old calf
(4) Multicentric lymphoma in a 5-year-old cow
(5) Cutaneous lymphoma in a 12-year-old horse

2. Which one of the following statements regarding persistent lymphocytosis in cattle is true?

(1) It is seen in most cattle infected with the bovine leukosis virus (BLV).
(2) It is composed of normal lymphocytes.
(3) It is most common in cattle with lymphoma.
(4) It is synonymous with lymphoblastic leukemia.
(5) It is a characteristic finding in cattle with the leukocyte adhesion deficiency.

3. Which one of the following statements regarding equine viral arteritis (EVA) is true?

(1) Efforts to prevent the spread of disease should focus on insect control.
(2) Anemia occurs due to immune-mediated hemolysis.
(3) Clinical disease is characterized by high morbidity and mortality.
(4) Subclinical infections in stallions are the most common source of infection.
(5) Horses should be vaccinated against this disease in preparation for interstate or international transport.

4. Which statement regarding water intoxication in cattle is true? Water intoxication:

(1) causes anemia through Heinz body formation.
(2) causes neurologic signs due to the rapid movement of sodium out of the brain.
(3) causes intravascular hemolysis and hemoglobinuria.
(4) should be treated aggressively to rapidly normalize serum electrolyte concentrations.
(5) reduces sodium concentrations in the cerebrospinal fluid (CSF) below the plasma sodium concentration.

DIRECTIONS: Each of the numbered items or incomplete statements in this section is negatively phrased, as indicated by a capitalized word such as NOT, LEAST, or EXCEPT. Select the ONE numbered answer or completion that is BEST in each case.

5. Infestation with which intracellular parasite is LEAST likely to respond to treatment with oxytetracycline?

(1) *Anaplasma marginale*
(2) *Babesia bigemina*
(3) *Eperythrozoon suis*
(4) *Ehrlichia equi*
(5) *Eperythrozoon wenyoni*

6. Which one of the following signs is NOT typical of the regenerative response to anemia?

(1) Basophilic stippling in cattle
(2) Polychromasia in cattle
(3) Macrocytosis in pigs
(4) Reticulocytosis in horses
(5) Marrow erythroid stem cell hyperplasia in horses

7. Which one of the following vector–pathogen associations is NOT correct?

(1) Biting flies—leptospirosis
(2) Biting flies—bovine leukosis virus (BLV)
(3) Ticks—anaplasmosis
(4) Biting flies—equine infectious anemia (EIA) virus
(5) Keds—eperythrozoonosis

8. An Arabian foal is suspected of having combined immune deficiency syndrome (CID). Which one of the following findings is NOT characteristic?

(1) Persistent lymphopenia
(2) Lymphadenopathy
(3) Abnormal lymphocyte function assays
(4) Absence of lymphoid germinal centers
(5) Low serum immunoglobulin M (IgM)

9. Several sheep in a flock are noted to have peripheral lymphadenopathy. Aspiration of an enlarged lymph node yields a thick white pus. Which one of the following statements is NOT an appropriate recommendation?

(1) Shearing equipment should be sanitized between sheep.
(2) Affected sheep should be isolated from the remainder of the flock.
(3) Sheep should be treated with a topical acaricide to eliminate keds.
(4) Facilities should be checked for hazards promoting skin trauma.
(5) Serologic testing could be performed to identify suspected carrier sheep.

10. A horse being treated with penicillin and phenylbutazone for respiratory infection develops mild anemia, peripheral edema, and petechiation of mucous membranes. Which choice would NOT be a logical course of action?

(1) Perform a Coggins test for equine infectious anemia (EIA).
(2) Perform a skin biopsy.
(3) Examine erythrocytes for autoagglutination.
(4) Discontinue penicillin administration.
(5) Vaccinate against *Streptococcus equi* infection.

11. Which one of the following morphological descriptions is NOT true?

(1) *Babesia equi*—Maltese cross in erythrocytes
(2) *Anaplasma centrale*—small bodies near the center of erythrocytes
(3) *Eperythrozoon ovis*—ring form in erythrocytes
(4) *Anaplasma marginale*—free organisms in plasma
(5) *Ehrlichia equi*—small bodies in neutrophils

12. A positive Coombs' test would NOT be likely for which one of the following causes of anemia in large animals?

(1) Neonatal isoerythrolysis
(2) Red maple toxicosis
(3) Penicillin-induced, immune-mediated hemolytic anemia
(4) Equine infectious anemia (EIA)
(5) Equine lymphosarcoma

ANSWERS AND EXPLANATIONS

1. The answer is 5 [III A 2 a (4)]. Cutaneous lymphoma in horses may exist in a nonaggressive form. Affected horses often live for years, while clinical signs wax and wane. In contrast, almost all cattle with lymphoma die within 30 days of the first apparent clinical signs. Spontaneous regression of cutaneous lymphoma in cattle has been reported, but affected animals frequently die of metastatic tumor masses within 6 months.

2. The answer is 2 [III A 1 b (1)]. Persistent lymphocytosis is composed of normal, non-neoplastic lymphocytes and is seen in a small subset (30%) of cattle infected with the bovine leukosis virus (BLV). It is an inconsistent finding in cattle with lymphoma. Persistent neutrophilia is the characteristic finding for cattle with the leukocyte adhesion deficiency.

3. The answer is 4 [II A 1 b (2), (4)]. Equine viral arteritis (EVA) is most commonly spread by aerosol or copulation with a carrier stallion. Insect transmission and immune-mediated hemolysis are characteristics of equine infectious anemia (EIA) but not viral arteritis. Viral arteritis is rarely fatal, and vaccination leads to antibody titers, which may preclude interstate or international transport.

4. The answer is 3 [I D 2 d (1) (a), (d)]. Water intoxication causes a rapid drop in plasma osmolality and osmotic intravascular hemolysis. Sodium concentration in the cerebrospinal fluid (CSF) is higher than that in the diluted plasma, leading to rapid movement of water into the brain, cerebral edema, and neurologic signs. Rapid administration of intravenous fluids can worsen clinical signs.

5. The answer is 2 [I D 2 a (2)]. Oxytetracycline is an effective antibiotic against rickettsial organisms of the genus *Anaplasma, Eperythrozoon,* and *Ehrlichia* but is not effective against the protozoon parasite *Babesia bigemina.* Imidocarb is the most frequently used babesicidal drug.

6. The answer is 4 [I A 2 d (1)]. Horses do not get reticulocytosis. In other large animal species, reticulocytosis, macrocytosis, polychromasia, and basophilic stippling all are seen in the peripheral blood of animals with regenerative anemia. In horses, the detection of erythroid stem cell hyperplasia in the bone marrow is often the only way to determine if anemia is regenerative.

7. The answer is 1 [I D 2 a (4)]. Leptospirosis is caused by the ingestion or inhalation of organisms. Arthropod transmission is not thought to occur or to be of major importance. Bovine leukosis virus (BLV) is thought to be spread iatrogenically in many cases, but it can be isolated from biting flies. Arthropod transmission is thought to be the major route for *Anaplasma, Eperythrozoon,* and the equine infectious anemia (EIA) virus.

8. The answer is 2 [IV A 2 d]. Combined immunodeficiency syndrome (CID) is caused by a defect in lymphocyte maturation, which leads to lymphopenia, low immunoglobulin production, abnormal function tests, and absence of germinal centers. Lymphadenopathy is not seen.

9. The answer is 3 [III B 2, 5, 6]. The most likely diagnosis is caseous lymphadenitis. Efforts should be made to prevent the transmission of organisms to uninfected sheep and to decrease skin trauma. Identification and separation of infected sheep aids in the prevention of new cases. Arthropods are not thought to be important vectors.

10. The answer is 5 [II A 1 a, b]. Clinical signs are compatible with vasculitis (as seen with EIA or EVA), immune-mediated anemia and thrombocytopenia, or purpura hemorrhagica. Purpura hemorrhagica can be diagnosed by a skin biopsy and may be exacerbated by exposure to streptococcal antigens.

11. The answer is 4 [I D 2 a (3) (a), (b)]. Of the important intraerythrocytic parasites, only *Eperythrozoon* organisms are found free in the plasma.

12. The answer is 2 [I D 1 c (1) (e)]. A positive Coombs' test suggests that erythrocytes are coated with antibody, which occurs with immune-mediated hemolysis. Hemolysis with red maple toxicosis is caused by oxidative injury to erythrocytes and is not immune-mediated.

Chapter 15

Diseases of the Urinary Tract and Kidney

John Pringle

I. RENAL DISEASE

A. Renal disease in horses

1. **Acute renal failure** is a sudden, theoretically reversible inability of the kidney to function in clearing nitrogenous wastes while maintaining fluid and electrolyte homeostasis.

   a. **Patient profile.** Acute renal failure can occur in horses of any age.

   b. **Clinical findings.** Signs of acute renal failure are nonspecific and are often related to concurrent disease (e.g., colitis, diarrhea, exertional rhabdomyolysis).

      (1) **Complaints** include **anorexia, depression, weakness,** and **decreased athletic performance.** There may be **abnormal frequency** or **volume of urination. Edema** and increased water intake can also occur.

      (2) **Oliguria** is a characteristic finding with hemodynamic causes, whereas **polyuria** may be evident with acute renal failure caused by aminoglycosides.

   c. **Etiology and pathogenesis**

      (1) **Etiology.** As in all species, the inciting cause of reduced kidney function in horses can be prerenal, renal, or post renal.

         (a) **Prerenal causes** are factors that decrease blood flow to the glomerulus. These factors include severe hypovolemia due to dehydration, endotoxemia, or cardiac failure; vascular injury due to endotoxin; or compromised autoregulation of renal blood flow by prostaglandin synthase inhibitors [i.e., nonsteroidal anti-inflammatory drugs (NSAIDs)]. Many compounds are considered potentially nephrotoxic, but the mechanisms are not well documented.

         (b) **Renal causes** directly damage the kidney tissue. Many toxins have a specific site of action, such as the glomerulus or the proximal tubules. However, there are no tests available to diagnose the site of damage, which could then lead to the early recognition and removal of toxin. Renal causes include:

            (i) **Nephrotoxic medications,** such as aminoglycosides, certain sulfonamides, polymyxin B, phenylbutazone or other NSAIDs, and menadione sodium bisulfite (vitamin K_3)

            (ii) **Endogenous pigments,** such as hemoglobin from acute intravascular hemolysis or myoglobin from a large release from muscle

            (iii) **Substances in various plants** (e.g., oak, wilted red maple leaves, wild onion, white snakeroot) and some **heavy metals** (e.g., mercury), which might be contained in some blistering agents

            (iv) **Cantharidin,** the toxin in **blister beetles** (signs of intestinal erosive disease overshadows any such accompanying toxicity)

         (c) **Postrenal** causes of renal failure impair the animal's ability to rid itself of the urine that has been produced. Postrenal causes in horses include mainly bladder rupture in newborn foals. Although uroliths can develop in adult horses, they less commonly cause urinary obstruction in contrast to other species.

      (2) **Pathogenesis.** Regardless of the cause, the common elements of acute renal failure include the accumulation of nitrogenous wastes in blood, with serum creatinine elevations above 170 mmol/L and blood urea exceeding 9 mmol/L. These changes do not occur until two-thirds to three-fourths of the nephrons are no longer functioning; therefore, lesser degrees of kidney damage do not result in detectable accumulations of nitrogenous wastes.

d. Diagnostic plan and laboratory tests

    (1) Laboratory tests

        (a) Elevated creatinine and **urea** reflect an inability to rid the body of nitrogenous wastes, but these results do not provide the localization of the problem or the cause. Serum electrolytes, including sodium, potassium, and chloride, are initially normal but can all decrease with diarrhea or polyuria.

        (b) Urinalysis. A urine sample should be obtained to ensure urine flow.

            (i) Urinalysis showing a **urine specific gravity** of less than 1.02 in the presence of clinical dehydration is suggestive of intrarenal disease.

            (ii) The **color of urine,** the presence of the heme pigments myoglobin or hemoglobin, and the presence of free red blood cells (RBCs) or protein can be used to indicate possible underlying causes.

            (iii) Sediment analysis normally reveals considerable mucus and calcium carbonate crystals, and casts are easily overlooked because they dissolve quickly in the normally alkaline urine of herbivores.

    (2) Renal ultrasonography may detect cystic or structural changes in the kidney or renal pelvis.

    (3) Nuclear medicine techniques, where available, measure the glomerular filtration rate.

    (4) Renal biopsy can be performed with ultrasound guidance or blindly, but, because there is the risk of serious hemorrhage, this test should be reserved for cases in which biopsy is an essential part of determining the prognosis.

e. Therapeutic plan

    (1) The **correction of fluid, electrolyte,** and **acid–base disorders** is essential. The amount of fluids required should be based on the state of hydration. The packed cell volume (PCV) and total protein (TP) measurements can be used to estimate the fluid deficit.

        (a) Oral fluids (e.g., water, isotonic saline, or a balanced electrolyte solution) are usually well tolerated, except in the case of acute renal failure associated with gastrointestinal disease (e.g., colitis). **Electrolytes** ideally should be tailored to the requirements identified by the serum electrolyte and blood gas analysis. Generally, a balanced electrolyte solution with a bicarbonate source, such as **lactated Ringer's solution,** is sufficient. Adult horses (400–500 kg) can be given 6–8 L of warm water or electrolytes every 30–60 minutes orally until rehydrated.

        (b) Intravenous therapy should be reserved for patients with gastrointestinal problems.

    (2) Furosemide, dopamine, or both are indicated in those horses that fail to begin passing urine. These horses have the anuric form of renal failure.

    (3) Underlying diseases, such as septicemia or rhabdomyolysis, **should be treated.**

    (4) Potentially nephrotoxic drugs (e.g., NSAIDs, aminoglycosides, sulfonamides), which can be far more nephrotoxic in the presence of dehydration, **should be discontinued.**

f. Prognosis for recovery is good but depends largely on the early detection of renal failure, appropriate treatment, and the ability to adequately treat concurrent disease.

g. Prevention includes providing adequate fluid therapy when there is circulatory compromise or exposure to potential nephrotoxins.

2. Renal dysfunction in the neonate is poorly understood.

    a. Some newborn foals may have **high serum creatinine levels** detected shortly after birth. Although this finding may indicate a renal disorder, high serum creatinine levels can also occur because of a placental problem in the mare. In these cases, the serum creatinine should become normal within several days after birth, and the foal requires no specific treatment.

    b. Newborn foals also can have **hyposthenuric urine** (1.006) for a short period after birth, which may only indicate renal immaturity.

3. **Chronic renal failure** is a progressive renal disease resulting from the continued loss of nephronal function or population reduction. This disorder may be a sequela to acute renal failure. There are two broad categories of chronic renal failure in horses: glomerulonephritis and tubulointerstitial disease.

   a. **Glomerulonephritis** is immunologically mediated and is the most common form of chronic renal failure in horses.

      (1) **Patient profile.** This disorder can occur in horses of any breed, age, or sex.

      (2) **Clinical findings.** The signs noted in horses depend on the stage and severity of the renal damage. **Chronic weight loss, anorexia,** and **polyuria** with the consumption of large quantities of water usually are key findings. Also, if there is major glomerular damage, there may be dependant edema due to massive urinary protein loss, which results in hypoproteinemia.

      (3) **Etiology**

         (a) The glomerular lesion is caused by circulating immune complexes to **viral** [e.g., **equine infectious anemia (EIA)**], **bacterial (streptococcal),** or **parasitic antigens** that deposit on the epithelial side of the glomerular basement membrane.

         (b) Although less common in horses, the glomerular damage can also be the result of **autoimmunity,** characterized by the formation of antibodies against the glomerular basement membrane.

      (4) **Pathogenesis.** The pathogenesis of both types of chronic renal failure involves a decreased glomerular filtration rate in which solutes that are normally filtered and secreted by tubules are retained. There is also a loss of plasma electrolytes (e.g., sodium, chloride, phosphate), which are normally retained in the body. In glomerulonephritis, autoimmune deposits and viral, bacterial, or parasitic deposits activate the complement system, which leads to cellular influx and increased vascular permeability of the glomerular basement membrane, allowing the leakage of large protein molecules (e.g., serum albumin).

         (a) Nephrons that can still function have to increase solute filtration. This excess solute flow results in inefficient water and electrolyte handling, which leads to **diuresis** and an observed **polyuria** with a compensatory **polydipsia.**

         (b) As a result of the reduced ability of the tubules to handle water and electrolytes, there is **increased sodium, chloride,** and **phosphate** in the urine. Decreased reabsorption of bicarbonate with decreased hydrogen ion excretion may also result in **acidosis.**

         (c) Despite the increased filtration by the nephrons, uremia occurs, and long-term effects cause a **moderate anemia, focal ulceration of oral and intestinal mucosa, uriniferous odor to the breath,** and **excessive dental tartar.**

      (5) **Diagnostic plan and laboratory tests**

         (a) **Laboratory findings**

            (i) **Moderate azotemia** and **isosthenuria** may be evident in affected horses with normal hydration.

            (ii) **Persistent proteinuria without hematuria** is specific to glomerulonephritis.

            (iii) **Specific urine protein testing** should be performed because the routine urine dipsticks often give a false-positive result for protein in alkaline or concentrated urine.

            (iv) **Hypoproteinemia** or **hypoalbuminemia** may also be found in the serum if there have been prolonged losses.

            (v) **Hypercalcemia** may be present, but this finding may indicate a diet high in calcium (e.g., alfalfa).

         (b) A **renal biopsy** can be taken but may not be warranted because of the risk of hemorrhage and the lack of contribution to therapy and prognosis.

      (6) **Therapeutic plan.** There is no effective treatment for glomerulonephritis because it is usually only recognized when permanent renal insufficiency has occurred. Usually, the disease progresses, and ultimately, the horse must be euthanized.

        (a) Corticosteroids may be administered to reduce the effects of the immune complex disease.

        (b) Diet. Horses that are stable and not markedly affected by the clinical effects of the disease can be managed with a high-quality carbohydrate diet and reduced protein (less than 10%) in feeds.

        (c) Plasma transfusions have been advocated to provide temporary relief of edema caused by hypoproteinemia.

    (7) Prevention is not possible because the reasons for a specific horse developing the disease are unknown.

  b. Tubulointerstitial disease

    (1) Patient profile. This disease can occur in horses of any age or breed and may be related to a history of prior acute illness that caused acute tubular necrosis.

    (2) Clinical findings

        (a) Signs are similar to chronic renal failure of glomerulonephritis [see I A 3 a (2)], with the exception of edema of hypoproteinemia. Affected horses also have **polyuria** or **polydipsia,** but in certain management situations where water consumption is not readily observed, this may go unnoticed.

        (b) On **rectal palpation,** the left kidney may be smaller than normal.

    (3) Etiology. Tubulointerstitial disease may be a sequela to acute tubular necrosis, with reported causes in horses including vitamin K_3 administration, aminoglycoside or mercury toxicity, pyelonephritis, hydronephrosis, myoglobinuria from acute myositis, or nephrolithiasis. Often, however, the cause is not determined.

    (4) Diagnostic plan and laboratory tests

        (a) Laboratory findings

            (i) Azotemia and **isosthenuria** without any clinical dehydration is evident. In tubulointerstitial nephritis, there is little protein in the urine.

            (ii) Electrolyte abnormalities of hyponatremia, hypochloremia, hypercalcemia, and hypophosphatemia may be evident.

        (b) Renal ultrasound can identify a renal mass or renal pelvis calculi.

        (c) A **renal biopsy** can be performed, but this test seldom provides information regarding the cause or directs treatment.

    (5) Therapeutic plan. Long-term treatment is unlikely to be successful, but, because these horses are not losing protein in large quantities, they can often be managed humanely by ensuring unlimited access to water, provision of a salt block, and good-quality feed with low calcium content (no alfalfa).

        (a) Any prerenal component to the renal failure (e.g., diarrhea, dehydration) or any acute exposure to nephrotoxic drugs or agents **should be corrected.**

        (b) Ancillary treatment may include **anabolic steroids** and **B vitamins. Periodic serum monitoring** of blood gases can be done, and if plasma bicarbonate drops below 18 mEq/L as a result of acid retention, the horse can be given **sodium bicarbonate** (225 g/day orally).

    (6) Prevention. Horses with acute renal failure, particularly of hemodynamic or toxic causes, should be treated early in the course of disease and with sufficient amounts of fluid support to prevent this permanent renal tubular damage.

4. Pyelonephritis

  a. Patient profile. Pyelonephritis mainly affects female animals. However, in certain circumstances (e.g., bladder paralysis), males may also develop pyelonephritis.

  b. Clinical findings. In horses, pyelonephritis is often subclinical, with the only detectable signs being frequent urination and pus in the urine.

  c. Etiology and pathogenesis

    (1) Etiology. Bacteria isolated from affected horses include coliforms and *Proteus* species.

    (2) Pathogenesis. In horses, this disorder can follow parturition, be associated with urinary bladder atony or ectopic ureters (see II D), or may occur without any identifiable risk factor.

(a) **Urine stasis,** which occurs in ectopic ureter or bladder atony, is a recorded risk factor.

(b) The **short urethra** in females predisposes them to the development of **ascending urinary tract infection,** which leads to pyelonephritis.

d. **Diagnostic plan and laboratory tests**

(1) **Laboratory tests**

(a) **Pyuria** is usually a hallmark of the disease and may be accompanied by **proteinuria** and **hematuria.** These urine changes can also be found in cystitis; however, evidence of renal involvement may be observed with systemic changes to blood samples (e.g., leukocytosis with a neutrophilia, hypergammaglobulinemia, high fibrinogen).

(b) **Azotemia** of renal failure may be noted but is not always present, because the infection may be restricted to the renal pelvis, may affect only one kidney, or may result in damage to less than two-thirds of the body's renal function.

(2) **Renal ultrasound** may be used to detect purulent debris in the renal pelvis or enlargement of the renal pelvis.

(3) **Urine culture** confirms the causative organism but does not indicate the extent of invasion in the urinary tract.

e. **Therapeutic plan**

(1) **Any predisposing factor,** such as ureteral ectopia or ascending urinary tract infection, **should be treated.** To assess the **response to treatment,** a catheterized urine sample can be submitted for culture and cytology 1 week following the cessation of therapy to ensure that the urinary tract has returned to its normally sterile condition.

(2) **Catheterization.** When bladder atony or paralysis is the cause, the bladder should be emptied frequently by catheterization. However, a return to normal bladder function is needed for long-term success in treatment.

f. **Prognosis.** The long-term survival of affected animals depends on early detection and appropriate treatment. The correction of any predisposing urinary tract abnormality that may result in continued urine stasis also influences long-term recovery.

B. Renal disease in cattle

1. **Acute tubular necrosis** is reported as the most common cause of renal failure in cattle in selected areas of the United States and may be related to the increased risk of plant toxicities in those regions.

a. **Patient profile.** Acute tubular necrosis usually affects adult cattle when related to plant toxicity, but this disease can occur in cattle of any age when associated with the administration of nephrotoxic drugs.

b. **Clinical findings**

(1) **Complaints** are nonspecific and include **mild depression, anorexia, dehydration,** and **decreased rumen motility** or rumen stasis.

(2) **Physical examination** reveals an elevated temperature, pulse, and respiratory rate.

(a) A **primary disorder** (e.g., sepsis, diarrhea) may be obvious, predisposing the animal to the development of acute tubular necrosis.

(b) A **bleeding diathesis** may be seen in uremic cattle, along with recumbency.

(c) On **rectal palpation,** the kidney is likely a normal size and consistency.

c. **Etiology and pathogenesis.** Acute tubular necrosis can be caused by **decreased renal blood flow,** the administration of **nephrotoxic drugs,** or the ingestion of **nephrotoxic plants.** The management systems of cattle production may expose cattle to all of these causes.

(1) **Decreased renal blood flow**

(a) **Hypovolemia.** Acute severe volume depletion may be caused by diseases such as neonatal calf diarrhea, lactic acidosis ("grain overload"), or abomasal torsion (in older cattle).

(b) Hemodynamically mediated diseases (e.g., endotoxemia of mastitis or metritis) can also cause decreased renal blood flow.

(c) Severe ruminal distention (e.g., bloat, vagus indigestion) is another cause of decreased renal blood flow.

(2) Nephrotoxic drugs can cause tubular damage.

    (a) The most commonly reported nephrotoxic reaction is **aminoglycoside toxicity** from **neomycin.**

    (b) Selected **sulfonamides** and the administration of outdated or excess doses of **tetracyclines** can also result in nephrotoxicity.

    (c) Acute intravascular hemolysis in cattle (or sheep) from **copper toxicity** results in tubular necrosis from endogenous pigment damage.

(3) Plant toxins that result in tubular necrosis include oak (*Quercus* species), which is particularly common in the southeastern United States, and oxalate-containing plants, such as redroot pigweed *(Amaranthus retroflexus).* The effect of any nephrotoxic agent is enhanced by decreased blood volume or electrolyte (sodium, potassium) depletion.

  d. Diagnostic plan and laboratory tests. Failure of renal function is usually diagnosed by laboratory evaluation because clinical signs are seldom diagnostic.

    (1) Serum creatinine and **urea** are increased, with urine specific gravity less than 1.022.

    (2) Proteinuria may be present. If the sample is analyzed rapidly before the destruction by alkaline urine, granular casts (an early finding in acute renal tubular necrosis) may be present.

    (3) Dehydration is suggested by the increased hematocrit and total plasma protein.

  e. Therapeutic plan

    (1) Fluid therapy. The main goal of treatment is providing intravenous fluid and electrolytes to restore and maintain circulating blood volume, which ensures renal perfusion. Fluids should be isotonic, containing sodium, potassium, chloride, and calcium. **Normal saline** with small quantities of added **potassium** and **calcium** can be used.

    (2) Other treatments include administering appropriate antimicrobial therapy (if there is ongoing sepsis), discontinuing any aminoglycoside, sulfonamide, or tetracycline therapy, and relieving any abdominal distention.

  f. Prognosis. Acute tubular necrosis is a highly reversible condition if detected early and treated appropriately, particularly if the condition is related to decreased renal blood flow. The prognosis is less favorable if there is sepsis associated with the tubular necrosis.

  g. Prevention of acute tubular necrosis in cattle includes avoiding the use of potentially nephrotoxic drugs and restricting access to pastures that may contain plant nephrotoxins (e.g., oak).

2. Amyloidosis

  a. Patient profile. Renal amyloidosis, although rare in horses, is sporadically diagnosed in cattle, particularly in those older than 4 years with chronic foci of inflammation. This disorder is also occasionally diagnosed in sheep and goats with paratuberculosis or visceral caseous lymphadenitis (CLA).

  b. Clinical findings

    (1) Complaints include ventral edema, chronic intractable diarrhea, and weight loss.

    (2) On **rectal palpation,** the kidneys are uniformly enlarged.

  c. Pathogenesis. Affected cows usually have a chronic bacterial infection (e.g., pericarditis, pulmonary abscessation, peritonitis, metritis). These bacterial infections lead to reactive systemic amyloidosis and the production of **amyloid ("AA") protein,** which is a β-pleated protein that is resistant to normal proteolytic digestion. Amyloid protein is deposited on the glomeruli and results in the gross enlargement of the kidneys. The cell of origin of amyloid protein is unknown.

    (1) Glomerular proteinuria results in hypoproteinemia with subcutaneous and visceral edema (e.g., ascites, pleural and pericardial effusion).

(2) Amyloid infiltration into the small intestine, resulting in gastrointestinal lymphangiectasis and edema, intestinal malabsorption, and gastrointestinal motility dysfunction, is responsible for the intractable diarrhea and weight loss.

d. Diagnostic plan and laboratory tests
  (1) Laboratory tests. Blood samples reveal azotemia with persistent and massive proteinuria. The hemogram is usually normal, but fibrinogen is elevated.
  (2) Liver function tests. Occasionally, there is liver involvement.
  (3) Biopsy of the kidney can be used to confirm the diagnosis.
e. Therapeutic plan
  (1) Dimethylsulfoxide (DMSO) administration has resulted in clinical improvement in humans, dogs, and hamsters.
    (a) The exact **mechanism of action** is unknown, although DMSO has been shown to prevent the precipitation of Bence Jones proteins and to solubilize suspensions of amyloid fibrils.
    (b) Approved uses. Because DMSO is not approved for parenteral use in food-producing animals, it should be reserved for the treatment of animals to allow for the harvesting of future genetic stock, such as semen or embryo production.
  (2) Broad-spectrum antibiotics can be used to treat any underlying bacterial infection.
  (3) Plasma transfusions and **diuretics** can be administered to temporarily alleviate signs of edema.
  (4) Euthanasia. Given the grave prognosis, most animals should be euthanized when the diagnosis is established.
f. Prevention. Because amyloidosis occurs sporadically, there are no recommended preventive measures.

3. Pyelonephritis
  a. Patient profile and history. Pyelonephritis usually occurs in adult dairy cows from November to May (i.e., during the time the cows are more likely to be stabled indoors). Recent urinary catheterization or artificial insemination may be found in the history.
  b. Clinical findings
    (1) Complaints. Affected cattle may have an acute **decrease in appetite and milk production,** show **reluctance to walk,** and may have **abdominal pain** that could be confused with an intestinal obstruction. Although these signs are very similar to traumatic reticuloperitonitis (TRP), affected animals resist a withers pinch (in contrast to those with TRP) and are not sensitive to pressure at the xiphoid region.
    (2) Physical examination findings
      (a) Urine. The urine initially has blood clots associated with short episodes of acute colic. As the disease progresses, frank pyuria may be present. Pollakiuria and hematuria are also seen.
      (b) On **rectal examination,** the kidneys may be enlarged with a loss of normal lobulation. More chronic cases also have ureteral enlargement that can be palpated rectally.
  c. Etiology and pathogenesis
    (1) Etiology. In cattle, *Corynebacterium renale* can cause pyelonephritis, sometimes in outbreaks. *C. renale* is found in clinically normal cattle, and the organism does not survive in the environment for a long period of time.
    (2) Pathogenesis
      (a) Transmission occurs via mechanical means, such as tail switching, urine splashing, and the use of contaminated equipment (e.g., catheters, specula).
      (b) Route of infection. When the organism gains entry, it ascends the urethra (not always bilaterally), invades the renal pelvis and medulla, and later invades the renal cortex, causing fibrosis.
      (c) Manifestations of disease include:
        (i) Toxemia and fever

      (ii) Uremia (with extensive bilateral involvement)

      (iii) Abdominal pain, caused by the obstruction of the ureter or renal calyx by pus or tissue debris

  d. Diagnostic plan and laboratory tests are the same as for horses (see I A 4 d).

  e. Therapeutic plan

    (1) Penicillin is the treatment of choice (30,000–50,000 IU/kg every 12 hours for at least 10 days). In well-established cases, prolonged therapy for up to 6 months may be necessary. To assess the **response to treatment,** a catheterized urine sample can be submitted for culture and cytology 1 week following the cessation of therapy to ensure that the urinary tract has returned to its normally sterile condition.

    (2) Nephrectomy may be necessary if the disease is unilateral.

  f. Prognosis is the same as for horses (see I A 4 f).

C. Renal disease in swine

1. **Patient profile.** Sows recently exposed to natural breeding are at risk for developing acute pyelonephritis.

2. **Clinical findings.** The disease is observed in sows or gilts post breeding. Initially, some sows may have a **vaginal discharge.** Affected animals become ill suddenly, show profound **depression** and **fever,** and can die within 12 hours of the onset of clinical signs. Most affected sows die without premonitory signs.

3. **Etiology and pathogenesis.** The causative organism is commonly *Eubacterium suis.* Infection may be introduced at mating or may be residual from the previous farrowing. The relationship between mating and pyelonephritis is well established in sows.

4. **Diagnostic plan and laboratory tests** are the same as for horses (see I A 4 d).

5. **Therapeutic plan.** Sows that show signs of urinary bleeding or dysuria after breeding should be treated prophylactically with **antibiotics.** To assess the **response to treatment,** a catheterized urine sample can be submitted for culture and cytology 1 week following the cessation of therapy to ensure that the urinary tract has returned to its normally sterile condition.

6. **Prognosis** is the same as for horses (see I A 4 f).

II. LOWER URINARY TRACT DISORDERS

A. Cystitis

1. **Patient profile.** In large animals, cystitis is sporadic and uncommon. This disorder occurs mainly in adult females and is associated with recent parturition or breeding.

2. **Clinical findings**
   a. **Pollakiuria** and the passing of small amounts of turbid urine containing blood, pus, or both may be evident.
   b. **Perineal scalding** with **alopecia** may be present if the process has been ongoing.
   c. **Rectal palpation** may detect **bladder thickening.**

3. **Etiology and pathogenesis**
   a. **Primary disease.** With the exception of cystitis caused by *Corynebacterium renale* in cattle and *Eubacterium suis* in pigs, cystitis is rarely a primary disease in large animals.
   b. **Secondary disease.** Cystitis most often occurs secondary to urine retention in diseases such as urolithiasis, bladder atony, paralysis, late pregnancy or dystocia, and Sudan grass myelomalacia (in horses). The ascending infection is usually associated with *Escherichia coli, Proteus* species, or *Actinomyces pyogenes.*

4. **Diagnostic plan and laboratory tests.** The key part of the diagnosis is to collect samples aseptically for cytologic and bacteriologic evaluation. A sterile catheter should be used.

a. On **sediment analysis,** there are high numbers of white blood cells (WBCs), desquamated epithelial cells, RBCs, and bacteria (free or intracellular).

b. The **complete blood cell count (CBC)** is usually normal.

5. **Therapeutic plan.** The goal in treatment is to identify and correct any underlying predisposing cause of cystitis, such as bladder atony or urolithiasis.

a. **Antibiotics** (e.g., penicillin, ampicillin, cephalosporins, trimethoprim-sulfas) can be used as initial treatment because they are well concentrated in the urine.

b. **Treatment duration** should last from 10 days to 1 month. However, this may not be scientifically valid because uncomplicated cystitis in humans can be cured with a single high dose of antibiotics.

B. **Urinary incontinence** is an uncommon problem in large animals and is associated with **neurologic diseases** (e.g., sacral fractures) in all species. In horses, urinary incontinence is associated with equine protozoal myelitis (EPM), equine herpes virus type 1 (EHV-1) infection, cauda equina neuritis syndrome, and sorghum or Sudan grass intoxication (see Chapter 11). Other causes of urinary incontinence are rare and sporadic, including **bladder tumors, estrogen-responsive incontinence** in mares, and **anatomic defects** (e.g., ectopic ureters; see II D).

C. **Patent urachus** is discussed in Chapter 18 VI B. The urachus serves as a connection between the fetal bladder and the allantoic cavity, which should spontaneously close at birth.

D. **Ectopic ureters**

1. **Patient profile.** This congenital problem has been reported only sporadically in horses. However, it may simply be overlooked in other large animal species that are under less intensive observation. Although ectopic ureters have been reported in both sexes, they may be more readily detected in females because of more obvious urine dribbling.

2. **Clinical findings.** Affected horses show urinary incontinence from birth but may appear able to void urine normally. Urine scald is evident around the perineum, but the horse may otherwise be clinically normal. In prolonged cases, ascending urinary tract infection may ensue, resulting in pyelonephritis and signs of systemic illness.

3. **Diagnostic plan**

a. The **clinical sign** of urine dribbling from birth is usually sufficient for a diagnosis.

b. **Cystoscopic observation** of the aberrant entry of ureters to the bladder neck, urethra, or even vagina can confirm the diagnosis.

c. **Retrograde urography** and **intravenous excretory urography** have been used effectively to determine the location of the ureters' entry into the lower urinary tract.

4. **Therapeutic plan.** When identified, the ectopic ureters should be surgically relocated to enter the bladder. If the ectopia is unilateral and the ipsilateral kidney is hydronephrotic, it can be removed surgically.

E. **Bladder rupture in horses**

1. **Patient profile.** Bladder rupture occurs most frequently in male foals, but it has been found in mares after dystocia and in other adult horses in isolated cases. In foals, the rupture is presumed to occur before or at parturition. This disorder is also increasingly recognized in recumbent newborn foals that require intensive care and may be a complication of iatrogenic increases in abdominal pressure while lifting or moving the foal.

2. **Clinical findings**

a. Foals appear normal at birth, with signs of **depression** beginning approximately 24–48 hours after birth.

b. Mild but progressive **abdominal enlargement** develops, with fluid accumulation and a reduced interest in suckling.

c. Foals may make **frequent attempts to urinate** but often pass only small amount of urine. These signs of straining may be mistaken for meconium impaction, but within several days, respiratory distress from the abdominal enlargement and severe depression from azotemia and fluid and electrolyte disturbances are evident.

    d. Patent urachus may be an accompanying abnormality.

  3. Etiology and pathogenesis

    a. With bladder rupture in **male foals,** the **small diameter** and **increased length of the urethra** allows pressure to build up within a distended bladder during foaling, causing the rupture of the dorsal body of the bladder (which is the weakest point).

    b. Some foals may also have a **congenital bladder wall defect** that predisposes to rupture during parturition, but there is little hemorrhage associated with the site of rupture.

  4. Diagnostic plan and laboratory tests

    a. The **history** and **clinical findings** are highly suggestive of bladder rupture.

    b. Abdominocentesis to confirm the presence of urine in the abdomen can also be performed.

      (1) Methylene blue can be instilled into the bladder. Its presence in a peritoneal fluid sample confirms the presence of urine in the abdomen.

      (2) Creatine level. Demonstration of an abdominal fluid creatine level that is at least two times higher than the serum creatine level also confirms the presence of urine in the abdomen.

      (3) Calcium carbonate crystals. In adult horses, calcium carbonate crystals (normally found in urine) can be detected in the affected animal's abdominal fluid.

    c. Laboratory studies. Characteristic changes on a **serum electrolyte panel** (e.g., severe **hyponatremia, hypochloremia,** and **hyperkalemia)** indicate uroperitoneum. The hyperkalemia can be severe enough to cause cardiotoxicity. **Azotemia** is a predictable finding in foals.

  5. Therapeutic plan

    a. Surgery. The tear or defect in the bladder requires surgical correction. However, because of the often profound fluid and electrolyte disturbances, initial correction of these metabolic abnormalities is essential before placing the animal under general anesthesia.

    b. Fluid drainage. The extravasated fluid in the abdomen, if causing severe abdominal distention, should be drained by a large-bore needle puncture to relieve the pressure on the diaphragm.

    c. Fluid therapy should be given in the form of normal saline to increase sodium and chloride levels. Dextrose (5%) should be added to help reduce the serum potassium. Additionally, foals may be acidotic and require sodium bicarbonate, which also helps reduce the serum potassium to less cardiotoxic levels.

F. Obstructive urolithiasis

  1. Obstructive urolithiasis in ruminants is likely the most common and clinically important urinary tract disease of ruminants. Clinical disease occurs when calculi lodge in the urethra and cause urinary tract obstruction. The highest incidence of clinical signs of urolithiasis in cattle and sheep is noted **during the early concentrate feeding period** (i.e., fall, winter) and during cold weather when water consumption decreases.

    a. Patient profile. Clinical disease is mainly seen in **castrated males** and is particularly common in feedlot and range-fed steers or wethers. Although bulls, cows, heifers, ewes, and rams also form urinary calculi, these cases less often develop into a clinical problem.

      (1) The female urethra is shorter and more able to pass urethral calculi than the male urethra.

      (2) In bulls, the urethra is up to 40% larger in diameter than in a similarly aged steer; therefore, bulls are less likely to become obstructed by uroliths.

    b. Clinical findings vary with the site and completeness of urinary tract obstruction.

      (1) Partial or incomplete obstruction. Urine dribbling from the prepuce ("dribblers") with **blood-tinged urine** surrounding the prepuce may be evident, with **white, powdery crystals** precipitating around the preputial orifice. These animals have prolonged, painful urination and may tramp or tread when attempting to pass urine.

(2) Complete urethral obstruction. Bladder rupture occurs after 48–72 hours if the obstruction is not relieved.
  (a) Inappetence, depression, and **colic signs** (with kicking at the abdomen) may be evident.
  (b) Treading. Steers shift their weight to opposing hind limbs (i.e., treading) and appear restless, getting up and down frequently.
  (c) Tenesmus may also be present, with palpable pulsations of the urethra and straining sufficient to prolapse the rectum.
  (d) The **preputial orifice hairs** are dry.
  (e) Sheep may also exhibit **tail wriggling.**
(3) Other signs can include grunting and grinding of the teeth (i.e., odontoprisis, bruxism).
(4) Rectal palpation may reveal a large and tightly distended urinary bladder.
c. Etiology and pathogenesis. The precipitation of urinary solutes around a nidus leads to the formation of calculi. This metabolic disorder is a combination of dietary, endocrine, and climatic factors.
  (1) Nidus formation. Factors involved in nidus formation include the administration of estrogen implants or the consumption of estrogenic feeds, vitamin A deficiency, or other factors that result in excessive urinary tract epithelial desquamation.
  (2) Urinary solute precipitation occurs for several reasons, including:
    (a) Increased phosphate or carbonate calculi formation in the presence of the alkaline urine of herbivores
    (b) Increased concentration of urine solutes as a result of water deprivation in cold weather
    (c) Heavy fluid loss, which may occur in hot weather
    (d) Excessive mineral intake (which often occurs in feedlots), particularly with respect to a high phosphate intake
  (3) Mucoproteins in the urine act as cementing agents to solidify the solutes that have precipitated around the nidus. Therefore, increased mucoprotein favors calculi formation. Heavy-concentrate and low-roughage feeding and the pelleting of rations (common practice in most feedlot feeding regimens) greatly increases the quantity of mucoproteins in the urine.
  (4) Calculi. Cattle usually have single, hard, discrete calculi, but there can be up to 200 calculi present in an individual animal's urinary tract.
    (a) Obstruction location
      (i) Cattle. Stones most often cause obstruction at the distal portion of the sigmoid flexure of the penis. There is a natural stricture at this site, which is where the retractor penis muscles attach.
      (ii) Sheep and **goats** tend to have fine, sand-like calculi, which are located throughout the urinary tract but most often block the vermiform appendage.
      (iii) With **massive urolithiasis,** obstruction may occur anywhere along the urethra in both cattle and sheep.
    (b) Types of calculi. Although several crystal types have been found in ruminant uroliths, the two main types are magnesium ammonium phosphate and silicate uroliths.
      (i) Magnesium ammonium phosphate calculi are found most commonly in feedlot cattle and sheep fed high-concentrate and low-roughage rations. These calculi are highly insoluble in alkaline urine (pH of 8.5–9.5); thus, they precipitate readily in the normally alkaline urine of herbivores. These calculi are usually small, smooth, and soft, with a high recurrence because there are many present.
      (ii) Silicate calculi occur in range-fed animals in the Great Plains regions, with grazing on mature prairie grasses or wheat or oat stubble (which can contain up to 2% silica). Water in these areas can also be high in silicates. Silicate calculi are rough and hard, usually forming only a single calculus. Given the high level of silica in both diet and water,

there can be outbreaks of urinary tract obstruction resulting from this calculi at any time of the year in any age and gender animals.

(c) Sequelae of urolithiasis include the rupture of the urethra, rupture of the urinary bladder, or both.

(i) Urethral rupture. The calculus lodges in the penile urethra, usually at the sigmoid flexure, and causes pressure necrosis of the urethral wall. Urine leaks into the subcutaneous tissue around the penis and accumulates in the subcutaneous connective tissue along the prepuce, resulting in extensive edema along the abdominal floor (extending from the sigmoid flexure to the umbilicus). Usually, the leakage of fluid relieves the acute pain of urinary bladder distention, but over time, this fluid can cause toxemia and tissue necrosis with sloughing of the skin of the ventral abdomen.

(ii) Bladder rupture. Abdominal pain is no longer present, and there is bilateral fluid-filled distention of the abdomen (a "pear-shaped" abdomen). In contrast to urethral rupture, there is little or no detectable ventral edema in the preputial or umbilical region. On rectal examination, the bladder is not palpable.

d. Diagnostic plan and laboratory tests

(1) The **clinical examination** often is sufficient to make a diagnosis of either urethral or bladder rupture.

(a) Urethral rupture

(i) The ventral abdominal edematous swelling that is associated with the prepuce caudally to the level of the scrotum, accompanied by pain at the sigmoid flexure, is usually sufficient to make the working diagnosis.

(ii) In sheep and goats, the vermiform appendage is usually blocked with sabulous material. Examination of the penis tip often reveals a turgid cyanotic vermiform appendage. Blockage further proximal in the penile urethra is usually present.

(b) Bladder rupture

(i) In the patient with abdominal swelling, the **five "Fs"** of abdominal distention should be considered: fat, fluid, feces, fetus, and flatus. A fluid wave can usually be balloted across the abdomen, and centesis of the abdomen with a large-bore needle readily yields a large amount of clear, acellular fluid.

(ii) Palpation of the penis at the sigmoid flexure may identify the site of obstruction, with pain induced on manipulation of the region.

(iii) On **rectal palpation,** the urinary bladder is usually nonpalpable. Although the abdomen is filled with fluid, this cannot be determined by per rectum palpation.

(2) Laboratory tests

(a) Serum biochemistry reveals an azotemic animal with a marked reduction in serum sodium and chloride. Potassium, however, does not increase markedly in ruminants with bladder rupture.

(b) An **abdominocentesis fluid sample** can be used to confirm uroperitoneum (see II E 4 b).

e. Therapeutic plan. The goals of treatment are to reestablish patent urethra and correct fluid, acid–base, and electrolyte imbalances.

(1) Cattle

(a) Medical therapy

(i) For early cases of urethral obstruction in which urethral or bladder rupture have not occurred, it is possible to attempt medical therapy by using **tranquilizers** (acepromazine at 20–40 mg/500 kg intramuscularly), **smooth muscle relaxants,** or **antispasmodics** (e.g., dipyrone). These agents can induce relaxation of the retractor penis muscle, which allows the sigmoid flexure to straighten, producing a wider, straighter urethra. Some reports suggest a 70% effectiveness in early cases.

      (ii) If there is no urine passage within 6 hours, these medications can be repeated, but surgery may be required. Rectal examination to assess bladder size and turgor can be used to assess the need for surgery.

  (b) Surgery. In the case of urethral or bladder rupture, surgical intervention (under epidural anesthesia) is required.

      (i) A **low urethrotomy** at the distal part of the sigmoid flexure can be performed to expose and remove the calculus, suturing the incision site if the stone has not caused extensive necrosis.

      (ii) A **high perineal urethrostomy** should be performed if local cellulitis or necrosis is present. The penis is transected proximal to the site of blockage and anchored to the skin. The more proximal urethra can be probed for evidence of additional calculi, but a urethral diverticulum at the level of the ischial arch usually prevents catheterization into the bladder. Tears in the bladder wall in bladder rupture usually heal spontaneously without requiring abdominal surgery.

      (iii) In both urethral and bladder rupture, **systemic antibiotics** post surgery are advised. The **correction of fluid** and **electrolyte losses** with isotonic sodium chloride is indicated but is seldom performed in field situations. Animals with urethral or bladder rupture should be sent to slaughter as soon as they are no longer uremic.

(2) Sheep and goats

  (a) Massaging the vermiform appendage free of the sandy debris should be attempted, but usually, the vermiform appendage needs to be amputated.

  (b) Catheterization. Sabulous debris in the more proximal penile urethra can be flushed out by passing a **catheter** up the penile urethra and instilling small amounts of saline periodically.

  (c) Surgery

      (i) Urethrostomy (as performed in steers) may be indicated if other treatments fail. Even after establishing urethral patency, the bladder may not spontaneously empty immediately because of chronic distention and atony.

      (ii) In the cases of urethral rupture with urine leakage in the subcutaneous tissues, small linear incisions in the overlying skin can be made to drain the urine that has collected and reduce the risk of extensive skin slough.

f. Prognosis. The survival rate for urethral rupture is approximately 90%, but for bladder rupture, the survival rate is 50%.

g. Prevention. Many dietary and management factors can affect the formation of urinary calculi and subsequent obstruction.

(1) Diet

  (a) For animals with **phosphate** or **magnesium ammonium phosphate calculi,** the diet can be assessed to ensure a calcium to phosphorus ratio of 2:1. Adding ground limestone to the diet can help avoid precipitation of excess phosphate in urine. Urine pH can be acidified (using ammonium chloride in the feed), increasing the solubility of the calculi.

  (b) For range-fed animals with **silicate calculi,** a common method of reducing problems with urinary blockage is to pasture only females or bulls on the high-risk pastures. Calculi still form but seldom result in urinary obstructive problems.

(2) Adequate water should be provided, particularly in cold weather when water sources may freeze.

(3) Increasing salt intake in the diet by up to 4% can also reduce calculi-related problems. Increased dietary salt forces diuresis (which prevents the concentration of urinary solutes). Furthermore, in the case of phosphate or magnesium ammonium phosphate crystals, sodium causes chloride to displace the magnesium and phosphate, preventing these minerals from being deposited around nidus of the calculus.

(4) Delaying castration of steers until after 6 months of age can allow the development of a larger urethral diameter, but this delay may not be practical in range or feedlot animals.

(5) Adequate vitamin A intake reduces nidus formation, and estrogenic implants can be avoided to reduce the mucoprotein content in the urine.

2. Obstructive urolithiasis in horses

a. Patient profile. Cystic calculi (stones in the bladder) are not common in horses and seldom cause acute clinical signs of obstruction. Some males may develop stones that lodge in the urethra.

b. Clinical findings. Persistent hematuria (or post-exercise hematuria) is often the only clinical sign. Otherwise, horses with cystic calculi can have mild recurrent colic, urine scalding of the perineum, stranguria, dribbling urine, or pollakiuria. Weight loss and a stilted gait have also been reported. These bladder stones are usually readily palpable on rectal examination.

c. Pathogenesis. Less is known about the formation of these calculi in horses than in ruminants, but the factors are likely similar because horses also have alkaline urine, which favors the deposition of carbonate and phosphate crystals. Calculi are usually solitary, large, and composed of calcium carbonate or phosphates. They tend to develop near the neck of the bladder.

d. Diagnostic plan and laboratory tests

(1) In addition to **clinical findings, cystoscopy** or **ultrasound** can be used to demonstrate or suggest the presence of a stone. Occasionally, calculi can be felt with a urinary catheter.

(2) Urinalysis reveals crystals, as well as free RBCs and WBCs. Concurrent cystitis is also a common finding.

e. Therapeutic plan. The stones can be removed surgically by either an abdominal approach or via urethrotomy in male horses. In mares, some stones can be removed manually through the urethra. Electrohydraulic lithotripsy has been used successfully in shattering the stones in situ for ease of removal.

f. Prognosis. Horses that have had cystic calculi may have problems with chronic cystitis even after stone removal, and the calculi may recur.

g. Prevention. In selected cases, diet supplementation with urinary acidifiers has helped prevent calculi formation.

DIRECTIONS: Each of the numbered items or incomplete statements in this section is followed by answers or by completions of the statement. Select the ONE numbered answer or completion that is BEST in each case.

1. Which one of the following statements regarding pyelonephritis is true?

(1) Cows that are housed during the winter develop pyelonephritis as a result of the infection by *Ureaplasma laidlawi* during natural breeding or artificial insemination.

(2) In horses, pyelonephritis is a sporadic occurrence with infection by coliforms such as *Proteus* species and is associated mainly with breeding trauma or urine pooling in mares.

(3) In pigs, the organism *Eubacterium suis* is a key cause of pyelonephritis, and clinical signs are insidious with pyuria and chronic weight loss.

(4) Sows develop pyelonephritis as a result of *Eubacterium suis* infection from recent farrowing or natural mating, with initial clinical signs highly different from those noted in cows or horses.

2. Which one of the following statements regarding horses with chronic renal failure is correct?

(1) Hypercalcemia may be present, but it appears to be dependent on diet because calcium levels can return to normal levels in low-calcium diets.

(2) In glomerulonephritis, the glomerular lesion is caused by autoimmunity to the glomerular basement membrane, or less commonly, circulating immune complexes to viral or bacterial (e.g., streptococcal) antigens.

(3) Chronic renal failure in horses is most commonly tubulointerstitial, rather than glomerulonephritis.

(4) When recognized, glomerulonephritis in horses is best treated with corticosteroids to reverse the immunologic damage to the glomerular basement membrane.

3. Acute renal failure in ruminants can be associated with which of the following?

(1) Neonatal calf diarrhea, abomasal displacement, and lactic acidosis ("grain overload") can be causes of acute renal tubular necrosis in cattle with their associated profound volume depletion.

(2) Although aminoglycosides can induce nephrotoxicity in all species, ruminants are usually spared from this risk because they rarely receive such drugs.

(3) Administration of outdated or excess doses of tetracyclines has resulted in renal failure in cattle.

(4) Copper toxicity in cattle and sheep causes acute renal tubular necrosis due to the cupric ion damage to tubular epithelium.

(5) Plant toxins that result in renal tubular necrosis in ruminants include oak (*Quercus* species) and Russian knapweed (*Centaurea repens*).

4. Which one of the following statements regarding urinary tract disorders in large animals is correct?

(1) Renal amyloidosis occurs with approximately equal frequency in both horses and cattle, with signs of ventral edema, chronic intractable diarrhea, and weight loss, with the kidneys often uniformly enlarged on rectal palpation.

(2) Cows affected by renal amyloidosis seldom have any other concurrent disease.

(3) Ectopic ureters in large animals is a congenital problem with signs of urine dribbling from birth. Although this disorder has been reported mainly in horses and in both sexes, it may be more readily detected in females with more obvious urine dribbling.

(4) Ectopic ureter of large animals is usually only corrected for aesthetic reasons because, apart from urine scald, the animals seldom have any other associated complications.

5. Which one of the following statements regarding foals with bladder rupture is correct?

(1) Bladder rupture occurs most frequently in female foals after dystocia or is otherwise most common in either sex foal that is stepped on by the dam.

(2) Foals appear normal at birth and within 6–12 hours become severely depressed because of azotemia and peritonitis.

(3) Foals develop progressive abdominal distention and show signs of straining, which may be mistaken for meconium impaction.

(4) If untreated, a main cause for mortality is the progressive azotemia.

(5) Tests to help confirm the presence of urine in the abdomen include the instillation of a positive contrast (such as barium) into the bladder and the demonstration of its presence in the abdomen either by radiography or a peritoneal fluid sample.

6. Which one of the following statements regarding the prevention of urolithiasis in ruminants is correct?

(1) For phosphate or magnesium ammonium phosphate calculi, the diet should have a calcium to phosphate ratio of 2:1, possibly by adding ground limestone to the diet, which can help avoid the precipitation of excess phosphate in the urine.

(2) For silicate calculi, the urine pH can be acidified using ammonium chloride in the feed because these calculi are also more soluble in acid urine.

(3) For silicate calculi that occur in range-fed animals, pasturing only females on the high-risk pastures is advised because the hormonal differences in the cows result in less risk of calculi formation.

(4) For urolithiasis of most types of calculi, the dietary salt intake should be reduced to prevent excess solutes in the urine.

(5) Delaying the castration of male animals until after 6 months of age can reduce the problem of urinary obstruction by stones because the testosterone influence prevents nidus formation.

7. Which one of the following statements regarding cystic calculi of horses is true?

(1) Clinical signs of bladder stones in horses are similar to those in ruminants, with blockage of the urethra the main clinical sign.

(2) The main type of stone in horses is silicate calculi, which results from high silicic acid on certain pastures and oat feedstuffs.

(3) Cystic or bladder stones are usually best diagnosed by urine crystal analysis.

(4) Finding high numbers of calcium carbonate crystals in the urine of horses without signs of urinary tract disease does not necessarily suggest the presence of a bladder stone.

ANSWERS AND EXPLANATIONS

1. The answer is 4 [I C 2]. Sows may die without premonitory signs. The causative organisms are coliforms and *Corynebacterium renale*. The high risk factors associated with pyelonephritis are commonly bladder paralysis, urine stasis, or ureteral ectopia. Signs in pigs are usually peracute with death.

2. The answer is 1 [I A 3 a (5)]. Hypercalcemia may be present, but it appears to be dependent on diet because calcium levels can return to normal levels in low-calcium diets. In glomerulonephritis, the glomerular lesion is caused by autoimmunity to the glomerular basement membrane or, more commonly, by circulating immune complexes to viral or bacterial (e.g., streptococcal) antigens. Chronic renal failure in horses is most commonly glomerulonephritis, rather than tubulointerstitial. Although corticosteroids have been advocated, they do not reverse the damages to glomeruli.

3. The answer is 3 [I B 1 c]. The administration of outdated or excess doses of tetracyclines has resulted in renal failure in cattle. Diarrhea and grain overload can induce volume depletion, but it usually requires a torsion of the abomasum for similarly severe vascular compromise. One of the most commonly drug-associated nephrotoxicities in the United States is from neomycin. Hopefully, this will soon be only a historical note with increased vigilance and care in medicating food-producing animals. Acute intravascular hemolysis that results in tubular necrosis from endogenous pigment damage. Although oak is toxic, ruminants can safely graze on pastures with Russian knapweed (see Chapter 11).

4. The answer is 3 [II D 1, 2]. Although ectopic ureter has been reported mainly in horses and in both sexes, it may be more readily detected in females with more obvious urine dribbling. The clinical signs are appropriate, but horses rarely develop renal amyloidosis. Cows affected by renal amyloidosis often have a chronic bacterial infection (e.g., pericarditis, pulmonary abscessation, peritonitis, metritis), leading to reactive systemic amyloidosis. Associated complications usually include urine reflux, the formation of hydroureter, and the predisposition of the animal to ascending urinary tract infection.

5. The answer is 3 [II E 2]. Foals develop progressive abdominal distention and show signs of straining, which may be mistaken for meconium impaction. Bladder rupture is more common in males, and the damage from the dam is not a recorded high risk factor. Signs usually take 24–48 hours to develop after birth, and peritonitis is not a big concern because the urine is sterile. Untreated animals get life-threatening hyperkalemia and severe electrolyte imbalances. Barium would be contraindicated and would cause an intense peritoneal inflammation.

6. The answer is 1 [II F 1 g]. For phosphate or magnesium ammonium phosphate calculi, the diet should have a calcium to phosphate ratio of 2:1. Silicate stones are not solubilized by an acidified pH change. Calculi still form in females but seldom result in urinary obstructive problems in cows. Salt in the diet, up to 4%, can reduce calculi-related problems by a forced diuresis that prevents concentration of urinary solutes. The development of a larger urethral diameter, not the influence of testosterone, reduces the risk of urinary obstruction.

7. The answer is 4 [II F 2]. Finding high numbers of calcium carbonate crystals does not necessarily suggest the presence of a bladder stone. Signs in horses are persistent hematuria or post-exercise hematuria. Horses have alkaline urine that favors the deposition of carbonate and phosphate crystals. Bladder stones are readily palpable on rectal examination, or they can be detected by cystoscopy or ultrasound.

Chapter 16

Dermatologic Diseases

Timothy H. Ogilvie

I. DIAGNOSTIC APPROACH TO DERMATOLOGIC DISEASE

A. **History and clinical findings.** Because an accurate history is often difficult to obtain, use of a detailed questionnaire is helpful. Important points to consider when obtaining the history include:

1. Age, breed, sex, and color of the animal

2. Duration, characteristics, and changes in the primary complaint

3. Presence or absence of pruritus

4. Seasonality of the condition

5. Type of housing

6. Other affected animals

7. Internal and external parasite control program

8. Systemic or topical medication used for skin conditions or recent problems

9. Other medical problems

B. **Physical examination.** The overall condition of the animal should be assessed.

1. **Lesions.** The **distribution** (e.g., generalized, localized, specific body regions) and **type** (e.g., primary, secondary) of skin lesions should be noted.
   a. **Primary lesions** include papules, macules, nodules, tumors, pustules, wheals, and vesicles.
   b. **Secondary lesions** include scales, crusts, excoriations, erosions, ulcers, lichenification, pigmentation changes, and fissures.

2. The **skin surface** should be palpated to determine features not easily visible (e.g., crusts beneath hair, dryness, ability to epilate hairs, presence of peripheral lymphadenopathy).

3. The **mucous membranes** should be examined.

C. **Differential diagnoses.** The skin can react to a variety of insults in limited ways. This may make reaching a diagnosis difficult. Lists of differential diagnoses are based on information gained from the history and physical examination. Several causes of the presenting complaint are usually considered, and the diagnosis is confirmed by either testing the hypothesis or measuring any response to a specific therapy.

D. **Diagnostic techniques**

1. **Skin scraping** is often used to demonstrate the presence of external parasites (e.g., mites, lice).
   a. **Materials** for skin scraping include a sterile container, mineral oil, a #10 scalpel blade, glass slides, and coverslips.
   b. **Procedure**
      (1) Areas with hair (e.g., fetlock) should be lightly clipped before scraping.
      (2) Multiple superficial scrapings covering a large surface area should be obtained. Skin scrapings should be deep enough to induce capillary oozing to recover deep skin-dwelling mites.
      (3) The collected material is placed in a container until a microscopic examination can be performed. The sample is then placed on a glass slide and finely dispersed in mineral oil to provide a confluent layer without air bubbles.

2. **Wood's lamp examination** is not useful in large animals. *Microsporum canis* is the only dermatophyte that fluoresces and then only 50%–60% of the time. This organism usually affects only dogs and cats. Horses and cattle are most commonly infected with *Trichophyton* species, which do not fluoresce. Therefore, a negative Wood's lamp examination does not rule out dermatophytosis.

3. **Dermatophyte culture.** Animals with focal or generalized alopecia with or without scaling or crusting are candidates for a dermatophyte culture.
    a. **Materials** for the test include a dermatophyte test medium, 70% isopropyl alcohol, mosquito forceps, a #10 scalpel blade, and sterile empty containers, such as evacuated blood collection tubes.
    b. **Procedure**
        (1) **Collecting the sample.** The forceps and each lesion to be sampled should be wiped gently with isopropyl alcohol and allowed to dry in order to remove as many bacterial and saprophytic contaminants as possible. Multiple, small, scaling and lightly crusted lesions should be sampled. Broken hairs, scales, and crusts from the periphery of the lesion are collected. A blade may be useful in scraping scales and debris from the skin surface. The forceps are used to pluck and sample broken hairs. Samples should be stored in separate sterile containers.
        (2) **Testing the sample.** Samples should be removed from containers with sterile forceps in a clean working area and gently pressed onto, but not buried beneath, the culture medium. The top of the culture dish should be loosely replaced to allow sufficient ventilation. Most dermatophytes grow at room temperature with the exception of *Trichophyton verrucosum,* which requires incubation at 37°C.
        (3) **Results.** The **dermatophyte test medium** is an amber-colored **Sabouraud's dextrose agar,** containing phenol red, a pH indicator, as well as several antibacterial and antifungal agents to inhibit the growth of contaminant organisms. Dermatophytes preferentially use the protein in the medium as they begin to grow, producing alkaline metabolites that cause the medium to turn red. The dermatophyte colony is typically a white-to-beige, powdery-to-fluffy growth. The **red color change** on Sabouraud's and colony growth characteristics should occur concurrently for positive identification.

4. **Potassium hydroxide (KOH) preparations** may permit the immediate diagnosis of a dermatophytosis. However, negative results do not rule out dermatophytosis. Examination of KOH preparations requires considerable expertise because fungal elements may be overlooked, and numerous artifacts (e.g., fibers, cholesterol crystals, oil droplets) may be confused with fungal elements. A dermatophyte culture should always be performed in conjunction with a KOH preparation.
    a. **Materials** for the test include mosquito forceps, a #10 scalpel blade, a sterile empty container, glass microscope slides, coverslips, a Bunsen burner, and the clearing solution.
    b. **Procedure.** Hairs and scales should be collected from the periphery of several lesions using the mosquito forceps and the blade. A drop of clearing solution is placed on a glass slide, hairs and scales are added to the solution, and a coverslip is placed over the material. The purpose of the **clearing solution** is to dissolve hard keratin and bleach the melanin of the hair shaft so that hyphae and arthroconidia can be identified more readily. Clearing solutions include **15% KOH** (heated for 15–20 seconds or allowed to stand at room temperature for 30 minutes) or a KOH and dimethyl sulfoxide (DMSO) solution, which permits immediate examination. The slide is scanned with the 10-times (10x) objective in search of abnormal hairs with a fuzzy internal structure. High-power examination of these hairs may demonstrate hyphae, which usually have uniform width and septae. Bead-like chains of arthroconidia may be seen as well.

5. **Acetate tape preparations** are used to diagnose *Oxyuris equi* or *Chorioptes equi* infestation.

a. **Materials** used include acetate (nonfrosted) tape, mineral oil, and glass microscope slides.

b. **Procedure.** A piece of tape is pressed onto several areas in the anal and perianal region and then removed and placed (adhesive side down) on a glass slide liberally coated with mineral oil (which will clear debris and facilitate the examination of the preparation).

6. *Dermatophilus* **preparation.** Crusted lesions accompanied by matting of the coat in horses and ruminants are clinical findings for dermatophilosis. Because suppuration underlies the crust, **direct smears** of the exudate must be made, stained, and examined on a glass slide for characteristic bacteria. Crusts can be removed from the patient, macerated with scissors, and mixed with several drops of water on a glass slide. After crusts have been softened in water, they should be crushed with the top of an applicator stick. Excess debris should be removed, the slide should be air dried, heat fixed, and then stained with Gram's, Giemsa, or Wright's stain.

7. **Biopsy for routine histopathology.** The types of lesions to be biopsied include suspect neoplastic lesions, persistent ulcers, dermatoses not responding to appropriate therapy, and any unusual or serious lesions. Fully developed primary lesions should be selected. Biopsy for histopathology is usually unrewarding for chronic (e.g., lichenified, hyperpigmented) lesions. If possible, multiple lesions should be biopsied.

   a. **Materials** for performing a skin biopsy include 6-mm and 4-mm biopsy punches, a #15 scalpel blade, sharp scissors, Adson forceps, needle holders, 2-0–3-0 nonabsorbable suture material, 2% lidocaine, a 3-ml syringe with a 22- to 25-gauge needle, a tongue depressor, gauze, and 10% buffered formalin.

   b. **Procedure**

      (1) **Preparation.** Surgical preparation (i.e., shaving and scrubbing) will remove crusts and epithelial tissue that are important for diagnosis and should not be performed. Local anesthesia is accomplished by inserting the needle at the margin of the lesion and infiltrating lidocaine subcutaneously.

      (2) **Biopsy techniques.** Excisional (either punch or elliptical) skin biopsy techniques can be used.

         (a) **Punch biopsies** are used to assess a single nodule. Most lesions can be sampled with a 6-mm disposable biopsy punch. When a biopsy has been obtained, the site can be sutured with simple interrupted sutures or a cruciate stitch. When obtaining biopsies of ulcerations, the biopsy should include normal tissue, the leading edge of the lesion, and abnormal tissue.

         (b) **Elliptical biopsies.** Punch biopsies are not appropriate for vesicular, bullous, or ulcerous lesions. Instead, an elliptical biopsy is preferred. Elliptical biopsies, which are obtained with a scalpel, should be mounted with gentle pressure on a small piece of tongue depressor or cardboard to prevent curling.

8. **Biopsy for immunofluorescence testing.** Immunofluorescence testing is used as an adjunct to conventional histology in patients with suspected immune-mediated skin disease (e.g., pemphigus foliaceus, bullous pemphigoid, discoid lupus erythematosus, systemic lupus erythematosus, some forms of vasculitis). The technique is similar to that used to obtain biopsies for histopathology, but other fixatives are used. The diagnosis of immune-mediated skin disease is made on the basis of both histologic and immunofluorescent findings.

9. *Onchocerca* **preparation.** Horses with lesions of alopecia and scaling (with or without pruritis) that include diffuse ventral midline dermatitis and/or facial, cervical, thoracic, or proximal forelimb lesions are candidates for *Onchocerca* infestation. Many horses will have microfilariae present in the dermal tissue without any evidence of skin disease. A positive preparation only suggests that *Onchocerca* organisms are the cause of the dermatitis.

    a. Sample. If possible, a lesion should be sampled in a region where microfilariae are not recovered in high numbers in normal horses (e.g., avoid the ventral midline). The sample should be obtained with a 10-mm punch biopsy and split in half. Half of the sample should be put in formalin, and the other half should be placed on a dampened gauze sponge in a tightly closed container until a preparation can be made.

    b. Preparation. A small piece of tissue that includes dermis is placed on a glass slide, minced with a scalpel, and a few drops of nonbacteriostatic saline are added. The slide is then incubated at room temperature for 15 minutes.

    c. Results. The slide is scanned with a microscope (4x objective) along the margins of tissue debris, searching for indications of motion in the saline. If the characteristic "whiplash" movement of the parasite is noted, a higher power objective should be used. Microfilariae are slender and delicate, measuring approximately 8 μm $\times$ 220 μm.

10. Bacterial culture. A bacterial culture should be requested when folliculitis or bacterial pyodermas are suspected. Normal skin is heavily contaminated by bacteria; therefore, cultures must be carefully taken and interpreted. Cultures of open, draining lesions generate misleading bacteriologic data.

    a. Samples

        (1) Intact samples. Intact nodules, pustules, and abscesses may be aspirated with a needle and syringe or punctured with a scalpel and swabbed with a culturette after gently cleaning the overlying skin with alcohol and allowing it to air dry.

        (2) Biopsy samples. When intact lesions containing pus are not available for sampling, a culture of surgical biopsy specimens is preferred. Papules, plaques, nodules, and areas of diffuse swelling may be surgically prepared and punch or excision biopsies taken with aseptic technique.

    b. Preparation. Samples for culture are routinely plated on blood agar and inoculated in thioglycolate broth to encourage the growth of any anaerobes.

II. ENVIRONMENTAL AND MECHANICAL DERMATOSES

A. **Frostbite** is a skin injury resulting from exposure to excessive cold.

    1. Patient profile and history

        a. Neonates and sick, debilitated, or dehydrated animals are most prone to frostbite injury.

        b. Lesions are seen on the extremities after cold weather.

    2. Clinical findings include erythema, scaling, and alopecia affecting the ears, tails, teats, scrotum, and feet. Severe cases are characterized by necrosis, dry gangrene, and sloughing. Affected skin usually lacks feeling.

    3. Pathogenesis. Frostbite is more common in animals with **poor circulation** (e.g., as seen with ergotism, fescue toxicosis, vasculitis) or in animals that are unable to seek shelter.

    4. Diagnostic plan. History and clinical signs determine the diagnosis.

    5. Therapeutic plan

        a. Mild cases. Treatment is unnecessary for mild cases.

        b. Severe cases. Rapid thawing in warm water (41°C–44°C) followed by the application of **bland, protective ointments** and **creams** is the treatment of choice for severe cases. Where there has been necrosis and sloughing of skin, topical **wet soaks** and **systemic antibiotics** should be used. **Surgical excision** should be postponed until an obvious boundary is present between viable and nonviable tissue.

6. **Prevention.** After it has been frozen, tissue may have an increased susceptibility to cold injury.

B. **Thermal injuries (burns).** Occasionally, burns are seen in large animals in association with barn fires, brush fires, electrocution, or lightening strike. The prognosis is poor for animals with burns covering more than 50% of the body surface. Treatment includes:

1. Cleansing with mild soap and water 2–3 times daily
2. Initial surgical debridement
3. Daily hydrotherapy
4. Topical antibiotics
5. Systemic nonsteroidal anti-inflammatory agents

C. **Primary irritant contact dermatitis**

1. **Patient profile and history.** The animal may present with dermatitis of the face, distal extremities, or ventrum.

2. **Clinical findings.** This dermatitis ranges in severity from erythema to papules, edema, scaling, vesicles, erosions, ulcers, necrosis, and crusts. Pruritus and pain are variable. Self-trauma resulting from the irritation can cause alopecia, lichenification, and scarring. Leukotrichia and leukoderma may be permanent sequelae.

3. **Etiology.** Primary irritants invariably cause dermatitis if they come into contact with skin in sufficient concentration for a long enough time. No sensitization is required. For example, leukoderma around the mouth of horses is commonly caused by the rubber bit.
   a. **Caustic substances** may be either acids or alkalis. Crude oil, diesel fuel, turpentine, leather preservatives, mercurials, blisters, and wood preservatives are all primary irritants.
   b. **Moisture** is an important predisposing factor because it decreases effectiveness of normal skin barriers. Causes for excessive moisture include body excretions (i.e., feces, urine), a damp environment, and wound secretions. Conditions that cause excessive moisture include:
      (1) Scalding of the perineum in diarrheic calves or foals
      (2) Flank or udder fold dermatitis in lactating dairy cows
      (3) Ovine fleece rot
   c. **Other causes** of primary contact dermatitis include improperly used topical parasiticides and irritating plants (e.g., sneezeweed, stinging nettle).

4. **Diagnostic plan.** The nature of any contact dermatitis can usually be inferred from the distribution of the lesions.
   a. **Muzzle or extremities**—plants and environmental substances (e.g., fertilizers)
   b. **Single limb**—irritating medications (e.g., blisters)
   c. **Face and dorsum**—sprays, dips, and wipes
   d. **Perineum and rear legs**—urine and feces
   e. **Tack-associated areas**—preservatives, dyes, and polishes
   f. **Ventrum**—bedding and filthy environment

5. **Laboratory tests.** A skin biopsy reveals varying degrees of superficial dermatitis (e.g., hyperplastic, spongiotic), with neutrophils or mononuclear cells predominating.

6. **Therapeutic plan.** Irritants should be identified and eliminated. Any residue should be removed with large amounts of water and gentle cleansing soaps. Astringent soaks (e.g., aluminum acetate, magnesium sulfate in water) are applied to moist, oozing lesions for 5–10 minutes three times daily. Topical antiseptics, antibiotics, and/or glucocorticoids may be considered in cases of severe or significant inflammation.

7. **Prognosis.** Removal of the irritant results in remarkable improvement of the dermatitis in 7–10 days.

D. **Chemical toxicosis.** Ingestion or exposure to some chemicals or agents produces skin disease.

  1. **Mercury** poisoning produces acute gastroenteritis and death if ingested in sufficient quantities. Mercury also causes alopecia with the loss of long hairs in the tail and mane if ingested in smaller quantities over a longer time.

  2. **Iodine** (or iodides) causes epiphora, nasal discharge, lacrimation, and seborrhea sicca with partial alopecia over the dorsum, head, neck, and shoulders. There is usually a history of sodium iodide or potassium iodide administration.

E. **Photodermatitis**

  1. **Sunburn**
     a. **Patient profile and history.** Sunburn produces a dermatitis of lightly pigmented skin (e.g., Saanen goats, white pigs).
     b. **Clinical findings** include erythema and scaling. Severe burning causes exudation, necrosis, and crust formation. Sunburn is common on the lateral aspects of the udder and teats of white goats that are turned out in summer and along the back and ears of white-skinned pigs.
     c. **Laboratory tests.** A skin biopsy reveals superficial perivascular dermatitis, dyskeratotic keratinocytes in superficial dermis, and basophilic degeneration of elastin.
     d. **Prevention.** As in all species, initial exposure to sunlight should be limited. Sunscreen may be applied to susceptible animals if warranted.

  2. **Photosensitization** is characterized by acute onset of erythema, edema, and variable degrees of pruritus and pain.
     a. **Clinical findings.** Cutaneous lesions are often restricted to unpigmented, sparsely-haired areas but may extend to dark-skinned areas in severe cases. The eyelids, lips, face, ears, perineum, and coronary band region are commonly involved. Vesicles and bullae develop that progress to oozing, necrosis, skin sloughing, and ulceration.
     b. **Pathogenesis**
        (1) There are **three basic features** for all types of photosensitization:
           (a) Presence of a photodynamic agent in the skin
           (b) Concomitant exposure to a sufficient amount of certain wavelengths of ultraviolet light (UVL)
           (c) Cutaneous absorption of UVL, which is facilitated by a lack of pigment in the haircoat
        (2) **Molecules** of photodynamic agents absorb light energy at a specific wavelength and enter a higher energy state. In the presence of oxygen, excited molecules produce free radicals, which cause structural damage of cell and lysosomal membranes. This in turn causes the release of hydrolytic enzymes and other chemical mediators of inflammation.
        (3) **Classification of photosensitization**
           (a) **Primary photosensitization.** The photodynamic agent is preformed or produced metabolically in the body and may be acquired by ingestion, injection, or contact (Table 16-1).

TABLE 16-1. Primary Photosensitization in Large Animals

Photodynamic Plant Species	Chemicals
St. John's-wort	Phenothiazine
Buckwheat	Thiazides
Spring parsley	Acriflavines
Perennial rye grass	Rose bengal
Burr trefoil	Methylene blue
	Sulfonamides
	Tetracyclines

      (b) **Hepatogenous photosensitization.** Phylloerythrin, a porphyrin compound formed by the microbial degradation of chlorophyll in the gut, is normally conjugated in the liver and excreted in the bile. Liver dysfunction, biliary stasis, or both may cause an accumulation of phylloerythrin in the blood and body tissues with resultant photosensitization.

      (c) **Photosensitization due to aberrant pigment synthesis (porphyria)** is characterized by an accumulation of photodynamic porphyrins in the blood and body tissues as a result of aberrant pigment synthesis.

      (d) **Photosensitization of unknown mechanism** is associated with the ingestion of lush pastures (e.g., clover, alfalfa, vetch, oats).

  c. Diagnostic plan. Diagnosis is based on a thorough clinical examination and history, including information on the diet, pasture, and any drug therapy. The number of animals at risk should be compared with the number of animals affected. If many animals are affected, this may indicate a photosensitivity, whereas one affected animal may suggest photoallergy. Liver tests should be performed when the clinician suspects hepatogenous photosensitization (see Chapter 5 I B 1).

  d. Therapeutic plan. Therapy should be aimed at the primary cause. The source of the photodynamic agent should be identified and eliminated, sunlight should be avoided, and symptomatic therapy should be provided for hepatic disorders.

    (1) **Glucocorticoids** or **nonsteroidal anti-inflammatory drugs (NSAIDs)** may be used to ameliorate signs.

    (2) **Systemic antibiotics** may be necessary if there is secondary pyoderma.

    (3) **Surgical debridement** may be employed for severe necrosis and skin sloughing.

  e. Prognosis. The prognosis is favorable for animals with primary photosensitization but is poor for those with hepatogenous photosensitization.

III.   NUTRITIONAL DERMATOSES

A. Ergotism

  1. Patient profile. This condition affects cattle, most commonly in the cooler months.

  2. Clinical findings. The two clinical syndromes of ergotism include **neurotoxicity** and a form of **chronic gangrene.** With the gangrenous form, early edema of the coronary regions (most often the hindlegs) progresses to an abrupt line of ischemic necrosis (i.e., dry gangrene), usually in the mid-metatarsus area. The distal limb is cold and insensitive and eventually sloughs. Occasionally, ear tips and the tail tip are affected. Severe diarrhea often accompanies necrosis of the extremities.

  3. Etiology and pathogenesis

    a. *Claviceps purpurea* is a fungus that infests many cereal grains and crops under warm, moist growing conditions. These harvested grains are then used in the winter stabling period, and animals (mainly cattle) become affected 2–4 months after exposure.

    b. Ergot alkaloids in fungus-contaminated feedstuffs cause vasoconstriction and capillary endothelial damage, with resultant ischemic necrosis and gangrene.

  4. Diagnostic plan and laboratory tests. The presumptive diagnosis is based on clinical signs, history, environment, and finding blackened, fungus-contaminated feed. The diagnosis is confirmed by necropsy of affected animals and the analysis of suspected feedstuffs.

5. **Differential diagnoses** for the clinical signs include **gangrene, frostbite,** and **trauma.**

6. **Therapeutic plan and prevention.** Treatment is rarely attempted, and affected animals usually are culled. Ergot-contaminated grains or feedstuffs should not be fed to cattle. As a general rule, grain should not contain more than 0.1% ergot-contaminated heads if it is to be used for animal feed.

B. **Fescue toxicosis (fescue foot)** is virtually identical to poisoning by *Claviceps purpurea,* but fescue foot occurs specifically in cattle or sheep that are grazing fescue grass (tall fescue) pastures contaminated with *Acremonium coeniaphilum.*

C. Zinc deficiency

1. **Patient profile.** Zinc deficiency is most often seen in cattle, sheep, and goats.

2. **Clinical findings**
   a. **Skin manifestations** include a dull, rough haircoat and parakeratosis with scaling, crusting, and alopecia, particularly over the face, ears, eyes, distal limbs, and mucocutaneous junctions.
   b. Generally, the animal has **poor growth, stiff** or **swollen joints,** and a **decreased resistance** to infections.

3. **Etiology.** A zinc-deficient diet or diets high in chelating minerals may cause this condition.

4. **Diagnostic plan and laboratory tests**
   a. **Response to therapy** is the best diagnosis.
   b. **Serum** and **hair levels** for zinc can be low or normal; thus, these tests are not diagnostic.
   c. A **skin biopsy** shows evidence of parakeratotic hyperkeratosis.

5. **Therapeutic plan.** Modern diets are usually well balanced for trace minerals such as zinc.
   a. **Cattle** should get 2–5 g zinc sulfate daily.
   b. **Sheep** should get 40 mg zinc sulfate daily.

D. Copper deficiency

1. **Patient profile.** Copper deficiency affects mainly cattle and sheep.

2. **Clinical findings**
   a. Affected animals have **stunted growth, diarrhea, anemia, infertility, lameness, loss of wool crimp (in sheep),** and **heart failure.**
   b. **Skin changes** include a rough, brittle, faded haircoat (speckled in appearance), which the animal itches and licks.
   c. Dark hairs may become light, particularly around the eyes, giving animals a **"spectacled" appearance.**

3. **Etiology and pathogenesis.** There is a dietary deficiency of copper or a secondary molybdenum excess. Copper is essential for the function of many oxidative enzymes, and evidence of dysfunction of these systems may be seen in the skin and haircoat (e.g., failure of pigmentation).

4. **Diagnostic plan and laboratory tests**
   a. **Serum copper levels** should be less than 0.7 μg/ml to be diagnostic but might often be normal in affected animals.
   b. **Liver copper levels** from a biopsy specimen seem to be more reliable and are evidence of herd copper status.

5. **Therapeutic plan and prevention.** Modern rations with attention to mineral supplementation should limit the likelihood of copper deficiencies.
   a. **Oral copper therapy.** Copper sulfate is administered once weekly for 3–5 weeks at the following levels. Be aware that **copper toxicity** may occur at these levels.

          (1) Calves—4 g
          (2) Cattle—6–10 g
          (3) Sheep—1.5 g
     b. Alternative forms of therapy and prevention include injections and slow-release oral, copper bullets.

E. Selenium toxicosis

    1. Clinical findings. Acute poisoning may result in sudden death, whereas chronic poisoning **(alkali disease)** produces hair loss and laminitis. Hair loss is most pronounced from the tail (in cattle and horses) and the mane (in horses).

    2. Etiology. Selenium poisoning is caused by the ingestion of toxic levels of inorganic or organic selenium. Sources include supplemented feeds and plants that concentrate selenium from soils (so-called **convertor** or **indicator plants,** such as *Astragalus* species and *Haplopappus* species).

IV. VIRAL DERMATOSES

A. Introduction

    1. Clinical findings. Many pox viruses that cause skin lesions begin as erythema and progress through papule, vesicle, pustule, and scab stages before resolving.

    2. Diagnostic plan and laboratory tests. Cutaneous lesions may be the only manifestation of viral infection. Guidelines for obtaining samples for examination are as follows:
      a. Samples should be stored at 4°C in a transport medium.
      b. Samples should be taken from more than one lesion in more than one animal.
      c. Areas for sample collection should be washed with water or saline but not with alcohol because it inactivates most viruses.
      d. Specimen collection of the skin and mucous membranes should be extended to the periphery and base of the lesion.
      e. Tissues should be submitted for both electron microscopy and virus isolation.

B. Specific conditions

    1. Cowpox is a benign but contagious skin disease.
      a. Clinical findings. This disease is characterized by typical pox-like lesions on the teats and udders of cows.
      b. Etiology. The source of infection may be infected cows or milkers that were recently vaccinated against smallpox (vaccinia virus). Pain from the lesions may cause failure of milk letdown and mastitis.
      c. Therapeutic plan. Treatment consists of the local application of soothing creams.

    2. Pseudocowpox is similar to cowpox but is more common and cycles in the herd with a prolonged clinical presentation and healing time (up to 18 months). It is caused by a parapoxvirus and seen primarily in lactating heifers. The infection is zoonotic and causes **milker's nodules** in humans.
      a. Clinical findings. Lesions are restricted to teats of lactating cows. Edema and erythema is followed by papules (within 48 hours), then a dark red scab that becomes raised by granulation tissue (the central area appears umbilicated). The center desquamates, leaving a raised ring of crust in the shape of a horseshoe. The granuloma may persist for months.
      b. Diagnostic plan and laboratory tests. Diagnosis is based on the clinical findings and history and supported by electron microscopy examination of vesicle fluid (which shows intracytoplasmic inclusions) or virus isolation.

      c. **Therapeutic plan and prevention.** Treatment of affected cows has little effect, but the spread of disease is lessened by milking affected cows last, using teat dips, and reducing teat trauma.

  3. Bovine ulcerative mammillitis is caused by **bovine herpesvirus type 2,** and the resulting lesion is ulcerative in nature.

      a. **Clinical findings.** The teats of young, milking animals are most often affected with painful edema, vesiculation, and skin sloughing. There is no systemic involvement, but mastitis occurs because of the very painful nature of the lesions and subsequent failure of milk letdown.

      b. **Diagnostic plan and laboratory tests.** The diagnosis is based on clinical signs and supported by virus isolation in a bovine tissue culture (either from vesicle aspirate or lesion biopsy). Histopathology of biopsy specimens shows intranuclear inclusion bodies in early lesions.

      c. **Therapeutic plan.** Treatment is nonspecific and focuses on softening and protecting the lesions from secondary infections through the use of antibiotic creams.

  4. Sheeppox and goatpox are contagious, pox-like dermatides that occur mostly outside of North America.

  5. Swinepox is a common benign disease that affects the ventral abdomen of pigs. The poxvirus is transmitted by lice and affects mainly young pigs. Mortality is negligible, and treatment is not practiced.

  6. Ovine viral ulcerative dermatosis is a venereal and skin disease caused by a poxvirus. This dermatosis is most common in the western United States during the breeding season. Lesions consist of granulating ulcers on the genitalia, lips, or legs. Treatment is nonspecific, and prevention focuses on hygiene management.

  7. Equine viral papular dermatitis is reported sporadically and produces asymptomatic papules over the body. The disease is self-limiting but must be differentiated from other conditions, such as furunculosis.

  8. Horsepox is rare and reported only in Europe.

  9. Contagious ecthyma (viral pustular dermatitis, sore mouth, orf) is a parapoxvirus that affects sheep and goats, and this disease may be transmitted to humans. The organism remains infectious in the environment for extended periods (i.e., years); thus, when a farm has been contaminated, all incoming naive animals are at risk of disease. There is high morbidity on the first exposure of a flock. Immunity is strong and usually lifelong, but passive transfer is not effective in protecting lambs born to previously infected ewes.

      a. **Clinical findings** include early papules followed by vesicles, which result in pustules and scabs on the lips, muzzle, and oral cavity in young animals. Lesions are painful, and animals are reluctant to eat. Debilitation due to starvation and secondary bacterial infection are the biggest dangers. Occasionally, ewes will have lesions on their udders.

      b. **Diagnostic plan and laboratory tests.** The diagnosis is made based on clinical signs and the submission of a biopsy specimen for fluorescent antibody testing. Virus isolation may be performed on the exudate.

      c. **Therapeutic plan.** Treatment includes supportive care, force feeding, and topical antibiotics.

      d. **Prevention.** Vaccines are available for use in endemic areas. Lambs and kids should be vaccinated 2 weeks after weaning, and all show animals should be vaccinated 1 month before showing.

  10. Equine coital exanthema. This is a sporadic venereal disease of horses that is characterized by necrotic, circumscribed lesions of the penis or vulva/perineum. **Equine herpesvirus type 3** infects animals, usually through breeding.

      a. **Clinical findings.** Lesions are initially vesicular but rapidly progress to a dry pustule and ulceration stage.

      b. **Diagnostic plan.** The diagnosis is confirmed by virus isolation from early vesicular lesions.

    c. Therapeutic plan. There is little effect on fertility, but secondary bacterial infections may occur. Affected stallions are treated with local application of antibiotic or steroid creams.

11. Systemic viral diseases with cutaneous manifestations
    a. Bovine viral diarrhea/mucosal disease (see Chapter 1)
    b. Malignant catarrhal fever (see Chapter 1)
    c. Bluetongue (see Chapter 1)
    d. Infectious bovine rhinotracheitis (see Chapter 6)
    e. Foot and mouth disease (see Chapter 1)
    f. Scrapie (see Chapter 11)
    g. Border disease
    h. Vesicular exanthema (see Chapter 1)
    i. Vesicular stomatitis (see Chapter 1)

V. BACTERIAL SKIN DISORDERS

A. Folliculitis and furunculosis

1. Patient profile. These conditions are most commonly presented in horses and goats.

2. Definitions
    a. Folliculitis—inflammation of the hair follicle
    b. Furunculosis—an inflammatory process that breaks through the hair follicle and extends to surrounding dermis and subcutis
    c. Carbuncle—coalescence of multiple areas of furunculosis in horses causing focal induration and fistulous tracts

3. Etiology. The major causative agents are the ***Staphylococcus* species.** Coagulase-positive staphylococci that are pathogenic in large animals include ***S. aureus, S. intermedius,*** and ***S. hyicus.*** Other agents include ***Streptococcus* species, *Corynebacterium pseudotuberculosis* (Canadian horsepox or contagious acne), *Corynebacterium equi,*** and ***Dermatophilosis congolensis*** (see V C, E). In goats, causative agents include ***Staphylococcus* species, *Actinomyces pyogenes,*** and ***Pseudomonas aeruginosa.***

4. Pathogenesis. Predisposing factors to folliculitis or furunculosis are mechanical trauma, insect bites, and moisture, combined with poor sanitation.

5. Specific conditions
    a. Staphylococcal folliculitis. Initially, erect hairs may be found overlying a 2-mm to 3-mm papule. Lesions regress or progressively enlarge to 6–10 mm in diameter and develop a central ulcer that discharges serosanguinous material and becomes encrusted. During healing, the lesion flattens and is accompanied by alopecia and scaling, resembling ringworm.
    b. Staphylococcal furunculosis. This disorder presents as a combination of nodules, draining tracts, ulcers, and crusts. Large lesions are edematous plaques that resemble urticaria. Scarring, leukoderma, and leukotrichia may follow.
    c. Pastern folliculitis (greasy heel complex). Lesions are found on the caudal aspect of pasterns or fetlocks of horses and may be caused by a variety of organisms singly or in concert.

6. Diagnostic plan. The diagnosis is based on a complete history, a physical examination, direct smears and a bacterial culture of the lesions, and a skin biopsy.

7. Laboratory tests
    a. A **bacterial culture** may reveal organisms in pure culture, but the interpretation may be difficult because of the normal occurrence on skin of some organisms (e.g., Staphylococci).

b. A **tissue biopsy** reveals perifolliculitis with both folliculitis and furunculosis. There are extensive tissue eosinophilia accompanying furunculosis. Gram-positive bacteria may be visible.

8. Therapeutic plan
  a. Mild cases often resolve spontaneously.
  b. Severe cases require topical cleansing, drying, and antibacterial therapy (aqueous iodophors or chlorhexidine daily for 5–7 days, then twice weekly until resolved). **Systemic antibiotics** are necessary in severe progressive cases (procaine penicillin G 22,000 IU/kg twice daily for 7–10 days). Many coagulase-positive staphylococci are resistant to penicillin but are sensitive to **erythromycin, trimethoprim-sulfamethoxazole,** and **aminoglycosides.** Long-acting **oxytetracycline** (10–20 mg/kg) may be used if daily treatment is impractical.

9. Prognosis. Although healing is usually complete in 7–10 days, severe cases may not respond to treatment.

B. **Ulcerative lymphangitis**

1. Patient profile. This sporadic disease is seen mainly in horses and is often associated with heavy populations of horses.

2. Clinical findings
  a. Lesions occur on the lower limbs of the horse, particularly of the fetlock and seldom above the hock. Lesions begin as hard, fluctuant nodules, which abscess, ulcerate, and develop draining tracts of creamy green pus. Individual ulcers heal in 2 weeks, but new lesions develop.
  b. Regional lymphatics are often corded, but there is no obvious lymph node involvement.
  c. Limb edema and **subsequent scarring** is common.

3. Etiology. *Corynebacterium pseudotuberculosis* is most commonly isolated (a gram-positive pleomorphic rod). Other isolates include: *Staphylococcus* species, *C. pyogenes, Rhodococcus equi, Pasteurella haemolytica, Fusobacterium necrophorum,* and *Actinobacillus equuli.* Infections usually arise from wound contamination and are more prevalent in stabled animals where there are crowded conditions and poor hygiene.

4. Diagnostic plan. The diagnosis is based on history, a physical examination, and direct smears and a culture of the lesions.

5. Differential diagnoses include glanders and other bacterial causes of lower limb cellulitis.

6. Therapeutic plan. Hydrotherapy, exercise, surgical drainage, and high doses of penicillin (20,000–80,000 IU/kg, twice daily) for prolonged periods (more than 30 days) should be used.

7. Prognosis. The prognosis is poor for horses with significant scarring because recurrences are common.

8. Prevention. Good management practices provide the best means of control. Improving hygiene and decreasing population pressures is recommended.

C. **Udder impetigo**

1. Etiology. This condition in cattle is caused by *Staphylococcus aureus.* The infection is spread by the milker's hands and is zoonotic.

2. Clinical findings. Infection results in multiple pustules on the teat and udder skin. Cattle experience discomfort and a decrease in herd milk production as the disease progresses through the herd.

3. Therapeutic plan. Treatment is with systemic antibiotics or antibiotic disinfectant creams.

4. Prevention. Good sanitation is necessary for control (e.g., udder and milking machine disinfection, the use of latex gloves for milking personnel). An autogenous bacterin produces immunity for approximately 6 months in problem herds.

D. **Bacterial abscesses** are very common in domestic animals following trauma and infection of deep tissues with staphylococci and a variety of other opportunistic organisms.

1. Chronic deep-seated pectoral abscesses (pigeon fever, pigeon breast, Wyoming strangles)

  a. Patient profile. Adult horses are affected in the southwestern United States primarily in the autumn. Prevalence may be associated with heavy rainfall or high insect populations.

  b. Clinical findings. Abscesses develop deep in the superficial musculature (most commonly in the pectoral region) and may measure 10–20 cm. The horse shows signs of fever, lameness, depression, anorexia, local edema, and pain with the rupture of the abscess within 2–4 weeks of identification.

  c. Etiology and pathogenesis. *C. pseudotuberculosis* is the causative organism. It is hypothesized that the organism is transmitted via insect bites.

  d. Diagnostic plan and laboratory tests. Diagnosis is based on clinical findings, characteristics of the purulent discharge, and the culture results.

  e. Therapeutic plan. Antibiotics (penicillin at 20,000 IU/kg intramuscularly, twice daily) are used following surgical drainage.

2. Caseous lymphadenitis (CLA)

  a. Patient profile. CLA is a common disease of adult sheep and goats that has a worldwide distribution.

  b. Clinical findings. The disease presents as abscessed lymph nodes (subcutaneous nodules) that eventually break open and drain a thick, green pus.

  (1) Abscesses are most common on the **head** and **neck.**

  (2) Abscesses may also be found in the **abdominal cavity** and cause chronic weight loss (this manifestation is called **visceral CLA** or **thin ewe syndrome).**

  (3) Abscesses may occur in **other locations** with clinical findings specific to the location (e.g., ataxia, pneumonia, renal disease).

  c. Etiology and pathogenesis. *C. pseudotuberculosis* (biotype ovine/caprine) is the causative organism.

  (1) **Direct** or **indirect transmission** of the organism occurs through **contamination of skin wounds.** Shearing or trauma allows the colonization of subcutaneous tissue and the abscessation of local lymph nodes. The organism persists in chronically draining lesions and in the soil.

  (2) The visceral form evolves from **hematogenous dissemination** from the superficial lymph nodes. The visceral form may exist independent of the subcutaneous form.

  d. Diagnostic plan and laboratory tests. For the subcutaneous form, the demonstration of abscessed lymph nodes with a high herd prevalence is highly suggestive of CLA. A **microbiologic culture** is diagnostic. Serology [e.g., enzyme-linked immunosorbent assay (ELISA)] identifies exposed animals but does not have good specificity.

  e. Therapeutic plan

  (1) **Surgical drainage** is the usual treatment of choice for individual animals but is often not attempted because locally abscessed lymph nodes cause few clinical problems. Lancing abscesses will only serve to contaminate the environment. Any surgical intervention must be linked with the isolation of the animal.

  (2) **Antimicrobials** (e.g., penicillin, tetracycline) often fail because of the protected environment of the organism within thick-walled abscesses.

  f. Prevention. The principles of prevention include:

  (1) **Culling** infected sheep or goats (identified by superficial palpation)

  (2) **Disinfecting** all common implements or tools (e.g., shears)

  (3) **Not purchasing** animals from contaminated herds or flocks

(4) Vaccinating animals with commercial toxoids or bacterins

E. **Actinomycotic infections**

1. **Actinomycosis (lumpy jaw; see Chapter 13 II B)**
   a. **Patient profile.** Actinomycosis is seen in adult cattle and sometimes in calves.
   b. **Clinical findings.** A bony enlargement over the mandible or maxilla is seen and may cause stertorous breathing or pressure necrosis of the skin. These abscesses eventually rupture, discharging a thick, clear, yellow pus containing small yellow-white **sulfur granules.** Emaciation and death eventually ensue because of the animal's inability to eat.
   c. **Etiology and pathogenesis.** The causative organism is *Actinomyces bovis,* which enters the subcutis through abrasions in the mouth.
   d. **Therapeutic plan.** In animals with advanced lesions, treatment is disappointing. Recurrence is common.
      (1) Early treatment consists of **sodium iodide** (1 g/12 kg body weight given intravenously once and repeated in 14 days).
      (2) Penicillin (22,000 IU/kg intramuscularly twice daily for 7 days) is efficacious if used before bony lesions develop.

2. **Dermatophilosis (streptothricosis, rainscald)**
   a. **Patient profile.** This disease may affect up to 80% of a herd or group of animals. It is most common in horses but can be seen in cattle, sheep, and goats. This condition is potentially zoonotic.
   b. **Clinical findings.** Early signs of infection include **follicular** and **nonfollicular papules** and **pustules** that **rapidly coalesce** and **become exudative.** These lesions cause groups of hairs to become crusted and matted together. Proximal portions of matted hair embedded in exudate results in the **"paintbrush effect."** White-skinned areas (e.g., the muzzle, distal limbs) are more severely affected and may exhibit severe erythema as a result of photodermatitis.
      (1) Distribution of lesions. Lesions occur primarily over the dorsum but are also seen on the scrotum, perineum, udder, and distal limbs.
         (a) The disease affects the ears and tail base of goat kids and causes wool-mats in sheep **(lumpy wool disease).**
         (b) The disease on coronary bands and carpi of sheep may be termed **strawberry foot rot.**
         (c) Exudative crusted lesions over the rump and top line may be referred to as **rainscald.**
         (d) Lesions involving the distal limbs (i.e., pasterns, coronets, heels) may be called **greasy heel**, **scratches,** or **mud fever**. Distal limb lesions may be associated with edema, pain, and lameness.
      (2) Epithelial defects. Removal of hair tufts from larger lesions over the back exposes ovoid, ulcerated, hemorrhagic, purulent, and painful epithelial defects. Active lesions contain thick, creamy, yellowish or greenish pus that adheres to the skin surface and undersurface of crusts. Acute, active lesions are painful but not pruritic.
   c. **Etiology and pathogenesis**
      (1) Causative agent. *Dermatophilus congolensis* is a gram-positive, facultative, anaerobic actinomycete. Clinically silent but chronically infected animals become a source of infection under favorable climatic conditions.
      (2) Predisposing factors
         (a) Skin damage. Crucial to development of dermatophilosis is skin damage (e.g., biting flies and arthropods, prickly vegetation, maceration).
         (b) Moisture, such as that occurring with heavy rainfall, is essential in the pathogenesis by allowing for the release of infective, motile zoospores.
         (c) Concurrent diseases and **immunosuppression** predispose animals to disease.

(d) **Other putative predisposing factors** include high ambient temperature, high humidity, poor nutrition, poor hygiene, and stress.

d. **Diagnostic plan.** A history and physical examination should provide the diagnosis, which is confirmed by laboratory tests.

e. **Laboratory tests**

(1) **Stains.** The diagnosis is confirmed by **direct smears** of pus or saline-soaked minced crusts stained with **new methylene blue stain, Diff-Quik,** or **Gram stains.**

(a) **Appearance.** *D. congolensis* appears as fine-branching, multiseptate hyphae that divide transversely and longitudinally to form cuboidal packets of coccoid cells arranged in two to eight parallel rows within branching filaments (i.e., a **railroad-track appearance**). In the chronic or healing phase of the disease, direct smears are rarely positive.

(b) **Negative results.** If a dermatophilus preparation is negative in a suspect case, the diagnosis should not be ruled out without submitting the crusts for microbiology.

(2) **Culture** is performed on blood agar in a microaerophilic atmosphere. *D. congolensis* is cultured only from integument and crusts in affected animals.

(3) A **skin biopsy** reveals folliculitis, intraepidermal pustular dermatitis, superficial perivascular dermatitis, and intracellular edema of keratinocytes. Surface crusts are composed of alternating layers of keratin and leukocytic debris. *D. congolensis* organisms are present in leukocytic debris and hair follicles.

f. **Differential diagnoses** include dermatophytosis, staphylococcal folliculitis and furunculosis, zinc-responsive dermatosis, and pemphigus foliaceus.

g. **Therapeutic plan. Healing** is characterized by dry crusts, scaling, and alopecia (ringworm-like lesions).

(1) **Systemic therapy** is needed for animals with severe, generalized, or chronic infections. Systemic antibiotic regimens include 22,000 IU/kg of procaine penicillin twice daily for 7 days.

(2) **Crust removal** and **topical treatment** will suffice for patients with less generalized dermatitis. Topical solutions should be applied as total body washes, sprays, or dips for 3–5 consecutive days and then weekly until healing. Treatments include iodophors (e.g., povidone iodine shampoo), 2%–5% lime sulfur, 0.5% zinc sulfate, 0.2% copper sulfate, or 1% potassium aluminum sulfate.

h. **Prognosis.** Most lesions regress in 4 weeks if the animals are kept dry.

i. **Prevention.** Previously infected animals do not develop significant immunity, so reinfection is always a possibility.

(1) Owners should be instructed to improve hygiene, nutrition, and management practices.

(2) Arthropod and insect control measures should be employed, and affected animals should be isolated.

(3) Measures should be taken to limit mechanical skin trauma.

F. Erysipelas

1. **Patient profile.** Erysipelas is a disease of growing or young adult swine (particularly young sows) and has a global distribution. Erysipelas is a zoonotic disease and people handling infected animals or carcasses are at increased risk of infection.

2. **Clinical findings.** There are two clinical expressions of the disease.

a. The **acute form** involves an **acute septicemia** that is characterized by sudden death or high fevers, depression, anorexia, and, in a subset of animals, classic **diamond-shaped, hyperemic plaques.**

(1) These **plaques** usually follow the other signs of septicemia and are most prominent on the underside of the pig or on the ears. The skin lesions are

often palpable before they can be visualized, and if the animal lives, these lesions may go on to coalesce.

(2) **Disease progression.** Pigs affected by the acute form die after exhibiting signs of dyspnea, cyanosis, and diarrhea. The mortality rate may be high (75%), but the mortality rate depends on the pathogenicity of the strain of the organism and the immunity of the herd. With pigs that recover, the skin lesions become dry, hard, and eventually slough.

b. A **chronic form** of the disease manifests as arthritis, endocarditis, or both. Lameness and stiffness is evident, particularly in the knee, elbow, hip, hock, and stifle. Animals may suffer chronic ill-thrift or may die suddenly due to the heart lesions.

3. **Etiology and pathogenesis.** *Erysipelothrix rhusiopathiae* is the causative organism. There are many different serotypes with varying degrees of virulence. The organism persists in the environment, which is contaminated from the feces of carrier pigs. Susceptible animals are most likely infected via the oral route.

4. **Diagnostic plan and laboratory tests.** Classic lesions, herd epidemiology, and necropsy findings (including bacterial culture of affected tissues) lead to the diagnosis.

5. **Differential diagnoses.** Diseases with similar clinical expressions include **hog cholera** and **salmonellosis.** Necropsy results rule out these diseases.

6. **Therapeutic plan.** The treatment of choice for **acutely affected pigs** is penicillin (50,000 IU/kg intramuscularly, once daily for 3 days). Pigs with the **chronic form** of the disease do not respond well to treatment.

7. **Prevention.** Vaccination is somewhat effective in controlling the disease, particularly if a booster is given 30 days after the initial vaccination. Vaccination should be coupled with increased attention to hygiene and biosecurity measures aimed at limiting access to facilities by pigs, personnel, feral animals, and equipment.

G. **Exudative epidermitis (greasy pig disease, exudative dermatitis)**

1. **Patient profile.** This disease is seen worldwide. Entire litters of nursing piglets may be affected. Usually, this disease is of less clinical importance as animals get older.

2. **Clinical findings**
   a. In **young piglets,** there is marked skin reddening with seborrhea and cutaneous pain. There is anorexia, depression, and dehydration leading to death despite therapy.
   b. **Older piglets** have the characteristic **greasy pig** expression with thick, brown seborrheic scabs that are most prominent around the head and face. The skin is thickened, and there is a characteristic odor. Piglets usually go on to recover if treated.

3. **Etiology.** The causative agent is *Staphylococcus hyicus* and is possibly spread by carrier sows. The organism gains entrance through abrasions, most often around the face and head. However, the disease is extremely infectious.

4. **Diagnostic plan and laboratory tests.** Diagnosis depends on clinical signs combined with a culture of the skin exudate and slide agglutination with *S. hyicus* antisera.

5. **Therapeutic plan and prognosis.** The organism is sensitive to most antibiotics (excluding sulfa drugs) if intervention occurs within 2 days of the development of clinical signs. After this time, the prognosis is poor.
   a. **Procaine penicillin** (20,000 IU/kg, intramuscularly daily for 3 days) has shown good efficacy.
   b. **Local treatment** with mild disinfectant or soapy rinses is also of value.

6. **Prevention.** Improvements in hygiene and biosecurity are recommended. After an outbreak, the premises should be disinfected and left vacant for 10–14 days. All

implements used in treating piglets (e.g., pliers, tattooing equipment) should be thoroughly disinfected.

VI. FUNGAL DERMATOSES

A. Introduction

1. **Definitions**
   a. **Mycosis** is a disease caused by a fungus.
   b. **Dermatophytosis** is the infection of keratinized tissues (i.e., nail, hair, and stratum corneum) by species of *Microsporum, Trichophyton,* or *Epidermophyton.*

2. **Hosts.** Dermatophytes may be transmitted from animals to man and vice versa. Zoophilic fungi prefer animals as hosts. These fungi rarely cause acute inflammation in animals but often cause severe inflammatory reactions when they invade humans.

B. Superficial mycoses. Dermatophytosis (dermatomycosis, ringworm, tinea, girth itch) occurs most commonly in young animals.

1. **Clinical findings**
   a. **Horses.** Lesions are common on the saddle and back areas, thorax, head, and shoulders. Lesions may be discrete, small (2–3 cm), round areas of erect hairs that progress to alopecia. Also, there may be **generalized scaling (seborrhea sicca)** without alopecia. Pruritus and pain vary from severe to absent. Lesions may be limited to the posterior pastern region (these lesions may be known as **scratches, mud fever, greasy heel-like**) and may wax and wane with stress, local irritation, moisture, and unsanitary conditions.
   b. **Cattle.** Affected areas are typically characterized by raised, grey, crusted lesions that begin as discrete areas of alopecia but rapidly become confluent. The neck, face, and head are most commonly affected, and the lesions are not pruritic. Lesions are described as **"asbestos-like" scales.**
   c. **Pigs.** Areas that are commonly affected include the topline and sides of the animal. Lesions appear as progressive rings of alopecia. The interior of the rings is scabby and alopecic.
   d. **Sheep and goats**
      (1) In **sheep,** the head is the most common site of involvement, with discrete, circular areas of alopecia. These lesions are covered with a grey crust.
      (2) In **goats,** there may be whole-body involvement.

2. **Etiology and pathogenesis**
   a. **Etiology.** Microsporum species and *Trichophyton* species are the most frequently isolated animal dermatophytes.
      (1) **Genera** are divided into **three groups** on the basis of natural habitat:
         (a) **Geophylic** organisms inhabit the soil (e.g., *Microsporum gypseum, Microsporum nanum, Trichophyton verrucosum, Trichophyton mentagrophytes*).
         (b) **Zoophilic** organisms prefer animals to humans (e.g., *Microsporum canis, Trichophyton equinum*).
         (c) **Anthropophilic** organisms prefer humans to other animals (e.g., *Microsporum audouinii*).
      (2) **Predisposing factors** for development of ringworm include:
         (a) **Age** (young animals are most susceptible)
         (b) **Immunity** (e.g., immunosuppression, reduced T-cell function)
         (c) **Environment** (e.g., contamination, crowding, high humidity, poor ventilation, darkness)
         (d) **Poor condition** (e.g., poor nutrition, debilitating diseases)
   b. **Pathogenesis**

(1) Transmission. The causative organisms are transmitted by direct contact with infected animals or fomites. The incubation period post-contact is 1–6 weeks, and fungal spores remain viable for years.

(2) Infection. Dermatophytes do not invade living tissue. The organisms invade the hair shaft, causing breaking and alopecia. These organisms elaborate toxins (irritants) or allergens that enter the dermis and evoke an inflammatory response.

(3) Host. Dermatophytes are adapted to survive on the skin of a particular host but cause violent responses in a host that is not adapted to its presence (e.g., zoophilic dermatophytes in humans).

c. **Diagnostic plan.** The condition is most commonly diagnosed by clinical findings and confirmed by laboratory tests.

d. **Laboratory tests.** For confirmation, microscopic examination of the hair and surface debris and a fungal culture are necessary.

(1) Microscopic examination. For **potassium hydroxide (KOH) preparation,** several drops of 20% KOH should be applied to a glass slide onto which hair and keratin have been placed. This should be heated gently for 20 seconds and then examined microscopically for arthrospores on or in hair shafts.

(2) Fungal culture media include:

(a) Dermatophyte test medium (DTM) plus 2 drops of injectable B vitamin complex

(b) Sabouraud's dextrose agar with cycloheximide and chloramphenicol

(3) A **Wood's lamp** test to produce fluorescence can be attempted, but this test usually is negative in large animals with dermatophytosis.

(4) Skin biopsy. If a skin biopsy is employed, histopathologic findings are variable but include:

(a) Perifolliculitis, folliculitis, and furunculosis

(b) Superficial perivascular dermatitis

(c) Intraepidermal vesicular or pustular dermatitis

(d) Septate fungal hyphae and spherical to oval conidia within the surface keratin and crust, within the hair follicles, or in and around the hairs

e. **Differential diagnoses** include staphylococcal dermatitis, dermatophilosis, demodicosis, zinc-responsive dermatosis (in ruminants), and pemphigus foliaceous (in horses).

f. **Therapeutic plan**

(1) Safety measures. Caution should be exercised during treatment because the disease is zoonotic.

(a) Animals that test negative for the disease should be **isolated,** and all **in-contact animals** should be treated.

(b) The **environment** and **fomites** should be disinfected, and all **infectious materials** (e.g., crusts, hair, bedding) should be disposed of.

(c) The **environment** can be treated with 5% lime sulfur, 5% sodium hypochlorite, 5% formalin, 3% captan, or 3% cresol.

(2) Topical antifungal agents. Treatments may differ depending on the species, label specifications, and animal use. Some topical antifungal agents include:

(a) 2%–5% lime sulfur

(b) 3% captan (1–2 ounces of a 50% powder in 1 gallon water)

(c) Iodophors

(d) 0.5% sodium hypochlorite once daily for 5 days as a body spray or dip, then once weekly until clinical cure is evident

(e) 1%–5% thiabendazole solution applied topically once every 3 days

(3) Systemic therapy is controversial but may be effective and necessary in some instances. Systemic treatments include:

(a) Oral thiabendazole (50–100 mg/kg)

(b) Sodium iodide (10%–20%) at 1 g/14 kg (repeat in 7 days)

(c) Griseofulvin is expensive, and its use is probably not warranted under usual circumstances.

        (i) Cattle: 5–7.5 mg/kg orally for 7–10 days
        (ii) Swine: 1 g/100 kg/day orally for 7–40 days
        (iii) Horses: 5–10 mg/kg/day orally for 7–10 days

g. Prognosis. Most lesions regress spontaneously in 2–3 months, particularly if the nutritional plane is good and the animal is exposed to sunlight. Dermatophytosis is normally self-limiting with spontaneous remission in 1–4 months.

h. Prevention. Control depends on reducing contagion to the environment, other animals, and humans while waiting for spontaneous remission.

C. **Subcutaneous mycoses**

  1. Equine sporotrichosis

    a. Clinical findings. Lesions are usually confined to the limbs, although occasionally they may be found on the upper body (i.e., shoulder, hip, perineal regions). Lesions are hard, subcutaneous nodules that develop progressively along lymphatics that may become corded. Large nodules may abscess, ulcerate, and discharge a small amount of thick, brownish red pus or serosanguinous fluid.

    b. Etiology and pathogenesis. The etiologic agent is ***Sporotrichum schenckii,*** a dimorphic fungus. This organism is a soil and vegetation inhabitant that has a worldwide distribution. *S. schenckii* enters the host via wound contamination (e.g., puncture wounds from thorns, wood slivers, bites).

    c. Diagnostic plan. Diagnosis is primarily based on history and physical examination findings; a skin biopsy may also be useful.

    d. Laboratory tests

      (1) A **skin biopsy** shows hyperplastic perivascular dermatitis early in the course of the condition. Later, there is diffuse or nodular dermatitis. *S. schenckii* present as round to oval cells producing buds ranging from 3–6 μm in diameter. Classic "cigar bodies" are less commonly observed. *S. schenckii* is often impossible to find in histologic sections.

      (2) Direct culture from exudate or tissues is reliable because the organism grows readily on Sabouraud's agar.

    e. Differential diagnoses include bacterial and fungal granulomatous disorders, such as glanders and ulcerative lymphangitis.

    f. Therapeutic plan. This is a zoonotic disease, so caution should be exercised when handling infected animals; care should be taken to avoid contact with discharge from nodules. Therapy is iodide administration.

      (1) Preparations

        (a) Oral inorganic iodides. A 20% solution of sodium iodide may be used intravenously at 40 mg/kg for 2–5 days. This is followed by potassium (orally, once daily) until the lesions regress.

        (b) Potassium iodide may be used at 1–2 mg/kg orally twice a day for 1 week, then decreased to 0.5–1 mg/kg orally once a day until 3–4 weeks after the lesions have resolved.

      (2) Side effects

        (a) Some horses may exhibit **iodism** (scaling, alopecia, depression, anorexia, fever, coughing, lacrimation, nasal discharge) with therapy. If side effects develop, the dose should be reduced, or treatment should be temporarily discontinued.

        (b) Systemic iodides may cause **abortion in pregnant mares.**

  2. Phycomycosis (pythiosis, Florida horse leeches)

    a. Patient profile. This condition affects horses in tropical or subtropical climates. In North America, the disease is most common along the Gulf of Mexico coast.

    b. Clinical findings. The lower limbs, abdomen, neck, and head may be affected by ulcerated, necrotic, yellow-gray, draining tracts. These lesions are pruritic and may appear similar to exuberant granulation tissue. Necrotic, organized cores within the masses give the disease the common name **leeches.**

    c. Etiology and pathogenesis. Several fungi within the class *Phycomycetes* may be responsible for the condition. The most common organisms are ***Hyphomyces destruens*** and ***Entomophthora coronata.*** These organisms may gain entrance to the horse through sites of trauma or skin barrier breakage (e.g., due to moisture).

    d. Diagnostic plan and laboratory tests. The diagnosis is confirmed by the histopathology of the lesion. A preparation cleared with KOH reveals hyphal elements.

    e. Therapeutic plan

        (1) Surgical debridement of lesions combined with **amphotericin B** injections has proven to be the most effective treatment. Amphotericin B (150 mg gradually increasing to 400 mg/450 kg) is nephrotoxic, so kidney function should be monitored via blood urea nitrogen (BUN) levels during treatment. Treatment may be necessary for up to 30 days.

        (2) Dimethylsulfoxide (DMSO) also has been beneficial when applied locally in certain cases.

    f. Prevention. Good hygiene and dry skin should be maintained when possible.

VII. PARASITIC DISEASES

A. **Introduction.** Parasitic diseases cause animal suffering through annoyance, irritation, pruritus, disfigurement, and secondary infection. There are also economic losses from decreased weight gain and milk production, hide damage, wool loss, death, and the financial burden of diagnostic, therapeutic, and preventative programs. Treatment of ectoparasitism is a complex issue because of:

    1. Regional differences in availability and control of therapeutic agents

    2. Species and age differences among hosts

    3. Meat and milk withdrawal time variability

    4. Safety issues in pregnant animals

B. **Mange**

    1. Psoroptic mange (sheep scab, ear mange)

      a. Patient profile and history. This intensely pruritic skin disease is seen in cattle, sheep, goats, and horses.

      b. Clinical findings

        (1) Cattle. Early lesions form as papules on the withers, neck, and tailhead. As these papules coalesce, hair is lost, and the skin becomes wrinkled and thickened. There is intense pruritus.

        (2) Horses may appear clinically normal or exhibit variable head shaking, ear scratching, and rubbing. Long-haired areas of the body (e.g., mane, tail) may also be affected, resulting in rubbing, thickened skin, and hair loss.

        (3) Sheep. Papules occur most commonly on the thorax. These lesions ooze serum, coalesce into scabs, and mat the fleece. The fleece is lost as the animals become itchy. Flocks may be less negatively affected if nutrition and management is good.

        (4) Goats. Although there may be whole-body involvement, the condition is most commonly one of scabs on the external ear canal. Lesions may range from mild scabs to large proliferative-looking scabs occluding the ear canal.

      c. Etiology and pathogenesis. *Psoroptes* **species** mites are nonburrowing but do cause skin excoriation. These parasites feed on both blood and tissue fluids. Transmission is via direct and indirect contact.

        (1) *P. ovis* is the only mite that affects sheep, but it may also be found on other species (e.g., cattle).

(2) *P. equi* occurs on horses.

(3) *P. cuniculi* is the ear mite of various animals.

d. **Diagnostic plan and laboratory tests.** Routine skin scrapings provide the diagnosis. Also, otoscopic examination may be performed to detect ear mites, followed by a microscopic examination of the material collected from deep within the ear canal.

e. **Differential diagnoses** include sarcoptic mange, chorioptic mange, psorergatic mange, lice, keds, and flybite dermatitis.

f. **Therapeutic plan**

   (1) Sheep may be treated with a whole-body dip of approved ascaricides (e.g., 0.01% diazinion, 0.5% malathion, 0.06% coumaphos). Retreatment according to label directions is necessary.

   (2) Cattle. Ivermectin (0.2 mg/kg subcutaneously) is efficacious for mites in cattle.

   (3) For **horses** or **goats** with ear mites, commercial dog and cat ear mite preparations are effective after a thorough cleaning of the ear with benzene hexachloride.

g. **Prevention.** Psoroptic mange may be a **reportable disease** in many countries; therefore, notification of federal authorities is indicated when the disease is suspected. Prevention of the disease in sheep requires a whole-body treatment (i.e., dipping) at least twice yearly. Mites survive off of the host for 2 weeks, so it is important to leave the environment unpopulated for this time period.

2. Sarcoptic mange (barn itch, scabies)

a. **Patient profile and history.** This parasitic condition is most common in pigs but all species of animals may be affected. The main complaint from owners is an intense pruritis in the animal. The most susceptible animals are those that are thin and in overcrowded conditions. The condition is most prevalent in the winter stabling period.

b. **Clinical findings** include an intense pruritus of face, neck, shoulders, and rump. Nonfollicular papules, crusts, excoriations, and alopecia are seen.

c. **Etiology and pathogenesis**

   (1) Etiology. Severe, chronic sarcoptic mange is associated with poor feeding, management, and hygiene practices on the farm. The causative agents are the *Sarcoptes* **species.**

   (2) Pathogenesis

      (a) Infection and life cycle. These organisms tunnel through epidermis to feed on tissue fluids and possibly epidermal cells. The parasite life cycle is completed in 2–3 weeks. Mites are susceptible to drying and survive only a few days when separated from the host.

      (b) Pruritus in scabies is caused by a **hypersensitivity reaction** to mite products. Piglets become infected from sows shortly after birth and develop the hypersensitivity reaction and pruritis 8–10 weeks later. The reaction is characterized by tissue eosinophilia, positive intradermal tests using mite antigen, and difficulty in detecting mites on skin scrapings.

d. **Diagnostic plan.** The history and a physical examination lead to a presumptive diagnosis because this parasite is the only mange mite that affects pigs. Response to therapy is useful for diagnosis in small groups of animals because mites are difficult to find. Laboratory testing confirms the diagnosis.

e. **Laboratory tests**

   (1) Positive skin scrapings confirm the diagnosis, but mites can be difficult to find. **Cerumen** gathered from the ear canal and pinnae are the most consistent source of ear mites in swine.

   (2) A **skin biopsy** shows a superficial, perivascular dermatitis with numerous eosinophils. Occasionally, mites are visible in parakeratotic scale crusts and subcorneal "tunnels."

f. **Differential diagnoses** include psoroptic mange, chorioptic mange, psorergatic mange, lice, keds and flybite dermatitis.

g. **Therapeutic plan.** This mange is a reportable condition to federal authorities in many constituencies. Cross-infections between humans and animals occur.
   (1) **Ivermectin** is the standard treatment, although insecticides may also be used.
   (2) **Dips** should be applied at least twice in a 14-day interval. Several agents are available (e.g., 0.5% malathion, 0.03% lindane, 0.06% coumaphos, 0.5% methoxychlor, 2% lime sulfur). **Insecticide sprays** should also be used in the surrounding stable unless the stable can be depopulated for 3 weeks.
   (3) **Nutrition** and the **general health** of the animals should be improved.

3. **Chorioptic mange (leg mange, tail mange, symbiotic scab, scrotal mange, foot mange)**
   a. **Patient profile.** This is the most common type of mange in cattle and horses. Horses with feathered fetlocks (i.e., draft horses) are prone to the condition.
   b. **Clinical findings**
      (1) **Horses** exhibit pruritus of the lower legs by stamping, rubbing, and stepping. Close examination may reveal scabs and a greasy dermatitis. Chorioptic mite infestation may be a component of **greasy heel.**
      (2) **Cattle** are affected by multiple small scabs along the udder, thighs, and perineum. In extreme cases, the coronet and muzzle may be affected. These lesions are not pruritic.
      (3) **Rams** exhibit a scrotal dermatitis.
   c. **Etiology and pathogenesis**
      (1) **Etiology.** The major causative species of mites is ***Chorioptes bovis,*** which can infect most domestic animals. Chorioptic mites are surface-inhabiting parasites that feed on epidermal debris. They do not affect humans.
      (2) **Pathogenesis**
         (a) **Transmission** is by direct contact or via common equipment (e.g., combs, brushes).
         (b) **Life cycles,** which span 3 weeks, are completed on the host. Mite populations are affected by the season and are heaviest at times of cooler temperatures and higher humidity. There is spontaneous disease regression in the summer because the mite population decreases.
         (c) The mites cause an **allergic dermatitis.**
   d. **Diagnostic plan and laboratory tests.** A combination of history, physical examination, and skin scrapings leads to the diagnosis. Mites may be demonstrated around the coronet and interdigitally during clinically inapparent periods.
      (1) **Microscopic findings.** Chorioptes mites are easy to demonstrate. Live mites may move fairly rapidly through the microscopic field, so a mixture of one-part rotenone to three-parts mineral oil is recommended.
      (2) A **skin biopsy** will show superficial perivascular dermatitis with numerous eosinophils. Mites are rarely found.
   e. **Therapeutic plan and prevention.** Infected and in-contact animals should be treated.
      (1) **Ivermectin** should be used at recommended dosages and repeated in 2 weeks.
      (2) **Other treatments** include the total body application of 0.5% malathion, 0.5% methoxychlor, 0.06% coumaphos, or 0.25% crotoxyfos, bearing in mind labeled clearances for the species of interest.
      (3) None of the treatments eliminate the infection from the herd or flock, and reinfections usually occur in subsequent years.

4. **Psorergatic mange (Australian itch, itch mite)**
   a. **Patient profile.** Psorergatic mange is a condition of sheep that has a worldwide distribution.
   b. **Clinical findings.** Affected animals rub and bite their flanks, thighs, and sides. Their wool becomes tattered and scaly. Usually only a small percentage of the flock is affected because young animals have not developed the disease yet and older animals may be the carriers.

c. **Etiology and pathogenesis.** *Psorergates ovis* completes its entire life cycle on the sheep in 4–5 weeks. The mite is active only in the superficial layers of skin, causing a mechanical irritation initially and, usually, a hypersensitivity reaction over time. Mite numbers are highest in the winter months.

d. **Diagnostic plan.** The clinical signs of disease appear similar to other external parasites, such as sheep keds. For diagnostic testing, animals with the appearance of scurfy skin should be selected and their skin scraped for mites along the ribs or shoulder.

e. **Therapeutic plan and prevention.** The condition is difficult to eradicate, but ivermectin and common insecticides are used.

5. **Demodectic mange**
   a. **Patient profile.** This type of mange affects all domestic animals but is most significant in goats.
   b. **Clinical findings.** Skin nodules (3 mm in size) are apparent on the face, neck, shoulders, and sides. Lesions are not pruritic and are more easily palpated than seen. These lesions form small caseated abscesses. There may be some minor alopecia and hyperkeratosis.
   c. **Etiology and pathogenesis.** *Demodex* **species** may be considered normal skin residents. Demodectic mites live in hair follicles and sebaceous glands and are host-specific. It is thought that clinical demodicosis occurs in immunocompromised animals or animals with concurrent diseases (e.g., ringworm). In herd outbreaks, genetic predisposition or endogenous/exogenous causes of immunosuppression should be considered.
   d. **Diagnostic plan.** History and physical examination findings are supported by skin scrapings of alopecic or scaly areas.
   e. **Laboratory tests**
      (1) **Skin scraping.** Affected areas should be squeezed firmly and scraped deeply until blood is drawn. Nodular lesions should be incised and manually evacuated to reveal exudate loaded with Demodex mites.
      (2) A **skin biopsy** shows follicular distention with mites accompanied by granulomatous/eosinophilic perifolliculitis, folliculitis, or furunculosis.
   f. **Therapeutic plan.** Ascaricides that are recommended for other mites may help control Demodex infection but will not be curative. **Ivermectin** (0.3 mg/kg administered by subcutaneous injection) has proven efficacious. A limited number of large, localized lesions in goats can be **incised, expressed manually,** and **infused with lugols iodine** or **rotenone in alcohol (1:3).**
   g. **Prevention.** Severely affected animals should be culled or not used for breeding stock because this disease is difficult to treat, and there is genetic predilection for disease susceptibility.

C. | Ked, louse, and tick infestation

1. **Sheep keds**
   a. **Patient profile and history.** Sheep keds has a global distribution. Heaviest infestations are seen during cool, wet times (winter).
   b. **Clinical findings.** The usual infestations are light to moderate, so clinical signs are limited to slight irritation and scratching. Self-trauma may cause wool damage. Heavier infestations result in ill-thrift and anemia. Keds are visible to the naked eye and measure 6–7 mm in length.
   c. **Etiology and pathogenesis.** *Melophagus ovinus* (wingless fly), an obligate parasite, lives its entire life cycle on sheep (occasionally on goats), feeding on blood.
      (1) The spread of this parasite is most likely by direct transmission. Females deposit single larvae and are not prolific (approximately 1 larva/week), so populations build slowly.
      (2) Adult sheep gradually build up resistance to the parasite.
      (3) Keds may also transmit the blue tongue virus.
   d. **Diagnostic plan.** Keds are readily seen on physical examination if the wool is parted.

e. Therapeutic plan. Shearing removes many keds, but these parasites are also susceptible to many ascaricides (e.g., organophosphates) and ivermectin.

2. Lice (pediculosis)

a. Patient profile. Any of the common domestic animals are susceptible to louse infestation.

(1) Heaviest infestations seem to occur on younger animals and those in the poorest condition.

(2) Animals unable to practice grooming are most often affected (e.g., stanchioned cattle).

(3) Lice infestation seems to occur more commonly in winter and is particularly common in goats. Lice populations are much higher in the winter because of lower skin, hair, or wool temperatures, overcrowding, poor nutrition, and the availability of moisture. High skin temperatures in the summer kill off lice; therefore, small populations survive only inside ears, between legs, and in tail switches.

b. Clinical findings. Affected animals suffer from skin irritation, a roughened hair coat, alopecia, and anemia. Lice may occur over the entire body in heavy infestations but are more common over the back, neck, brisket, tail head, and any long-haired part of the body.

c. Etiology and pathogenesis

(1) Etiology. Lice can be classified as **sucking lice** or **biting lice.** Within each category, species are host specific.

(a) Biting lice include *Damalinia bovis, Damalinia ovis, Damalinia caprae, Damalinia limbata,* and *Damalinia crassipes.*

(b) Sucking lice

(i) Cattle: *Hematopinus eurysternus, Haematopinus quadripertusus, Linognathus vituli, Solenopotes capillatus*

(ii) Sheep: *Linognathus pedalis, Linognathus ovillus*

(iii) Goats: *Linognathus stenopis*

(iv) Horses: *Damalinia equi, Haematopinus asini*

(2) Pathogenesis

(a) The **life cycle** of lice is completed from egg to adult on the host and takes 2–4 weeks. Lice can survive for up to 7 days away from the host.

(b) Transmission is by direct contact or fomites.

(c) Sucking lice may cause anemia through blood removal. **Biting lice** mainly cause **skin irritation** because they feed on epithelium and cutaneous debris.

d. Diagnostic plan. Demonstration of lice and the eggs (nits) is definitive. However, careful examination is necessary to visualize the lice, particularly on a dark haircoat or in a dark environment. The hair should be parted and a flashlight used to look for the pale-colored (almost transparent) biting louse or the blue-grey sucking louse. Nits are attached to the hair shaft.

e. Therapeutic plan

(1) Products effective in horses, cattle, goats, sheep and swine include many **organophosphates** and **synthetic pyrethroids.** The efficacy of these products is enhanced by the removal of long hair (e.g., shearing in sheep, clipping in cattle). Resistance to these products can occur if used singly over time.

(2) Ivermectin may also be used (200 μg/kg) and is extremely effective against sucking lice. It is also reported to be effective against biting lice. All animals in the group should be treated, although lice may only be seen on one animal (old or sick).

f. Prevention. Improved hygiene and nutrition are important control measures. The environment should be kept clean, and animal crowding should be decreased.

3. Ticks. Heavy infestations of ticks **limit weight gains** and **productivity** in animals because of irritation and annoyance.

a. **Patient profile.** Ticks are parasitic on all domestic animals and have a global distribution.
b. **Clinical findings.** Ticks may be found in the ear canal or on the body.
   (1) **Anemia.** Many tick species are bloodsuckers and can cause profound anemia.
   (2) **Paralysis** or other **central nervous system (CNS) signs** may occur because of a toxin elaborated by the salivary glands of female ticks.
c. **Etiology and pathogenesis**
   (1) **Etiology.** The most common ticks in North America are the *Dermacentor, Boophilus, Amblyomma, Otobius,* and *Ixodes* **species.**
   (2) **Pathogenesis**
      (a) **Life cycles** are variable. Some species are obligate parasites of a single host, whereas other species have various and successive hosts. Generally, eggs are laid in the soil, and larvae attach to passing hosts. The larvae mature to adults. Females feed on blood and drop to the ground to lay eggs.
      (b) The **blood-feeding phase** of the cycle promotes infection with various bacterial, viral, and rickettsial diseases that are dependant on the location and epidemiology of the disease.
      (c) **Other diseases** found in North America related to tick infestation include:
         (i) **Babesiosis**
         (ii) **Tularemia**
         (iii) **Anaplasmosis**
         (iv) **Caseous lymphadenitis**
         (v) **Epizootic bovine abortion**
         (vi) **Lyme disease**
d. **Diagnostic plan.** Diagnosis is based on observation and the identification of the tick.
e. **Therapeutic plan and prevention**
   (1) **Insecticides.** Treatment with insecticides is the usual course of action. Various agents (such as pyrethroids, organophosphates, or ivermectin) may be used through sprays, dips, or powders. A regular, consistent program must be employed. However, resistance may develop and can be a problem in any control program.
   (2) **Control** is difficult because of the life cycle of the tick off of the animal and its ability to live for extended periods of time away from its hosts. Consequently, not many tick control programs have been successful.

D. **Fly-related dermatoses**

1. **Hypoderma infestation (warbles, grubs).** This infestation, if heavy, may worry the cattle and cause production losses. Other significant losses are caused by carcass and hide depreciation and the cost of control programs.
   a. **Patient profile and history.** Hypoderma infestation is most common in beef cattle, although it may be seen in dairy cattle raised in feedlot conditions and occasionally in horses in poor condition raised in close proximity to cattle. Young cattle are most severely affected.
   b. **Clinical findings**
      (1) Small numbers of **painful subcutaneous nodules,** each with a breathing pore, are seen over the withers of young cattle in the spring. Occasionally, nodules can be extremely numerous.
      (2) **Other clinical findings** are associated with reactions to larvae, interrupted migration, or aberrant migration of larvae. All of these secondary reactions are relatively infrequent.
         (a) **Bloat.** An inflammatory reaction may occur around larvae in the submucosa of the esophagus, causing esophageal obstruction and a buildup of rumenal gases.

(b) **Paralysis** results from an inflammatory reaction surrounding dead larvae in the spinal column (in cattle and horses).

(c) **Intracranial myiasis** (in unusual hosts such as horses, goats, humans, or sheep). Larvae may migrate aberrantly and do not complete their life cycle but cause neurologic signs if an inflammatory reaction to dying larvae occurs intracranially.

(d) **Anaphylactic reaction.** This reaction is associated with the rupture of L_3. The therapeutic destruction of L_2 has also been recorded as a cause of anaphylactic reaction (in cattle).

c. **Etiology and pathogenesis**

(1) **Etiology.** *Hypoderma bovis* and *Hypoderma lineatum* are the adult flies of the pathogenic larvae.

(2) **Pathogenesis**

(a) The **adult flies** are active in the summer and fix eggs to hairs on the legs of cattle. Larvae that hatch penetrate the skin and migrate through subcutaneous tissues toward the diaphragm.

(b) **Larvae** then find their way to the submucosa of the esophagus (*H. lineatum*) and the spinal cord or epidural fat (*H. bovis*).

(c) **Warble stage.** During January and February, larvae migrate to the dorsum of the body and reach subcutaneous tissues of the back, where they create a breathing hole and molt (L_2 and L_3). This time period may vary and is often earlier in lower latitudes. This "warble stage" lasts approximately 30 days.

(d) In the **spring, mature larvae** wriggle out of the cystic nodules and fall to the ground to pupate.

d. **Diagnostic plan.** The history, physical examination findings, and the demonstration of larvae confirm the diagnosis.

e. **Therapeutic plan**

(1) Most commonly, a **topical organophosphate preparation** is applied to kill migrating larvae in the early stages. This timing varies, depending on the geographical location. Later dosing runs the risk of being ineffective against L_3 larvae or causing reactions to the dead parasite in sensitive locations (spinal cord, esophagus).

(2) **Ivermectin** has also proven to be very effective.

2. **Screwworm infestation**

a. **Patient profile.** Screwworms are seen in all domestic animals in range or extensive management conditions in subtropical or tropical climates. Infestation occurs most commonly when fly numbers are highest in the spring, summer, and fall.

b. **Clinical findings** include extensive damage to skin, subcutaneous tissue, and muscle, accompanied by a copious amount of brown discharge and a foul odor. Animals are initially irritated by the fly strike, and then they become pyrexic, anorexic, and depressed. Death may ensue.

c. **Etiology and pathogenesis**

(1) **Etiology.** Larvae of *Cochliomyia hominivorax* and *Chrysomyia bezziana* cause screwworm disease.

(2) **Transmission.** These flies lay eggs at the site of fresh wounds (e.g., from trauma, castration, dehorning) or at sites of soiling and moisture (e.g., eyes, perineum).

(3) **Life cycle.** Larvae hatch and mature in 1 week, fall to the ground, and pupate.

(4) **Disease progression.** At the site of the wound, maturing larvae feed and burrow into living tissue, producing a pronounced liquefactive, necrotic defect. Secondary bacterial infection and simultaneous fly strike with other maggots occur. Animals die from this profound tissue necrosis and secondary bacterial infection with accompanying toxemia and dehydration.

    d. Diagnostic plan. The diagnosis is made on clinical examination; however, the condition may be well advanced before it is noticed because of coat (wool) cover.

    e. Therapeutic plan. Infestation with screwworms is a federally reportable disease in the United States.

        (1) Early treatment of individuals is necessary and consists of clipping and debridement of affected areas, cleansing the area, and applying insecticide preparations and antiseptic creams to the site of infestation. Many insecticides are effective and should coat the site to provide residual activity.

        (2) Symptomatic therapy also may be necessary (e.g., antibiotics, fluids).

    f. Prevention. The United States has mounted a very successful screwworm eradication program based on the sterilization and subsequent release of male flies to copulate with females that mate only once. (Sterilization of male flies is accomplished by using cobalt 60.) Consequently, *C. hominivorax* has been eliminated.

        (1) Delaying surgical procedures until after fly season should be considered.

        (2) Prophylactic wound dressings (insecticidal and antiseptic) should be used on surgical sites.

        (3) Animals should be observed closely after surgeries or during calving or lambing seasons.

        (4) Ivermectin should be used at the time of surgery.

3. Cutaneous myiasis (blowflies)

    a. Patient profile. The disease is relatively minor in North America but causes significant animal suffering and economic losses in the major sheep-rearing areas of Australia and New Zealand.

    b. Etiology and pathogenesis

        (1) Etiology. Flies lay eggs on animals in areas of moisture and warmth (e.g., the perineum) or decaying flesh. Flies of highest concern are ***Calliphora, Lucilia* species,** and ***Phormia* species.**

        (2) Pathogenesis. Eggs hatch, and larvae feed mainly on tissue debris and decaying matter but also release proteases that allow the penetration of epidermis, leading to the extension of the wound bed and tissue damage. Secondary bacterial invasion and fluid loss occur. Larvae pupate on the ground or on carcasses or in wool.

    c. Diagnostic plan. Diagnosis is based on observation and examination.

    d. Therapeutic plan. Treatment includes clipping or shearing affected sites, cleaning up the wounds, and debridement of necrotic tissue. Insecticides, antibiotic creams, and lotions should be applied.

    e. Prevention revolves around preventing the matting of haircoats with moisture and debris, delaying surgeries until after fly season, and practicing fly control.

E. | **Helminth infestation**

1. Habronemiasis (summer sores)

    a. Patient profile. Habronemiasis is a skin condition of horses and is seen sporadically in the spring and summer. This disease is most common in adult animals inhabiting warm climates.

    b. Clinical findings. Skin lesions (single or multiple) are characterized by granulomatous inflammation, ulceration, intermittent hemorrhage, serosanguinous exudate, and exuberant granulation. There is mild to severe pruritis. Small (1 mm in diameter), yellowish granules are seen in diseased tissue; these granules represent necrotic calcified foci surrounding the larvae. Lesions are found on the legs, ventrum, prepuce, and in the urethral fossa and medial canthus of the eye.

        (1) If found in the **urethral process,** habronemiasis may cause dysuria or pollakiuria.

        (2) If found in the **conjunctival sac,** yellowish, gritty plaques on the palpebral and bulbar conjunctivae, eyelid granulomas, and blepharitis are present.

(3) Gastric and **pulmonary locations** for *Habronema* species are asymptomatic.

c. Etiology and pathogenesis

(1) Etiology. *Habronema muscae* and *Draschia megastoma* are the adult worms of the major pathogenic larvae.

(2) Pathogenesis

(a) Adults normally inhabit the equine stomach.

(b) Eggs and **larvae** are passed in the feces and are ingested by maggots of intermediate hosts (e.g., *Musca domestica, Stomoxys calcitrans*). Infectious larvae are deposited on the horse, particularly in moist areas or open wounds while flies are feeding.

(i) Larvae that are deposited near the mouth are swallowed and complete the life cycle in the stomach.

(ii) Those deposited on the nose migrate to the lungs.

(iii) Larvae deposited in wounds or moist areas of the body produce both a local inflammatory and allergic reaction.

d. Diagnostic plan. The diagnosis is aided by a complete history and a physical examination.

e. Laboratory tests

(1) Deep scrapings or **smears** of lesions, particularly if yellow granules are retrieved, may reveal larvae with numerous surrounding eosinophils and mast cells. However, smears are often negative.

(2) Biopsy reveals a diffuse dermatitis with eosinophils and mast cells. There will be a multifocal coagulation necrosis, containing few to many nematode larvae.

f. Differential diagnoses include bacterial or fungal granulomas, equine sarcoid, squamous cell carcinoma, and exuberant granulation tissue. Also, *Habronema* and *Draschia* larvae will invade secondarily sarcoid, squamous cell carcinoma, and other infective granulomas, which may cause errors in diagnosing the primary skin disorder.

g. Therapeutic plan. Local and systemic therapy should be combined.

(1) Local therapy

(a) Surgery. Massive or refractory lesions should be surgically debulked. Cryotherapy should be employed using a double freeze–thaw cycle.

(b) Topical therapy includes combinations of larvicidal, antimicrobial, anti-inflammatory, penetrating, and protective agents that are applied daily under bandages. An example would be 0.03% echothiophate (phospholine iodide) with ophthalmic ointment (maxitrol) containing neomycin, polymyxin, and dexamethasone.

(2) Systemic therapy involves:

(a) Organophosphates (trichlorfon 22 mg/kg intravenously in 1 L of 5% dextrose, repeated in 2 weeks)

(b) Ivermectin (200 μg/kg orally)

(c) Glucocorticoids. Prednisone or prednisolone (1 mg/kg orally once daily) results in resolution in 7–14 days and are useful adjuncts.

h. Prevention. Fly control, including the prompt removal and disposal of manure and soiled bedding, is essential. Adult *Habronema* should be eliminated from the stomach by using injectable ivermectin. Any wounds should be treated symptomatically and early.

2. Onchocerciasis

a. Patient profile. This condition is seen most commonly in horses 4 years and older. The infestation is nonseasonal but occurs more severely in warm weather.

b. Clinical findings

(1) Lesions occur on the face and neck (particularly near the mane), the ventral chest, and the abdomen. Lesions vary from focal annular alopecia, scaling, and crusting to widespread alopecia, erythema, ulceration, oozing, crusting, and lichenification.

(2) **Seborrhea sicca** may be seen in some horses. Pruritus varies from mild to severe.

(3) **Leukoderma**, premature graying, and alopecia may be permanent sequelae.

c. **Etiology and pathogenesis**

(1) **Etiology.** *Onchocerca cervicalis* infests horses throughout the world.

(2) **Pathogenesis**

(a) **Adult worms** inhabit the ligamentum nuchae. Microfilariae are numerous on the ventral midline, face, and neck.

(b) **Hosts.** *Culicoides* **species,** gnats, and possibly mosquitos are intermediate hosts.

(c) **Reactions.** Most horses have resident populations of *O. cervicalis,* but only certain horses develop clinical signs, suggesting that cutaneous onchocerciasis is a hypersensitivity reaction to microfilarial antigens. Dead or dying microfilariae provoke the most intense inflammatory reactions in both eyes and skin.

d. **Diagnostic plan and laboratory tests**

(1) A **physical examination** will aid in the diagnosis.

(2) A **skin biopsy** is diagnostic and will show superficial to deep perivascular to diffuse dermatitis with eosinophils. Numerous microfilariae surrounded by degranulating eosinophils are visible. Because microfilariae can be found in normal equine skin, pathogenicity must be evaluated in the light of microfilariae numbers and the inflammatory reaction present.

e. **Differential diagnoses.** The condition may appear similar to dermatophytosis, fly-bite dermatoses (because of the seasonal incidence), sarcoptic mange, psoroptic mange, and food hypersensitivity.

f. **Therapeutic plan**

(1) **Ivermectin** (200 μg/kg orally) usually produces clinical remission of the skin lesions in 2–3 weeks. Some horses require one or two additional treatments. Ivermectin is not an adulticide, so periodic retreatment is necessary.

(2) **Concurrent systemic glucocorticoids** for the first 5 days of microfilarial treatment suppress much of the inflammatory reaction (and hence clinical signs) associated with the dead and dying microfilariae.

3. **Oxyuriasis (pin worms, thread worms)**

a. **Patient profile.** Stabled horses are affected most often.

b. **Clinical findings** include broken hairs on the tail and a "rat tail" appearance.

c. **Etiology and pathogenesis.** *Oxyuris equi* infests the cecum and colon. Adult females leave the anus and lay eggs on the perineal skin, causing variable degrees of pruritis. This irritation causes the affected animal to rub the tail base, resulting in broken hairs and excoriation (i.e., "rat tail").

d. **Diagnostic plan.** The diagnosis is made by viewing the egg clusters on the anus or by applying clear acetate tape to the anus and looking for the eggs under a microscope. The ova of *O. equi* have an operculum (a cap located on the one end) and measure approximately 90 μm $\times$ 40 μm.

e. **Differential diagnoses.** This condition may appear similar to insect hypersensitivity, pediculosis, chorioptic mange, food hypersensitivity, drug eruption, or self-mutilation.

f. **Therapeutic plan.** Therapy is instituted by routine deworming with benzimidazoles, ivermectin, or pyrantal pamoate.

4. **Bovine stephanofilariasis**

a. **Patient profile.** Cattle (particularly beef) in the western and southwestern United States are affected. Patients range in age from 6 months to adults.

b. **Clinical findings.** Papules and nodules are found as early lesions on the ventral midline. Lesions become ulcerated and crusted, and these lesions cause alopecia and leukoderma. Mild pruritus is evident.

c. **Etiology and pathogenesis.** Clinical signs are caused by ***Stephanofilaria stilesi,*** a filarid worm. Adults form cyst-like structures at the base of hair follicles.

TABLE 16-2. Reported Causes of Urticaria in Domestic Animals

Causes	Examples
Dermatographism	Pressure, brushing, rubbing
Contact allergies	Saddle, soap, tack
Environmental	Cold, exercise
Venoms	Insect bites, spider bites, snake bites
Medications	Penicillin, phenylbutazone, iron dextrans
Topical treatments	Parasiticides
Foods and plants	Stinging nettle
Biologicals	Strangles vaccine, tetanus or botulinum toxoids
Systemic bacterial infections	Strangles
Dermatitis	Dermatophytosis, hypodermiasis
Inhalants	Pollens, molds, chemicals

These structures become surrounded by microfilariae. ***Hematobia irritans*** and other flies are intermediate hosts.

d. **Diagnostic plan.** Crust scrapings reveal parasites (parts of adults and microfilariae).

e. **Therapeutic plan.** Ivermectin is an effective microfilaricide and reduces the numbers of adults.

VIII. IMMUNOLOGIC SKIN DISEASES

A. Urticaria (hives, heat bumps, feed bumps)

1. **Patient profile.** Urticaria seems to be most common or most often recognized in horses.

2. **Clinical findings.** Urticarial reactions are acute in onset and are characterized by localized or generalized discrete (0.5–5.0 cm) edematous swellings with a flattened top (i.e., **wheals**). Lesions usually last only a few days, but clinical signs may persist due to the emergence of fresh wheals.

3. **Etiology and pathogenesis.** Urticaria may have a distinct and specific cause (e.g., penicillin allergy) or be part of a systemic event (e.g., strangles). There are a variety of triggers (Table 16-2) for the immunologic event (type I or III hypersensitivity). Triggers may be allergic or nonallergic.

4. **Diagnostic plan and laboratory tests.** The clinical findings are relatively obvious, but a detailed history and physical examination are necessary to establish the precipitating cause.

   a. A **skin biopsy** interpreted by a referral institution may be helpful. Specific patterns relative to causative agents may be identifiable.

   b. In particularly stubborn cases, **serum tests** for immunoglobulin E (IgE) antibody to some common allergens may prove beneficial. These tests are available commercially.

5. **Therapeutic plan.** Any identifiable or offending agent should be removed. Follow up with symptomatic treatment with any or a combination of the following agents:

   a. **Glucocorticoids** are recommended (e.g., 0.1–0.2 mg/kg dexamethasone or 0.5–1.0 mg/kg prednisone/prednisolone).

   b. **Nonsteroidal anti-inflammatory agents (NSAIDs)** include aspirin (5 mg/kg orally), phenylbutazone (2.2–4.4 mg/kg/orally), flunixin meglumine (1 mg/kg orally or intravenously), or diethylcarbamazine (100 mg/kg orally).

   c. **Antihistamines** are rarely beneficial but may be indicated if pruritis is involved. Also, hydroxyzine HCl (400 mg orally three times daily to effect, for a 500-kg horse) may be effective in horses with chronic urticaria, which is refractory to steroids. The dose may be reduced gradually over time.

   d. **Epinephrine** (3–5 ml of 1:1000 solution, administered subcutaneously or intramuscularly) is indicated for life-threatening **angioedematous reactions.**

  6. Prevention. If the etiologic agent or risk factors can be established, recommendations regarding prevention are relatively straightforward. If an allergen can be identified, subsequent **hyposensitization** may be attempted.

B. **Equine insect hypersensitivity (sweet itch, Queensland itch)**

  1. Patient profile. This pruritic dermatitis of horses seems to worsen with age. It is seen in the warmer months, usually when animals are on pasture (paralleling fly exposure). Certain breeds may be more severely affected.

  2. Clinical findings. Signs may include an initial intensely pruritic papular dermatitis of the head, ears, withers, back, croup, ventral midline, and tailhead. Lesions may extend to involve the legs, groin, axillae, intermandibular space, and ventral thorax. The intense pruritis causes excoriations, crusting, and lichenification of the papules. In severe cases, alopecia and pigment disturbances occur. "Rat tail" (disheveled tail hairs) and a "buzzed-off" mane are common.

  3. Etiology and pathogenesis. The cause of this disease is a type-II hypersensitivity reaction to salivary antigens from ***Culicoides* species** (gnat), ***Simulium* species** (blackfly), ***Stomoxys calcitrans*** (stable fly), and possibly ***Haematobia irritans*** (horn fly). The distribution of lesions reflects the feeding areas of the flies.

  4. Diagnostic plan. A presumptive diagnosis is made subjectively based on a combination of the history, physical examination, and response to therapy.

  5. Laboratory tests

   a. A **skin biopsy** is very helpful because it reveals superficial or deep perivascular dermatitis with eosinophils. Also, focal areas of epidermal necrosis may be seen.

   b. A **complete blood cell count (CBC)** may show a peripheral eosinophilia.

   c. **Intradermal skin testing** may be employed. Aqueous preparations of whole-insect antigens can be used but are not widely available. Testing can evoke immediate or delayed reactions.

  6. Differential diagnoses. Other conditions that may appear similar are ectoparasitisms and other hypersensitivity dermatoses.

  7. Therapeutic plan

   a. **Insect control.** Flies should be kept out of the stables by better manure control and the use of screens sprayed with residual insecticide. Insecticide control should be applied to affected horses. Recommended insecticides include:

    (1) Weekly permethrin or organophosphate sprays

    (2) Ear tags sold for cattle use (cypermethrin) attached to halter or braided into mane and tail

   b. **Systemic antipruritic agents.** If insect control is not effective, any or a combination of the following should be used:

    (1) **Prednisone** or **prednisolone** (1 mg/kg orally) is given once daily until pruritis is controlled, then the dosage is tapered to the lowest effective alternate-day dose.

    (2) **Hydroxyzine** (200–400 mg/kg orally 2–3 times daily) is effective in some horses. The dose may later be tapered or discontinued after fly season.

    (3) **Hyposensitization.** The use of commercial aqueous whole-flea antigen (flea antigen 1:1000 weight/volume) has been successful. One ml is administered intradermally until effective (3–8 weeks). Booster injections are given as needed every 1–2 months.

    (4) **Antihistamines, diethylcarbamazine,** and **tranquilizers** have not proven effective.

C. **Pemphigus foliaceous**

1. **Patient profile.** Pemphigus has been reported in goats and horses (particularly in Appaloosa horses).

2. **Clinical findings**
   a. **Lesions** begin on the face (especially at mucocutaneous junctions) and extremities, then become widespread. In some horses, the disease affects only the coronary bands. Transient vesicles or pustules are followed by crusting, scaling, and oozing and annular erosions bordered by epidermal colarettes. Signs of pain or pruritis are variable.
   b. There may be concurrent signs of **systemic illness** (e.g., pyrexia, depression, anorexia, weight loss) in 50% of affected animals.

3. **Etiology and pathogenesis.** This autoimmune disease of the skin is characterized histologically by intraepidermal acantholysis and immunologically by autoantibody against the glycocalyx of keratinocytes. The result is the detachment of epidermal cells.

4. **Diagnostic plan.** Physical examination findings are suggestive, but the diagnosis depends on laboratory confirmation.

5. **Laboratory tests**
   a. **Direct smears from intact vesicles or pustules** reveal numerous acanthocytes, nondegenerate neutrophils or eosinophils, and no intracellular bacteria. Occasional acanthocytes are seen in any suppurative condition, but when numerous and present in clusters, they are strongly indicative of pemphigus.
   b. **Skin biopsy of intact pustules or vesicles** reveals subcorneal acantholysis with resultant cleft, vesicle, or pustule formation. Within vesicles, cells from the stratum granulosum are seen attached to overlying stratum corneum. Neutrophils or eosinophils predominate in vesicles or pustules.
   c. **Direct immunofluorescence testing** reveals diffuse intercellular deposition of immunoglobulin, complement in the epidermis, or both. Glucocorticoid therapy can cause false-negative results. False-positive results can occur in equine dermatophilosis.
   d. **Indirect immunofluorescence testing** for pemphigus-like antibodies is frequently positive (titers 1:10 to 1:8000). However, titers can also be demonstrated in the serum of normal horses and horses with dermatophilosis or lymphosarcoma.

6. **Differential diagnoses** include dermatophytosis, dermatophilosis, bacterial folliculitis, and sarcoidosis.

7. **Therapeutic plan.** Therapy is expensive and may have to be maintained for life.
   a. **High doses of systemic glucocorticoids** is the initial treatment of choice (0.2 mg/kg dexamethasone intramuscularly as an initial treatment followed by 1 mg/kg prednisone or prednisolone orally, twice daily). Control may be obtained in 7–10 days, then alternate morning therapy should be started with the lowest dose of oral glucocorticoid possible for the elimination of clinical signs.
   b. It may be necessary to add or substitute **immunomodulating drugs** if glucocorticoids prove unsatisfactory. An example is **aurothioglucose** (i.e., gold therapy) with the recommended regimen of:
      (1) Two intramuscular test doses 1 week apart (5 and 10 mg for goats; 20 and 40 mg for horses), plus systemic glucocorticoids
      (2) Followed by aurothioglucose (1 mg/kg) given weekly until there is a response (6–12 weeks)
      (3) Followed by monthly aurothioglucose administration
   c. **Adverse effects of chrysotherapy** in humans include dermatitis, stomatitis, blood dyscrasia, and proteinuria. There are no reported side effect in horses or goats; however, the hemogram should be checked biweekly and urinalysis checked weekly during induction, then every 2–3 months during maintenance.

IX. **ENDOCRINE DERMATOSES.** Endocrine diseases that have cutaneous manifestations are discussed in Chapter 10.

X. **MISCELLANEOUS DERMATOSES** disorders include dermatoses for which the etiology and pathogenesis are unknown or multifactorial.

A. Equine eosinophilic granuloma with collagen necrosis (nodular necrobiosis, nodular collagenolytic granuloma, acute collagen necrosis, eosinophilic granuloma)

1. **Patient profile.** This condition is described in horses, usually during the warm months of the year.

2. **Clinical findings.** Single or multiple lesions (2–10 cm in diameter) affect the neck, withers, and back. Lesions are rounded, well circumscribed, firm, nonalopecic, nonulcerative, and are not painful or pruritic. Occasionally, cystic or plaque-like lesions are seen and may discharge a central, grayish white caseous core.

3. **Etiology and pathogenesis.** The cause is unknown. This disorder is likely a hypersensitivity reaction, but the insulting cause is highly speculative (e.g., antigens such as insect bites or trauma caused by saddle and girth).

4. **Diagnostic plan and laboratory tests.** The history and physical examination is supported by a skin biopsy, which shows multifocal collagen degeneration with granulomatous inflammation containing eosinophils. Older lesions have marked, dystrophic mineralization.

5. **Therapeutic plan**
   a. With **solitary** or **few lesions,** surgical excision or sublesional glucocorticoids are recommended. The steroids used are triamcinolone acetonide (3–5 mg/lesion) or methylprednisolone acetate (5–10 mg/lesion).
   b. With **multiple lesions,** prednisone or prednisolone (1 mg/kg orally, once a day for 2–3 weeks) is administered.
   c. **Relapses** occur periodically, and older, mineralized lesions respond poorly to glucocorticoids and have to be excised.

B. Equine pastern dermatitis (greasy heel, scratches, mud fever, verrucous dermatitis)

1. **Clinical findings.** Lesions are bilaterally symmetrical and begin on the caudal aspect of the pastern, particularly of the hind limbs. Erythema and edema progress to exudation and crusting. Secondary bacterial infection and seborrhea are common complications. Pain and pruritus are variable. In chronic cases, thickening of skin, fissures, exuberant granulation tissue, severe limb edema, and lameness may be seen.

2. **Etiology and pathogenesis.** Equine pastern dermatitis is not a specific disease; rather, it is a cutaneous reaction pattern of multifactorial etiology. The condition may be associated with several of the following conditions:
   a. **Staphylococcal folliculitis**
   b. **Dermatophilosis**
   c. **Dermatophytosis**
   d. **Chorioptic mange**
   e. **Primary irritant contact dermatitis**
   f. **Contact hypersensitivity**
   g. **Photosensitization**
   h. **Pemphigus foliaceus**

3. **Therapeutic plan.**
   a. **Symptomatic treatments** include gentle clipping and cleansing, topical application of astringent or antiseptic soaks (if the skin is already moist), or emollient ointments and creams (if the skin is dry and thickened).

    b. Definitive treatment. The specific causes, if identifiable, should be treated.

      (1) Topical treatments include povidone–iodine rinses and metronidazole.

      (2) Other treatments include systemic antibiotics, systemic glucocorticoids, NSAIDs, and environmental hygiene.

      (3) Surgery. Occasionally, the condition is chronic and nonresponsive to therapy. Chronic cases with exuberant granulation tissue may require surgical excision.

XI. NEOPLASTIC DISEASES

A. Introduction

1. **Patient profile.** Generally, the risk of developing cutaneous neoplasia increases with age, except in horses. Specific sex and species predilections for neoplasms exist in large animals. Examples include:

    a. Udder papillomatosis, squamous cell carcinoma in female goats

    b. Squamous cell carcinoma in female sheep

    c. Scrotal hemangiosarcoma in male swine

    d. Mastocytoma in male horses

2. **Types of cutaneous neoplasms.** The most common cutaneous neoplasms (listed by the animal affected and in the approximate descending order) are:

    a. Cattle: papilloma, squamous cell carcinoma, melanoma, mast cell tumor

    b. Horses: sarcoid, papilloma, squamous cell carcinoma, melanoma

    c. Swine: melanoma, hemangioma, squamous cell carcinoma

    d. Sheep: squamous cell carcinoma, papilloma

    e. Goats: squamous cell, papilloma, melanoma

3. **Clinical findings** vary with the type and location of the tumor.

4. **Diagnostic plan and laboratory tests.** In general, the diagnosis of cutaneous neoplasia is based on the history and clinical signs, exfoliative cytology (aspiration and impression smears), excisional biopsy, and histopathology.

5. **Therapeutic plan.** Clinical management may include surgery, cryosurgery, electrosurgery, hyperthermia, radiation therapy, chemotherapy, immunotherapy, or combinations of these treatments.

B. Epithelial neoplasms. Papillomatosis (fibropapillomatosis, warts) generally is seen in young animals (less than 18 months old). An exception is warts appearing on the teats of cows; these warts increase in prevalence with age. Warts are unsightly and of concern in show animals. They may also interfere with normal body functions if prominent (e.g., breeding, eating, milking).

1. **Clinical findings**

    a. Cattle, sheep, and goats

      (1) Location. Warts are found most commonly on the head, neck, and shoulders. Warts on the teats are usually multiple, small, and in various shapes. Warts may also be found in the perineal or genital area. There is an alimentary form that can affect the mouth, esophagus, and rumen.

      (2) Appearance. Warts may be 1 mm to more than 1 cm in diameter and have a dry, grey, proliferative appearance. Warts may be attached to the skin by a wide base or with a pedunculated stem. They are uncommon in sheep.

    b. Horses. In animals less than 3 years of age, multiple verrucous lesions are common on the muzzle and genitalia. Aural plaques (papillary acanthoma, hyperplastic dermatitis) are also found. These are bilateral lesions located on the inner surface of the ear, and, less commonly, around the vulva and anus. These lesions progress from small, smooth depigmented papules and plaques to larger, hyperkeratotic plaques.

2. Etiology and pathogenesis
   a. Etiology. Papova viruses (PVs) are the demonstrated causes of warts in all species but goats and swine. PVs are generally host-specific. Bovine papova virus (BPV) 1, 2, and 5 can cause fibropapillomas and fibroblastic skin tumors. BPV 3–6 cause epithelial papillomas.
   b. Pathogenesis
   (1) Transmission. Papillomatosis is infectious and is transmitted by direct and indirect contact (i.e., animal to animal or via implements such as tatooing instruments or ear-tagging pliers). Infection requires damaged skin (from trauma, ectoparasites, UV light). In the specific case of aural plaques in horses, it is assumed that transmission is by blackfly bites.
   (2) Disease progression. The virus attacks the basal cells of the epithelium and causes hyperplasia of epithelial tissue (papilloma) or proliferation of connective tissue (fibropapilloma). Fibropapillomas are the common form of papillomatosis in cattle, whereas papillomas are the common form of warts in horses.

3. Diagnostic plan
   a. The **presumptive diagnosis** is made on the clinical picture and confirmed by histopathology if any doubt exists with the clinical picture.
   b. Histopathology. If there is only epithelial proliferation, squamous papilloma (e.g., a typical equine papilloma) should be considered. With equine aural plaques, there is concurrent epidermal hypomelanosis.

4. Therapeutic plan. Aural plaques are persistent and, because of conformation and location, do not lend themselves to removal. For other warts that persist or in cases where a more rapid resolution is desired, consider:
   a. Cryosurgery or surgical excision. This approach may also stimulate regression in warts that are not excised.
   b. Podophyllum 50% (applied daily until remission)
   c. Intradermal injections of autogenous or commercial wart vaccines. The response of the low, flat warts without stalks (particularly if located on the teats) is poor.

5. Prognosis. Typical papillomatosis in horses, cattle, and sheep, and papillomatosis of the head, neck, and forelegs in goats regress spontaneously in 1–6 months. Warts in other locations (e.g., glans penis or alimentary tract) carry a much less favorable prognosis. The prognosis is also poor if more than 20% of the body is affected.

6. Prevention. Although warts are difficult to prevent, some recommendations include isolating affected animals, decreasing cutaneous environmental injuries, and disinfecting the environment and equipment using formaldehyde or lye.

C. Squamous cell carcinoma (SCC)

1. Patient profile. SCC is a tumor that affects all large animals except swine. Usually seen in mature animals, this disease is of significant economic importance in cattle because of the relative frequency with which it occurs around the eye of range cattle (see Chapter 12 III B). It is also one of the more frequently diagnosed tumors of the skin of horses.

2. Clinical findings
   a. Horses. SCCs commonly occur on the head, at mucocutaneous junctions, and on male and female genitalia. Tumors begin as solitary lesions, usually as nonhealing, enlarging, granulating erosions (or ulcers) or as proliferative, cauliflower-like masses. Necrosis and a foul odor is common. Tumors are usually slow growing and invade rather than metastasize; up to 80% may regress. SCCs of the equine penis or prepuce are more aggressive and metastasize early.
   b. Cattle. The most common SCC in cattle is the ocular form (i.e., **cancer eye**). Early lesions are grey-white plaques of tissue on the conjunctiva or nictitating

membrane. The majority of these lesions may regress, but many develop into papillomas of the orbit, eyelids, or periorbital skin. These are firmly and widely attached and result in irritation and lacrimation. They may become secondarily infected.

3. **Etiology and pathogenesis.** SCCs develop from squamous epithelium, and their genesis is related to chronic exposure of poorly pigmented, poorly haired skin to UV radiation. There may also be genetic factors (e.g., Herefords with cancer eye). Papilloma virus may be associated with the development of SCC because the virus has been found in SCC precursor lesions. Also, DNA of the papilloma virus has been identified in the tumors of cattle with SCCs.

4. **Diagnostic plan and laboratory tests.** Exfoliative cytology from smears of the tumor is helpful. A tumor biopsy reveals irregular masses or cords of epidermal cells that proliferate downward and invade the dermis. Other findings include keratin formation, horn pearls, intercellular bridges, and mitoses.

5. **Therapeutic plan** (see also Chapter 12 III B 4)
   a. **Surgical excision** of the lesions, **cryosurgery,** or both is the treatment of choice. Hyperthermia (commercial portable units are available and affordable) has proven to be very useful.
   b. **Immunotherapy.** Surgical procedures may be combined with immunotherapy, such as repeated intratumor injection (every 2–3 weeks) of the bacillus of Calmette-Guérin (BCG) or a vaccine (see Chapter 12) of fresh tumor extract. Because there is a risk of anaphylaxis with repeated injections of BCG, the patient should be pretreated with flunixin meglumine immediately before intralesional injection.

6. **Prevention.** For cancer eye in cattle, a breeding program should be established to increase pigmentation around the eyes of susceptible cattle (e.g., Herefords).

D. | **Mesenchymal tumors (equine sarcoid)**

1. **Patient profile. Equine sarcoid** can affect any age and breed of horse, but the majority of affected horses (70%) are younger than 4 years old. Appaloosa, Arabian, and Quarter horses are overrepresented and may have a genetic predisposition. There also may be a genetic predilection associated with the major histocompatibility complex.

2. **Clinical findings.** Sarcoid is the most common neoplasm of the horse. Sarcoids usually occur on the head (periocular, pinnae, comissures of lips), legs, and ventral trunk. In many horses (30%–50%), they are multiple. There are five basic gross types of sarcoids:
   a. **Verrucous (warty):** may be sessile or pedunculated
   b. **Fibroblastic (proud flesh-like):** sessile or pedunculated
   c. **Mixed type:** verrucous/fibroblastic
   d. **Occult (flat):** annular areas of alopecia with scaling and crusting
   e. **Subcutaneous nodules:** usually located around the genitalia

3. **Etiology and pathogenesis.** Equine sarcoid is caused by a virus, possibly a PV (the type is yet undetermined). The lesions are moderately malignant but may remain static for years before undergoing a spurt of growth. These lesions do not metastasize but are locally invasive.

4. **Diagnostic plan and laboratory tests.** Histopathology is often necessary to achieve a final diagnosis and will reveal fibroblastic proliferation, epidermal hyperplasia, and dermoepidermal activity.
   a. **Collagen fibers** and **fibroblasts in the dermis** are whorled, tangled, or occasionally in a herringbone pattern.
   b. **Tumor cells** are spindle-shaped, fusiform to stellate, often with hyperchromasia, atypia, and mitoses.
   c. **Fibroblasts at the dermoepidermal junction** orient perpendicularly to basement membrane in a picket fence pattern. Overlying epidermis is hyperplastic and hyperkeratotic.

5. **Differential diagnoses.** The clinical expression of the sarcoid may appear similar to many cutaneous masses in the horse.
   a. **Verrucous sarcoid**—papilloma, SCC
   b. **Fibroblastic sarcoid**—SCC, exuberant granulation tissue, habronemiasis, infectious granulomas (e.g., pythiosis, zygomycosis, bothriomycosis, mycetoma)
   c. **Occult sarcoid**—dermatophytosis, dermatophilosis, demodicosis, staphylococcal folliculitis, onchocerciasis
   d. **Subcutaneous nodules**—folliculitis, nodular necrobiosis

6. **Therapeutic plan**
   a. **Immunotherapy** with commercial BCG vaccine (a mycobacterial cell wall preparation in oil) has been very effective for sarcoids, especially with periocular lesions.
      (1) The vaccine is administered intralesionally every 2–3 weeks for approximately four treatments. Necrosis and the ulceration of lesions may occur following treatment.
      (2) **Side effects** include an occasional malaise or anorexia. Fatal anaphylaxis has also been reported following repeated injections of commercial BCG, so pretreatment with flunixin meglumine and prednisolone are recommended.
   b. **Cryosurgery, radiotherapy,** and **hyperthermia** are also advocated for sarcoid treatment and have met with favorable results, particularly with singular lesions. Static occult and verrucous sarcoids are best left alone because the trauma of biopsy or surgical excision often causes increased growth and aggressive behavior of the tumor.

E. **Melanocytic neoplasms. Melanomas** are most common in aged horses (particularly Arabians and Percherons with a gray coat color) and certain breeds of swine (e.g., Sinclair miniature, Duroc-Jersey).

1. **Clinical findings.** Horses present with solitary or multiple, dermoepidermal or subcutaneous masses. Firm and nodular, these masses may also be alopecic, ulcerated, and grossly hyperpigmented. They are most often present on the perineal region, undersurface of the tail, the pinnae, the periocular region, and distal limbs.

2. **Pathogenesis.** Melanomas may exhibit one of three growth patterns:
   a. Slow growth for years without metastasis
   b. Slow growth for years with sudden rapid growth and malignancy
   c. Rapid growth and malignancy from the onset

3. **Diagnostic plan.** The diagnosis is confirmed by a biopsy and the histopathology of a suspect lesion.

4. **Therapeutic plan**
   a. **Early radical surgical excision** or **cimetidine** (2.5 mg/kg orally, three times daily for 3 months), an H_2 histamine antagonist, has been used for the clinical management of melanomas. Tumors may reduce in size by up to 50%. Treatment should be given for 2–3 weeks after there has been no further measurable decrease in the tumor size. Treatment is most helpful if used before or in conjunction with surgical management.
   b. **Intralesional cisplatin** has also been used and is usually successful only in the reduction of tumor size.

XII. **HEREDITARY DERMATOSES.** A partial list of hereditary conditions that affect the skin of domestic animals follows. Readers are invited to review other texts for complete description of clinical findings.

A. **Bovine porphyria** is a congenital defect of porphyria metabolism, resulting in the accumulation of porphyrins in all tissues. High levels in the skin result in a photosensitivity dermatitis.

B. **Bovine protoporphyria** is similar to bovine porphyria but is a milder disease.

C. **Hypotrichosis** is a congenital condition of cattle, sheep, and pigs that causes partial or complete hair loss. There may be other associated defects (e.g., hypothyroidism, seborrhea, anodontia, poor growth rates).

D. **Reticulated leukotrichia of horses** is likely hereditary and is seen usually in yearling Quarter horses. Linear crusts on the back line result in the characteristic crosshatched patterns of alopecia.

E. **Ichthyosis** has been recorded as a hereditary and a congenital disease in certain cattle (e.g., Holstein). This disease is characterized by alopecia and a scaled skin appearance. Most animals with this disease are euthanized.

F. **Epitheliogenesis imperfecta** has been recorded in calves, lambs, pigs, and foals. An inherited and congenital absence of skin causes death in affected animals.

G. **Epidermolysis bullosa** is a congenital disease of sheep and cattle that is characterized by the development of epidermal bullae in young animals.

H. **Baldy calf syndrome (inherited epidermal dysplasia)** is an inherited, congenital defect of the Holstein breed. The disease is characterized by alopecia and the failure of horn growth. The condition is fatal because affected animals fail to grow.

I. **Dermatosparaxis** is an inherited disorder of cattle, horses, and sheep. The disease is characterized by increased skin and connective tissue fragility. The skin of affected animals is very vulnerable to trauma.

J. **Dermatosis vegetans of swine** is an inherited disorder of the skin and coronets of the feet in young pigs. Clinical signs include erythema, edema, and crustiness. Some pigs may recover, but many affected pigs die from an associated giant-cell pneumonitis.

STUDY QUESTIONS

DIRECTIONS: Each of the numbered items or incomplete statements in this section is followed by answers or by completions of the statement. Select the ONE numbered answer or completion that is BEST in each case.

1. Which one of the following statements regarding primary contact dermatitis is true? Primary contact dermatitis:

(1) requires previous sensitization to the offending agent.
(2) often develops at body locations which trap moisture.
(3) is invariably pruritic.
(4) is treated with corticosteroids as a first order of treatment.
(5) will not resolve even after removal of the offending agent.

2. The cellular damage that is produced in cases of photosensitization is caused by:

(1) molecular excitation.
(2) sunburn.
(3) high levels of cellular chlorophyll.
(4) lack of skin pigmentation.
(5) renal disease.

3. A dairy herd presents with papules, scabs, and granulomas on the teats of the cows. The condition appears to be chronic. The most likely diagnosis is:

(1) horsepox.
(2) bovine ulcerative mammillitis.
(3) pseudocowpox.
(4) contagious ecthyma.
(5) bovine mucosal disease.

4. Staphylococcal organisms may be implicated in which grouping of skin infections?

(1) Purpura hemorrhagica, folliculitis, furunculosis, acne
(2) Udder impetigo, pastern folliculitis, furunculosis, abscesses
(3) Greasy heel, pigeon breast, purpura hemorrhagica, acne
(4) Pigeon breast, caseous lymphadenitis, udder impetigo, lumpy jaw
(5) Lumpy jaw, caseous lymphadenitis, pastern folliculitis, Canadian horsepox

5. Which of the following statements regarding dermatophilosis is true? Dermatophilosis is:

(1) a synonym for dermatophytosis.
(2) extremely pruritic in its early active stage.
(3) most prevalent in dry, arid environments.
(4) diagnosed by microscopic examination of stained smears from active lesions.
(5) best treated with topical fungicides.

6. Which statement regarding ringworm infection in sheep is true?

(1) Limbs are the most common site for the lesions.
(2) Reinfection is common.
(3) Young animals in confinement are most commonly affected.
(4) Diagnosis is confirmed by use of a Wood's lamp.
(5) There is little zoonotic potential compared to other species.

7. Which one of the following statements regarding external parasitism of domestic animals is true?

(1) Psoroptic mange is painful rather than pruritic.
(2) Mite populations are highest in the summer.
(3) *Chorioptes* species are the only mange mites of pigs.
(4) *Melophagus ovinus* lives its entire life on the skin of sheep.
(5) Tick populations are controlled with applications of organophosphates on infested animals.

8. Which statement regarding habronemiasis of horses is true? Habronemiasis of horses:

(1) is also known as "leeches" of horses in the tropics.
(2) is characterized by yellowish granules within inflammatory lesions.
(3) produces gastrointestinal signs more commonly than a dermatitis.
(4) causes pruritis of the perineal area.
(5) is transmitted by mosquitoes.

413

9. Which one of the following statements regarding papillomatosis in horses and cows is true?

(1) Warts on the face of horses and teats of cows are most common in young animals.
(2) Aural plaques should be removed.
(3) Warts typically regress in 1–6 months.
(4) The most common form of warts is fibropapilloma.
(5) Commercial wart vaccines hasten a response.

10. Which one of the following statements regarding melanomas is true? Melanomas:

(1) are seen most commonly in aged cattle.
(2) are the most common neoplasia in horses.
(3) are caused by a virus.
(4) are treated successfully with intralesional bacille Calmette-Guérin (BCG).
(5) may grow very slowly for years.

DIRECTIONS: The numbered item in this section is negatively phrased, as indicated by a capitalized word such as NOT, LEAST, or EXCEPT. Select the ONE numbered answer or completion that is BEST.

11. Which one of the following procedures should NOT be employed when taking a specimen for a suspected viral dermatitis?

(1) Samples should be taken from more than one animal or more than one location in any individual animal.
(2) The site should be aseptically prepared with a betadine scrub and alcohol.
(3) Tissues should be submitted for both direct electron microscopy and virus isolation.
(4) The sample should include the periphery of the lesion.
(5) Samples should be protected by cool storage (4°C) in transport media.

1. The answer is 2 [II C 3 b]. Moisture is an important predisposing factor to the development of primary contact dermatitis. Previous sensitization to the agent is not necessary. Development of sensitivity is a function of concentrations and exposure to the agent. The dermatitis may or may not be pruritic or painful. Corticosteroids may be indicated in long-standing cases, but the first line of treatment is the elimination of the agent and the washing and rinsing of the area. Resolution usually occurs 7–10 days after the removal of the irritant.

2. The answer is 1 [II E 2 b]. Cellular damage occurs when photodynamic agents that have been deposited in the skin absorb ultraviolet (UV) light and become excited, causing cellular damage. Although a lack of skin pigmentation may increase effects of photosensitization, it is not directly causative of cellular destruction. Chlorophyll found in plants must be converted to phylloerythrin before this agent acts as a photodynamic agent. Liver disease, not renal disease, may result in photosensitization.

3. The answer is 3 [IV B 2]. This clinical description best fits pseudocowpox. As named, horsepox affects only horses and is a rare disease not seen outside of Europe. Bovine ulcerative mammillitis produces ulcers and teat skin sloughing. Contagious ecthyma is a disease of sheep and goats, affecting the mucous membranes of the nose and mouth. Bovine mucosal disease affects the oral cavity and the gastrointestinal tract.

4. The answer is 2 [V A–C]. The skin conditions in which *Staphylococcus* species are implicated are udder impetigo, pastern folliculitis (greasy heel), furunculosis, acne, and many abscesses. Purpura hemorrhagica is a urticaria that is seen most commonly as secondary to *Streptococcus equi* infections. Pigeon breast, caseous lymphadenitis, and Canadian horsepox are corynebacterial infections. Lumpy jaw is an actinomycotic infection.

5. The answer is 4 [V E 2 d, e]. Dermatophilosis is a bacterial skin infection that is found most frequently under moist, humid conditions. The condition is characterized by painful (not pruritic), crusty lesions, which leave a moist, denuded area when removed. Stained impression smears of these moist lesions or the underside of the scabs will be diagnostic for the classic appearance of the bacteria. Because this is a bacterial disease, topical fungicides have no place in the therapeutic plan.

6. The answer is 3 [VI B 2]. Dermatomycosis (ringworm) is most common in the young of any species under confinement conditions. In sheep, the head is the most likely area to be involved. Reinfection in any species is not common. Many dermatophytes do not fluoresce under a Wood's light. Sheep are no different than other species in terms of the potential to spread the condition to humans. Ringworm is a zoonosis.

7. The answer is 4 [VII C 1 c]. The sheep ked, *Melophagus ovinus,* is an obligate parasite of the host. Psoroptic mange is very pruritic and *Chorioptes* species infest a wide variety of hosts. Mite populations are usually highest at times of cool, moist conditions, usually when animals are housed in the winter months. Tick populations cannot be controlled by treatment of the host alone because these parasites live off the host for a portion of their life cycle.

8. The answer is 2 [VII E 1 b]. The ulcerative granulomatous skin lesions that are seen with the infestation by *Habronema* or *Draschia* larvae are characterized by yellow granules in diseased tissue. "Leeches" is the common name for phycomycosis. Although *Habronema* and *Draschia* normally inhabit the equine stomach, they do not cause clinical symptoms. *Oxyuris equi* causes perineal pruritus, whereas Onchocerca microfilariae may be transmitted by mosquitos.

9. The answer is 3 [XI B 1]. Although warts are usually most common in young animals, an exception to this includes warts on the teats of cattle. It is not recommended that aural plaques be removed because of their location over the cartilaginous pinnae. In horses, the most common form of warts is fibropapilloma, whereas papillomas are the most common form in cattle. Low, flat warts respond poorly to vaccination; therefore, vaccination is not correct in all instances.

10. The answer is 5 [XI E 2]. Melanomas are seen most commonly in aged horses. Sarcoids are seen most often in aged cattle. Sarcoids are caused by a virus and are treated with the intralesional instillation of bacille Calmette-Guérin (BCG).

11. The answer is 2 [IV A 2 c]. A diagnostician should not aseptically prepare the site before sampling it for virus isolation because disinfectants and alcohol may inactivate the virus. Samples should be taken from more than one animal or more than one location in any individual animal. The sample should include the periphery of the lesion. Samples should be protected by cool storage (4°C) in transport media. Tissue should be submitted for both direct electron microscopy and virus isolations.

Chapter 17

Mastitis
Timothy H. Ogilvie

I. BOVINE MASTITIS

A. Overview

1. **Definitions**
   a. **Clinical mastitis** is inflammation of the mammary gland characterized by changes in milk color and consistency.
   b. **Subclinical mastitis** produces no noticeable udder inflammation or milk abnormalities but results in a high somatic cell count (SCC).
   c. **Peracute mastitis** is a severe inflammation of the udder with a marked systemic reaction.
   d. **Acute mastitis** is a severe inflammation of the udder with a mild to moderate systemic reaction.
   e. **Subacute mastitis** is a mild inflammation of the udder with persistent milk abnormalities, such as changes in consistency, color, or milk production.
   f. **Chronic mastitis** is defined as recurrent attacks of udder inflammation with little noticeable change in the milk between attacks.

2. **Patient profile and history**
   a. Almost all clinical mastitis occurs during **lactation,** and 60% of cases occur during the first 6 weeks of lactation.
   b. Mastitis is the **most costly disease** in North American animal agriculture, with an estimated 50% of dairy cows affected to some degree. However, most cases are nonclinical or subclinical, and cows vary in susceptibility.

3. **Etiology and pathogenesis**
   a. **Etiology.** Most cases of mastitis are caused by microbial infection. **Sources** of infection include the udder, skin, and environment.
   b. **Pathogenesis**
      (1) In most cases, causative organisms enter the teat duct through the streak canal, multiply there, and progress upward into the lactiferous sinus, collecting ducts, and alveoli.
      (2) The invading organisms cause an **inflammatory response** following leukocyte migration to the udder and edema.
      (3) **Resolution** of the infection may result in fibrosis, abscess formation, or glandular atrophy.

4. **Laboratory tests.** Milk cultures should be obtained before initiating therapy so that alternate plans may be made in case of treatment failure. The culture results from a single case (e.g., *Escherichia coli*) might not reflect herd status (e.g., *Staphylococcus aureus*).

5. **Therapeutic plan**
   a. A commercially available and proven **intramammary medication for nonlactating cows** should be used on all quarters of all cows at the end of lactation (drying off).
   b. Cows with clinical signs should be treated promptly with a proven **intramammary medication for lactating cows.** Exceptions to this may be staphylococcal mastitis and other causes of mastitis nonresponsive to antibiotics (e.g., yeasts, fungi, *Mycoplasma* species, *Nocardia asteroides*). Treated cattle should be identified so that milk-withholding requirements can be respected.
   c. Treatment for **acute clinical cases** should include the **manual removal** of as much milk as possible from infected quarters (i.e., stripping).

6. Prevention. The goal in most dairies is to maintain a herd incidence of less than or equal to 3% clinical infection, zero colony-forming units/ml on bacteriology of a bulk milk tank sample, and an SCC of 100,000–250,000 cells/mm^3. An effective mastitis control program includes:

  a. Hygiene

    (1) Post-milking teat sanitation with commercially available and proven products reduces infection from contagious pathogens.

    (2) Premilking teat sanitation with commercially available and proven products reduces the likelihood of mastitis due to environmental pathogens (e.g., coliforms).

    (3) Management practices that improve overall hygiene of the environment should be employed, allowing cows to be clean, dry, and comfortable.

  b. Milking procedures and machine function

    (1) Milking machines should be installed and maintained according to the manufacturer's instructions.

    (2) Inflations and hoses should be changed on a regular basis.

    (3) Teats should be disinfected and dried with individual paper towels or washcloths before milking machine placement.

    (4) Teat cup sanitation should be practiced between cows.

  c. Accurate and up-to-date **records** should be maintained, and **cull** cows with chronic mastitis.

B. | **Subacute mastitis**

  1. Streptococcal

    a. *Streptococcus agalactiae* mastitis

      (1) Patient profile and history

        (a) History. This organism was the primary cause of mastitis in North America before antibiotic therapy, machine milking, universally accepted prevention techniques, and improved hygiene practices. It is still an important and relatively common pathogen exceeded in prevalence only by *Staphylococcus aureus*. Therefore, owners should be warned not to become complacent about the organism as a cause of mastitis because it may still result in major losses of milk.

        (b) Susceptibility. The disease is often introduced into the herd by infected cows. Cows have varying susceptibilities within herds. Also, cows exhibit an increased susceptibility with age. This phenomenon, although unexplained, likely results from increased teat sphincter patency with age.

      (2) Clinical findings

        (a) Glands. Mastitis caused by *S. agalactiae* is usually nonclinical with periodic clinical flare-ups. The affected mammary gland will evidence heat, pain, and swelling. Inflammation may be mild except following the initial exposure to the organism, in which case the inflammatory reaction of the gland is moderate (subacute mastitis). If an animal is untreated, clinical cases persist with recurrent flare-ups.

        (b) Milk. Although milk from affected glands may appear normal between mastitis episodes, examination of the milk during clinical periods reveals clots ("ropey" milk) in watery foremilk. Total milk yield per lactation is reduced with each recurrent bout.

      (3) Etiology and pathogenesis

        (a) Etiology. *S. agalactiae* causes a highly contagious, obligate infection of the mammary gland.

        (b) Pathogenesis

          (i) Transmission. This organism may survive outside of the mammary gland for a short time; therefore, it may be transmitted from cow to cow via **fomites** (e.g., milker's hands, multi-use towels, milking machines). The organism colonizes the teat, and infections of the mammary gland occur following passage of the organism through the teat canal.

(ii) **Inflammation.** The organism does not invade the glandular tissue but remains on the epithelial surface of acini and ducts, where it causes tissue damage by lactic-acid production. This **epithelial inflammation** results in fibrosis of interalveolar tissue and involution of the acini. Further flare-ups produce more lobular fibrosis and loss of secretory function and, thus, a decreased milk yield. **Glandular atrophy** is the eventual outcome.

(iii) **Milk clots.** As inflammation subsides during each episode, the epithelial lining of the acini and ducts sloughs. This inflammatory debris and other somatic cells result in the clinical appearance of stringy or ropey clots in the milk.

(4) Diagnostic plan

(a) Clinical mastitis is diagnosed by **clinical findings** and supported by **tests** that qualify and quantify udder inflammation in the individual. Bacterial isolation and identification confirm *S. agalactiae* as the causative organism.

(b) For a **herd diagnosis,** bulk tank SCC and microbiology of composite bulk milk tank samples aid in making the diagnosis.

(5) Laboratory tests

(a) **Routine milk culture** demonstrates relatively pure cultures of *S. agalactiae.* However, bacterial isolation from the milk of individual cows may be negative during the invasive phase of the initial infection or during clinical flare-ups when cell counts are high. **Bulk milk samples** are often used for isolation of the organism to identify or monitor herd problems.

(b) **Indirect tests** to measure increased cellularity of the milk are also used. The **California mastitis test (CMT)** [which measures cell nuclear protein], individual cow SCCs, and bulk tank SCCs are used to confirm and quantify udder inflammation.

(6) Therapeutic plan

(a) **Lactating cows.** Commercially available **procaine penicillin G** intramammary infusions are used for lactating animals (100,000 units/gland for one daily infusion for 3 days). This treatment often results in a high cure rate (90%).

(b) **Unresponsive cows.** If the cow does not respond with 3 days of therapy, consider that there might be a resistant strain of *Streptococcus,* a mixed bacterial infection, or the attainment of ineffective levels of antibiotic in the milk of a high-producing cow.

(i) **Resubmission** of samples for culture and sensitivity is then necessary.

(ii) **Alternative therapies** include increasing intramammary penicillin dosage, changing antibiotics, or using the parenteral route. With these alternative therapies, labeled recommendations for antibiotic residues in the milk will not be valid, and milk must be discarded for more time before it is fit for human consumption.

(c) **Dry cows.** Dry cow therapy with commercial nonlactating cow products also is effective to eliminate the organism from the gland. However, this treatment usually is not necessary because of the efficacy of lactating cow therapy.

(7) Prevention. Eradication of herd infection is possible through a dedicated program of improved hygiene and intramammary infusion therapy of all cows. A mastitis control program (see I A 6) should be employed for this disease for the general production of high-quality milk. Dedication to hygiene and prevention is necessary to maintain freedom from new infections.

b. Other streptococcal causes of mastitis

(1) Patient profile and history. Mastitis caused by miscellaneous streptococci is of great concern as control procedures for mastitis caused by *S. agalactiae* and *S. aureus* grow more common.

(2) Clinical findings. These streptococci may produce acute clinical mastitis with severe udder swelling and clots in the milk. There are associated but moderate systemic signs of fever, anorexia, and depression. Alternatively, infections may be subacute to subclinical.

(3) **Etiology and pathogenesis.** The causative organisms are considered environmental pathogens and are not contagious like *S. agalactiae* or *S. aureus.*

   (a) *Streptococcus dysgalactiae* is similar to *S. agalactiae,* but the organism does not spread as readily from cow to cow. Infection is associated with teat lesions and faulty milking techniques, and clinical disease usually occurs early in lactation.

   (b) *Streptococcus uberis* may be ubiquitous in the environment and is a common inhabitant of the mucous membranes, gastrointestinal tract, udder, and skin of cows. Consequently, the possibility of sample contamination must be considered following isolation of the organism from a milk sample. This organism causes all types of mastitis and is often introduced during the dry period, particularly if cows have not been treated with dry cow therapy. New infections often follow teat injuries.

   (c) *Streptococcus viridans, Streptococcus zooepidemicus, Streptococcus pyogenes,* and *Streptococcus pneumoniae* do not commonly produce mastitis in cows, but when they do, these organisms may cause peracute to chronic mastitis. Infection may be introduced from other species (e.g., humans), and if infection is herd-wide, it may be difficult to eradicate.

(4) **Diagnostic plan and laboratory tests.** Clinical findings are nonspecific for the etiologic agent and must be supported by culture of milk specimens and sensitivity patterns of microbiological isolates.

(5) **Therapeutic plan**

   (a) *S. dysgalactiae* and *S. uberis* infections usually respond well to penicillin but require dry cow treatment if established in a herd.

   (b) *S. zooepidemicus* infection does not respond well to antibiotics, so culling of affected animals should be considered.

   (c) *S. pyogenes, S. pneumoniae,* and *S. viridans* infections must be treated with systemic antibiotics and supportive care. Loss of function of the gland is common.

(6) **Prevention.** An established mastitis control program similar to that for other organisms limits the incidence of infection (see I A 6). In the case of *S. uberis,* blanket dry cow therapy should be considered because of increased incidence of infection during the dry period.

2. Staphylococcal

  a. *Staphylococcus aureus* is likely the most economically important cause of mastitis since better control of *S. agalactiae* has developed.

(1) **Patient profile and history.** The disease tends to peak in younger cattle, but there is no true age susceptibility to infection.

(2) **Clinical findings.** Expression of clinical signs may depend on the stage of lactation when infection occurs.

   (a) In early lactation, a **peracute form** may occur (see I C 2).

   (b) The **chronic form** of **subacute mastitis** is the most common clinical presentation. There is persistent inflammation of the gland, but the signs of development may be so subtle that they can be missed. There is a slowly developing induration, fibrosis, and atrophy with occasional clots in the milk. There is usually less milk production loss than with *S. agalactiae,* but the infection is more difficult to treat and control.

(3) **Etiology and pathogenesis**

   (a) **Etiology.** *S. aureus* is not an obligate parasite of the mammary gland but is a contagious pathogen.

   (b) **Pathogenesis**

     (i) **Transmission.** Infected cattle serve as sources of infection. Organisms are transmitted by fomites [see I B 1 a (3) (b)].

     (ii) **Route of infection.** Infection is via the teat canal. Bacteria colonize the teat sinus often following injury or improper milking technique. *S. aureus* proliferates in the collecting ducts and the alveoli, invades tissue, and produces tissue destruction. β-Toxins and α-toxins may be involved in this tissue destruction, but this pathogenesis is debatable.

  (iii) This **tissue necrosis** evolves to connective tissue proliferation, fibrosis, abscessation, and glandular atrophy. *S. aureus* persists in the environment, on teats and mucous membranes as well as in walled-off glandular abscesses.

(4) Diagnostic plan. A definitive diagnosis depends on the laboratory tests.

(5) Laboratory tests

  (a) **Milk culture.** Bacterial isolation and identification may be accomplished through culturing milk from affected cows. A culture reveals *S. aureus*, a coagulase-positive, hemolytic *Staphylococcus*.

  (b) **SCC and CMT.** As with other causes of mastitis, individual cow SCCs quantify udder inflammation. The CMT also may be used to detect infected cows.

(6) Therapeutic plan

  (a) **Antibiotic therapy.** *S. aureus* is often sensitive in vitro to many antibiotics. However, treatment during lactation is often disappointing and results in recurrences because the organism is inaccessible to antibiotics when within glandular abscesses or obstructed, fibrotic glandular tissue.

  (b) **Lactation therapy** may be instituted in clinical cases if economics warrant this decision. Examples of when lactation therapy may be warranted include if treatment occurs early in lactation before milk is suitable for human consumption or when milk must be discarded for some other reason.

  (c) **Dry cow therapy** is recommended in chronically or subclinically affected cattle (based on SCC and bacteriology). Products are specifically manufactured for use in the dry period and have slow-release or long-acting intramammary formulations (e.g., cloxacillin, novobiocin).

(7) Prevention

  (a) **Eradication** of the organism is difficult because of the rigorous nature of the program necessary to both reduce and eliminate infections. Cost and benefit analyses may reveal that a 10% new quarter infection rate may be acceptable and justifiable to producers who are unable to comply with efforts required for eradication.

  (b) **Immunization.** Some success has been reported with the use of an autogenous or commercially available *S. aureus* bacterin, particularly a bacterin containing *S. aureus* capsular antigen.

  (c) **Control** and prevention is the aim of a mastitis program similar to that which may be introduced for control of *S. agalactiae*. This program includes:

    (i) Maintenance of strict milking hygiene
    (ii) Dry cow therapy
    (iii) Maintenance of proper milking machine function
    (iv) Rigorous identification of infected animals through routine composite milk culturing of all cows annually
    (v) Segregation of animals into an infected and noninfected string
    (vi) Culling of infected animals
    (vii) Environmental sanitation (including teat dipping)
    (viii) Monitoring of procedure results and ongoing prevalence of mastitis

b. Other staphylococcal causes of mastitis

(1) Clinical findings. Staphylococci other than *S. aureus* usually produce a subclinical mastitis. In the occasional clinical case, there are mild clinical signs of udder warmth and clots or flakes in the milk.

(2) Etiology and pathogenesis. Causative organisms are coagulase-negative staphylococci (e.g., *Staphylococcus epidermidis*). These organisms colonize the teat, orifice, and teat canal.

(3) Diagnostic plan and laboratory tests. Increased herd level SCCs or CMTs may prompt further microbiological investigation. Staphylococci may contaminate milk samples (individual cow or bulk tank), and this should be accounted for when interpreting culture results.

(4) **Therapeutic plan.** Staphylococci usually are eradicated by standard lactational or dry cow therapy.

(5) **Prevention.** Isolation of these organisms may indicate poor milking hygiene (e.g., udder wash, teat dipping). Therefore, a mastitis control program that focuses on hygiene and accepted udder health care procedures is recommended.

C. **Acute and peracute mastitis.** Many of the organisms that cause acute and peracute mastitis reside in the environment, and most are not inhabitants of the udder.

1. **Coliform mastitis (acute mastitis, acute coliform mastitis, environmental mastitis).** Coliform organisms are the most common cause of fatal mastitis and approximately 50% of cows die or are culled because of the disease. The gram-negative organisms are opportunistic and contaminate the teat between milkings.

   a. **Patient profile**
      (1) Coliform mastitis occurs **most commonly** within a few days of calving (0–6 weeks) and usually involves one or two quarters of the mammary gland. This disease may be seen in recumbent cattle (e.g., parturient paresis, downer cow).
      (2) **Susceptibility.** Low levels of somatic cells in the bovine udder may increase the susceptibility of cows to coliform mastitis.
      (3) **Incidence.** Disease usually occurs sporadically, but a high herd incidence can be 25%. There may be higher incidence in older cows, higher producing cows, or in herds that practice stringent control for subclinical mastitis. Coliform mastitis is most common in larger herds and herds experiencing heavy population pressures, crowding, and poor hygiene or management practices.

   b. **Clinical findings.** Coliform mastitis causes peracute or acute clinical signs. Rarely does the disease progress to a prolonged course of chronic mastitis.
      (1) **Systemic signs** may occur before changes are evident in the milk. The disorder is characterized by the sudden onset of agalactia and toxemia. Cows exhibit anorexia, severe depression, trembling, tachycardia, tachypnea, and fever or a subnormal temperature in advanced cases. Cows are weak and recumbency is common. Often, there is concurrent diarrhea and dehydration.
      (2) **Affected quarters** are warm and swollen but are not gangrenous or cold as in some other peracute mastitis conditions. Affected glands secrete a serous fluid with small flakes that are best seen by using a strip cup.

   c. **Etiology and pathogenesis**
      (1) **Etiology.** *E. coli*, *Klebsiella* species, and *E. aerogenes* are discussed together and, for the purposes of this section, are collectively called coliforms.
      (2) **Pathogenesis.** These organisms are transferred from the environment to the cow and produce similar (indistinguishable) clinical signs. Even though they produce acute and often fatal clinical signs, many infections by these organisms are subclinical and self-limiting.
         (a) **Source.** Bedding and feces, usually under wet conditions, are primary sources of contamination. *Klebsiella pneumoniae* has most specifically been associated with sawdust and wood shavings bedding.
         (b) **Predisposing factors.** Coliform bacteria on the teat end are usually transitory because the teat most often provides an effective barrier to infection. However, improper milking machine function, teat injuries (stepping or crushing), teat sphincter relaxation with older cows, and the use of teat dilators may allow penetration by environmental pathogens. Infection also can occur in the very late dry period just before parturition. The mammary gland is most prone to infection by these organisms in early lactation and more resistant in later lactation.
         (c) The **systemic effects** of this condition result from the elaboration of **endotoxin** from the organism or from the recruitment of host mediators, such as eicosanoids, prostaglandins, and thromboxanes. Endotoxin causes in-

creases in vascular permeability (edema) and neutrophil "pooling" in the udder. The systemic effects may lag behind the growth of the organism in the udder and parallel the massive release of endotoxin as the organisms die off.

(d) **Host defense. Neutrophils** may be ineffective in eliminating organisms but will limit bacterial invasion, and in the case of an adequate host response, the infection is limited to mammary sinuses with no secretory tissue involvement. The gland usually returns to normal function if the animal recovers.

d. Diagnostic plan. The diagnosis is based on the patient profile, history, clinical signs, and milk findings. Milk culture and sensitivity help define the pathogen, although it must be recognized that occasionally samples are negative depending on the effectiveness of neutrophils in clearing the organism.

e. Laboratory tests

  (1) **Hematology** shows a severe leukopenia, neutropenia, and a degenerative left shift due to massive neutrophil pooling in the affected gland.

  (2) **Serum chemistry** often reveals hypocalcemia.

  (3) **Culture** results are positive for the coliform organism except in those cases where neutrophils have cleared the organism from the milk. This may occur in less acute cases.

  (a) **Rapid-response culture** media are available for differentiation of gram-positive and gram-negative organisms causing clinical mastitis (Hy-Mast Mastitis Screening Test, Pharmacia & Upjohn Animal Health, Orangeville, Ontario, Canada).

  (b) Results of **milk culture** may be available in 12–24 hours and allow more informal decisions to be made regarding use of intramammary antibiotic therapy.

f. Differential diagnoses include other causes of acute and peracute mastitis, parturient paresis (see Chapter 9), and other causes of septicemia or toxemia, such as salmonellosis (see Chapter 3).

g. Therapeutic plan. Acute coliform mastitis should be considered an **emergency** situation and treatment instituted accordingly.

  (1) **Antibiotic therapy** is somewhat controversial.

  (a) Studies have shown that by the time clinical signs occur, most of the organisms have been cleared from the mammary gland by the neutrophils. Also, a major die-off of bacteria in response to antibiotic use causes a further release of endotoxin, which exacerbates clinical signs.

  (b) Others argue that antibiotics are necessary in cases in which neutrophils have not countered the infection or when organisms may have moved into the blood stream (bacteremia).

  (c) When used, appropriate **systemic antibiotics** include gentamicin (2–5 mg/kg intravenously, twice daily), amoxicillin and clavulanic acid combinations, and cephalosporins.

  (2) **Other common treatments** include:

  (a) **Stripping** the affected quarter hourly

  (b) **Oxytocin** (30 IU), which may aid in milk letdown

  (c) **Fluid and electrolyte therapy**—balanced electrolyte solution (40–60 L during the first 24 hours) or hypertonic saline (7.5%) combined with oral fluids

  (d) **Anti-inflammatory agents**
    (i) **Corticosteroids:** 1 mg/kg intravenously twice during the first day of treatment only
    (ii) **Flunixin meglumine:** 0.25–1.1 mg/kg intramuscularly or intravenously twice daily

  (e) **Intramammary antibiotics**—commercially available and may be used at night after the last stripping but show little experimental efficacy

  (f) **Calcium,** which should be administered carefully if necessary (perhaps subcutaneously)

    (g) Nursing care, such as rolling the cow periodically from side to side to prevent muscle necrosis, bedding the animal on a firm but cushioned surface (e.g., manure pack), and bathing and massaging the udder

  h. Prevention and control of coliform mastitis within a herd includes:

    (1) Improving milking and premilking hygiene

    (2) Encouraging environmental hygiene and clean bedding

    (3) Considering other types of bedding (e.g., sand) if sawdust or shavings are incriminated

    (4) Keeping bedding dry and avoiding overcrowding

    (5) Keeping cows standing for a time after milking

    (6) Controlling parturient diseases (e.g., milk fever, downer cows)

    (7) Providing calving and maternity pens to help decrease udder trauma at calving

    (8) Administering a coliform subunit (core) bacterin against a variety of gram-negative organisms at drying off, 3–4 weeks later, and again at or near freshening

2. Peracute staphylococcal mastitis

  a. Patient profile and history. The most common presentation of staphylococcal infection of the mammary gland is as a chronic subclinical mastitis. Occasionally, infection presents as a peracute or acute mastitis seen in early lactation. In its peracute form, this infection is often fatal.

  b. Clinical findings

    (1) There is a sudden and severe **systemic reaction.** The cow's temperature may be 41°C–42°C but becomes subnormal as the condition progresses. There is tachycardia, anorexia, depression, and muscular weakness resulting in recumbency, and the case may appear similar to coliform mastitis.

    (2) The **affected quarter** is swollen, hard, and sore, causing lameness in ambulatory animals.

    (3) Discoloration of the udder may be evident early (blue-black gangrene). The development of a gangrenous udder is unique to *Staphylococcus* and *Clostridium* infections. Within 24 hours, the gangrenous areas turn black and ooze serum, and subcutaneous emphysema may be evident. The milk secretion is scant with bloody, serous fluid and occasional gas. Toxemia is profound, death is rapid, and even in animals that recover, the quarter is lost. The affected quarter sloughs over time in a messy manner.

  c. Etiology and pathogenesis. *S. aureus* is the most common cause of peracute staphylococcal mastitis. The pathogenesis is as in subacute staphylococcal mastitis, but the peracute nature of the disease is likely the result of an infection in early lactation with a large inoculum of organism.

  d. Diagnostic plan. The diagnosis of peracute mastitis is made on clinical findings. The definitive diagnosis is supported by laboratory tests and culture of *S. aureus.*

  e. Laboratory tests

    (1) Hematology shows an inflammatory leukogram.

    (2) Clinical biochemistry indicates a severe, systemic state (shock). Fibrinogen is elevated.

    (3) Milk culture is positive for *S. aureus,* but the information is of little relevance because of the peracute nature of the disease.

  f. Differential diagnoses include parturient paresis, coliform mastitis, *A. pyogenes* mastitis, and clostridial infection of the udder.

  g. Therapeutic plan. Generally, treatment is very expensive, and cows that recover are often culled because only three viable quarters remain. The life of the animal may be saved with **early** and **aggressive therapy.** The following treatments can be considered:

    (1) Intravenous crystalline penicillin or tetracycline followed by subsequent intramuscular treatment

    (2) Intravenous fluids

    (3) Frequent massage, bathing, and milk stripping from the affected quarter (Note: oxytocin has little effect on milk letdown in this instance.)

    (4) Amputation of the quarter, which is usually a final and heroic attempt to save the cow's life

    (5) Intramammary antibiotic infusions have little effect because of the edema, swelling, and gangrenous necrosis of the udder.

  h. Prevention. Little can be done to prevent this condition other than maintenance of udder health as recommended in I B 2 a (7).

3. Acute streptococcal mastitis

  a. Etiology and clinical findings. Infection with *S. dysgalactiae, S. uberis, S. viridans, S. pyogenes, S. pneumoniae,* and other streptococci nonagalactiae organisms may produce an acute mastitis with swelling of the individual quarter. There may be a moderate systemic reaction, and milk secretion is abnormal with evidence of flakes and clots. Specifically, *S. pneumoniae* will produce a peracute mastitis.

  b. Therapeutic plan. The disease should be treated like other cases of acute mastitis (see I C 1 g).

4. *Actinomyces pyogenes* mastitis

  a. Patient profile and history

    (1) *A. pyogenes* mastitis can occur in any cow but is distinguished from other types of mastitis because it usually occurs in **dry cows** or **pregnant heifers.** Mortality is high in cattle, and glandular function is lost.

    (2) This infection is seen most commonly in **Europe** during **summer** months (hence the name *summer mastitis*) and in extensive dairy production areas (e.g., New Zealand, Australia). The disease is seen in North America if seasonal calving is practiced in dairy operations.

    (3) This sporadic form of mastitis occurs most often in **pastured cattle** under conditions of wet summers, high fly populations, and poorly observed animals.

  b. Clinical findings

    (1) This peracute mastitis causes **severe, systemic reactions.** The cow's fever reaches 40°C–41°C. There is tachycardia, anorexia, depression, and weakness. Abortions may occur.

    (2) The **udder** is hard, swollen, and painful. An initial watery secretion becomes purulent and foul smelling. This secretion is subjectively diagnostic for the disease.

    (3) In cows that survive the initial systemic reaction, the quarter becomes very hard, and abscesses develop, which rupture at the supramammary lymph nodes or at the base of the teat. Gangrene does not occur, but the quarter sloughs.

  c. Etiology and pathogenesis. *A. pyogenes* may act alone or with other organisms to produce a suppurative mastitis. The organism is thought to be spread by flies and introduced via the teat canal.

  d. Diagnostic plan and laboratory tests. Clinically, the disease is distinctive, and the causative organism can be recovered on milk culture.

  e. Therapeutic plan. Therapy has little effect in clinical cases. If considered, treatment should include:

    (1) The systemic use of broad-spectrum antibiotics

    (2) Stripping the affected quarter every 1–2 hours in the initial phase of the disease

    (3) Supportive care (e.g., fluid therapy, rolling, deep bedding)

  f. Prevention. In places where the disease is prevalent (e.g., New Zealand, Australia), dry cow treatment may need to be performed 2–3 times during the dry period. There must be strict attention to fly control and closer observation of cows on pasture.

5. *Nocardia* mastitis

  a. Patient profile. This is a relatively uncommon type of mastitis but has been isolated periodically in herds. This disease is usually sporadic and most common in early lactation.

  b. Clinical findings

    (1) With infection **early** in lactation, there is severe systemic involvement often resulting in death of the cow. If not fatal, the infection may resolve to chronic mastitis and udder fibrosis with draining, suppurative sinus tracts.

(2) Infection **later** in lactation may produce acute inflammation with only moderate systemic involvement. There is still glandular fibrosis with the presence of discrete nodules discernable on palpation of the gland. The milk appears greyish with clots, white granules, or both.

(3) **Subclinical infections** may occur but do not differ significantly from other types of subclinical mastitis.

c. **Etiology and pathogenesis.** Nocardia asteroides, the causative organism, is a common soil contaminant. If disease is a herd problem, there is likely a common method of introduction (e.g., multi-injection mastitis preparations, cracked milking machine liners). When the gland is invaded by the organism, extensive glandular destruction and fibrosis occur. Local invasion of other tissues may occur (lymph nodes). There is eventual loss of production, and the cow is invariably culled if she survives.

d. **Diagnostic plan.** Clinical findings are highly suggestive of the condition, and the causative organism is confirmed by microbiology.

e. **Therapeutic plan.** Therapy is unrewarding. Long-term treatment (1–2 weeks) of erythromycin and miconazole would be necessary but is of limited value. The organism is specifically resistant to neomycin-based intramammary products.

f. **Prevention.** Milking and environmental hygiene is all that can be recommended for the herd. Culture-positive cows should be culled.

6. *Mycoplasma* **mastitis**
    a. **Patient profile and history**
        (1) Cows at any age or stage of lactation may be affected, but those in early lactation show the most severe systemic signs. The disease occurs worldwide and is most common in large, intensively managed herds with constant movement of cattle onto the premises.
        (2) Historically, incidence of disease was thought to be associated with the use of multi-dose vials of intramammary products. Now, disease is thought to occur in association with shedder cows or outbreaks of pneumonia, urogenital disease, and polyarthritis in heifers and calves.
    b. **Clinical findings**
        (1) In **lactating cows,** a sudden drop in milk production and a painless udder swelling occur (edema). Supramammary lymph nodes may enlarge. All four quarters may be affected.
            (a) **Systemic findings.** A mild fever and anorexia is seen with cows in early lactation; otherwise, there may be little systemic involvement.
            (b) The **udder secretion** appears normal in the early course of disease, but if left to stand, a fine, grainy or flaky precipitate settles to the bottom of the sample container. As the disease progresses, the milk assumes a cheesy consistency in chronic cases.
            (c) **Duration.** Cases may persist for weeks. Depending on the type of *Mycoplasma* involved, the gland may atrophy for the current and subsequent lactations or return to normal function.
        (2) **Dry cows** show little udder swelling.
        (3) **Other cows** or **young dairy animals** in the herd may show arthritis or pneumonia.
    c. **Etiology and pathogenesis**
        (1) **Etiology.** Many species of *Mycoplasma* may produce mastitis, but *Mycoplasma bovis* is the most common causative agent.
        (2) **Pathogenesis**
            (a) **Source.** M. bovis produces a purulent interstitial mastitis. It may be introduced to a herd or survive in shedder cows that have recovered from disease. The source of shedding may be from the udder, vagina, or upper respiratory tract.
            (b) **Route of infection.** M. bovis may reside on mucous membranes and gain entrance to the gland via the teat canal or systemically through aerosol,

spreading hematogenously. If the organism invades the udder via the teat, the infection may spread to other quarters and sites hematogenously.

d. **Diagnostic plan.** The specific clinical findings related to the udder, other clinical findings in the herd (e.g., pneumonia, arthritis, vaginitis), and laboratory results collectively form the diagnosis.

e. **Laboratory tests.** *Mycoplasma* species can be cultured from the milk of affected quarters, but this test is not routinely performed by many laboratories. In individually affected animals, there is a marked leukopenia and a very high SCC (more than 20 million/ml).

f. **Therapeutic plan**

(1) **Systemic antibiotics.** Therapy is unrewarding, but attempts to cure the condition may be made with systemic antibiotics (e.g., tetracycline, erythromycin, tylosin). Residue avoidance and labeled restrictions for use in dairy animals must be considered.

(2) **Response to therapy.** It is difficult to advise on the eventual course of the disease because outcomes are variable. While individual animals may recover health and function, many other cows fail to recover. Also, herd outbreaks occur, which necessitates culling many animals.

g. **Prevention** includes closing the herd, establishing a routine udder health and mastitis control program, and monitoring incidence of infection via bulk milk tank culture. Some practitioners advocate the use of an autogenous vaccine in chronically affected herds.

D. **Other causes of mastitis**

1. *Mycobacterium bovis.* Mastitis resulting from *M. bovis* infection is a **public health hazard** because contaminated milk may be macroscopically normal but can act as a source of human tuberculosis. Fortunately, many jurisdictions are free of this disease because of active regulatory efforts (i.e., identification and slaughter) carried out in the past. *M. bovis* (the causative agent for **tuberculosis** in cattle) causes a hard, swollen udder and, on occasion, enlarged, supramammary lymph nodes. This disease occurs with other systemic findings (e.g., pneumonia, chronic ill-thrift).

2. **Fungi and yeasts.** Yeasts are more common than fungi, and *Candida* species are the most often implicated. Infection may persist for weeks and may resolve or produce udder damage, resulting in cullage of the affected individual.

a. **Clinical findings**

(1) There is little **systemic reaction** with this mastitis, although there may be some fever and anorexia.

(2) The **udder inflammation** is acute, with marked swelling of the affected quarters and enlargement of the supramammary lymph nodes.

(3) **Milk.** There is a significant drop in milk production, and the milk appears viscous, white-grey, and mucoid in consistency.

b. **Etiology and pathogenesis.** *Cryptococcus neoformans* and *Aspergillus fumigatus* are other reported yeasts causing mastitis. The use of contaminated infusion material or overzealous use of intramammary antibiotic therapy may result in herd outbreaks. Also, there is a growing body of subjective evidence that implicates yeast contamination of the udder from growth in bedding during periods of moisture and warmth.

c. **Therapeutic plan.** The best advice is to discontinue all antibiotic therapy and strip out the quarter four times daily.

(1) Yeast mastitis is not responsive to therapy, but the infection is self-limiting in some cows in 30–60 days, particularly those animals infected with *Candida* species.

(2) The use of **intramammary antibiotics** is contraindicated in this condition.

3. **Algae**

a. **Clinical findings and etiology.** *Prototheca trispora* and *Prototheca zopfii* have been identified as causing chronic, clinical mastitis in cattle. The organisms are isolates from the environment and produce glandular swelling, decreased milk

production, and large clots in watery milk. There is a progressive abscessation of the gland, and the cow must be culled.
   b. **Therapeutic plan.** There is no successful treatment.

4. *Pseudomonas aeruginosa*
   a. **Clinical findings and pathogenesis.** This organism may produce either an acute mastitis with a systemic reaction or a chronic mastitis. Glandular function may be lost. Usual sources of infection include contaminated infusions or environmental sources (e.g., contaminated udder wash water).
   b. **Therapeutic plan.** Third-generation cephalosporins are recommended for treatment, but success may be limited.

5. **Bacilli**
   a. **Clinical findings and etiology. *Bacillus cereus* and *Bacillus subtilis*** may cause an acute hemorrhagic mastitis. Teat and udder trauma are precipitating events for the introduction of the organism spores. Proliferation of the organisms produces a peracute, toxic mastitis. Gangrene follows, with eventual loss of the quarter if the cow lives.
   b. **Therapeutic plan.** Treatment must be intensive and heroic, consisting of intravenous fluids, broad-spectrum antibiotics, anti-inflammatory agents, udder massage, and frequent quarter stripping. Results are often disappointing.

6. *Clostridium perfringens*
   a. **Clinical findings and etiology. *C. perfringens* type A** may produce a peracute, highly fatal toxic mastitis, which is characterized by gangrene and a thin, brown glandular secretion accompanied by gas.
   b. **Therapeutic plan.** Early treatment with intravenous crystalline penicillin may be successful.

II. EQUINE MASTITIS.
Mastitis in mares is rare. What is more common is swelling and soreness of the udder due to failure of the foal to nurse. A lower incidence of mastitis in mares as compared with dairy cows may be explained by the smaller size of the udder and teats. In addition, there is less exposure to physical trauma, milking machines, and contaminated fomites, and the gland is emptied relatively often because of the frequent nursing of the foal.

A. Clinical findings. The udder is enlarged, warm, firm, and painful on palpation. Both halves of the udder are often affected simultaneously. The milk is abnormal (thin, discolored and with clots). Glandular edema may extend forward along the ventral abdomen.

B. Etiology. When mastitis does occur (e.g., at foal weaning), culture may reveal a causative organism. *S. zooepidemicus* is the most common isolate, but many other pathogens, including gram-negative organisms, have been isolated in cases of mare mastitis.

C. Differential diagnoses should include mammary gland neoplasia.

D. Therapeutic plan. Response to therapy is usually good. Therapeutic measures include systemic antibiotics (if the mare is ill), warm udder compresses, frequent stripping using oxytocin, and hydrotherapy.

1. The choice of **antibiotic therapy** should be made on the basis of milk culture and sensitivity. In the absence of this information, **broad-spectrum antibiotics** should be used.

2. **Bovine intramammary antibiotic infusions** may be used in cases of mild to subacute infections.

III. **OVINE AND CAPRINE MASTITIS.** Subacute and chronic forms of mastitis are most common, but acute types of the disease have the most clinical importance.

A. **S. aureus mastitis.** *S. aureus* is the most common cause of mastitis in sheep and goats.

  1. **Patient profile and history.** This disease is most common in animals on pasture and is identical with the bovine peracute form.

  2. **Clinical findings** include systemic signs: watery, bloody-brown secretion, udder edema, and gangrene.

  3. **Pathogenesis.** The organism usually gains access via teat injuries from suckling lambs or kids. The source of infection is contaminated pastures or bedding.

  4. **Therapeutic plan.** Treatment is unrewarding, and the mortality rate is high in affected animals. Methods of treatment are identical to those used for cows with peracute mastitis (i.e., fluids, broad-spectrum antibiotics, frequent stripping).

  5. **Prevention** consists of culling affected ewes and pasture rotation. Also, in areas where small ruminant dairying is of economic importance, vaccination with a staphylococcal bacterin and drying-off therapy with intramammary antibiotics may be of value.

B. *Mycoplasma* **mastitis** is known as **contagious agalactia.** This disease is seen in southern Europe and northern Africa. Causative agents include *M. agalactiae* and *M. mycoides* var *mycoides* in goats. Infection causes mastitis, arthritis, ophthalmitis, and abortion. The mortality rate is high (10%–30%), and the udder is permanently damaged.

C. *Pasteurella hemolytica* **mastitis**

  1. **Patient profile and history.** Mastitis caused by *P. hemolytica* is common in ewes, although it is sporadic in occurrence. The disease is peracute, gangrenous, and likely results from teat injuries from suckling lambs.

  2. **Clinical findings.** Glandular swelling and toxemia are cardinal signs. Hind limb lameness may be an early and diagnostic sign. The udder is initially hot, swollen, and painful but rapidly becomes cold, blue, and gangrenous. Death occurs due to toxemia. If the animal survives, the udder will slough. Pneumonia may occur concurrently in the lambs.

  3. **Pathogenesis.** Transmission is from infected soil or bedding but does not seem to be related to poor hygiene. There is evidence that some ewes may act as chronic carriers for *P. hemolytica*.

  4. **Therapeutic plan.** Broad-spectrum antibiotics may be an effective treatment if administered early.

  5. **Prevention.** Control procedures include culling recovered ewes, autogenous vaccination, and pasture rotation.

D. *S. agalactiae* **mastitis** in sheep and goats is similar to that in cows (see I B 1 a).

E. **Caprine arthritis encephalitis mastitis.** Udder changes are part of the viral disease syndrome known as caprine arthritis encephalitis (CAE) [see Chapter 13 III D]. CAE is associated with a hard udder developing soon after kidding. No milk can be expressed. Recovery is incomplete with this chronic disease syndrome.

IV. **PORCINE MASTITIS**

A. **Patient profile**

  1. Mastitis occurs in sows at **farrowing** and is most common in mature sows that are

raised in intensive husbandry situations (e.g., farrowing crates). The condition is sporadic, and although mortality in sows is low, piglet losses are high because of starvation and crushing.

2. **Risk factors** include increasing age, overnutrition, confinement housing, poor sanitation, and large litters.

B. **Clinical findings**

1. **Appearance**

   a. The **sow** may appear normal immediately post farrowing, but she soon loses interest in the piglets and will lie in sternal recumbency rather than adopting a nursing posture. The sow may appear nervous and agitated.

   b. The **piglets** are restless and squealing, and they wander about the pen and drink surface water. If allowed by the sow to suckle, piglets will nuzzle the udder but are unsuccessful in nursing.

2. **Systemic findings.** Sows are anorexic and feverish (39.5°C–41°C). The condition is commonly associated with constipation. Despite the historical name for this condition (mastitis-metritis-agalactiae or MMA), metritis is not a feature. The mucoid, white vaginal discharge, which is present in most sows post farrowing, is a normal occurrence. The glands are mottled red and yield very little milk on manual expression.

3. **Local findings.** Most of the mammary glands are swollen, painful, and hot.

C. **Etiology and pathogenesis**

1. **Etiology.** The majority of cases are caused by **coliform organisms** (e.g., *E. coli*, *K. pneumoniae*).

2. **Predisposing factors.** The likelihood of disease may include thyroid dysfunction, failure of prolactin release, or eclampsia.

3. **Pathogenesis. Endotoxin release** from the dying organisms in the udder is postulated to produce the clinical signs similar to acute coliform mastitis in dairy cattle (see I C 1).

D. **Diagnostic plan.** The condition is unique and diagnosed on clinical findings. Laboratory diagnostics are not commonly used in practice.

E. **Differential diagnosis.** First-litter gilts may present with glandular changes similar to those of mastitis, but the swelling is associated with agalactiae only, and the gilt is not systemically ill.

F. **Therapeutic plan**

1. **Sow.** Treatment consists of **systemic antibiotics, oxytocin,** and **corticosteroids.** Antibiotics should be chosen for their broad-spectrum activity, but in practice, even penicillin (20,000 IU/kg intramuscularly twice daily) has proved effective when combined with oxytocin (20–40 IU intramuscularly) and dexamethasone (20 mg intramuscularly) for 3 days.

2. **Piglets** may need **supplemental nutrition,** such as milk or electrolytes plus glucose, if treatment is delayed, but response of the sow is often rapid enough to allow the piglets to be successful at nursing if treatment is instituted early.

G. **Prevention** should center on cleanliness of the farrowing environment and of the sow before farrowing.

1. **Crates** should be disinfected between farrowings and the sow washed with soap and water as she is moved into the farrowing crate. Allow the sow ample time (1 week) to become used to her environment before farrowing, and do not institute major feeding changes.

2. **Prophylactic antibiotics** may be necessary and effective in herds with ongoing problems.

DIRECTIONS: Each of the numbered items or incomplete statements in this section is followed by answers or by completions of the statement. Select the ONE numbered answer or completion that is BEST in each case.

---

1. The majority of clinical mastitis cases in dairy cattle in North America are:

(1) acute or peracute in clinical expression.
(2) seen in the first 6 weeks of lactation.
(3) seen in heifers.
(4) caused by trauma.
(5) associated with low somatic cell counts (SCCs).

2. An accepted program of mastitis control and prevention includes:

(1) dry cow therapy for all cows at the end of lactation.
(2) parenteral antibiotics for all fresh cows.
(3) conversion to "automatic take-off" milking machines.
(4) rinsing the udder immediately before teat-cup placement.
(5) vaccination of cows with a *Escherichia coli* subunit bacterin at freshening.

3. Which one of the following terms fits the definition of a mastitis that causes a severe inflammation of the udder with a marked systemic reaction?

(1) Acute mastitis
(2) Chronic mastitis
(3) Subacute mastitis
(4) Peracute mastitis
(5) Subclinical mastitis

4. Which one of the following statements regarding *Streptococcus agalactiae* is true?

(1) It is an environmental pathogen that causes mastitis.
(2) It most often causes acute clinical mastitis.
(3) It does not invade glandular tissue.
(4) When established in a herd, it requires dry cow therapy for elimination.
(5) It has been eradicated from most dairy herds in North America.

5. Which one of the following statements regarding coliform mastitis is true?

(1) It is a contagious mastitis spread from cow to cow.
(2) It results from exotoxins elaborated by coliform bacteria.
(3) It produces signs of toxemia and gangrene of the mammary gland.
(4) It produces a thick, purulent udder secretion.
(5) It may resolve with little damage to the udder.

6. In animals with peracute staphylococcal mastitis, the affected mammary gland:

(1) is hard, painful, and discolored.
(2) secretes caseous, purulent material.
(3) rapidly infects the other three quarters.
(4) returns to full function after recovery.
(5) responds to stripping aided by oxytocin.

7. Which one of the following statements regarding peracute staphylococcal mastitis is true?

(1) It is best diagnosed by milk culture.
(2) It is the most common presentation of intramammary infection with *Staphylococcus aureus* .
(3) It is a disease of dry cows.
(4) It is best treated with intravenous antibiotics and electrolytes.
(5) It is usually spread from cow to cow through pulmonary secretions.

8. Which one of the following statements regarding summer mastitis is true?

(1) It is a disease of housed dairy cattle.
(2) It is most commonly transmitted by milking machines.
(3) It is a disease of dry cows caused by *Actinomyces pyogenes.*
(4) It is a subclinical mastitis of goats.
(5) It is seen most often in young mares.

9. Yeasts and algae are opportunistic pathogens that may cause mastitis. How are these pathogens similar?

(1) Both produce a severe systemic reaction.
(2) Neither has any effect on milk production.
(3) Both produce ropey clots in watery milk.
(4) Neither causes any external glandular reaction.
(5) Neither is responsive to antibiotic therapy.

10. Which one of the following statements regarding equine mastitis is true?

(1) It should be treated with frequent stripping of the affected glands.
(2) It is a common disease.
(3) It is caused most commonly by *Streptococcus equi* .
(4) It causes little observable udder change.
(5) It most commonly causes a thick, purulent glandular discharge.

11. Which one of the following statements regarding *Pasteurella hemolytica* mastitis is true?

(1) It is the most common cause of mastitis in sheep and goats.
(2) It is transmitted from lambs to ewes through suckling and teat injuries.
(3) It is known as contagious agalactiae.
(4) It produces a chronic, subacute mastitis.
(5) It is a federally reportable disease.

12. Which one of the following statements regarding mastitis in sows is true? Porcine mastitis

(1) is of little clinical importance.
(2) occurs most commonly at weaning.
(3) is treated with intramammary antibiotics.
(4) is similar in many respects to coliform mastitis of cattle.
(5) occurs concurrently with metritis.

ANSWERS AND EXPLANATIONS

1. The answer is 2 [I A 2 a]. Most cases of clinical mastitis are seen in multiparous cows early in lactation. Subclinical mastitis is of greatest prevalence, but of the clinical presentations, the order of occurrence (greatest to least) is subacute, acute, peracute. Mastitis is almost invariably caused by pathogenic bacteria and is associated with high cell counts in the milk of affected cows.

2. The answer is 1 [I A 4, 5]. Blanket dry cow therapy is recommended to treat pathogens causing clinical and subclinical mastitis (e.g., *Staphylococcus aureus*). Also, dry cow therapy reduces the risk of introducing new infections during a susceptible period of the mammary gland. Treatment of fresh cows with antibiotics is not recommended for control of mastitis. Automatic take-off milking machines afford no better control of mastitis than use of any regularly maintained, properly functioning milking system. Cows' udders should be dry before placement of teat cups to limit bacterial spread from contaminated teat ends. There are some vaccines that have proven efficacious in the prevention and control of mastitis, but an *Escherichia coli* subunit bacterin should be administered in three doses (two at and during the dry period) to allow adequate immunity to develop.

3. The answer is 4 [I A 1]. Peracute mastitis is a mastitis that causes a severe inflammation of the udder with a marked systemic reaction.

4. The answer is 3 [I B 1 a (3) (b) (ii)]. *Streptococcus agalactiae* does not invade glandular tissue, but through the effects of the lactic acid that it produces, it does produce epithelial destruction, resulting in lobular fibrosis and glandular atrophy. It is an obligate, contagious pathogen of the bovine udder and is most often expressed clinically as a subacute mastitis. It is still a relatively common mastitis pathogen (second only to *Staphylococcus aureus*) but can be eradicated through lactational therapy and strict hygienic and control measures.

5. The answer is 5 [I C 1 c]. This environmental mastitis results from contamination of the teat end by feces and contaminated bedding. The teat has often suffered damage that al-

lows entry of the organism. The udder becomes warm and swollen, but not gangrenous, and secretes a thin, watery fluid. There is little quarter damage, and most of the systemic disease is caused by endotoxins (cell-wall lipopolysaccharides) released as bacteria die.

6. The answer is 1 [I C 2 b (3)]. The gland is hard, painful, swollen, discolored, and gangrenous. It secretes a thin, brown fluid often accompanied by gas. A single gland is usually affected, and infection remains limited to that gland. Because of the necrotizing effects of the *Staphylococcus* toxins, the affected gland does not return to function even if the cow survives. Stripping is a recommended therapy, but the cow does not respond to oxytocin because of the morphologic changes induced by the toxins on the glandular tissue of the udder.

7. The answer is 4 [I C 2 g]. The peracute nature of the disease demands a diagnosis be made based on clinical signs so that treatment can be instituted promptly. It requires vigorous treatment with intravenous fluids (balanced electrolytes) and antibiotics. It is a sporadic disease of lactating cows, with the most common manifestations of *S. aureus* mastitis appearing as subclinical and then subacute mastitis. The organism is transmitted via fomites (e.g., milking machines), with the source often being mastitic glands of other cows in the herd.

8. The answer is 3 [I C 4 c]. *Actinomyces pyogenes* mastitis (summer mastitis) is a disease of dry cows in herds raised extensively (i.e., on pastures with limited observation). The organism is transmitted by flies, so fly control and hygiene are important methods of prevention.

9. The answer is 5 [I D 2, 3]. Neither organism is responsive to antibiotic therapy; in fact, antibiotics are contraindicated. There is little systemic reaction with either disease. Although algae usually produce large milk clots in watery milk, yeasts produce viscous, mucoid secretion. Both organisms cause a significant glandular reaction, and both cause a significant drop in milk production.

433

10. The answer is 1 [II D]. Mastitis is a relatively infrequent occurrence in mares. When it does occur, it produces glandular swelling and a thin, discolored discharge. Frequent stripping and systemic or intramammary therapy is recommended. *Streptococcus equi* causes "strangles," whereas *S. zooepidemicus* is a common isolate in cases of mare mastitis.

11. The answer is 2 [III C]. *Pasteurella hemolytica* is most often associated with pneumonia but may act as a cause of mastitis when transmitted from lambs to ewes through teat injuries from suckling. It is less common as a cause of mastitis than *Staphylococcus aureus* but produces an acute gangrenous mastitis.

Mycoplasma organisms produce the mastitis known as contagious agalactiae.

12. The answer is 4 [IV C 2]. The causative agents are most commonly coliforms, which produce signs of endotoxemia similar to that in dairy cattle. Mastitis is a clinically important disease in terms of the health of the sow and her piglets, who do not receive adequate nutrition during the mastitis episode. This disease most frequently occurs during early lactation and requires systemic therapy with antibiotics, corticosteroids, and oxytocin. Although metritis was once thought to be part of the mastitis complex, it is no longer considered to be involved.

Chapter 18

Neonatal Conditions, with Emphasis on the Equine Neonate

Jeanne Lofstedt

I. INTRODUCTION

A. Goals. Until recently, the focus of equine neonatology was on saving the critically ill foal. The emphasis has now shifted to evaluation of fetoplacental well-being during late gestation, with the goal being **early identification and appropriate intervention in the case of an abnormal pregnancy or periparturient event.** Owners, farm managers, and veterinarians should be cognizant of the findings that may indicate that the neonatal foal is at risk for future problems (Table 18-1) because early recognition and aggressive treatment of such foals generally improves their prognosis for survival and future athletic performance while at the same time decreasing overall treatment costs. If possible, high-risk mares should receive late-term fetal monitoring and be assured of an attended delivery with adequate resuscitation and stabilization of the foal after birth.

B. Recognition of high-risk pregnancies. Maternal conditions associated with a high-risk pregnancy are presented in Table 18-2. Mares experiencing problem pregnancies can usually be assigned to one of three categories:

1. Mares with histories of abnormal pregnancies, deliveries, or newborn foals

2. Mares at risk with the current pregnancy as the result of a systemic illness or a reproductive abnormality

3. Mares with no apparent risk factors that experience an abnormal periparturient event

C. Outcomes for foals admitted to neonatal intensive care units

1. **Short-term outcomes** have improved dramatically in the last two decades. Before 1980, fewer than 25% of foals presented to referral institutions for treatment were discharged alive. Foal units today quote overall success rates of greater than 70% for sick neonatal foals.
   a. Diseases associated with particularly favorable short-term survival rates include hypoxemic–ischemic encephalopathy [HIE, neonatal maladjustment syndrome (NMS)], uroperitoneum, infectious and noninfectious diarrhea, and noninfectious musculoskeletal diseases (e.g., angular limb deformities, flexural deformities).
   b. Diseases associated with poor short-term survival rates include established sepsis, sepsis accompanied by bacterial meningitis, septic arthritis, and septic osteomyelitis.

2. **Long-term outcomes.** One of the major problems in conducting long-term follow-up is finding an appropriate population for statistical comparison. Most often, comparisons are made with half or full siblings, or to the patient population at a referral hospital; however, neither of these populations are representative of the general population.
   a. Most of the common foal diseases seem to have little impact on the foal's ability to perform as an adult. Examples of diseases that appear to have little impact on future foal performance are HIE, severe bacterial lung disease, infectious and noninfectious diarrheas, uncomplicated umbilical diseases (e.g., omphalitis, patent urachus) and uroperitoneum.
   b. There are three disease categories that negatively impact the long-term performance of surviving foals:
      (1) Noninfectious orthopedic diseases

TABLE 18-1. Abnormalities Warranting Closer Evaluation of the Neonate

Abnormalities of Labor and Delivery	Abnormalities in the Neonate
Premature parturition or abnormally long gestation	Meconium-stained neonate
	Twins
Prolonged labor	Orphaned foal
Dystocia	Dysmaturity or prematurity
Induced labor	Delay or failure of colostrum ingestion
Cesarean section	Trauma (birth, dam, predators)
Premature placental separation	Adverse environmental conditions
Umbilical cord abnormality	Congenital anomalies
Placental abnormality (placentitis, edema, villous atrophy)	Weakness
	Failure to stand and nurse within 2–3 hours

  (2) Prematurity characterized by small stature and noninfectious orthopedic disorders (e.g., angular limb deformities, tarsal bone collapse)
  (3) Septic arthritis and osteomyelitis

II. PREMATURITY OR DYSMATURITY

A. Introduction

  1. **Terminology.** The literature abounds with terms for the neonatal foal with physical characteristics of immaturity: premature, immature, dysmature, intrauterine growth–retarded (IUGR), small for gestational age (SGA), ready or unready for birth, and viable or nonviable.

  2. **Criteria**
     a. **Gestational age.** Although most authors define a foal born before 320 days' gestation as premature (the mean gestation length of a Thoroughbred is 340 days), gestational age is only one of many criteria used to assess readiness for birth. Because gestation of mares is extremely variable, a 335-day fetus may be

TABLE 18-2. Maternal Conditions Associated With a High-Risk Pregnancy

Past History	Systemic Diseases	Reproductive Problems
Foals with NI, NMS, or congenital problems	Severe malnutrition	Severe endometrial fibrosis
Premature, septic, or hypoxic foals	Fever, endotoxemia, severe systemic infection	Hydrops allantois or hydrops amnii
Dystocia or premature placental separation	Severe anemia or hypoproteinemia	Purulent vaginal discharge
Foal rejection	Gastrointestinal crises	Prepubic tendon rupture or abdominal hernia
Exposure to infectious diseases known to cause abortion (e.g., EHV-1, EVA)	Laminitis	Poor colostral quality or premature lactation
	Musculoskeletal or CNS problems causing prolonged recumbency	Pelvic injuries

CNS = central nervous system; EHV-1 = equine herpesvirus-1; EVA = equine viral arteritis; NI = neonatal isoerythrolysis; NMS = neonatal maladjustment syndrome.

TABLE 18-3. Clinical Findings Suggestive of Immaturity

Gestation length less than 320 days

Weak suckle reflex, failure to nurse within 3 hours of birth

Failure to stand within 2 hours of birth

Low birth weight (less than 45 kg in Thoroughbreds or less than 10% of the dam's weight in other breeds)

Short, silky haircoat

Pliant ears and soft lips

Bulging, prominent forehead and eyes (especially in equine twins and other growth-retarded newborn foals)

Generalized weakness ("floppiness")

Increased passive range of motion of limbs

Marked flexor tendon laxity in the rear limbs

Hypothermia and difficulty thermoregulating

Intolerance to enteral feeding (abdominal pain)

Progressive tachypnea after birth with evidence of respiratory distress

Poor ossification of cuboidal bones in the carpi and tarsi

completely unprepared for birth if its normal gestational length was intended to be 365 days.

b. **Endocrine maturation**

(1) **Normal physiology.** The fetal pituitary–adrenal axis controls the final maturation of various organ systems, including the pulmonary system.

(a) **Cortisol.** The fetal adrenal gland is poorly responsive to adrenocorticotropic hormone (ACTH) throughout most of pregnancy, but in the last 3–5 days of gestation, its sensitivity changes, resulting in a significant increase in fetal cortisol 24–48 hours before birth. This cortisol surge causes maturation of the hematopoietic system, resulting in a total white blood cell (WBC) count of more than 5000 cells/μL in the healthy term foal immediately after birth.

(b) **Thyroid hormone.** The triiodothyronine (T_3) concentration in the healthy term foal is 10–20 times that of an adult horse. Thyroid hormone in the neonatal foal is required for thermogenesis, skeletal maturation, and may act synergistically with cortisol to cause normal lung maturation.

(2) **"Unready for birth" foals.** Foals removed suddenly from the uterus before final endocrine maturation has taken place (e.g., by a poorly timed cesarean section) have low serum concentrations of cortisol and thyroid hormone and, when challenged with exogenous ACTH, do not respond with appropriate increases of cortisol. They have incomplete body system maturation and generally adjust poorly to extrauterine life.

(3) **"Immature but ready for birth" foals.** Maturation is often hastened in foals exposed to chronic *in utero* stress (e.g., chronic placentitis) during gestation. Despite having characteristics of physical immaturity, foals stressed *in utero* have adequate pulmonary and hematologic function and cope well with extrauterine life.

B. **Clinical findings** are summarized in Table 18-3.

C. **Complications**

1. **Respiratory difficulties** are attributed to a number of factors, including dependent lung atelectasis caused by lung and chest wall immaturity, *in utero*–acquired pneumonia, and lack of mature surfactant.

2. Abnormal glucose homeostasis. Premature foals have a significantly lower blood glucose concentration than full-term foals and are less able to maintain stable glucose concentrations in the first 2 hours postpartum. Low hepatic glycogen stores, immature glycogenolytic mechanisms, and a blunted insulin response all contribute to abnormal glucose homeostasis in the premature newborn.

3. Angular limb deformities. Because ossification of the cartilaginous cuboidal bone precursors to the carpal and tarsal bones occurs in the last 2–3 weeks of gestation, the premature or dysmature foal that ambulates may experience collapse of these bones, which may in turn result in angular limb deformities.

4. Corneal ulceration. Entropion, leading to corneal irritation and ulceration, is a common complication experienced by the premature or immature foal.

5. Patent urachus. In the fetus, the urachus drains urine from the bladder into the allantoic sac. In late gestation, some urine is diverted to the amniotic sac via the urethra, and at the time of delivery (immediately after umbilical cord rupture), the abdominal musculature around the umbilicus contracts, resulting in cessation of urine flow from the urachus. Failure for this closure to occur in the immediate postpartum period leads to the development of a congenital patent urachus.

D. **Therapeutic plan.** Frequent and comprehensive clinical and laboratory evaluation of all body systems is required to detect and address deterioration in neurologic status, cardiorespiratory function, and renal function of the immature neonatal foal. **General supportive care** is necessary.

1. Prevention of decubital ulcers and scalding
   a. An air mattress or cushions help prevent decubital ulcers. A foal that is unable to maintain sternal recumbency or stand should have an attendant present to keep it in sternal recumbency, turn it from side-to-side every 2 hours, and assist it in standing as needed.
   b. Scalding by feces and urine can be minimized by covering the bedding with absorbent pads.

2. Prevention of nosocomial infection. Foals should be separated from the adult horse population and high-traffic areas, and strict hygiene and cleanliness should be maintained in the foal ward to decrease the risk of nosocomial infections.

3. Prevention of hypothermia. The ambient temperature can be increased using radiant heat lamps, hot water pads, blankets, and warmed intravenous fluids.

4. Nutritional support. Premature or dysmature foals are often unable to suckle from the mare and have to be fed via a bottle, bucket, or nasogastric tube.
   a. **Frequency and amount.** It is important to remember that the healthy foal nurses as frequently as 7 times/hour and consumes 16%–28% of its body weight/day (155 ml/kg/day) in milk. Initially, the premature foal should receive 10% of its body weight in milk, divided into at least 12 feedings over 24 hours; if the foal tolerates this amount, the volume fed can be increased gradually until the foal receives 20%–25% of its body weight in milk. Unfortunately, many immature foals do not tolerate large volumes orally (i.e., they develop colic or diarrhea) and partial or total parenteral nutrition may have to be implemented.
   b. **Methods**
      (1) **Bottle feeding.** A lamb nipple can be used to bottle feed a foal. A foal with a weak suckle reflex should never be bottle fed because aspiration pneumonia and malnutrition may ensue. Mare's milk is the optimal milk source. There are a number of commercially available mare milk replacers and many foals appear to thrive on goat milk. Hypoglycemic foals (i.e., those with a glucose concentration of less than 40 mg/dl) should receive intravenous dextrose (5%–10%) in addition to oral alimentation.
      (2) **Nasogastric intubation.** A small-diameter nasogastric tube is placed in the distal esophagus. The foal can nurse from the mare while the tube is in place.
      (3) **Bucket feeding.** Foals are easily taught to drink milk from a shallow pan or bucket. The foal should be encouraged to suckle a clean finger which is then gradually lowered into the bucket containing the milk.

    (4) Parenteral nutrition. Essentially, parenteral nutrition involves constant intravenous infusion of a hypertonic solution containing various concentrations of dextrose, amino acids, lipids, electrolytes, and vitamins.

      (a) Parenteral solutions should be mixed under a hood wearing sterile gloves and a mask to prevent contamination. They are generally administered via a nonthrombogenic jugular catheter and a dedicated line. Fluid administration rates are carefully controlled and fluid lines and hanging bags are changed daily.

      (b) Patients receiving parenteral nutrition should continue to receive small-volume enteral feeding if at all possible.

      (c) The patient should be monitored frequently to detect complications. Potential complications include hyperglycemia, hyperlipidemia, metabolic acidosis, hypokalemia, and infection at the catheter site.

5. Immunologic support. Failure of passive transfer (FPT) of colostral immunoglobulins (see IV) is a common occurrence in the premature or dysmature foal. Good-quality colostrum should be fed within 6 hours of birth, and passive transfer status should be assessed when the foal is 18–24 hours old. Plasma should be transfused if the immunoglobulin G (IgG) concentration is less than 800 mg/dl.

6. Antimicrobial treatment. Many premature births are associated with infections acquired *in utero*. Broad-spectrum bactericidal antimicrobials should be used prophylactically in all premature foals (see V E 2).

7. Cardiovascular support
    a. Dehydration and hemoconcentration. Foals should be treated intravenously with an isotonic balanced electrolyte solution (e.g., lactated Ringer's solution, 40–60 ml/kg/day).
    b. Acidemia is defined as a blood pH of less than 7.3. Foals with acidemia should be adequately ventilated and receive 1.3% (isotonic) sodium bicarbonate intravenously.

8. Respiratory support. Most immature foals have some pulmonary dysfunction.
    a. Atelectasis (as a result of lung and chest wall immaturity) can often be managed by simply maintaining the foal in sternal recumbency, turning it frequently, and encouraging lung expansion through stimulating deep breathing or coughing.
    b. Hypoxia is defined as an arterial oxygen tension (Pao_2) of less than 70 mm Hg with a normal arterial carbon dioxide tension ($Paco_2$). Hypoxic foals often benefit from humidified oxygen administered via face mask or nasal insufflation at a rate of 5–10 L/min.
    c. Hypercapnia is defined as a Pao_2 of less than 65 mm Hg and a $Paco_2$ of greater than 65 mm Hg. Hypercapnic foals benefit from assisted or controlled ventilation via orotracheal or nasotracheal intubation.
    d. Lack of surfactant. Surfactant replacement has been utilized in an attempt to increase survivability of the premature foal with immature lung surfactant. There are anecdotal reports that this treatment modality is beneficial, but large-scale controlled studies have not been undertaken.

9. Musculoskeletal support
    a. Foals with radiographic evidence of **incomplete carpal and tarsal bone ossification** should be housed in a small stall to restrict exercise.
    b. Excessive flexor tendon laxity can be managed with physical therapy and the application of heel extensions to the bottom of the foot. Support wraps should be light and used sparingly because they may exacerbate tendon laxity.

10. Treatment of other complications
    a. Corneal ulcer. Affected foals should be treated with topical antibiotics, mydriatics, and vertical mattress sutures to evert the eyelid.
    b. Patent urachus. Treatment includes chemical cautery or surgical excision (see VI B 4).
    c. Adrenal insufficiency. Treatment is controversial and reserved for those foals with laboratory evidence of adrenocortical insufficiency.

      (1) Physiologic doses of glucocorticoids (e.g., 50 mg of hydrocortisone succinate) have been used.

      (2) Administration of long-acting synthetic ACTH at a total intramuscular dose of 0.4 mg, followed by a 0.2-mg dose 6 and 12 hours later, has been advocated as well.

E. **Prognosis.** The periparturient history, laboratory testing, and observation of clinical progression over the first 2 days can be used to develop a prognosis for the premature or immature foal.

1. **Periparturient history**

    a. Foals delivered early and abruptly by induction of parturition, cesarean section, or because of severe systemic maternal illness in the mare generally have a poor prognosis. They do not experience the endocrinologic events required for normal maturation, are "unready for birth," and the prognosis for survival is poor (survival rate of 20%–25%).

    b. Foals delivered naturally, but prematurely, by a healthy mare usually have a fair prognosis. With appropriate supportive care, survival rates as high as 70% are possible. Close inspection of the placenta from these deliveries may reveal villous atrophy or placentitis. Placental pathology is thought to interfere with uteroplacental blood flow, imposing chronic *in utero* stress, maturation of the fetal pituitary–adrenal axis, and "readiness for birth."

2. **Laboratory testing** can be used to assess readiness for birth.

    a. Assessment of electrolyte concentrations in prepartum mammary secretions. The electrolyte concentrations in prepartum mammary secretions change dramatically shortly before the mare foals down. A **calcium concentration greater than 40 mg/dl** is a reasonable indicator of readiness for birth and can be used to determine if the time is appropriate for elective induction or a cesarean section.

      (1) At term, **calcium** and **potassium** concentrations in mammary secretions increase to greater than or equal to 40 mg/dl and 35 mEq/L, respectively, whereas the **sodium** concentration decreases to less than or equal to 30 mEq/L.

      (2) Before 310 days' gestation, elevated milk calcium levels indicate placental pathology, not fetal maturity. Changes in milk sodium and potassium concentrations do not occur in mares with placentitis; therefore, **fetal maturation is most accurately assessed by measuring concentrations of all three electrolytes.**

    b. Routine laboratory testing

      (1) Complete blood count (CBC)

        (a) Foals with a **total WBC count** of greater than 5000 cells/μL on day 1 of life (or a low WBC count on day 1 that increases to greater than 5000 cells/μL on day 2 or 3) generally have a favorable prognosis.

        (b) Foals with a **neutrophil–lymphocyte ratio** that is greater than 2 on day 1, or low on day 1, but increases to greater than 2 on day 2 or 3, have a fair prognosis.

        (c) Persistent leukopenia and **neutropenia** usually indicate that the foal is endocrinologically immature and will be a nonsurvivor in the postnatal period.

      (2) Fibrinogen concentration. A plasma fibrinogen concentration that exceeds 400 mg/dl at birth is generally associated with a favorable prognosis. It suggests that an *in utero* infection caused the premature delivery. As mentioned previously, foals stressed *in utero* generally adjust better in the early neonatal period.

      (3) Blood gas analysis. Nonviable premature foals usually have a metabolic acidosis with a blood pH persistently less than 7.3.

    c. Endocrinologic testing

      (1) Serum cortisol. A plasma cortisol concentration of 120–140 mg/ml within 2 hours of birth indicates readiness for birth, whereas a value of less than 30 mg/ml suggests poor adrenal function and an unfavorable prognosis.

(2) **ACTH response test.** Foals that are endocrinologically mature respond with a two-fold increase in plasma cortisol and a widening of the neutrophil–lymphocyte ratio in response to the administration of short-acting exogenous ACTH (0.125 mg, intramuscularly).

3. **Careful assessment of clinical progression** over the first 2 days of the immature foal's life can also be used to formulate a prognosis:
   a. In "unready for birth" foals, the first 12–18 hours after resuscitation are deceptively uneventful. However, progressive deterioration in neurologic function and an inability to maintain homeostasis soon develop. Death is certain without aggressive intensive care and the prognosis is poor. Some of the abnormalities exhibited by these foals are:
      (1) Systemic weakness, depression, and seizures
      (2) Intolerance to enteral feeding, resulting in abdominal distention, colic, and enterogastric reflux
      (3) Declining pulse quality, subcutaneous edema, and oliguria
      (4) Respiratory distress leading to respiratory acidosis
   b. A "ready for birth" foal that is born prematurely following exposure to chronic *in utero* stress usually progresses as follows:
      (1) The foal is weak initially and requires assistance to stand.
      (2) The foal's suckle reflex and appetite are reduced and it must receive milk and colostrum via a nasogastric tube.
      (3) The foal has difficulty regulating its blood glucose level and body temperature.
      (4) After 24 hours of supportive care, the foal gains strength, its mentation improves, and its appetite for milk often exceeds that of the normal foal.

4. **Other factors influencing outcome** include the **actual birth weight of the foal** (generally, the lower the birth weight, the poorer the prognosis), the **presence of other complicating factors in the perinatal period** (e.g., *in utero*–acquired infection or peripartum asphyxia), and the **resources available for treatment.**

III. ACUTE PERINATAL ASPHYXIA

A. Introduction

1. **Asphyxia** is defined as **decreased tissue oxygenation** and can be caused by **hypoxemia** (decreased blood oxygen content) or **ischemia** (decreased blood flow).

2. Acute perinatal asphyxia is a **multisystemic disease,** affecting the nervous, cardiovascular, gastrointestinal, and renal systems of the neonate. Because central nervous system (CNS) signs are noticed first and are the most overt, perinatal asphyxia initially was not recognized for the multisystemic disease that it really is. A variety of terms were used to describe the disease in affected foals based on the most salient neurologic deficits (e.g., barkers, wanderers, dummies, convulsives). In 1968, the term **"neonatal maladjustment syndrome"** (NMS) was coined to describe foals exhibiting gross behavioral disturbances and failure to adapt in the perinatal period. Ischemic–hypoxemic brain damage was suspected to be the cause of NMS.

B. Clinical findings. Perinatal asphyxia produces an array of clinical abnormalities. The clinical picture is influenced by the maturity of the foal at birth and the severity and duration of the asphyxial episode. Neurologic signs predominate; however, careful assessment usually reveals involvement of other organ systems.

1. **Neurologic signs**
   a. Affected foals often appear outwardly normal for the first 12–24 hours. Loss of dam recognition, loss of suckle reflex, aimless wandering, and head pressing are the first signs observed in asphyxiated neonatal foals.

b. Severely affected foals may exhibit bruxism; abnormal vocalization; hyperexcitability; extensor spasms of the limbs, neck, and tail; and convulsions alternating with a semicomatose unresponsive state. Dysphagia, central blindness, anisocoria, nystagmus, head tilt, proprioceptive deficits, and spasticity have also been reported.

2. Respiratory signs. Foals with respiratory dysfunction exhibit varying degrees of tachypnea and dyspnea. Erratic, abnormal breathing patterns are also observed with some frequency.

3. Cardiovascular signs. Dysfunction may manifest as tachycardia, signs of hypotension, or murmurs associated with valvular insufficiency.

4. Renal signs include oliguria and peripheral edema if fluid therapy is not adjusted for decreased urine output.

5. Gastrointestinal signs are ileus, poor feeding, colic, lethargy, abdominal distention, delayed gastric emptying, gastric reflux, and diarrhea. Reflux fluid and feces often test positive for occult blood. Colic, hemorrhagic diarrhea, and sudden death have been reported in severe cases.

C. **Etiology and pathophysiology**

1. Etiology. A variety of fetal and maternal conditions are associated with perinatal asphyxia.
   a. Fetal factors include **twinning, meconium aspiration, sepsis, prematurity or dysmaturity**, and **severe anemia**.
   b. Maternal factors include **conditions that cause hypotension or impaired tissue oxygenation** (e.g., endotoxemia, anemia, hemorrhagic shock), **maternal surgery** or **cesarean section**, and **placental abnormalities** (e.g., those caused by ingestion of endophyte-infested fescue during pregnancy, placental infection, or premature placental separation).

2. Pathophysiology
   a. Shunting. Initially, the fetus responds to asphyxia by shunting blood away from nonvital organs (e.g., the gut, kidneys, bone, muscle, and skin) to vital organs (e.g., the brain, heart, and adrenal gland).
      (1) Mild asphyxia causes a mild decrease in heart rate and a slight increase in blood pressure, but little change in cardiac output.
      (2) With severe asphyxia, the heart rate, cardiac output, and blood pressure decrease as oxidative phosphorylation fails and energy reserves in cardiac muscle are depleted.
   b. Metabolic derangements. Without sufficient energy, cellular ion pumps in various body tissues eventually fail, resulting in intracellular accumulation of sodium, chloride, water, and calcium and extracellular accumulation of excitatory neurotransmitters in the brain (e.g., glutamate).
      (1) Glutamate accumulation in the brain after an ischemic event apparently causes excessive stimulation of cell surface receptors, eventually resulting in neuronal death.
      (2) Intracellular free calcium accumulation causes cell death in several ways, including activation of enzyme systems that attack the structural integrity of the cell and impairment of mitochondrial function.
      (3) Oxygen free radicals are generated during the reperfusion phase that follows a hypoxemic–ischemic insult. Oxygen free radicals cause membrane fragmentation by attacking the lipids in cell membranes and are in part responsible for the increased capillary permeability, edema formation, and tissue damage that occur following restoration of blood flow to previously ischemic tissues.
   c. Sequelae
      (1) **Neurologic effects.** In the brain, asphyxia can lead to HIE accompanied by edema, necrosis, and hemorrhage.
      (2) **Cardiac effects.** The effects of perinatal asphyxia on myocardial function can be profound. Decreased myocardial contractility and congestive heart failure

(CHF) are common sequelae and may be associated with infarcts in myocardial and papillary muscles. The systemic hypotension caused by these lesions further contributes to tissue hypoxia, development of metabolic acidosis, and decreased renal perfusion in the asphyxiated neonate.

(3) **Pulmonary effects.** The neonatal pulmonary system responds to hypoxemia and acidosis by reflex vasoconstriction, which, in turn, causes an increase in pulmonary vascular resistance, pulmonary hypertension, and increased right atrial pressure.

    (a) If pulmonary arterial pressure exceeds systemic pressure, right-to-left flow through the ductus arteriosis and foramen ovale may result in reestablishment of persistent fetal circulation characterized by severe hypoxemia unresponsive to oxygen therapy.

    (b) Decreased pulmonary blood flow may cause decreased delivery of lipid precursors to the lung, resulting in decreased surfactant production.

    (c) Meconium aspiration, a common sequela of birth asphyxia, usually initiates a chemical pneumonitis that can further compromise pulmonary function.

    (d) Perinatal asphyxia may decrease the responsiveness of respiratory centers in the brain, causing periods of apnea or abnormal breathing.

(4) **Renal effects.** Redistribution of blood flow away from the kidneys causes decreased renal perfusion and, frequently, acute renal tubular necrosis and oliguria.

(5) **Gastrointestinal effects.** Reduced intestinal blood flow during an asphyxial episode causes variable degrees of bowel ischemia.

    (a) Mild signs of gastrointestinal dysfunction are commonly exhibited by asphyxiated foals, including meconium impactions and intolerance to enteral feeding manifested as abdominal distention, colic, diarrhea, or delayed gastric emptying.

    (b) Severe ischemia causes total loss of bowel integrity, resulting in overwhelming bacteremia and septic shock.

(6) **Other effects.** Severe asphyxia may lead to anoxic liver damage, necrosis and dysfunction of endocrine organs, and coagulopathy. To date, these disorders have not been described in asphyxiated equine neonates.

D. Diagnostic plan

1. **Physical examination.** An in-depth physical examination is indicated for all recumbent foals to:
   a. Provide baseline information against which foal progress can be compared
   b. Aid in the identification of subtle but important abnormalities that may be overshadowed by grossly obvious clinical signs, such as seizures

2. **Baseline clinicopathologic information should be gathered.** A CBC and blood culture should be ordered, and passive transfer status should be assessed. A sepsis score (see V D 3) should be calculated.

3. **Specific assessments**
   a. **Neurologic assessment.** Neurologic signs caused by HIE need to be distinguished from those caused by meningitis, hypoglycemia, or congenital anomalies.
       (1) **Cerebrospinal fluid analysis** allows differentiation of meningitis and HIE (meningitis is characterized by an increased leukocyte count and protein concentration).
       (2) **Imaging techniques,** such as **computed tomography (CT)** and **magnetic resonance imaging (MRI),** are being used with increasing frequency to document location, severity, and progression of brain injury in asphyxiated large animal neonates.
   b. **Respiratory assessment**
       (1) **Arterial blood gas analysis** usually reveals hypoxemia, hypercarbia, and acidemia. These are typical findings in a foal with hypoventilation; affected foals usually respond dramatically to nasal oxygen insufflation. In contrast, foals with persistent fetal circulation do not respond to inspired oxygen.

      (2) Thoracic radiography is always indicated for foals with birth asphyxia.

        (a) In cases of pulmonary hypertension, thoracic radiographs may reveal pulmonary hypoperfusion (clear lung fields with decreased pulmonary vascular markings).

        (b) Surfactant deficiency results in diffuse lung atelectasis and a diffuse reticulogranular radiographic appearance with air bronchograms.

        (c) Meconium aspiration results in patchy perihilar infiltrates, focal areas of atelectasis, and hyperaeration.

  c. Cardiovascular assessment

      (1) Electrocardiography and **echocardiography** may be indicated in foals with murmurs or cardiac dysrhythmias. Echocardiography may reveal persistent fetal circulation.

      (2) Determination of cardiac isoenzyme activities is necessary to detect myocardial necrosis.

  d. Renal assessment. Renal function is assessed by measuring **urine output,** performing a **urinalysis,** and assessing the results of a **biochemistry profile.** Typical findings include oliguria (a urine output of less than 2 ml/kg/hr), azotemia, and electrolyte disturbances such as hypocalcemia, hyponatremia, hypochloremia, and hyperkalemia.

  e. Gastrointestinal assessment. Gastrointestinal dysfunction is primarily diagnosed based on clinical signs. The most severe form of gastrointestinal dysfunction associated with birth asphyxia, necrotizing enterocolitis (NEC), can be diagnosed radiographically based on the presence of submucosal gas accumulation in the bowel wall (pneumatosis intestinalis).

E. **Differential diagnoses.** Conditions such as neonatal sepsis, meconium aspiration, prematurity, and hypoglycemia can mimic perinatal asphyxia. Perinatal asphyxia can also be a complicating factor in many of these conditions.

F. **Therapeutic plan.** Therapeutic goals are numerous and address the multiple organ failure that is present.

1. Treatment of CNS dysfunction includes seizure control, nursing care to prevent trauma, fluid therapy, nutritional support, and control of cerebral edema.

  a. Seizure control

      (1) Diazepam (0.11–0.44 mg/kg intravenously) has a rapid onset of action and is used for initial seizure control.

      (2) Pentobarbital (2–10 mg/kg intravenously every 12 hours) can be used to manage severe or repeated seizures. Serum concentrations of pentobarbital should be monitored.

      (3) Xylazine and acepromazine should not be used to control seizures. Xylazine causes transient hypertension and may exacerbate cerebral hemorrhage, and acepromazine lowers the seizure threshold.

  b. Control of cerebral edema. Cerebral edema occurs in some asphyxiated foals and is treated with **dimethylsulfoxide (DMSO;** 0.5–1.0 g/kg administered over 1–2 hours as a 10%–20% solution) and/or **mannitol,** an osmotic diuretic (0.25–1.0 g/kg given as a 20% solution slowly over 1–2 hours). Mannitol may exacerbate CNS hemorrhage; therefore, it should be used with extreme caution in asphyxiated neonates.

  c. Prevention of trauma. Leg wraps, a padded helmet, and a padded stall may be required to protect the asphyxiated neonate from self trauma.

2. Treatment of respiratory dysfunction includes **maintenance of oxygenation and ventilation** of the patient.

  a. Treatment of hypoxia. Hypoxia is usually corrected by administering **humidified oxygen** (3–10 L/min) **via nasal insufflation** and keeping the foal in **sternal recumbency.**

  b. Treatment of hypercapnia. Respiratory center depression can cause hypercapnia, characterized by a Pao_2 of less than 65 mm Hg and a $Paco_2$ greater than 65 mm Hg.

(1) **Positive-pressure ventilation** may be required for treatment of recurrent apnea, severe respiratory center depression, or diffuse pulmonary atelectasis caused by surfactant deficiency.

(2) If respiratory center depression is causing inappropriate control of breathing, **methylzanthines** (e.g., theophylline or caffeine) can be used to stimulate respiratory neuronal activity and increase responsiveness to hypercapnia.

    (a) The recommended dose of caffeine is a loading dose of 10 mg/kg and a maintenance dose of 2.5 mg/kg/day.

    (b) Methylxanthines have a narrow therapeutic range and they should be discontinued if signs of toxicity are noted (e.g., agitation, seizures, tachycardia, hypotension, colic, diarrhea).

  c. **Treatment of pulmonary atelectasis.** Intratracheal surfactant administration has been recommended by some authors.

3. **Treatment of cardiac dysfunction** revolves around judicious use of intravenous fluids (see III F 6 a) and the administration of inotropes.

  a. **Dopamine** or **dobutamine** (infused at a rate of 2–10 μg/kg/min) may be used to increase cardiac output and improve tissue perfusion.

  b. **Diuretics** (e.g., **furosemide**) may be used to treat the edema associated with cardiac failure.

  c. **Digoxin** (0.02–0.035 mg/kg orally every 24 hours) should be used if there is evidence of cardiac failure.

4. **Treatment of renal dysfunction** involves judicious use of intravenous fluids, diuretics, and administration of low doses of dopamine to stimulate dopaminergic receptors. Fluid input and urine output should be carefully monitored to avoid overhydration.

  a. **Dopamine infusions** (2–4 μg/kg/min) have been advocated to improve renal blood flow and urine output.

  b. **Diuretics.** Serum electrolyte concentrations should be carefully monitored during diuretic therapy.

    (1) **Furosemide infusions** of 0.25–2.0 μg/kg/min have been used successfully to treat oliguric renal failure in asphyxiated foals. Furosemide acts synergistically with dopamine to produce renal vasodilation and diuresis.

    (2) **Mannitol therapy** may be added if oliguria persists after dopamine and furosemide administration.

  c. **Dobutamine therapy** should be instituted if cardiac dysfunction appears to be causing systemic hypotension and renal hypoperfusion.

5. **Treatment of gastrointestinal dysfunction.** Gastrointestinal dysfunction is treated with decompression, the use of prokinetic agents, or both.

  a. **Nasogastric decompression.** If the foal has delayed gastric emptying and decreased intestinal motility, nasogastric decompression can be used to relieve fluid and gas accumulation. Severe, persistent large bowel distention may respond to **percutaneous trocarization** using sterile technique and a 16- or 18-gauge catheter.

  b. **Prokinetic agents,** such as **metoclopramide** (0.25–0.3 mg/kg by intravenous infusion) or **erythromycin** (5–10 mg/kg orally or by intravenous infusion) may improve gastric emptying and small intestinal motility.

6. **General supportive care**

  a. **Fluid therapy.** Polyionic isotonic fluids should be used to correct dehydration and expand blood volume. To avoid overhydration, asphyxiated foals should be carefully monitored using clinical assessment of hydration and monitoring of body weight changes and urine output. Normal urine output is 6–7 ml/kg/hr; measures should be introduced to improve urine output if it decreases to less than 2 ml/kg/hr.

    (1) Patients with metabolic acidosis should receive supplemental bicarbonate based on results of blood gas analysis. Caution should be exercised when bicarbonate is given to foals with severe respiratory compromise, because in

these foals, bicarbonate can worsen the acidosis because of carbon dioxide retention.

(2) Specific electrolyte abnormalities should also be corrected with fluid therapy.

b. Immunologic support. The plasma immunoglobulin concentration should be measured and colostrum or plasma administered if the foal's serum IgG levels are less than 800 mg/dl.

c. Nutritional support
(1) Nasogastric tube. Foals that are unable to nurse from the mare or a bottle should be tube fed using the recommendations given in II D 4.
(2) Parenteral nutrition. If gut function is questionable, parenteral nutrition should be employed. To minimize the risk of NEC, foals that have suffered severe asphyxia complicated by hypotension or hypothermia should not receive any enteral feeds until their vital signs are stable.
(3) Enteral feeding should be initiated gradually and mare's colostrum or milk should be fed preferentially.

d. Antibiotic therapy. Broad-spectrum bactericidal antimicrobial therapy should be given to all asphyxiated foals because sepsis commonly accompanies ischemic bowel damage.

e. Antiulcer medication (e.g., ranitidine, sucralfate) is recommended for asphyxiated foals because gastric ulceration is a common complication.

G. Prognosis

1. The prognosis is usually good for a term foal delivered without obvious complications, particularly if the foal was able to stand for period of time after delivery and had a normal immunoglobulin concentration at 18–24 hours of age. Approximately 75% of foals with good prognostic signs recover with intensive nursing care. In survivors, the clinical signs usually stabilize at 48–72 hours and their condition is significantly improved by 72–96 hours of age. Full recovery can take as long as 2 weeks.

2. The following findings are associated with a poor prognosis:
a. Concurrent septicemia
b. Failure to show any improvement in neurologic function by 5 days of life
c. A persistent comatose state or severe, recurrent seizures

3. Rare long-term neurologic sequelae may include unusually docile behavior as an adult, prolonged vision impairment, residual spasticity, or recurrent seizures.

IV. FAILURE OF PASSIVE TRANSFER (FPT)

A. Introduction

1. Incidence. FPT (i.e., inadequate transfer of colostral immunoglobulin) is widespread in both equine and bovine neonates, with reported prevalences of 2.9%–25% and 15%–68%, respectively. FPT also occurs in lambs, goat kids, and piglets, but the exact prevalences are unknown.

2. Neonatal immunity, colostrum production, and absorption of immunoglobulin. Neonates are capable of mounting an immune response at birth, but it is a primary response characterized by a prolonged lag period and production of low concentrations of antibody. Leukocytes of newborn animals exhibit reduced phagocytic and bactericidal activity as a result of fetal glucocorticoid production shortly before birth. Furthermore, the neonate's serum is deficient in some complement components, resulting in poor opsonic activity. Placental transfer of immunoglobulin does not occur to any extent in neonatal ungulates; therefore, they rely on colostral transfer of immunoglobulin to protect them against infectious disease early in the neonatal period. **Colostrum** is composed of immunoglobulins, immunologically active cellular components (lymphocytes, macrophages, polymorphonuclear cells) and nonspecific immune factors (lactoferrin, lysozyme, and complement).

a. **Colostral immunoglobulin secretion** occurs primarily via receptor-associated selective uptake of IgG from the maternal blood stream, transcellular transport, and release into lacteal secretions via the mammary epithelium. Colostral secretion takes place during the last 2–4 weeks of gestation and is regulated by hormonal changes that take place in late gestation.

b. **Colostral absorption.** Because of the low proteolytic activity in the digestive tract of newborns and the presence of trypsin inhibitors in the colostrum, colostral proteins are not degraded as a food source. Instead, they reach the small intestine, where the colostral immunoglobulins and other macromolecules are actively absorbed by specialized enterocytes through the process of pinocytosis.

   (1) The "window" of gut absorptive capacity for macromolecules is narrow, lasting from birth to 18–24 hours of age with a significant decline after 6 hours of age. Reduced absorptive capacity after 6 hours is attributed to shedding of the specialized enterocytes and replacement by mature cells incapable of pinocytosis.

   (2) Peak serum immunoglobulin concentrations are achieved 12–24 hours after birth; after this period, passively acquired antibody concentrations decline through normal catabolic processes.

3. **General causes and consequences**

   a. **Causes.** FPT usually is attributed to one of three factors:

      (1) **Poor colostral quality or quantity** (i.e., the failure of the dam to produce colostrum in sufficient amounts or of sufficient quality)

      (2) **Ingestion failure** (i.e., the failure of the neonate to ingest sufficient amounts of colostrum early in the neonatal period)

      (3) **Absorption failure** (i.e., failure of the neonate to absorb adequate amounts of colostrum from the gastrointestinal tract into the systemic circulation)

   b. **Consequences of FPT**

      (1) **Increased infectious disease morbidity and mortality.** FPT generally increases morbidity and mortality associated with infectious disease (e.g., septicemia, diarrhea, pneumonia) in cattle herds, and it is generally accepted that foals with FPT are at a higher risk of developing septicemia.

         (a) The consequences of FPT depend on the pathogen load in the environment and whether specific antibody to offending pathogen is present. Considerable confusion was created by one equine study where no association between FPT and morbidity/mortality was demonstrated in foals in the first 3 months of life. The results of this study were later attributed to a scrupulous environment and the fact that the mares were allowed time to adjust to the broodmare farm environment prior to foaling.

         (b) In herds with a high prevalence of septicemia, predisposing factors that should be considered in addition to FPT include unhygienic management practices, the presence of virulent pathogens, concurrent stress or disease, and lack of specific antibody.

      (2) **Increased duration of pathogen shedding.** FPT may increase the duration of pathogen shedding in calves with diarrhea.

      (3) **Decreased weight gain.** FPT has been shown to decrease weight gain of heifers up to 180 days of age.

      (4) **Starvation.** Because ovine colostrum supplies a considerable amount of energy, lambs that fail to ingest colostrum may starve to death rather than exhibit signs of septicemia.

      (5) **Decreased milk production.** FPT has been shown to affect milk production of heifers into their first lactation.

B. Etiology

1. **FPT in foals**

   a. **Poor colostral quality or quantity**

      (1) **Maternal age.** The foals of dams older than 15 years are at increased risk for FPT as a result of poor colostral quality.

      (2) **Leakage of colostrum (premature lactation)** results in decreased colostral IgG

concentration. Factors leading to premature lactation are poorly understood, but twinning, premature placental separation, and placentitis have been incriminated.

(3) Severe maternal illness and the **ingestion of endophyte-infested fescue** have been associated with decreased colostral volume, quality, or both.

(4) Premature foaling (either from natural causes or induction) can lead to colostrum of insufficient quantity, quality, or both, because time and hormonal preparation for colostrum production were inadequate.

   b. Ingestion failure

     (1) Foal rejection of the mare (e.g., as a result of maternal illness or poor mothering ability) results in delayed colostral ingestion.

     (2) Neonatal weakness or **musculoskeletal problems** (e.g., flexural deformities) can make it difficult for the foal to ambulate and ingest adequate amounts of colostrum within the appropriate time frame.

   c. Absorption failure. FPT is common in **premature foals,** even when they receive sufficient amounts of good-quality colostrum in the early postpartum period. Inefficient immunoglobulin absorption from the immature gastrointestinal tract, distribution and catabolism of IgG in foals that are already septic, and exposure to increased concentrations of exogenous or endogenous glucocorticoids (which would accelerate enterocyte maturation) have been incriminated as factors leading to FPT in these foals.

2. FPT in calves

   a. Poor colostral quality or quantity

     (1) First lactation. It is generally accepted that heifers in their first lactation produce less total colostrum containing less total immunoglobulin than cows in later lactations.

     (2) Holstein breed. Colostral quality may be affected by breed. Beef cattle generally produce colostrum with a high immunoglobulin concentration and Jersey cows have excellent colostral quality. In contrast, Holstein cows have notoriously poor colostral quality.

     (3) Colostral volume greater than 8.5 kg at first milking. In general, the larger the volume of colostrum produced, the lower the immunoglobulin concentration. If the first-milking colostra of dairy cows that produce more than 8.5 kg of colostra is discarded, more than 77% of the remaining colostra will have sufficient IgG to ensure adequate passive transfer (if sufficient volumes are fed in a timely fashion).

     (4) Premature calving or induction of parturition. Because colostrum secretion only occurs in the last month of gestation under hormonal influence, premature parturition or a shortened dry period fail to allow for optimum colostrum production. Premature induction of parturition may also decrease colostral quality. Prostaglandin administration reduces the IgG concentration, and glucocorticoids apparently decrease the volume of colostrum that is produced.

     (5) Premilking or premature lactation. The mammary gland only secretes a finite amount of colostrum; therefore, prepartum loss of colostrum via premilking or premature lactation will likely reduce postpartum colostral quality.

     (6) Delay in obtaining first-milking colostrum. If milking of colostrum from the mammary gland is delayed after calving, the colostrum will be diluted by secretion of milk into the mammary gland and have a low immunoglobulin concentration.

     (7) Colostral handling (pooling, repeated freezing and thawing).

       (a) Colostral pools created by mixing colostrum from different dams generally have lower immunoglobulin concentration than fresh colostrum and calves fed from these pools frequently do not achieve satisfactory passive transfer. There are several explanations for this:

         (i) It is likely that colostra from the second milking and beyond is contributed to the colostral pool.

         (ii) Colostra from cows producing large volumes of inferior quality colostrum are more likely to be added to the pool.

    (b) Processing of colostrum may affect the quality. Repeated freezing and thawing cycles or overheating of colostrum during the thawing process can denature immunoglobulins and affect the quality.

b. Ingestion failure

    (1) Poor udder or **teat conformation** or **poor mothering ability** make it difficult for the calf to ingest adequate amounts of colostrum in a timely fashion.

    (2) Maternal periparturient disease (e.g., milk fever, calving injury) interferes with timely consumption of adequate amounts of colostrum, particularly in an unsupervised range environment.

    (3) Poor neonatal vigor. The time for the calf to stand, find the teat, and suckle successfully varies between breeds. Holstein calves are well known for their poor neonatal vigor and FPT is almost certain if they are left on their own to suckle from the dam. Therefore, tube feeding of colostrum with an esophageal feeder within hours of life should be standard practice on most large dairy farms.

    (4) Congenital musculoskeletal abnormalities (e.g., arthrogryposis, contracted tendons) prevent successful teat seeking and/or suckling and such calves should receive colostrum via a bottle or esophageal feeder.

c. Absorption failure

    (1) Neonatal asphyxia (dystocia). Severe or prolonged dystocia can produce neonatal asphyxia, which has adverse affects on multiple organs, including the gastrointestinal tract. Associations between postnatal acidosis and FPT have been reported in calves.

    (2) Method of feeding affects passive transfer of immunoglobulin. Efficiency of absorption is higher with natural suckling than with bottle feeding or use of an esophageal feeder; however, in Holstein calves with poor neonatal vigor, the advantages of using an esophageal feeder far outweigh the disadvantage of less efficient immunoglobulin transfer.

    (3) Extremes in environmental temperatures apparently affect the efficiency of immunoglobulin transfer across the intestinal epithelium because FPT is more prevalent during such environmental extremes.

    (4) Absence of dam. There is evidence that calves will ingest more, and achieve higher serum immunoglobulin concentrations, if they are fed in the presence of their dams.

    (5) Other factors that may affect efficiency of absorption include **prematurity** (immature gastrointestinal tract) and **genetic variation in the efficiency of immunoglobulin transfer.**

C. Diagnostic plan and laboratory tests

1. Indications for testing

    a. Individual testing is often part of routine screening of all newborn animals, and is a common practice on stud farms. It is also used for evaluation of a sick neonatal animal presented for treatment.

    b. Herd testing. Tests for FPT can also be employed at the herd level to determine if FPT is contributing to unacceptably high morbidity and mortality in a herd. Immunoglobulin concentrations usually reflect passive transfer until the neonate is 8 days old; therefore, herd screening can be carried out on all animals younger than 8 days of age.

2. Timing

    a. Traditional testing. Testing is most commonly conducted when the calf or foal is 18–24 hours of age. If FPT is detected at this stage, it can only be rectified by the intravenous administration of plasma or whole blood.

    b. Early testing. If the foal suckled by 2 hours of age, passive transfer status can be assessed 8–12 hours after birth, prior to gut closure. If FPT is detected at this stage, an alternative source of colostrum can be administered in an attempt to achieve adequate passive transfer. Passive transfer status should be reassessed when the foal reaches 18–24 hours of age.

3. Laboratory tests used to screen for FPT
   a. Immunoglobulin concentration
      (1) Traditional testing
         (a) Calves. The IgG concentration that is generally considered protective in calves raised under average management conditions is 1000 mg/dl; therefore, FPT is diagnosed if the IgG concentration of a calf is less than 1000 mg/dl.
         (b) Foals. There are two cutoff points for FPT: one for foals that are sick at the time of testing and are being admitted to a referral center (less than 800 mg/dl), and one for foals that are healthy at the time of testing and are being screened on the farm (less than 400 mg/dl).
      (2) Early testing. In foals, an IgG concentration of less than 200 mg/dl at 8–12 hours of age is considered presumptive evidence of FPT.
   b. Single radial immunodiffusion (SRID) test. SRID represents the **"gold standard"** for assessing passive transfer in both horses and cattle and is the yardstick to which all other tests are compared. It is technically difficult to perform and results are not available for 24 hours; therefore, it is generally not used in the field.
   c. Total serum protein (TSP) or **Total solids (TS) test.** This test is a useful and inexpensive way of assessing passive transfer status in calves, but its utility has been questioned in foals. A TS concentration of less than 5.0 g/dl generally indicates FPT in the calf. TS concentration should be interpreted with caution in the dehydrated calf; a TS greater than 5.0 g/dl in a dehydrated animal may in fact indicate FPT.
   d. Globulin concentration from a biochemistry profile can serve as an indicator of immunoglobulin concentration. Approximately 1.5 g/dl of the globulin measurement represents the nonimmunoglobulin component and the remainder represents the immunoglobulin fraction. Therefore, in a calf with a globulin concentration of 1.8 g/dl, the immunoglobulin fraction is approximately 0.3 g/dl (1.8–1.5), or 300 mg/dl, and likely indicates FPT.
   e. Zinc sulfate turbidity (ZST) test. The ZST test is used in both cattle and horses. A commercial test kit is available for horses or the reagent can be prepared. Zinc ions in the zinc sulfate solution combine with immunoglobulins to form a precipitate in serum; the more the precipitate at a given concentration of zinc sulfate, the higher the immunoglobulin concentration.
   f. Sodium sulfite turbidity (SST) test. This test operates on the same principle as the ZST test, but is used primarily in calves.
   g. Glutaraldehyde coagulation (GCT) test. This test is used in both calves and foals and is based on the ability of glutaraldehyde to react with gamma globulin, forming a solid clot. Serum or whole blood may be used, depending on the test kit. Unfortunately, test sensitivity and specificity are low when this test is performed on whole blood in the bovine species, probably because fibrinogen and other clotting factors interfere with test accuracy. Therefore, the GCT cannot be endorsed as a screening test.
   h. Enzyme-linked immunosorbent assay (ELISA) is designed for the semi-quantitative measurement of IgG in foal serum or plasma. The test uses a color spot with calibration standards corresponding to 200, 400, and 800 mg/dl of IgG. The assay takes 15 minutes to perform and results correspond well to those obtained with SRID.
   i. Latex agglutination test. A commercial latex agglutination test is available for horses. The degree of agglutination between IgG in serum or blood and latex beads coated with antibody to equine IgG is used to estimate the IgG concentration.
   j. γ-Glutamyl transferase (GGT) activity is used as an indicator of passive transfer status in the calf. Colostral GGT concentration in the bovine is about 300 times the serum GGT concentration. GGT from colostrum is absorbed along with other macromolecules during the period when the gut is open. GGT activity is at its peak when the calf is 24–48 hours of age; a GGT value of greater than 300 IU/L indicates that the calf has consumed colostrum.

4. Assessing colostral quality. Colostrometers (modified hydrometers) are available to assess colostral quality in both horses and cattle. There is an excellent correlation between colostral specific gravity and colostral immunoglobulin concentration in horses, but the strength of this association in cattle is weak.

 a. **Bovine colostrum.** The literature and companies that manufacture colostrometers for commercial purposes state that bovine colostrum with a specific gravity greater than 1.050 is of satisfactory quality (i.e., the IgG concentration should be greater than 50 mg/ml). Recently this criteria has been shown to be inaccurate; the colostrometer will classify nearly 75% of low-quality colostra as satisfactory using this standard.

 b. **Equine colostrum** with a specific gravity of 1.060 (using the equine colostrometer) is usually classified as satisfactory, whereas samples with a specific gravity of greater than 1.090 are ideal. It is important to recognize that milk has a specific gravity of 1.040.

D. Therapeutic plan

 1. **Diagnosis within 12 hours of birth.** If FPT is diagnosed or suspected less than 12 hours after birth, **oral supplementation** of IgG is indicated.

 a. **Foals.** All foals receiving oral supplementation should be retested at 24 hours of age.

 (1) **Equine colostrum** from a colostrum bank should be used. Banked colostrum should have a minimum specific gravity of 1.060 (and ideally, a specific gravity greater than 1.090) and the foal should receive 1–2 L in 500-ml increments administered 1 hour apart via nurse bottle or nasogastric feeding tube. Administering colostrum in this way should provide at least 1 g/kg of immunoglobulin to the foal.

 (2) **Alternative sources of immunoglobulin** include bovine colostrum, equine plasma or serum, and commercially available lyophilized or concentrated IgG products.

 (a) **Bovine colostrum** can be safely administered to foals; usually 4 L is administered in the first 24 hours of life. Bovine immunoglobulins have a very short half-life in the foal and may not protect the foal against pathogens unique to the equine environment (e.g., *Actinobacillus equuli*). However, most colostrum-deprived foals that receive bovine colostrum do not succumb to sepsis.

 (b) **Equine plasma and serum** have very low immunoglobulin concentrations, so extremely large volumes are required to achieve adequate passive transfer.

 (c) **Commercial products.** If the foal is treated with a concentrated commercial product, it should receive at least 1 g/kg of IgG (i.e., approximately 40 g, for the average 40-kg foal).

 b. **Calves** should be fed fresh or frozen first-milking colostrum from a third or greater lactation cow.

 (1) **Holstein calves.** At least 2.8 L of colostrum should be administered via esophageal feeder in the first feeding.

 (2) **Other breeds.** Calves should receive colostrum in amounts equal to 10% of their body weight in the first 24 hours, with at least 2 L being fed in the first 6 hours of life.

 2. **Diagnosis 18 or more hours after birth.** If FPT is diagnosed 18 or more hours after birth, **intravenous supplementation** of IgG is indicated.

 a. **Foals**

 (1) **Sources of immunoglobulin**

 (a) **Commercial products.** Advantages of commercial products are that they are free of alloantibodies and infectious agents and generally provide a known quantity of IgG. Some products originate from horses immunized with endotoxin or with specific pathogens (e.g. *Rhodococcus equi*). The major disadvantage of commercial products is that they may lack antibodies specific to pathogens in the foal's environment.

 (b) **Plasma harvested from a local donor.** Harvested plasma provides specific protection to local pathogens, but harvesting is time consuming. Donors should test negative for equine infectious anemia and should be screened by a blood-typing laboratory to ensure that they are negative for Qa/Aa alloantibodies and alloantigens.

(2) Administration

    (a) The **volume of plasma required** depends on the magnitude of the immunoglobulin deficiency, the weight of the foal, and the immunoglobulin concentration in the donor plasma. Preexisting sepsis dramatically alters the distribution and catabolism of antibody in plasma and generally increases the amount required to achieve adequate passive transfer.

        (i) A general guideline is to administer 200–400 mg IgG/kg; for plasma of average quality, this translates to 20–40 ml/kg. In a healthy foal of average weight, administration of 20 ml/kg of plasma (1 L) will raise the IgG concentration by approximately 200 mg/dl.

        (ii) The highest concentrations of IgG are attained 1–3 hours posttransfusion, but it is best to assess the effects of plasma administration 24 hours posttransfusion, after redistribution has occurred to extravascular sites.

    (b) Plasma should be administered through an **in-line filter.** The first 50 ml is administered slowly and the foal is closely monitored for tachypnea, tachycardia, or altered behavior. If no adverse reactions are observed, plasma is administered at a rate of 20 ml/kg/hour (1 L/hour for a 50 kg foal).

  b. Calves

    (1) Sources of immunoglobulin include plasma and whole blood. Whole blood transfusions are frequently used in calves because whole blood is easier and less expensive to harvest than plasma.

    (2) Administration. The principles of administration are the same as for foals. The recommended volume of blood to administer is 2.5 L for the average calf with FPT.

  c. Lambs, piglets, and goat kids. Bovine colostrum is frequently used to supplement immunoglobulin in lambs, piglets, or goat kids if dam colostrum is not available. Anemia is occasionally reported in lambs fed bovine colostrum; the anemia has been attributed to immune complex attachment to the lamb's erythrocytes, resulting in the removal of the erythrocytes from the circulation.

E. Prevention

1. Foals

  a. Prophylactic treatment. Colostral IgG content should be evaluated using a colostrometer to predict the risk of FPT in the foal. If the colostral specific gravity is less than 1.060, some degree of FPT can be anticipated and should be corrected prophylactically by either providing additional high-quality colostrum or by transfusing the foal with plasma.

  b. Good management practices. Some of the factors predisposing to FPT can be circumvented by early intervention and careful management. Measures include identifying mares that dripped colostrum prior to parturition, attending foaling to ensure colostral ingestion by 2–3 hours of age, and screening of high-risk foals with doubtful nursing histories.

  c. Establishment of a colostrum bank. A colostrum bank should be established by collecting 200–250 ml of colostrum from the mare within the first 3 hours of foaling, after the foal has suckled several times. Colostrum for the colostrum bank should be collected from the teat opposite to the one first nursed by the foal.

    (1) Ideally, banked colostrum should have a high IgG concentration (i.e., a specific gravity greater than 1.090) and be free of anti–red cell antibodies to avoid neonatal isoerythrolysis.

    (2) Colostrum can be stored frozen for 18 months without losing significant amounts of antibody.

2. Calves

  a. Force-feeding of colostrum. Producers should be encouraged to observe early natural suckling or to force-feed colostrum in the first 6 hours of life. The calf should receive at least 10% of its body weight in colostrum in the first 24 hours of life and ideally, 2 liters should be consumed in the first feeding.

  (1) Holstein calves. It is common practice to feed Holstein calves 2.8–3 liters of colostra via esophageal feeder in the first 2 hours of life.

  (2) Calves on farms with unacceptably high infectious disease prevalence should be force fed colostrum and screened to quantify passive transfer status.

  b. Although the colostrometer has been used in the past to select colostra with a specific gravity of 1.050, the accuracy of this method has recently been questioned. Current recommendation is to discard colostra from cows producing more than 8.5 kg in their first milking.

  c. Because pooled colostrum is notoriously low in immunoglobulin concentration, the practice of feeding pooled colostrum to calves should be discouraged.

V. SEPTICEMIA AND FOCAL INFECTION

A. **Introduction.** Septicemia and focal infection are major causes of morbidity and mortality in neonatal foals and calves. FPT and unsanitary management practices are important factors predisposing the neonatal foal or calf to septicemia. The early signs of neonatal septicemia are subtle and nonspecific and are often missed by the owner of the foal or calf. Consequently, many septicemic neonates are presented with well-established infections involving multiple organ systems; these animals have a poor prognosis.

B. **Etiology, pathogenesis, and predisposing factors**

  1. Etiology. Gram-negative aerobic bacteria are the predominant cause of septicemia in neonatal foals and calves; however, **aerobic gram-positive** infections and **anaerobic infections** have been documented.

  a. *Escherichia coli* is the bacterial agent isolated most frequently from septicemic foals and calves.

  b. Other commonly isolated bacterial agents include *Actinobacillus* species (foals), *Pasteurella* species (calves and foals), *Klebsiella* species (calves and foals), and *Salmonella* species (calves and foals).

  c. In addition, there are sporadic reports of the following agents being recovered: *Pseudomonas* species, *Listeria monocytogenes, Clostridium perfringens, Clostridium septicum, Streptococcus* species, and *Staphylococcus aureus.* In foals, streptococci are usually recovered in conjunction with gram-negative bacteria, but have been isolated in pure culture from foals with septic physitis, osteomyelitis, and large subcutaneous abscesses. Polymicrobial infections are documented with some frequency in calves.

  2. Pathogenesis. Most neonatal infections are caused by opportunistic bacteria residing in the genital tract, on the skin, or in the environment of cattle and horses.

  a. *In utero*–**acquired infections** may ascend from the vagina, occur via hematogenous spread, or spread directly from the uterine wall. Clinical signs are evident during the first 24 hours of life.

  b. **Infections acquired during delivery** usually occur in stressed foals and should be suspected when meconium-contaminated amniotic fluid or a meconium-stained foal is observed. Portals of entry include the respiratory and digestive tract or the umbilicus.

  c. **Infections acquired after birth** usually manifest themselves when the neonate is 48–96 hours old and are the result of inadequate passive transfer of colostral immunoglobulin, poor husbandry practices, endemic infectious disease on the farm, or predisposing disease conditions.

  3. Predisposing factors. There are a number of periparturient factors that increase the risk of septicemia in the neonate.

    a. Bacterial placentitis is an important risk factor in horses. Premature lactation, purulent vaginal discharge, premature delivery, and an abnormal placenta should alert the clinician that bacterial placentitis may be present. The foal may acquire infection from the mare with bacterial placentitis transplacentally, or from contaminated discharge present in the birth canal. In addition, premature lactation associated with bacterial placentitis results in poor colostral quality and low serum immunoglobulin concentrations in the foal.

    b. Perinatal stresses (e.g., chronic *in utero* hypoxia, acute birth asphyxia, prematurity, dystocia) also increase the susceptibility of the neonate to infection. Compromised foals may be unable to stand and nurse causing a delay in colostral ingestion, low serum immunoglobulin concentrations, and an increased susceptibility to infection.

    c. Overcrowding, poor ventilation, and **contamination of the environment** with pathogenic bacteria (e.g., *Salmonella* species) also predispose the neonate to infection.

C. Clinical findings

1. Septicemia. Clinical signs of septicemia in the neonate vary according to the stage of disease and the site of localized infection.

    a. The **early signs of septicemia** in neonatal calves and foals are vague and nonspecific and are often indistinguishable from noninfectious diseases or focal infections (e.g., diarrhea). Early clinical signs may include depressed mentation (lethargy, poor suckle reflex, weakness, recumbency), diarrhea, and dehydration.

    b. Body temperature abnormalities may include fever or hypothermia; however, a normal rectal temperature should not be used to exclude a diagnosis of septicemia.

    c. Abnormal mucous membranes are usually present in septicemic neonates. Coloration may range from a muddy red-gray, to mottled, pale, or cyanotic. A toxic line rimming the incisors is occasionally observed in foals. The capillary refill time is usually delayed (>2 seconds) and scleral injection is common. Careful inspection may reveal petechiation of the ears, sclera, vulvar, or buccal membranes and suggests presence of disseminated intravascular coagulation (DIC).

2. Localized infection. Localization of infection in various organs of septicemic neonates can cause a variety of clinical signs.

    a. Pneumonia may occur as a complication of septicemia. Cough, nasal discharge, tachypnea, dyspnea, and fever support the diagnosis, but in many septicemic neonates, respiratory rates and lung sounds are normal despite extensive lung pathology. Therefore, chest radiographs are indicated in all septicemic neonates.

    b. Diarrhea may occur secondary to septicemia or enteritis caused by enteropathogens. Enteritis may provide a portal of entry for opportunistic bacteria.

    c. Septic meningitis is a common complication of septicemia in the neonatal animal. Early signs include lethargy, depression, aimless wandering, and abnormal vocalization. Signs usually progress to diffuse cranial nerve deficits; apparent blindness; truncal and limb ataxia; weakness; recumbency; and coma, seizures, or both.

    d. Septic arthritis and **osteomyelitis** are common, debilitating sequelae of neonatal septicemia. Acute lameness, periarticular edema, joint capsule distention, or physeal pain in a farm animal neonate should alert the clinician to the possibility of bone or joint infection.

    e. Uveitis is diagnosed based on the presence of hyphemia, hypopyon, or the accumulation of fibrin in the anterior chamber of the eye. Additional clinical manifestations include blepharospasm, photophobia, excessive tearing, miosis, and ciliary and episcleral injection.

    f. Omphalitis is characterized by heat, pain, swelling, and purulent discharge from the umbilicus (see also VI A). However, the absence of external signs of umbilical involvement should not preclude a diagnosis of omphalitis (ultrasonographic evaluation of the umbilical structures and deep abdominal palpation will confirm involvement of internal structures).

3. **Septic shock.** Neonatal animals frequently present in septic shock.
   a. The **early stage** of septic shock **(hyperdynamic septic shock, septicemia without circulatory collapse)** is characterized by injected mucous membranes, a normal capillary refill time and blood pressure, and warm extremities. Localizing signs of infection may or may not be present. Prompt and aggressive intervention at this time can result in a favorable outcome.
   b. The **late stage** of septic shock **(hypodynamic septic shock)** is characterized by tissue hypoperfusion. Clinical signs include cold extremities, sluggish capillary refill, hypotension, pale gray mucous membranes, and markedly altered mentation. At this stage, multiorgan failure is present and therapeutic intervention is often futile.

D. Diagnostic plan

1. **Routine laboratory testing**
   a. **Leukogram** abnormalities are commonly encountered in septicemic neonates. The white blood cell (WBC) count may be normal early in the course of sepsis, but an increase in the number of band neutrophils or toxic changes in neutrophils (e.g., Döhle's bodies, toxic granulation, vacuolization) are usually present. Neonatal farm animals with well-established septicemia generally have a profound leukopenia and neutropenia accompanied by toxic changes in their neutrophils.
   b. **Fibrinogen concentration** can be used to determine whether infection was acquired pre- or postnatally. A foal infected *in utero* may have a fibrinogen concentration as high as 1000 mg/dl at birth. Moderate increases in fibrinogen concentration (to approximately 400–500 mg/dl) are expected in neonates with early postnatal infections, but with chronicity, or well-established focal infection, the concentration increases dramatically.
   c. **Blood glucose.** Hypoglycemia is a common finding in the neonate with septicemia and has been attributed to decreased feed intake, low hepatic glycogen stores, and abnormal glucose metabolism caused by endotoxemia (depressed hepatic gluconeogenesis and increased peripheral uptake of glucose).
   d. **IgG determination** should be carried out in all neonatal farm animals suspected of being septicemic because there is a strong association between poor passive transfer of colostral immunoglobulin and septicemia.
   e. **Arterial blood gas analysis** is an important component in the evaluation of a septicemic foal or calf. Hypoxemia and a metabolic acidosis are frequently present.
   f. **Serum biochemistry profile.** Biochemical abnormalities that are detected with some frequency in the septicemic neonate are azotemia, which is attributed to poor renal perfusion, and hyperbilirubinemia, which is usually ascribed to endotoxin-induced cholestasis. In addition, foals or calves with severe diarrhea may exhibit electrolyte abnormalities (e.g., hyponatremia, hypochloremia, hypokalemia).

2. **Cultures**
   a. **Blood cultures.** A positive blood culture is required for a definitive antemortem diagnosis of septicemia, but it may take as long as 48–72 hours before a culture can be determined to be positive. Blood cultures should be repeated in any hospitalized foal that deteriorates clinically, has a fever spike, or exhibits a dramatic change in its WBC picture.
      (1) **Technique.** Blood cultures are easy to perform, but attention should be paid to sterile technique. The hair should be clipped and the venipuncture site surgically prepared. Depending on the culture type, a set amount of blood is withdrawn and transferred in an aseptic manner to the culture bottle or vial. A clean needle should be used to transfer the blood into the bottle.
         (a) Aerobic and anaerobic cultures are often performed.
         (b) Some authors recommend that at least two cultures spaced 1 hour apart be performed to maximize the chances of obtaining a positive result. However, in human neonates, a single culture has been shown to detect the presence of bacteria in the blood 91.5% of the time.
      (2) **Sensitivity.** Although previous antimicrobial use may cause false-negative blood culture results, the sensitivity of blood cultures in foals has been remarkably good, ranging from 61%–80%.

b. Culture from sites of focal infection. Bacterial cultures can also be performed on fluid obtained from sites of focal infection (e.g., cerebrospinal fluid, joint fluid, peritoneal fluid, tracheal fluid). In foals with *in utero*–acquired infections, blood cultures are frequently negative because infection occurs via inhalation or ingestion. In such cases, it may be useful to culture the pharynx, trachea, external ear canal, and stomach contents.

(1) Culture of the same pathogen from more than two sites of focal infection supports a diagnosis of bacteremia.

(2) Recovery of the same pathogen from blood and a site of focal infection lends support to the contention that the pathogen recovered from blood is in fact significant.

3. Sepsis scoring systems. Because no single laboratory test has emerged as being completely reliable for the early diagnosis of septicemia in farm animal neonates, various scoring systems and predictive models using easily obtainable historic, clinical, and clinicopathologic data have been developed for this purpose. In general, the goal of these mathematical models is to identify septicemic neonates early in the course of disease when appropriate therapeutic intervention would most likely result in a favorable outcome.

a. Laboratory parameters incorporated in these models include neutrophil count, band neutrophil count, toxic changes in neutrophils, fibrinogen concentration, blood glucose, and IgG determination.

b. Clinical parameters that appear in most of these models are scleral injection, fever or hypothermia, and evidence of focal infection (e.g., uveitis, diarrhea, respiratory distress, joint effusion).

c. Historic data incorporated in some of the models include history of vaginal discharge, systemically ill mare, general anesthesia in the mare, induction of parturition, and premature birth (i.e., less than 320 days' gestation).

E. Therapeutic plan

1. General supportive care

a. Respiratory support. Hypoxemia must be corrected and respiratory failure treated, if present (see II D 8).

b. Fluid resuscitation. Hypovolemic shock and hypoglycemia should be treated with appropriate warmed intravenous fluids.

(1) Alternating lactated Ringer's solution with 5% dextrose, or administering 2.5% dextrose and 0.45% saline, is often sufficient.

(2) If metabolic acidosis is severe, or uncorrectable by volume expansion with balanced polyionic solutions, intravenous infusion of isotonic (1.3%) sodium bicarbonate solution may be required.

c. Intravenous plasma should be administered to restore circulating blood volume, osmotic pressure, and immunoglobulin concentrations.

d. Positive inotropic agents. For circulatory embarrassment that persists after rehydration, positive inotropes should be administered. **Dopamine** (2–5 μg/kg/min by infusion) is the drug of choice because it increases cardiac output and causes splanchnic and renal vasodilation.

e. Nonsteroidal anti-inflammatory drugs (NSAIDs) have been shown to counteract a number of the clinical and laboratory changes associated with endotoxemia, including decreased cardiac output and hypotension. **Flunixin meglumine** (0.25–1.1 mg/kg, intravenously or intramuscularly every 8 hours) has been recommended.

f. Nutritional support. Foals that are unable to nurse should be fed via a nasogastric tube using the recommendations given in II D 4. Total or partial parenteral nutrition is indicated in foals that cannot be fed orally.

2. Control of generalized infection

a. General principles

(1) **Antibiotic selection.** When possible, antibiotic selection is made **based on the results of blood culture and sensitivity testing.** However, because blood culture results are not returned for several days, and the offending agent may

not be recovered, empiric therapy is usually initiated and modified later if needed. **Broad-spectrum bactericidal drugs** are indicated in the treatment of septicemic neonates for the following reasons:
  (a) Gram-negative and polymicrobial infections should be anticipated
  (b) Septicemia in neonates is rapidly progressive
  (c) Many septicemic neonates are neutropenic
  (d) Immune function in neonates is usually compromised by stress and FPT
  (2) Antibiotic administration. Initially, the **intravenous route** is preferred for antibiotic administration because peripheral circulation may be compromised, making absorption from other routes inconsistent.
  (3) Duration of therapy. The recommended duration of therapy for suspected but undocumented sepsis is 7–10 days. Neonates with positive blood cultures and no evidence of focal infection should be treated for at least 2 weeks, and those with localized infections should be treated for 3–4 weeks.
b. Antibiotic therapy in foals. Selection of antimicrobials should be based on the results of an antimicrobial susceptibility pattern; however, until culture results are returned selection of drugs will be somewhat empirical.
  (1) A combination of a *β*-**lactam antibiotic** (e.g., penicillin, ampicillin) and an **aminoglycoside** (e.g., gentamicin, amikacin) usually provides good broad-spectrum coverage. Many clinicians prefer amikacin because it is less nephrotoxic and is less likely to be associated with development of resistant bacterial infections. If possible, peak and trough serum concentrations of aminoglycosides should be monitored to ensure that the drug dose and dosing interval are appropriate. General doses are as follows:
    (a) Gentamicin: 2.2 mg/kg, intramuscularly or intravenously, every 8–12 hours or 3.3 mg/kg, intramuscularly or intravenously, every 12 hours
    (b) Amikacin: 7 mg/kg, intramuscularly or intravenously, every 8–12 hours or 10 mg/kg, intramuscularly or intravenously, every 12 hours
  (2) Cephalosporins. Cefotaxime or ceftiofur can be used in the empiric treatment of septic neonates. General doses are as follows:
    (a) Cefotaxime: 20–30 mg/kg, intravenously or intramuscularly, every 8 hours
    (b) Ceftiofur: 2.2–6.6 mg/kg, intramuscularly or intravenously, every 8–12 hours
  (3) Other drugs. The following drugs are also listed for the treatment of septicemic foals.
    (a) Trimethoprim–sulfonamide combinations: 15 mg/kg, intravenously or orally every 12 hours (resistance to this drug is wide spread)
    (b) Chloramphenicol: 25–50 mg/kg, intravenously or orally, every 6 hours
    (c) Ticarcillin–clavulanate: 50 mg/kg, intravenously, every 6–8 hours
c. Antibiotic therapy in calves is simplified by the limited number of choices available.
  (1) Ceftiofur (5 mg/kg, administered intravenously or intramuscularly every 8–12 hours) is widely used to treat calf septicemia, as are the **potentiated sulfonamides** (15 mg/kg administered orally, intramuscularly, or intravenously every 12 hours).
  (2) In Canada, **ampicillin sulbactam** (6.6 mg/kg administered intramuscularly every 12–24 hours) has been used successfully to treat neonatal calf septicemia.
  (3) Aminoglycosides are generally avoided because of prolonged tissue residues (18 months in the kidney) and because their use is **not endorsed by the National Cattlemens Association.** However, some clinicians still use gentamicin (3–5 mg/kg, administered intravenously or intramuscularly every 12 hours) if they can obtain assurance from the client that the animal in question will not enter the food chain for at least 18 months.
  (4) Fluoroquinolones are **banned for use in cattle in the United States,** but enrofloxacin (2.5–5 mg/kg orally every 24 hours) is used widely in other countries to treat septicemia in neonatal calves.

(5) Tetracyclines and **sulfonamides** are used by producers, but resistance to these drugs is widespread.

3. Treatment of focal infections

a. Septic meningitis (see also Chapter 11 I E)

(1) Antibiotic therapy

(a) Septic meningitis is treated with bactericidal **antimicrobials that penetrate the blood–brain barrier** (e.g, **trimethoprim–sulfonamide combinations** or **third-generation cephalosporins**).

(b) Combination therapy using a **β-lactam antibiotic** or **trimethoprim–sulfonamide** with an **aminoglycoside** is also beneficial as a result of synergistic interactions, despite poor penetration of aminoglycosides into the CSF.

(c) Although chloramphenicol readily crosses the blood–brain barrier, it is bacteriostatic against gram-negative enteric bacteria and is not recommended for the treatment of bacterial meningitis.

(2) Anticonvulsants (e.g., diazepam, phenobarbital) and NSAIDs (e.g., flunixin meglumine) may also be indicated.

b. Septic arthritis or osteomyelitis. Therapeutic measures include:

(1) Systemic antibiotic therapy

(2) Assurance of adequate serum immunoglobulin concentrations

(3) Analgesic therapy

(4) Drainage and removal of debris from the joint and adjacent tissues (lavage with sterile polyionic fluids)

(5) Articular rest

(6) Exogenous sodium hyaluronate or **polysulfated glycosaminoglycan therapy**

(7) Surgical debridement, installation of a sterile drain, and **immobilization of the limb** with a Robert-Jones splint bandage (in cases of osteomyelitis with evidence of bone sequestration or osteolysis)

c. Uveitis. Treatment should include **systemic antimicrobial therapy** and **local therapy** to prevent permanent ocular damage. A mydriatic (e.g., atropine), topical ophthalmic corticosteroid, systemic NSAID, and broad-spectrum ophthalmic preparation are indicated.

d. Omphalitis. Treatment is discussed in VI A.

F. **Prognosis**

1. The **overall survival rate** for septicemic neonates is less than 60%, but early recognition of sepsis and appropriate and aggressive intervention improve the outcome.

a. A septicemic large animal neonate with FPT and evidence of multiple organ involvement should always be given a guarded prognosis.

b. A neonate with a negative blood culture but evidence of focal infection (e.g., pneumonia, diarrhea) has a more favorable prognosis.

c. Appropriate and early therapeutic intervention in foals with *in utero*–acquired infections often results in a favorable outcome: survival rates greater than 75% have been quoted for this group.

2. The **long-term prognosis for future athletic performance** is guarded if multifocal bone or joint disease is diagnosed.

G. **Prevention.** Management of the mare with placentitis can decrease the risk of premature delivery and postnatal infection. *Aspergillus* species, β-hemolytic streptococci, and *E. coli* are the organisms isolated most frequently from mares with placentitis. **Treatment of placentitis** includes the use of antimicrobial agents, anti-inflammatory drugs, progestins, and stall rest.

1. Antimicrobial agents are usually selected based on results of culture and sensitivity. **Trimethoprim–sulfonamide** (25–35 mg/kg every 12 hours) is a good antimicrobial to start with because high concentrations are achieved in the placenta, allantoic fluid, amniotic fluid, and fetal serum.

2. NSAIDs, such as **phenylbutazone** (4 mg/kg orally every 24 hours) or **flunixin meglumine** (1 mg/kg orally, intravenously, or intramuscularly every 12 hours) may reduce uterine inflammation and uterine production of prostaglandin F2α, thereby decreasing the risk of premature delivery.

3. **Supplemental progestin therapy** with **altrenogest** (0.044 mg/kg every 24 hours) has been employed to maintain pregnancy in mares with placentitis. Although this progestin will maintain pregnancy in ovariectomized mares, the efficacy of this regimen in late-term mares with high-risk pregnancy is unknown.

VI. UMBILICAL ABNORMALITIES

A. **Umbilical remnant infections.** Infection may involve the urachus, umbilical veins **(omphalophlebitis)**, one or both umbilical arteries **(omphaloarteritis)**, or many structures **(omphalitis, umbilical abscess).**

1. **Clinical findings** may include umbilical enlargement, pain on palpation, patent urachus (common in foals, rare in calves), or purulent discharge. The internal or intra-abdominal umbilical structures may be the only structures affected in foals, making infection difficult to detect on physical examination.
    a. As with most neonatal infections, the first signs noted are decreased suckling and depression. Other abnormalities may include fever, dysuria, pollakiuria, and tenesmus.
    b. Deep abdominal palpation can be used to evaluate the internal umbilical structures, particularly in calves. Enlargement of the umbilical vein may be palpable coursing cranially toward the liver; enlarged umbilical arteries may be palpable coursing caudally toward the bladder. Palpation may elicit a grunt and abdominal splinting may be noted in calves with a septic umbilicus and associated peritonitis.

2. **Pathogenesis.** Infection may originate following contamination of the external umbilicus after birth or result from seeding from other sites during periods of septicemia. Bacteria may localize in the umbilical vessels, urachus, bladder, or interstitial tissues and the infection may extend into the peritoneal cavity or progress to a generalized septicemia. Urachal abscessation can cause the previously closed urachus to become patent externally or allow urine to leak subcutaneously or into the peritoneal cavity.

3. **Diagnostic plan and laboratory tests**
    a. **Routine laboratory tests.** Clinicopathologic alterations usually include neutrophilia with toxic changes in neutrophils and hyperfibrinogenemia.
    b. **Blood culture.** Because of the association of umbilical remnant infections with septicemia, blood cultures should always be performed.
    c. **Ultrasonography** should be used to evaluate the extent of involvement of internal umbilical structures. An increased diameter, thickened wall, or abscesses may be visible. The procedure is usually carried out with the foal in lateral recumbency and the calf standing.
        (1) In foals, the umbilical arteries and vein can be followed from the external umbilical stump to the cranial aspect of the bladder and liver, respectively. The urachus can usually be visualized along with the umbilical arteries just caudal to the umbilical stump.
        (2) In calves, the umbilical arteries retract into the abdominal cavity and thus should not be identifiable in the umbilical stalk; they are most easily located along the apex of the urinary bladder. The umbilical vein of calves is scanned from the umbilical stalk to the liver along the right ventral abdomen. Urachal remnants can usually not be identified in normal calves.

4. **Therapeutic plan.** The treatment options for umbilical remnant infections are medical management or surgical resection.
    a. **Medical therapy** consists of prolonged antibiotic administration (see V E 2) and encouragement of drainage. In one study, 50% of foals responded to medical therapy alone.

(1) Frequent ultrasound examinations should be carried out to evaluate progress in all neonates treated medically.

(2) Risks associated with not removing infected remnants are the development of septic arthritis, pneumonia, peritonitis, or uroperitoneum from urachal rupture.

b. Surgery. Evidence of multisystemic infection, umbilical vein involvement, uroperitoneum from urachal rupture, or failure to respond to medical therapy are all indications for surgery.

5. Prevention

a. Adequate passive transfer and a **clean environment** should be ensured to minimize the chances of septicemia and seeding of the umbilicus.

b. Proper postpartum care of the umbilical remnant decreases the chance of bacterial colonization. The following solutions have been used for dipping the umbilicus: **2% iodine, 1% povidone–iodine,** and **0.5% chlorhexidine.**

(1) In one study. chlorhexidine therapy caused the lowest bacterial counts on the umbilicus immediately posttreatment. Chlorhexidine also binds to the stratum corneum and has a longer residual effect than other treatments.

(2) The use of 7% iodine should be discouraged. Local tissue necrosis associated with application of 7% iodine may actually increase the prevalence of infection.

B. Patent urachus (see also II B 5)

1. Etiology and pathogenesis

a. Congenital patent urachus. The exact pathophysiologic mechanisms leading to the development of a congenital patent urachus have not been established. One theory is that excessive torsion of the umbilical cord *in utero* causes urachal obstruction, urine retention in the bladder, distention of the proximal urachus, and interference with urachal involution.

b. Acquired patent urachus. Reestablishment of urine flow after a normal urachal closure at birth is termed acquired patent urachus. Any insult that causes tension on the abdominal wall (e.g., prolonged recumbency, tenesmus, abdominal distention) or umbilical inflammation (e.g., omphalitis) may lead to the development of an acquired patent urachus.

2. Clinical findings

a. A diagnosis is usually made when urine is observed dribbling or flowing from the umbilical stump. Dermatitis may develop on the hindlimbs and ventral abdomen from urine scalding.

b. Fever, purulent discharge, and pain on palpation of the umbilicus suggest that the patent urachus is a sequela of an umbilical remnant infection.

3. Diagnostic plan

a. Contrast cystography can be used to confirm the diagnosis in cases where a patent urachus is suspected, but where urine is not obviously dribbling from the umbilical stalk.

b. CBC. A CBC should be performed to determine if there is intercurrent infection (findings would include leukocytosis and hyperfibrinogenemia).

c. Serum IgG concentration should be measured to determine if FPT is present.

d. Ultrasonography can be used to determine if the urachal patency is associated with infection of the umbilical remnants.

4. Therapeutic plan

a. Conservative management is used in cases of uncomplicated patent urachus occurring in foals younger than 5 days.

(1) Local therapy and **removal of predisposing conditions** are necessary.

(2) Cauterization of the urachus with **silver nitrate sticks, 2% iodine,** or **local injection of procaine penicillin** has been advocated to speed healing. These treatments should not be applied beyond the abdominal wall because they may cause urachal abscessation or cystitis.

(3) Careful monitoring of patients is indicated to identify infection.

    b. Surgical management is indicated for the following patients:
        (1) Patients with persistent urine dribbling in spite of cauterization and resolution of predisposing factors (e.g., recumbency)
        (2) Patients with involvement of other umbilical structures (demonstrated by ultrasound)
        (3) Patients with subcutaneous or intra-abdominal urine accumulation resulting from a rent in the urachus

5. Prevention
    a. The umbilicus should be allowed to rupture spontaneously.
    b. Critically ill neonates should be restrained to prevent excessive tension on the ventral abdomen.

C. **Excessive bleeding from the umbilicus.** Bleeding from the umbilicus may occur, particularly if it was cut or ligated. Occasionally, hemorrhage is severe enough to necessitate a blood transfusion. Rarely, hemoperitoneum will result from hemorrhage from an intra-abdominal umbilical vessel.

STUDY QUESTIONS

DIRECTIONS: Each of the numbered items or incomplete statements in this section is followed by answers or by completions of the statement. Select the ONE numbered answer or completion that is BEST in each case.

1. Which of the following conditions affecting neonatal foals is usually associated with a favorable long term outcome (i.e., a satisfactory performance animal)?

(1) Hypoxemic–ischemic encephalopathy (HIE)
(2) Prematurity with tarsal bone collapse
(3) Septic arthritis
(4) Twinning
(5) Septic physitis

2. Which of the following historic or laboratory findings would indicate that a prematurely delivered foal is endocrinologically mature ("ready for birth")?

(1) Cesarean section at 322 days' of gestation
(2) Total white blood cell (WBC) count less than 5000 cells/μL on day 3
(3) A neutrophil–lymphocyte ratio greater than 2 at birth
(4) A plasma fibrinogen concentration of 200 mg/dl on day 1
(5) No change in the neutrophil–lymphocyte ratio in response to adrenocorticotropic hormone (ACTH) administration

3. The bacterial agent that is cultured most frequently from neonatal calves and foals with septicemia is:

(1) *Actinobacillus equuili.*
(2) *Staphylococcus aureus.*
(3) *Klebsiella pneumoniae.*
(4) *Listeria monocytogenes.*
(5) *Escherichia coli.*

4. Which one of the following antibiotics, or combination of antibiotic drugs, would be a rational first choice for treatment of a foal with clinical and laboratory findings indicating a diagnosis of septicemia?

(1) Chloramphenicol
(2) Oxytetracycline
(3) Penicillin and amikacin
(4) Lincomycin and spectinomycin
(5) Ampicillin

5. Which one of the following antibiotics would be a rational first choice for treatment of a calf with clinical and laboratory findings indicating a diagnosis of septicemia?

(1) Chloramphenicol
(2) Oxytetracycline
(3) Enrofloxacin
(4) Ceftiofur
(5) Erythromycin

6. In a study conducted in foals, which one of the following disinfectants was shown to cause the greatest decrease in bacterial count at the end of the umbilicus immediately post-dipping?

(1) Dilute sodium hypochlorite
(2) 0.5% Chlorhexidine
(3) 7% Tincture of iodine
(4) 2% Iodine
(5) 1% Povidone–iodine

7. How much milk should a healthy 1-week-old foal weighing 60 kg consume in a 24-hour period?

(1) 12 liters
(2) 6 liters
(3) 4 liters
(4) 2 liters
(5) 24 liters

8. Which one of the following statements pertaining to the feeding of bovine colostrum to neonatal foals is true?

(1) Bovine colostrum should never be fed to foals because it causes severe bloating and diarrhea.
(2) Bovine colostrum should never be used in foals because it often causes an immune-mediated hemolytic anemia.
(3) Bovine colostrum prevents septicemia caused by *Actinobacillus equuli*, but not septicemia caused by *Escherichia coli*.
(4) Bovine antibodies have a short half-life, but will protect the foal against septicemia most of the time.
(5) Bovine colostrum cannot be used in foals because unrealistically large volumes are required to provide adequate protection.

9. Which one of the following laboratory findings likely indicates adequate passive transfer on routine screening of a healthy 2-day-old calf?

(1) Total serum protein (TSP) concentration of 6.2 g/dl
(2) Immunoglobulin G (IgG) concentration of 400 mg/dl
(3) γ-Glutamyl transferase (GGT) activity of 23 IU/L
(4) IgG concentration of 800 mg/dl
(5) TSP concentration of 4.9 g/dl

10. Which one of the following drugs is contraindicated in treating a neonatal foal with coma, intermittent seizures, and oliguria following an acute asphyxial episode at birth (premature placental separation)?

(1) Diazepam
(2) Dimethylsulfoxide (DMSO)
(3) Acepromazine
(4) Furosemide
(5) Dopamine

ANSWERS AND EXPLANATIONS

1. The answer is 1 [I C 2 a]. With appropriate care foals with hypoxemic-ischemic encephalopathy survive, and in the long term, this condition has little impact on performance. In contrast, foals with infectious or noninfectious orthopedic diseases have poor long term prognoses. Products of a twin pregnancy also have a grim prognosis as performance animals because they are small in stature and often suffer from noninfectious orthopedic conditions (e.g., tarsal collapse).

2. The answer is 3 [II A 2, E 2 b–c]. A neutrophil–lymphocyte ratio that is greater than 2 by 3 days of age indicates maturity of the adrenal–pituitary–hypothalamic axis and readiness for birth. In contrast, a white blood cell (WBC) count less than 5000 cells/μL in the first 3 days of life and no widening of the neutrophil–lymphocyte ratio in response to adrenocorticotropic hormone (ACTH) administration indicates immaturity of the endocrine system and unreadiness for birth, as does a cesarean section performed at 322 days' of gestation. A fibrinogen concentration of less than 400 mg/dl at birth suggests that chronic *in utero* stress due to placentitis was probably not the cause of the premature delivery and, therefore, the fetus was probably not ready for birth.

3. The answer is 5 [V B 1 a]. *Escherichia coli* is the pathogen cultured most frequently (representing more than 50% of isolates) from septicemic farm animal neonates. *Staphylococcus aureus*, *Klebsiella pneumoniae*, and *Listeria monocytogenes* are isolated sporadically from septic calves and foals. *Actinobacillus equuli* is usually only found in foals.

4. The answer is 3 [V E 2 b (1)]. Both penicillin and amikacin are bactericidal drugs and the combination provides broad-spectrum coverage. Amikacin is preferred over gentamicin by many clinicians because it is less nephrotoxic and also because resistance is less likely. Chloramphenicol provides broad-spectrum coverage, but it is bacteriostatic and therefore not ideal for treating a rapidly progressing infection in a neonatal animal with an immature immune system. Resistance of septicemia pathogens to ampicillin and oxytetracycline is widespread.

5. The answer is 4 [V E 2 c]. Ceftiofur is a broad-spectrum bactericidal drug and many clinicians use it for the treatment of septicemia in neonatal calves. It is illegal to use chloramphenicol in cattle; therefore, this antibiotic would not be a good choice. Oxytetracycline is bactericidal but resistance is widespread. It is illegal to use enrofloxacin in cattle in the United States and there are some concerns that this antibiotic may cause joint cartilage abnormalities in rapidly growing young animals. Erythromycin is bacteriostatic and has a gram-positive spectrum of activity, so this drug would not be a good choice in a neonatal calf with a rapidly progressing gram-negative bacterial infection.

6. The answer is 2 [VI A 5 b]. In a study conducted in foals, application of 0.5% chlorhexidine to the umbilicus was shown to cause the lowest bacterial count on the umbilicus immediately post-treatment. The use of 7% tincture of iodine is discouraged; local tissue necrosis associated with the application of 7% iodine may actually increase the prevalence of infection.

7. The answer is 1 [II D 4 a]. A healthy newborn foal usually consumes approximately 20%–25% of its body weight in milk over a 24-hour period. Therefore, a healthy 1-week-old foal weighing 60 kg should consume 12 liters of milk over a 24-hour period (0.20 x 60 = 12).

8. The answer is 4 [IV D 1 a (2) (a)]. Although the immunoglobulins in bovine colostrum are rapidly catabolized in foals, bovine colostrum does provide protection against most pathogens capable of causing septicemia, with the exception of *Actinobacillus equuli*, a pathogen unique to the equine environment. Bovine colostrum is well-tolerated by foals and only occasionally causes diarrhea. There are no reports of hemolytic anemia in foals fed bovine colostrum, although anemia has been reported to occur in lambs The volume of bovine colostrum required to confer protection in foals is approximately 4 liters, a volume that is easily achieved.

9. The answer is 1 [IV C 3]. A TSP concentration greater than 5.0 g/dl generally indicates adequate passive transfer. A healthy 2-day-old calf with a total serum protein (TSP) concentration of 6.2 g/dl has adequate passive transfer. An immunoglobulin G (IgG) concentration of greater than 1000 mg/dl indicates adequate passive transfer, as does γ-glutamyl transferase (GGT) activity greater than 300 IU/L.

10. The answer is 3 [III F 1 a (3)]. Acepromazine, which may lower the seizure threshold and cause systemic hypotension, further decreasing renal perfusion, is contraindicated in a neonatal foal with neurologic signs following an acute asphyxial episode at birth. Diazepam is frequently used for seizure control and dimethylsulfoxide (DMSO) is employed by many clinicians to treat cerebral edema. Furosemide is indicated as a diuretic in oliguric asphyxiated foals and dopamine infusion is advocated to increase renal blood flow.

Comprehensive Exam

QUESTIONS

DIRECTIONS: Each of the numbered items or incomplete statements in this section is followed by answers or by completions of the statement. Select the ONE numbered answer or completion that is BEST in each case.

1. A herd of cattle is experiencing production losses characterized by chronic diarrhea, poor growth rates, and lower than expected reproductive performance. Secondary haircoat changes include generalized hair loss, a brittle texture, and changes to the hair color (lightening). What would be the most likely diagnosis?

(1) Ergot alkaloid contamination of feed
(2) Iodism
(3) Selenium toxicosis
(4) Molybdenum deficiency
(5) Copper deficiency

2. A farmer who manages a veal operation has had a series of calves exhibiting anorexia, fever, and drooling. The examination of affected calves reveals fevers, puffy cheeks, and a foul odor to the breath. The most likely diagnosis is:

(1) actinobacillosis.
(2) oral necrobacillosis.
(3) actinomycosis.
(4) vesicular exanthema.
(5) bovine papular stomatitis.

3. Which one of the following etiologic agents is most likely to cause bacterial endocarditis (BE) in a pig less than 1 year of age?

(1) *Actinobacillus* species or *Staphylococcus aureus*
(2) *Actinomyces pyogenes* or *Streptococcus* species
(3) *Streptococcus* species or *Erysipelothrix rhusiopathiae*
(4) *Staphylococcus aureus* or *Actinomyces pyogenes*
(5) *Streptococcus* species or *Actinobacillus* species

4. The polyuria seen in animals with equine Cushing's disease may result from:

(1) pyelonephritis.
(2) excessive cortisol secretion.
(3) nephrosis.
(4) glomerulonephritis.
(5) polydipsia.

5. A female goat has been losing weight for 6 weeks. This is the only animal affected out of a flock of 75 does, although the owner remembers one or two similar does last year that went on to die. Postmortem examinations were not performed. The clinical examination rules out dental disease, primary undernutrition, arthritis, and diarrhea. Two other differential diagnoses high on your list include:

(1) Johne's disease and coccidiosis.
(2) Johne's disease and visceral caseous lymphadenitis (CLA).
(3) gastrointestinal helminths and visceral CLA.
(4) abomasal emptying defect and coccidiosis.
(5) gastrointestinal helminths and abomasal emptying defect.

6. In a horse that has an acute onset of blepharospasm, tearing, and photophobia in one eye, what is the most appropriate approach to further evaluation and treatment?

(1) Apply fluorescein to the eye; if possible for corneal ulcer, treat with topical antibiotics and corticosteroids.
(2) Apply a topical anesthetic stain to the conjunctiva, flush the cornea with saline, and then treat the eye with a topical triple antibiotic ointment.
(3) Apply a topical anesthetic to the conjunctiva followed by fluorescein to the eye; if no ulcer is present, treat with topical antibiotics and antiviral agents.
(4) Apply fluorescein stain to the eye; if negative, treat with a topical triple antibiotic ointment.
(5) Apply fluorescein stain to the eye; if positive, treat with antibiotics and a cycloplegic.

7. The following laboratory findings are present in an 11-year-old Thoroughbred gelding with chronic, intermittent abdominal pain: marked increases in γ-glutamyl transferase (GGT) and alkaline phosphatase (AP) activity, a mild increase in sorbitol dehydrogenase (SDH) activity, a conjugated bilirubin level that is greater than 30% of total bilirubin, marked bilirubinuria, leukocytosis, and hyperfibrinogenemia and hyperglobulinemia. What is the most likely diagnosis?

(1) Theiler's disease
(2) Tyzzer's disease
(3) Mesenteric abscess
(4) Thromboembolic colic
(5) Cholelithiasis

8. Which one of the following statements is correct when examining a horse with abdominal pain?

(1) Sedate the horse immediately and before any clinical examination so that the examination may be carried out in a routine, logical fashion.
(2) Be aware that some colics responsive to medical therapy may present with severe pain and anxiety.
(3) Omit a rectal examination if gastric reflux has been demonstrated on gastric intubation.
(4) Remember that abdominal distention will be present with small intestinal obstruction.
(5) Be aware that high rectal temperatures are associated with colics in which surgical intervention should be considered.

9. A 4-year-old Holstein cow calved 3 days ago. This morning, she is completely anorexic and her milk production has decreased from 25 kg last evening to 3 kg this morning. She is passing scant amounts of feces. Physical examination findings include a temperature of 39.0°C, a heart rate of 120 bpm, and a respiratory rate of 40 breaths/min. The cow's eyes are sunken and her oral mucous membranes are tacky. Simultaneous auscultation and percussion reveals a large, gas-filled viscus on the right side that extends from the eighth intercostal space to the mid-right paralumbar fossa. The viscus can also be palpated per rectum in the right abdomen. What is the best set of differential diagnoses for this cow's condition?

(1) Traumatic reticuloperitonitis (TRP), abomasal displacement
(2) Cecal torsion, abomasal volvulus
(3) Cecal displacement, right abomasal displacement
(4) Gas in the spiral colon, acute diffuse peritonitis
(5) Rumen tympany, abomasal torsion

10. Which one of the following statements regarding microcytosis is true? Microcytosis is:

(1) most commonly seen after acute blood loss.
(2) a predisposing factor for red maple toxicosis.
(3) most commonly associated with iron deficiency.
(4) most commonly seen in large animals with intraerythrocyte parasite infestations.
(5) determined by calculating that mean corpuscular volume (MCV) is abnormally high.

11. Coccidiosis is a disease common to many domestic animals. Which of the following statements is correct?

(1) Coccidiosis is usually associated with high mortality rates but low morbidity rates.
(2) *Eimeria* species are the pathogenic organism in all domestic animals.
(3) Treatment with coccidiostats during episodes of clinical disease is the best course of action.
(4) Nervous system signs may be seen in individual cattle.
(5) Diagnosis depends on the demonstration of organisms in the feces.

12. One of your colleagues asks you for a consultation on the serum chemistry profile of a 2-day-old embryo-transfer calf that has been slightly weak since birth. The calf was born in posterior presentation and had to be delivered by forced extraction. Your colleague tube-fed the calf with 2 L of colostrum immediately after delivery, and although the calf was unable to nurse from the cow, it readily suckled colostrum offered by nurse bottle after that time. The calf is normal on physical examination. You notice that the γ-glutamyl transferase (GGT) activity of this calf is 996 IU/L. A chart in a clinical pathology text states that the normal GGT activity of cattle is less than 31 IU/L. How would you interpret this laboratory finding?

(1) The calf has bile duct atresia.
(2) The calf ingested adequate amounts of colostrum.
(3) The calf is septicemic.
(4) The calf is in renal failure.
(5) The calf may be suffering from Tyzzer's disease.

13. Hyperkalemic periodic paralysis (HYPP) is a heritable disease in:

(1) horses and humans.
(2) horses and cattle.
(3) cattle and pigs.
(4) humans and pigs.
(5) sheep and goats.

14. In a "typical" outbreak of pleuropneumonia caused by *Actinobacillus pleuropneumonia* :

(1) all foals die within 2 weeks of contracting the disease.
(2) cows are unaffected, but calves develop enzootic pneumonia.
(3) all exposed sheep and goats suffer high mortality rates.
(4) broodmares suffer signs of upper respiratory disease and those in foal, abort.
(5) growing pigs are most severely affected, with a high morbidity rate and variable mortality rate.

15. A dairy farmer has cases of swollen, abscessed mandibles in a few of his heifers. The abscesses discharge a thick, yellowish material and do not resolve with antibiotic treatment. The most likely diagnosis is:

(1) osteosarcoma.
(2) actinomycosis.
(3) osteodystrophy.
(4) osteoporosis.
(5) osteomalacia.

16. A swine farmer has a group of feeder pigs that are off-feed. Many of these pigs have high fevers and some exhibit reddened, raised lesions with a diamond shape. The most likely diagnosis is:

(1) erysipelas.
(2) exudative dermatitis.
(3) ringworm.
(4) sporotrichosis.
(5) sarcoptic mange.

17. A farmer describes an outbreak of mastitis that caused a sudden drop in milk production and a painless udder swelling of all four quarters in affected cows. New animals recently have been introduced to this large herd, and there is a concurrent problem with pneumonia and lameness in the heifers. Milk secretion looks relatively normal, but if a sample is left to stand, a fine grit settles to the bottom of the sample cup. The most likely diagnosis is:

(1) *Actinomyces pyogenes* mastitis.
(2) *Mycoplasma* mastitis.
(3) *Nocardia* mastitis.
(4) *Streptococcus uberis* mastitis.
(5) *Staphylococcus epidermidis* mastitis.

18. A 4-year-old mare with acute colitis develops head edema, a painful neck, depression, and anorexia on the fourth day of intravenous fluid and plasma therapy. What is the most likely diagnosis and its treatment?

(1) Jugular vein thrombosis is the diagnosis and should be treated with catheter removal, topical dimethylsulfoxide (DMSO) or hydrotherapy, and systemic antibiotics.
(2) Congestive heart failure (CHF) is the diagnosis and should be treated with diuretics and positive inotropic agents, such as digoxin, and reduce sodium in the diet.
(3) Electrolyte deficiencies causing cardiac arrhythmias is the diagnosis and should be treated with the correction of the underlying electrolyte imbalance, lidocaine for ventricular arrhythmias, or quinidine for atrial fibrillation if arrhythmia persists after electrolyte replacement.
(4) Acute equine purpura hemorrhagica is the diagnosis and should be treated with hydrotherapy, diuretics, nonsteroidal anti-inflammatory drugs (NSAIDs), and penicillin.
(5) CHF is the diagnosis, but due to poor prognosis for return to function, euthanasia is recommended.

19. A veterinarian is consulted regarding a 4-year-old horse with a fleshy mass on the eyelid. The owner noticed the mass in February. What should be on the veterinarian's list of differential diagnoses?

(1) Habronemiasis
(2) Sarcoid
(3) Squamous cell carcinoma (SCC) and habronemiasis
(4) Sarcoid, SCC, and habronemiasis

20. Which one of the following statements regarding acute renal failure in horses is correct?

(1) Causes of acute renal failure in horses include the administration of nephrotoxic medications [e.g., menadione sodium bisulfite (vitamin K_3)], the consumption of red maple leaves, and the accidental consumption of mercury.
(2) Adult horses that develop uroliths usually show signs of renal failure because of post renal urinary obstruction.
(3) Urine sediment analysis in horses with suspected renal tubular disease that shows only a large amount of calcium carbonate crystals in alkaline urine is most suggestive of uroliths because the absence of tubular casts rules out tubular disease.
(4) A high serum creatinine level combined with low urine specific gravity in a foal 2 days old that has few other clinical signs suggests an underlying congenital renal disorder.
(5) Because many toxins have a specific site of action, such as glomerular or proximal tubular damage, the best test on horses is a renal biopsy to diagnose the site of damage, leading to the early recognition and removal of the toxin.

21. A veterinarian is consulted regarding transient bouts of loose feces in a 6-year-old riding horse. On examination of the horse, no definitive findings are noted, and the veterinarian recommends routine deworming, vaccinations, and dental care. Four months later, the horse appears to be thin and has a plaque of ventral, midline edema. Upon questioning, the owner reports that the horse's feces also continue to be nonformed. What is the most likely diagnosis?

(1) Granulomatous enteritis
(2) Equine monocytic ehrlichiosis (Potomac horse fever)
(3) Chronic impaction of the small intestine
(4) Gastric ulceration
(5) Equine pancreatitis

22. Which one of the following statements regarding anhidrosis in horses is correct? Anhidrosis:

(1) can be diagnosed with serum sodium measurements.
(2) is a genetic condition.
(3) may be complete or partial.
(4) is seen most commonly in obese mares.
(5) is treated most commonly with thyroxine and calcium salts.

23. A veterinarian is called to examine a small flock of sheep with swelling and stiffness of the limbs, ventral abdominal distention, and depression. Two young sheep have died. A postmortem examination reveals dilated right and left ventricles of the heart, acute congestion of the liver, and significant pleural, pericardial, and peritoneal fluid. The sheep were fed a 3-kg mixture of 50:50 oat hay and alfalfa hay, 1-kg of a 16% grain mix labeled for sheep, and they had free access to a 22% protein/trace mineral supplement labeled for beef cattle. Vaccination and deworming prophylaxis appeared adequate. What is the most likely diagnosis and how should this diagnosis be confirmed?

(1) Chronic parasitism confirmed by intestinal parasites found in fecal flotations
(2) Congestive heart failure (CHF) due to toxic exposure (most likely gossypol toxicosis) confirmed by free gossypol found in the protein and mineral supplement and concentrate mix
(3) Acute hepatotoxicity due to plant toxicity confirmed by pathognomonic lesions or rumenotomy found in a liver biopsy
(4) Ovine progressive pneumonia serology or viral isolation from blood
(5) Liver flukes confirmed by a Baermann float of feces

24. Blindness can be associated with a variety of conditions in domestic animals. Which conditions often result in blindness?

(1) Leptospirosis in horses, vitamin D toxicosis in cattle
(2) Polioencephalomalacia in calves, lead poisoning in cattle
(3) Lead poisoning in cattle, listeriosis in sheep
(4) Leptospirosis in horses, listeriosis in sheep
(5) Vitamin D toxicosis in cattle, polioencephalomalacia in calves

25. Which one of the following pairs describing the etiologic agent and treatment of liver abscesses in cattle is correct?

(1) *Escherichia coli* —gentamicin
(2) *Salmonella typhimurium* —trimethoprim–sulfamethoxazole
(3) *Actinomyces bovis*—tilmicosin
(4) *Fusobacterium necrophorum*—penicillin
(5) *Aspergillus* —thiabendazole

26. Which one of the following is most likely to cause intravascular hemolysis in cattle?

(1) *Anaplasma marginale*
(2) *Eperythrozoon wenyoni*
(3) Cobalt deficiency
(4) Onion toxicosis
(5) *Babesia bigemina*

27. A client has a 9-day-old Standardbred filly foal that has had diarrhea of 1 day's duration. The veterinarian examines the foal and finds no abnormalities other than watery feces. What is the appropriate next measure?

(1) The owner should apply petroleum jelly to the perineum and call the veterinarian if the diarrhea persists for more than another 48 hours.
(2) The owner should consider having a galactose tolerance test run on the foal.
(3) Flunixin meglumine and lincomycin should be administered to the foal.
(4) The owner should observe the foal for 2 more days. The mare and foal should be separated, except for two daily feedings.
(5) An enema should be administered to treat meconium impaction.

28. An 8-year-old horse has a persistent cough when stabled but is otherwise afebrile and maintains a good appetite and demeanor. Which one of the following statements apply to this case?

(1) The cough is usually an immunologic reaction to airborne allergens, and cellular infiltration of the lower airways is a neutrophilic type because of secondary bacterial colonization.
(2) Finding eosinophils in the lower airways is highly consistent with a diagnosis of allergic lower airway disease, such as chronic obstructive pulmonary disease (COPD) or heaves
(3) Using the atropine challenge test for a diagnostic test, failure to relieve the signs suggests that clinical signs are caused by a disease other than COPD.
(4) After changing management practices to reduce the dust in the environment and using corticosteroids to reduce airway irritation, both treatments can be eliminated gradually as clinical signs abate.
(5) Other signs might include exercise intolerance and abdominal muscle hypertrophy, with changes in intrapleural pressure larger than 10 mm Hg.

29. A 4-year-old Jersey cow was examined because of weight loss, decreased milk production, and inappetence. Findings on clinical examination included tachycardia, distention of the jugular and mammary veins, edema of the submandibular area, jugular vein pulsation, and a right-sided heart murmur. Common causes of this set of clinical findings include:

(1) aortic valve insufficiency, cor pulmonale, and myocardial lymphosarcoma.
(2) aortic valve insufficiency, pyrrolizidine alkaloid toxicity, and acute grain overload.
(3) cor pulmonale, bacterial endocarditis, and pyrrolizidine alkaloid toxicity.
(4) myocardial lymphosarcoma, acute grain overload, and septic pericarditis.
(5) bacterial endocarditis, septic pericarditis, and myocardial lymphosarcoma.

30. A producer is faced with sudden deaths in some of his growing lambs. The lambs are unvaccinated and being fed a high-energy ration. There were no presenting clinical findings that the owner noticed prior to death. The most likely diagnosis is:

(1) salmonellosis.
(2) pulpy kidney disease.
(3) shipping fever.
(4) abomasal emptying defect.
(5) coccidiosis.

31. A veterinarian is called to examine a 1-day-old Standardbred colt with a history of lethargy and inappetence. The colt was delivered at 339 days' gestation. The mare dripped colostrum prior to giving birth. Second-stage parturition lasted 10 minutes and the delivery was unassisted. The foal was meconium-stained after birth. The foal was standing by 6 hours of age and was first observed to nurse by 8 hours of age. The foal weighs 32 kg, has lax flexor tendons, a silky hair coat, and a bulging forehead. Which one of the following most accurately describes the risk factors present in this foal?

(1) Dystocia; fetal distress/anoxia *in utero* ; prolonged labor; delayed colostral intake
(2) Poor colostral quality; prolonged gestation; fetal distress/anoxia *in utero* ; delayed colostral intake
(3) Poor colostral quality; delayed colostral ingestion; premature delivery; dystocia
(4) Prolonged labor; fetal distress/anoxia *in utero* ; dysmaturity; exposure to infectious disease
(5) Poor colostral quality; fetal distress/anoxia *in utero* ; delayed colostral intake; dysmaturity

32. Which one of the following statements regarding *Mycobacterium paratuberculosis* infection is true?

(1) It may be acquired from clinically or subclinically affected animals.
(2) It can occur at anytime past 1 year of age in cattle, pigs, and small ruminants.
(3) It is limited in effect to the large intestine.
(4) It is invariably fatal in cattle.
(5) It generally causes diarrhea in cattle and small ruminants.

33. A veterinarian is called to a dairy farm to attend to three sick calves. These are 3 of 20 calves that are ages 4–6 months and were turned out to pasture yesterday. On physical examination, these calves are recumbent and unable to stand but appear bright and alert. The calves have increased heart and respiratory rates. The most likely diagnosis is:

(1) paralytic myoglobinuria.
(2) white muscle disease.
(3) tying-up syndrome.
(4) blackleg.
(5) osteomyelitis.

34. A mature Jersey cow on pasture has a yellow-orange bilateral nasal discharge, irritation and pruritus of the nasal cavity, and is sneezing. What is the most likely diagnosis?

(1) Ethmoid carcinoma
(2) Nasal bot fly infestation
(3) Bovine malignant catarrh (BMC)
(4) Chronic infectious bovine rhinotracheitis (IBR) infection
(5) Allergic rhinitis

35. A 6-week-old dairy calf is exhibiting periodic episodes of convulsions and opisthotonos, interspersed with relatively normal periods characterized by hyperesthesia and a hyper-alert attitude. The calf is not blind and is fed primarily a whole-milk diet. The veterinarian's primary differential diagnosis is:

(1) polioencephalomalacia.
(2) hypomagnesemic tetany.
(3) lead poisoning.
(4) tetanus.
(5) nervous ketosis.

36. Which one of the following disorders causes primary equine hyperparathyroidism?

(1) Nutritional imbalances
(2) Mineralization of soft tissues
(3) Hyperplasia or neoplasia of the parathyroid glands
(4) Renal disease
(5) Excessive corticosteroid administration

37. Which one of the following neoplastic diseases is thought to have a viral etiology?

(1) Multicentric lymphoma in a 5-year-old cow
(2) Cutaneous lymphoma in a 1-year-old calf
(3) Thymic lymphoma in a 9-month-old calf
(4) Cutaneous lymphoma in a 12-year-old horse
(5) Multicentric lymphoma in a 6-month-old calf

38. Endotoxemia occurs with various disease processes. Of the following disease processes, which might you expect to be associated with endotoxemia?

(1) Strangles, dermatophilosis, salmonellosis
(2) Salmonellosis, strangles, neonatal septicemia
(3) White muscle disease, dermatophilosis, proximal enteritis
(4) Laminitis in horses, white muscle disease, clostridiosis
(5) Proximal enteritis, neonatal septicemia, laminitis in horses

39. Enzootic pneumonia as a clinical condition is described as existing in:

(1) dairy cows, foals, and piglets.
(2) dairy calves, lambs, and feeder pigs.
(3) dairy cows, lambs, and foals.
(4) broodmares, dairy calves, and piglets.
(5) feeder pigs, broodmares, and mature goats.

40. Knowing that mixed infections occur frequently in neonatal calf diarrhea and serve to confound and diminish the usefulness of etiologic diagnoses, a veterinarian often makes recommendations to an owner prior to receiving laboratory results regarding fecal pathogens. Which recommendation is most appropriate?

(1) Decrease contamination in the calving area by improving hygiene
(2) Vaccinate any cows remaining to freshen during the last 10 days of gestation
(3) Treat calves at birth with twice the dose of oral antibiotics at twice the recommended frequency
(4) Decrease the amount of milk fed to normal calves during the first 7 days of life
(5) Mix oral electrolytes with water when feeding calves

41. A horse recently developed fever, a serous nasal discharge, a cough, stiffness, and transient limb edema. These signs were followed by the development of a cardiac arrhythmia. What is the most likely diagnosis?

(1) Equine adenovirus infection complicated by myocarditis
(2) Equine influenza virus infection complicated by myocarditis and myositis
(3) Equine herpes rhinopneumonitis or neurologic disease
(4) Respiratory and cardiac form of equine viral arteritis (EVA)
(5) Strangles followed by *Streptococcus*-associated myocarditis

42. Which statement regarding equine tying-up syndrome is correct? Equine tying-up syndrome:

(1) is a vitamin E- or selenium-responsive condition.
(2) is a synonym for equine laminitis.
(3) is confined to young, rapidly growing animals.
(4) may cause brown-colored urine.
(5) results from chronic liver disease.

43. An 8-year-old Holstein cow is seen by a veterinarian for the complaint of ventral abdominal distention and decreased milk production. Physical examination reveals muffled heart sounds, mild tachycardia (heart rate is 84 beats/min), ascites, and brisket edema. The lung sounds are dull cranioventrally. Rectal examination reveals enlarged mesenteric lymph nodes. Complete blood cell count (CBC) reveals anemia and lymphocytosis with a normal fibrinogen concentration and neutrophil count. What is the most likely diagnosis and how should this diagnosis be confirmed?

(1) Bacterial endocarditis (BE) confirmed by blood cultures
(2) Reticulopericarditis confirmed with radiographs of the cranial abdomen to look for wire
(3) Lymphosarcoma caused by bovine leukemia virus (BLV) confirmed by viral isolation from the buffy coat of white blood cells and by locating a neoplastic mass on the right atrium with echocardiography
(4) Myocarditis caused by *Borrelia burgdorferi* confirmed by finding the tick
(5) High altitude disease (cor pulmonale) confirmed by elevated pulmonary artery (PA) pressures found by cardiac catheterization

44. A dairy client has an unacceptable prevalence of *Staphylococcus aureus* mastitis. Which one of the following statements is the best advice?

(1) Treat all cases of clinical mastitis with intramammary penicillin during lactation.
(2) Cull animals with *S. aureus* or segregate and milk separately.
(3) Immediately cease milking all culture-positive cows and dry teat.
(4) Treat all culture-positive cows with intramuscular penicillin.
(5) Strip out affected quarters from culture-positive cows every 2 hours.

45. In a pig barn with problems of low-grade cough, prolonged time to reach market weight, and some carcasses showing cranoventral lung consolidation and peribronchial lymphoid cuffing, what is the most likely diagnosis?

(1) Porcine reproductive and respiratory syndrome (PRRS)
(2) Enzootic pneumonia caused by inadequate ventilation
(3) Chronic form of *Actinobacillus* (*Hemophilus*) *pleuropneumonia*
(4) Swine influenza followed by secondary *Pasteurella multocida* pneumonia
(5) *Mycoplasma hypopneumoniae* infection in the herd

46. Hypomagnesemic tetany of ruminants also may be known as:

(1) milk fever, grass staggers, or alkali disease.
(2) grass tetany, milk fever, or alkali disease.
(3) "downer cow" syndrome, wheat pasture poisoning, or grass tetany.
(4) lactation tetany, grass staggers, or wheat pasture poisoning.
(5) "downer cow" syndrome, lactation tetany, or eclampsia.

47. In ruminants with obstructive urolithiasis, which one of the following clinical scenarios is most likely?

(1) In cases of complete urethral obstruction with bladder rupture, there is inappetence, depression and colic signs with kicking at the abdomen.
(2) Straining to urinate may be sufficient to prolapse the rectum, and obstructed sheep may also show tail wriggling.
(3) For early cases in which urethral or bladder rupture have yet to occur, it is possible to attempt medical therapy by passing a catheter retrograde into the bladder.
(4) If the bladder is ruptured, surgical closure of the defect is usually required for the steer to resume urine flow.
(5) In sheep and goats, the obstruction at the vermiform appendage is often a solitary calculus that can be crushed to allow the free flow of urine.

48. A veterinarian is called to examine a 19-year-old, grey, Hunter-type gelding because the owner had noticed that the horse had been losing weight over the past 2 months. Clinical examination reveals the horse to be severely underweight, but there are no other abnormal findings. Weight loss without other abnormal findings could be caused by:

(1) chronic obstructive pulmonary disease (COPD), liver flukes, or lymphosarcoma.
(2) lymphosarcoma, squamous cell carcinoma of the stomach, or COPD.
(3) liver flukes, malnutrition, or intestinal clostridiosis.
(4) squamous cell carcinoma of the stomach, malnutrition, or granulomatous enteritis.
(5) intestinal clostridiosis, lymphosarcoma, or squamous cell carcinoma of the stomach.

49. A 4-day-old calf has stopped nursing during the previous 12 hours, is depressed, lacks a menace reflex, has a rectal temperature of 39.9°C, and is showing signs of a stiff neck. The calf had a normal birth and suckled well on the first day. Which one of the following statements is correct?

(1) If this were a foal, the signs are typical for neonatal maladjustment syndrome (NMS).
(2) Intrauterine bovine virus diarrhea (BVD) infection at mid-gestation could explain these signs.
(3) An important part of the diagnostic regimen is a cerebrospinal fluid (CSF) sample and test for passive transfer.
(4) The depression and lack of menace reflex suggest hydrocephalus or hydranencephaly; therefore, there is no treatment for this calf.

50. The proper treatments for sole ulcer include:

(1) corrective trimming, pressure bandaging, and claw elevation (block).
(2) systemic antibiotics, corrective trimming, and footbaths.
(3) claw elevation (block), systemic antibiotics, and footbaths.
(4) corticosteroids, pressure bandaging, and corrective trimming.
(5) tetracycline sprays, systemic antibiotics, and pressure bandaging.

51. Which one of the following statements regarding bovine leukosis is true?

(1) It is spread primarily via aerosol infection.
(2) It may produce signs of spinal cord disease.
(3) It is preventable through vaccination.
(4) It manifests as lymphosarcoma in most patients.
(5) It has been proven to be a zoonosis.

52. Which one of the following conditions would likely cause abdominal pain in foals?

(1) Meconium impaction, gastric ulceration, cryptosporidiosis
(2) Gastric ulceration, granulomatous enteritis, ascarid impaction
(3) Meconium impaction, intussusception, ascarid impaction
(4) Intussusception, cryptosporidiosis, abdominal hernias
(5) Abdominal hernias, granulomatous enteritis, small intestinal volvulus

53. In the late summer, a 6-month-old Holstein heifer has had signs of depression and recumbency over the last 24 hours. Two other calves (of a group of 10) have died in the past week. The owner thinks the animals may have convulsed before they died. The other calves had loose, bloody stools and were being treated for presumed coccidiosis with amprolium, as well as with oral trimethoprim-sulfa and a multivitamin complex.

On physical examination of this 6-month-old calf, all vital signs are mildly elevated. The animal is depressed, is in left lateral recumbency, and has its head back (i.e., opisthotonos). Reflexes are intact, but the calf will not support itself in sternal recumbency. Menace reflex is absent bilaterally, but pupillary light reflexes are intact, and there is a dorsomedial strabismus. The state of hydration and mucous membranes are normal, feces appear to be formed, and there is normal rumen motility. What is the most likely diagnosis?

(1) Lead toxicity
(2) Polioencephalomalacia
(3) Nervous coccidiosis
(4) Thromboembolic meningoencephalitis (TEME)
(5) Vitamin A deficiency

54. Of the following treatments, the best therapy for acute coliform mastitis is:

(1) intramammary treatment with gentamicin.
(2) oral fluids.
(3) stripping the affected quarters frequently.
(4) intravenous calcium.
(5) 500 mg of dexamethasone twice daily for 7 days.

55. A veterinarian auscultates a 2-month-old calf that is small for its age. On auscultation, the veterinarian hears a grade III pansystolic murmur on both sides of the chest. When a cardiac catheterization is performed, elevated cardiac pressures, particularly in the right ventricle, are found. The most likely heart defect is:

(1) patent ductus arteriosus (PDA).
(2) ventricular septal defect (VSD).
(3) vegetative endocarditis involving the right atrioventricular (AV) valve.
(4) right AV valvular insufficiency.
(5) aortic insufficiency.

56. A veterinarian is called to examine an 8-year-old Thoroughbred mare with a 12-hour history of anorexia, depression, and the voidance of reddish brown urine. Physical examination reveals a rectal temperature of 39.8° C, a heart rate of 80 beats/min, and a respiratory rate of 30 breaths/min. The horse's mucous membranes are pale and her sclerae are icteric. Laboratory findings include a packed cell volume (PCV) of 16.2% and red-tinged plasma. The discoloration of the plasma remains after centrifugation. The urine is positive for occult blood and protein. Based on the clinical and laboratory findings, what is the most likely set of differential diagnoses?

(1) Acute glomerulonephritis, equine infectious anemia (EIA), anaplasmosis, red maple leaf toxicosis
(2) Babesiosis, EIA, red maple leaf toxicosis, autoimmune hemolytic anemia
(3) Babesiosis, equine exertional rhabdomyolysis, phenothiazine toxicosis, anaplasmosis
(4) Equine exertional rhabdomyolysis, pyelonephritis, EIA, phenothiazine toxicosis
(5) Babesiosis, autoimmune hemolytic anemia, pyelonephritis, equine exertional rhabdomyolysis

57. A 4-year-old Standardbred horse with a history of hind limb ataxia for 1 month exhibits muscle atrophy to the left gluteal region. The same sign is exhibited in 15 other horses, including brood mares and foals, none of which have had any recent signs of illness. Which one of the following statements is correct?

(1) A cerebrospinal fluid (CSF) sample should be obtained and assessed for evidence of sarcocystic neuron exposure.
(2) Cervical radiographs with myelography are the most likely method of diagnosis.
(3) Green pasture and fodder with supplemental vitamin E might have prevented this problem.
(4) A CSF sample of high protein with the lack of inflammatory cells will likely be found given this history.
(5) Finding eosinophils in the CSF is highly suggestive of equine protozoal myeloencephalitis (EPM).

58. Examination of the right rear foot of a mature dairy cow reveals warmth and swelling of the coronet. Also, there is a moist, red fissure in between the claws and a foul odor to the foot. The most likely diagnosis is:

(1) infectious pododermatitis.
(2) stable foot rot.
(3) laminitis.
(4) greasy heel.
(5) underrun sole.

59. Crushing deaths of piglets often may be related to:

(1) lactation tetany of sows.
(2) liver disease of piglets.
(3) vitamin E and selenium deficiency of piglets.
(4) hypothermia and hypoglycemia of piglets.
(5) iron deficiency of piglets.

60. Which one of the following statements regarding cryptosporidiosis is true?

(1) It is a skin disease of horses.
(2) It is a secretory diarrhea of calves.
(3) It is a pyogranulomatous lung infection of pigs.
(4) It is a foot (hoof) disease of sheep.
(5) It is an arthritis of goats.

61. Neonatal isoerythrolysis is diagnosed in a mule foal with acute hemolytic anemia. Which one of the following transfusion treatments would be the most appropriate?

(1) Whole blood from a male horse related to the dam
(2) Whole blood from the (horse) dam
(3) Washed erythrocytes from the (donkey) sire
(4) Plasma from a horse lacking the Aa or Qa blood group antigens
(5) Washed erythrocytes from an unrelated male donkey

62. A 15-year-old Arabian mare is brought to a veterinarian because of recurrent episodes of colic. Differential diagnoses would include which of the following?

(1) Enterolith, pedunculated lipoma, salmonellosis
(2) Enterolith, *Dictyocaulus arnfieldi* infestation, thromboembolic infarction
(3) Pendunculated lipoma, parasitic larval migration, intestinal foreign body
(4) Thromboembolic infarction, salmonellosis, sand impaction
(5) Sand impaction, *D. arnfieldi* infestation, feed impaction

63. Which set of signs is most consistent with lead toxicity in large animals?

(1) The chronic form is reported in horses and can manifest as paralysis of the recurrent laryngeal nerve and the pharynx, resulting in recurrent choke, regurgitation of food, and aspiration pneumonia.
(2) The acute form often shows a sudden onset and short duration of disease occurring within 12–24 hours.
(3) In the subacute form, in addition to neurologic signs of depression and blindness with nonreactive pupils, there are also signs of gastroenteritis (e.g., ruminal atony accompanied by constipation in the early stages), followed by fetid diarrhea (caused by abomasitis from lead salts).
(4) A key clinical sign to differentiate from polioencephalomalacia (PEM; a major differential diagnosis) is rumen motility, which is only mildly reduced in lead toxicity. The rumen is often fluid filled and atonic in PEM due to the diet change.

64. A veterinarian examines a 22-hour-old Thoroughbred filly that was born on a farm with above-average to excellent management conditions. The foal is vigorous and in excellent health as far as the veterinarian can ascertain. Because the mare reportedly leaked some colostrum immediately prior to foaling, the veterinarian decides to evaluate the foal's immunoglobulin concentration using an enzyme-linked immunosorbent assay (ELISA) test. The immunoglobulin G (IgG) concentration is greater than 400 mg/dl, but less than 800 mg/dl. Based on this result, the veterinarian should:

(1) supplement the foal with additional mare colostrum.
(2) supplement the foal with bovine colostrum.
(3) administer 2 L of commercial plasma intravenously.
(4) treat the foal with broad-spectrum antibiotics.
(5) not do anything.

DIRECTIONS: Each of the numbered items or incomplete statements in this section is negatively phrased, as indicated by a capitalized word such as NOT, LEAST, or EXCEPT. Select the ONE numbered answer or completion that is BEST in each case.

65. An effective intestinal parasite control program for sheep in North America would NOT include:

(1) prelambing deworming of adults with ivermectin.
(2) deworming of lambs in the spring before turning them out on pasture.
(3) raising lambs indoors and feeding hay from elevated racks.
(4) use of pastures grazed by cattle for rotation into sheep grazing.
(5) deworming of feeder lambs every 3 weeks during the winter with thiabendazole.

66. Which one of the following does NOT typically cause regenerative anemia?

(1) Postparturient hemoglobinuria
(2) Acute blood loss
(3) Iron deficiency
(4) Onion toxicosis
(5) *Anaplasma marginale* infection

67. Clinical findings with dental disease in horses include all of the following EXCEPT:

(1) quidding.
(2) eating hay in preference to grain.
(3) slow, painful mastication.
(4) weight loss.
(5) choke.

68. A dairy cow in the second week of lactation is noted to have pale mucous membranes, tachycardia, weakness, and hemoglobinuria. Which one of the following would NOT be a logical course of action?

(1) Increase efforts to control arthropods.
(2) Examine the phosphorous content of the ration.
(3) Examine urine by dark-field microscopy.
(4) Check the animal's diet for oxidant-containing plants.
(5) Examine erythrocytes for rickettsial organisms.

69. All of the following patients should undergo surgical repair for patent urachus EXCEPT:

(1) A hospitalized foal younger than 5 days old with a normal rectal temperature, normal results on a complete blood count (CBC), and a normal fibrinogen concentration.
(2) A foal with urine continuing to dribble from the urachus 1 week following cauterization with silver nitrate.
(3) A foal in which ultrasound examination of the umbilicus reveals urachal abscess.
(4) A foal with an umbilicus that is hot and painful on palpation and exuding a purulent discharge.
(5) A foal that has evidence of subcutaneous fluid accumulation in the area of the external umbilical remnants.

70. A Holstein calf is suspected of having bovine leukocyte adhesion deficiency (BLAD). Which one of the following findings is NOT characteristic of BLAD?

(1) Persistent neutropenia
(2) Lymphadenopathy
(3) Gingivitis
(4) Fever
(5) Bronchopneumonia

71. Several weanling beef calves die from excessive hemorrhage after dehorning. The farmer has additional calves to dehorn. Which one of the following recommendations would NOT be correct?

(1) Determine that the prothrombin time is normal before dehorning more calves.
(2) Only feed sweet clover as silage.
(3) Analyze feed for dicoumarol or related compounds.
(4) Treat calves with vitamin K_1.
(5) Discard all moldy sweet clover hay.

ANSWERS AND EXPLANATIONS

1. The answer is 5 [Chapter 16 III D 2]. This clinical picture best fits primary copper deficiency or molybdenum excess. Ergot (*Claviceps purpura*) contamination of feed results in gangrene of the extremities. Chronic selenium toxicosis results in laminitis and hair loss, which is usually most prominent on the tail. Iodine toxicity clinically presents as increased lacrimation, epiphora, nasal discharge, seborrhea, and hair loss.

2. The answer is 2 [Chapter 1 I I 1]. The set of clinical findings best describes oral necrobacillosis (necrotic stomatitis). Actinobacillosis involves the tongue, whereas actinomycosis is an osteomyelitis usually of the mandible. Vesicular exanthema is a disease of swine. Bovine papular stomatitis produces only mild clinical signs with oral papules or coalescent lesions on the muzzle and oral mucous membranes.

3. The answer is 3 [Chapter 8 II B 6 c]. Bacterial endocarditis (BE) in swine is frequently caused by either *Streptococcus* species or *Erysipelothrix rhusiopathiae*. *Actinobacillus equuli* is one of the two common organisms associated with the disease in horses. *Actinomyces pyogenes* is frequently isolated from affected cattle.

4. The answer is 2 [Chapter 10 III A 3 b (1)]. In equine Cushing's disease, polyuria may result from excessive cortisol secretion. Excessive cortisol secretion results from chronic adrenocorticotropic hormone (ACTH) release by the pituitary gland. High cortisol levels may block antidiuretic hormone (ADH) or its effect on the kidney. Also, the hyperglycemia resulting from excessive corticosteroid levels may cause an osmotic diuresis.

5. The answer is 2 [Chapter 4 II B 1, 2]. Both Johne's disease and visceral caseous lymphadenitis (CLA) cause chronic weight loss in adult goats. Coccidiosis causes diarrhea in young ruminants, whereas gastrointestinal helminths usually produce a herd level problem with poor growth rates and poor performance. Abomasal emptying defect is a specific condition reported only in Suffolk sheep.

6. The answer is 5 [Chapter 12 I A 3–4]. In a horse with the acute onset of blepharospasm, tearing, and photophobia in one eye, fluorescein dye should be applied to the cornea to detect any ulcers. If ulcers are present, correct therapy entails the administration of antibiotics and cytoplegics. Antiviral agents have not been employed with any reliability and in this case, the lesion is only in one eye, decreasing the likelihood of a systemic viral event, which more commonly results in bilateral lesions. Broad-spectrum antibiotics are not necessary if there is no ulcer or severe conjunctivitis present. If overused, broad-spectrum antibiotics may lead to mycotic superinfection.

7. The answer is 5 [Chapter 5 II A 3 a (2), d (2)]. Recurrent abdominal pain, obstructive icterus (as evidenced by the increased serum levels of cholestatic enzymes, conjugated bilirubinemia, and bilirubinuria), and an inflammatory leukogram are most consistent with a diagnosis of cholelithiasis. Theiler's disease does not present as recurrent abdominal pain, or with laboratory evidence of obstructive icterus. Tyzzer's disease is a disease of young foals, not adult horses. Horses with either thromboembolic colic or a mesenteric abscess will present with recurrent abdominal pain and an inflammatory leukogram, but not with signs of obstructive icterus.

8. The answer is 2 [Chapter 2 I A 2]. Some colics that respond to medical management, such as those due to gastric dilatation, present with severe pain and anxiety. Clinical examinations should be performed as much as possible without sedation of the animal so as not to mask clinical findings. Rectal examinations should always be performed as part of the complete physical examination when presented with a horse exhibiting abdominal pain. Abdominal distention is not present in cases of small intestinal obstruction because any distention is restricted by the thoracic cage. High rectal temperatures are most often associated with non-surgical conditions, such as bacterial infections.

9. The answer is 2 [Chapter 3 I C 2]. Cecal torsion or abomasal volvulus are the most likely causes of this cow's distress. The gas-filled viscus on the right side of a mature cow must be either the cecum or the abomasum. This cow is clearly in shock, suggesting that circulation to the viscus must be compromised. Therefore, the viscus is most certainly twisted (as a result of torsion or volvulus), rather than simply displaced or distended. A diffuse peritonitis may produce auscultable abdominal gas, but the ability to detect the displaced viscus via rectal palpation defines the involvement of the abomasum or cecum.

10. The answer is 3 [Chapter 14 I A 2 c (1)]. Compared with human beings and small animal species, all large animals, particularly small ruminants, have relative microcytosis. True microcytosis is most commonly seen with iron deficiency, when erythrocytes contain less hemoglobin than normal.

11. The answer is 4 [Chapter 11 II D 2]. Individual cattle may exhibit nervous signs (convulsions) with coccidiosis. Coccidiosis is most commonly a disease associated with high morbidity rates (i.e., many animals are affected) but low mortality rates (i.e., few animals die). Although *Eimeria* species are commonly pathogenic to ruminants, *Isospora* species cause disease in pigs. Treatment of individuals is less rewarding than prevention, which is carried out through a combination of coccidiostats and improvements in hygiene. Animals may exhibit disease (diarrhea) prior to the passage of oocysts in the feces, but healthy animals can also shed fecal oocysts.

12. The answer is 2 [Chapter 18 IV C 3 j]. γ-Glutamyl transferase (GGT) activity greater than 300 IU/L usually indicates that a calf has consumed adequate amounts of colostrum. Colostral GGT concentration in the bovine is approximately 300 times the serum GGT concentration. Diagnoses of septicemia or liver involvement are unlikely in a calf that appears systemically healthy. Renal failure should not cause an increase in GGT activity in serum.

13. The answer is 1 [Chapter 9 II B]. Hyperkalemic periodic paralysis (HYPP) is described as a heritable muscle disease of horses (Quarter horses, Appaloosas, American point horses, and Quarter horse crosses) and humans. In humans, it is referred to as HYPP or adynamia episodica hereditaria. Defective sodium channels in the nervous system remain open after membrane depolarization, allowing excessive inward sodium movement and heightened membrane depolarization. Simultaneously, normal sodium channels may be in-

activated, preventing the development of normal action potentials and leading to muscular weakness. Affected horses exhibit muscle fasciculations and spasms of the face, jaws, and legs, followed by weakness and recumbency.

14. The answer is 5 [Chapter 7 I B 4 b]. *Actinobacillus pleuropneumonia* causes porcine pleuropneumonia. When introduced into naive herds, the bacteria cause signs of pneumonia (fever, coughing, abnormal respiratory patterns). Morbidity and mortality rates are usually highest in the feeder pig population.

15. The answer is 2 [Chapter 13 II B 2, 5]. This set of clinical findings (i.e., swollen abscesses on the mandibles that discharge a thick, yellowish material and do not resolve with antibiotic treatment) best describes actinomycosis (lumpy jaw). Cancerous, degenerative, or nutritional deficiencies do not match the clinical findings or subjective information presented.

16. The answer is 1 [Chapter 16 V F 2]. Diamond-shaped skin lesions occurring in pigs that are anorexic and feverish are most likely caused by *Erysipelas*. Exudative dermatitis or greasy pig disease is a seborrheic skin condition. Ringworm is not accompanied by systemic signs. Sporotrichosis is a nodular disease of horses. Sarcoptic mange affects pigs, but the primary clinical finding is pruritus.

17. The answer is 2 [Chapter 17 I C 6 b]. The set of clinical findings (i.e., sudden drop in milk production, painless udder swelling of all four quarters in affected cows, concurrent problems with pneumonia and lameness, fine grit in the bottom of the sample cup) best fits the pattern of disease experienced with an outbreak of *Mycoplasma* mastitis.

18. The answer is 1 [Chapter 8 II C 2, 5]. The horse is suffering from jugular vein thrombophlebitis. The horse has several of the predisposing factors for the development of this condition, including protracted duration of catheter indwelling (more than 3 days), possible endotoxemia or septicemia from colitis leading to a coagulopathy, and administration of plasma and other fluid products through the catheter. Physical examination findings (i.e., a painful neck, head edema, depression, reluctance to put its head down to eat) support the diagnosis. Treatment includes the removal of the catheter, topical hydrotherapy or hot packs, topical anti-inflammatory agents such as dimethyl sulfoxide (DMSO), and appropriate antibiotics. Congestive heart failure (CHF) should not cause a painful neck and is not a likely consequence of acute colitis. Purpura hemorrhagica causes a vasculitis, usually resulting in leg and ventral abdominal edema, in addition to bottle jaw. A history of respiratory disease is usually present. Cardiac arrhythmias due to electrolyte imbalances do not result in a painful neck. Signs of CHF (such as head edema) are a late sequelae to cardiac arrhythmias, and other clinical signs should be apparent at that time (e.g., jugular vein distention, jugular pulses, ascites).

19. The answer is 4 [Chapter 12 III A 4]. Sarcoids, squamous cell carcinomas (SCCs), and habronemiasis have similar clinical presentations and often cannot be diagnosed definitively without the aid of histopathology. A biopsy with histopathologic examination is suggested to rule out other types of tumors and habronemiasis.

20. The answer is 1 [Chapter 15 I A 1 c]. Causes of acute renal failure in horses include the administration of nephrotoxic medications, the consumption of red maple leaves, and the accidental consumption of mercury. Obstruction does not commonly occur in horses. Calcium carbonate crystals are normally found in horse urine, and the alkaline urine readily dissolves casts. Some normal foals can have serum creatinine elevations temporarily after birth, and foals also have dilute urine at this time. Biopsy is not of value and poses a risk to the patient.

21. The answer is 1 [Chapter 2 III A]. The 6-year-old riding horse most likely has granulomatous enteritis (lymphocytic-plasmacytic enteritis), an immune-mediated disorder that causes a malabsorption syndrome. Characteristic findings include a chronic, nonresponsive diarrhea and possibly ventral edema. Equine monocytic ehrlichiosis (Potomac horse fever) is characterized by acute, watery diarrhea that lasts approximately 10 days in most horses. Gastric ulceration is associated with recurrent abdominal pain more often than diarrhea, and there is usually a history of nonsteroidal anti-inflammatory drug (NSAID) use. Chronic impaction of the small intestine would more likely be associated with colic than diarrhea.

22. The answer is 3 [Chapter 10 VII C 2]. Horses with anhidrosis may be completely un-

able to sweat or exhibit only partial sweating. Serum sodium levels are not affected, and the condition is not known to be genetic. There is no age, breed, or sex predilection. Anhidrosis is diagnosed by clinical findings, and treatment is symptomatic.

23. The answer is 2 [Chapter 8 V B 1]. Sheep and goats (particularly young animals) are more susceptible to the signs of gossypol toxicosis than cattle. Adult ruminants are able to detoxify gossypol by forming stable complexes with soluble proteins in the rumen. The 22% protein/trace mineral supplement labeled for beef cattle, which was being fed, revealed high amounts of free gossypol/kg in the supplement, and there were also high amounts of gossypol in the concentrate mix. Gossypol toxicosis results in cardiomyopathy by inactivating enzymes that are important in allowing myocardial cells to respond to oxidative stress. The sheep were adequately dewormed, so chronic parasitism or liver flukes were unlikely. Acute hepatotoxicity usually results in gastrointestinal or neurologic signs before causing congestive heart failure (CHF). Ovine progressive pneumonia virus infection usually results in pneumonia in older goats or may be a cause of ill thrift or mastitis.

24. The answer is 2 [Chapter 11 II C 1 b (1), 2 b (1) (b)]. Blindness is a finding in calves with polioencephalomalacia and in cattle with lead poisoning. Recurrent uveitis (blindness) in horses often develops as a sequela to systemic leptospirosis; however, neither listeriosis in sheep nor vitamin D toxicosis in cattle have blindness associated with the clinical picture.

25. The answer is 4 [Chapter 5 III A 1 c, e]. The organism most often responsible for causing liver abscesses is *Fusobacterium necrophorum*. Long-term penicillin or tetracycline therapy is indicated for the treatment of individual affected animals.

26. The answer is 5 [Chapter 14 I D 2 a (2) (c), (d)]. The intraerythrocytic protozoon of genus *Babesia* commonly cause intravascular hemolysis, whereas rickettsial organisms and oxidative agents frequently cause extravascular hemolysis. Cobalt deficiency is associated with depression anemia but not hemolysis.

27. The answer is 1 [Chapter 2 II B 1]. The most likely diagnosis in this case is foal heat diarrhea. These patients require symptomatic and supportive care only (e.g., application of petroleum jelly to the perineum). Other tests and treatments are only warranted if clinical signs deteriorate or if the condition persists. Observing the foal closely is valuable advice but separating the foal and the mare and providing for only two daily feedings would surely limit calorie intake for the foal. Meconium impaction is seen in younger foals presenting with straining, inappetence, abdominal distention, and an inability to pass feces.

28. The answer is 5 [Chapter 7 I F 2 b]. The clinical description best fits chronic obstructive pulmonary disease (COPD). The cough reflects a pulmonary hyperreactivity to airborne antigens, and the lower airway cytology will be neutrophilic because of immune, rather than bacterial, stimulation. Failure of the atropine challenge test reflects a chronic, irreversible bronchospasm, which indicates limited value of bronchodilator therapy. Management practice to reduce environment dust and pollution must be continuous and permanent. Likewise, low-dose corticosteroids may be instituted as long-term therapy in the chronically affected horse. Finally, nondegenerative neutrophils in the bronchoalveolar exudate is suggestive of COPD.

29. The answer is 5 [Chapter 8 II B 6 e]. The clinical findings best support a diagnosis of right-sided heart failure and tricuspid regurgitation. Right-sided heart failure and tricuspid regurgitation may be caused by bacterial endocarditis, septic pericarditis, and myocardial lymphosarcoma, as well as by cor pulmonale. Aortic valve insufficiency produces a left-sided heart murmur with subsequent signs of congestive heart failure (CHF). Pyrrolizidine alkaloid toxicosis produces hepatic dysfunction with resultant liver, central nervous system (CNS), gastrointestinal, or skin disease. Acute grain overload causes bloat, depression, dehydration, acidemia, diarrhea, and death.

30. The answer is 2 [Chapter 4 II A 3]. Pulpy kidney disease (enterotoxemia, overeating disease) is caused by *Clostridium perfringens* type D. The most common manifestation is sudden death in growing sheep on high-energy (fattening) diets. Salmonellosis usually presents as fever, depression, and hemorrhagic diarrhea. Shipping fever is a disease of beef cattle characterized by pneumonia. Abomasal emptying defect, a condition of Suffolk sheep, causes signs of anorexia and

chronic wasting. Coccidiosis causes a severe, watery diarrhea in lambs.

31. The answer is 5 [Chapter 18 III C 2 c (3) (c); IV A 2 b (1), B 1 a (2); Table 18-3]. The risk factors present in this foal are poor colostral quality, fetal distress/anoxia *in utero*, delayed colostral intake, and dysmaturity. The mare leaked colostrum prior to delivery, therefore, colostral quality is probably poor. Meconium staining indicates that fetal distress/anoxia was present during the birth process. Colostral intake was delayed; foals should start suckling no later than 3 hours after birth. Although the foal was not born prematurely by most definitions, it has many characteristics indicating dysmaturity, including a silky haircoat, lax flexor tendons, and a domed forehead.

32. The answer is 1 [Chapter 3 II B 2 e (3) (c); Chapter 4 II B 1]. Both clinically and subclinically affected animals will shed *Mycobacterium paratuberculosis*, which may then be ingested by susceptible animals. *M. paratuberculosis* infection, also known as Johne's disease or paratuberculosis, can affect cattle and small ruminants, but is not known to infect pigs. Infection initially causes histologic lesions in the small intestines and associated mesenteric lymph nodes and later affects the large intestine. *M. paratuberculosis* is not invariably fatal. There is evidence that the organism may be acquired and eliminated by many animals. Although diarrhea occurs in diseased cattle, in small ruminants (i.e., sheep and goats) it is more common to find emaciation without diarrhea.

33. The answer is 2 [Chapter 13 I A 2 a (2) (a)]. White muscle disease is the most likely condition given the set of clinical findings. Paralytic myoglobinuria occurs in older, heavily muscled animals. Tying-up syndrome is a condition of horses, and blackleg of cattle results most commonly in sudden death of older animals. With osteomyelitis, there should be evidence of a swollen, painful lesion usually over a joint.

34. The answer is 5 [Chapter 6 I B]. The Jersey cow has clinical signs that are typical for allergic rhinitis (i.e., characteristic color to the nasal discharge, bilateral nature of the discharge, nasal pruritus). The discharge from ethmoid carcinoma is more often unilateral and signs of blocked nasal passages are prominent, with no sneezing or nasal pruritus. Nasal bot flies are not known to affect cattle. Malignant bovine catarrh (MBC) is a systemic disease with far more severe signs, such as erosion of the nares, fever, and lymphadenopathy. Infectious bovine rhinotracheitis (IBR) does not present with signs specific to nasal irritation.

35. The answer is 2 [Chapter 9 I I 2 b]. Dairy calves on whole-milk diets are able to absorb less magnesium as they age. This set of clinical findings best fits a diagnosis of hypomagnesemic tetany. With polioencephalomalacia and lead poisoning, calves are blind or apparently blind. Tetanus presents with more tetanic signs, and nervous ketosis is a disease of early lactation mature cows.

36. The answer is 3 [Chapter 10 VI A 3]. In horses, primary hyperparathyroidism is the result of parathyroid hyperplasia or neoplasia.

37. The answer is 1 [Chapter 14 III A 1 b (1)]. Multicentric lymphoma in adult cattle (older than 3 years) is almost always associated with infection with the bovine leukosis virus (BLV). None of the other forms of lymphoma in horses or cattle is thought to have a viral etiology.

38. The answer is 5 [Chapter 2 I B 4 c (2)]. Laminitis (caused by gastrointestinal disease), neonatal septicemias (many of which are caused by gram-negative infections), and proximal enteritis (believed to be associated with gram-negative overgrowth) can all be associated with endotoxemia. Endotoxin (lipopolysaccharide endotoxin) is the cell wall of dying gram-negative organisms. Therefore, strangles (*Streptococcus equi* infection) clostridiosis, and dermatophilosis (*Dermatophilus congolensis* infection)—conditions produced by gram-positive organisms—do not result in endotoxemia. White muscle disease is a vitamin E/selenium deficiency of calves.

39. The answer is 2 [Chapter 7 I A 3–4, B 4 a]. Clinically, enzootic pneumonia is described in calves, growing (feeder) pigs, sheep (particularly lambs), and kids. Enzootic pneumonia is a chronic, nonprogressive pneumonia characterized by a low mortality rate but producing significant growth retardation in affected animals. It is most prevalent under conditions of overcrowding and intensive management. In calves, the disease process may begin as a viral respiratory infection that may

resolve or become complicated by bacterial infection, mycoplasmal infection (e.g., *Mycoplasma bovis, Mycoplasma dispar, Mycoplasma bovirhinis, Ureaplasma*), or both (multifactorial). *Mycoplasma hyopneumoniae* is the most common causative organism in feeder pigs. In lambs, infections caused by *Mycoplasma ovipneumonia, Bordetella parapertussis, Chlamydia*, and some viruses are believed to predispose the lung to invasion by *Pasteurella haemolytica*, resulting in pulmonary damage.

40. The answer is 1 [Chapter 3 II B 3]. Although there are many possible, rational recommendations a veterinarian can make regarding prevention of neonatal calf diarrhea, the only sound one in this subset of selections is to decrease contamination in the calving area by improving hygiene. Vaccination of cows must occur at a time prior to production of colostrum to ensure adequate levels of maternal antibody (i.e., 8 weeks prior to parturition). Oral antibiotics have not been shown efficacious in the treatment of enterotoxigenic *Escherichia coli* (ETEC) and are certainly of no value against viral pathogens. Limiting the amount of milk fed to healthy calves has not been shown to prevent diarrhea and there is a growing body of literature that recommends maintaining scouring calves on at least some milk. Milk should never be mixed with oral electrolytes for feeding.

41. The answer is 2 [Chapter 6 II A 3 a (3) (d) (ii), (4) (c)]. Respiratory signs may be accompanied by stiffness and transient limb edema. Myocarditis, which would account for the arrhythmia, may develop in complicated cases of equine influenza virus infection. Equine adenovirus infection is associated with only mild signs of respiratory disease, and no other complications. Equine rhinopneumonitis, caused by a herpesvirus, is unlikely to result in muscle damage. Equine viral arteritis (EVA) is unlikely to cause stiffness and is not associated with myositis or myocarditis. The clinical signs described are not consistent with strangles.

42. The answer is 4 [Chapter 13 I B 2 b]. Degenerating muscle cells release myoglobin at levels that exceed renal threshold and color the urine brown. Tying-up syndrome is not caused by vitamin E or selenium deficiency. It is seen in all ages of horses, and although this syndrome may be an inherited disorder of glycogen storage, it is not associated with liver disease.

43. The answer is 3 [Chapter 8 V A 1 b; V A 5 a (3); V A 5 b]. Bovine leukemia virus (BLV) sporadically causes multicentric lymphosarcoma. The right atrium is one of four common sites of neoplastic infiltration, including the uterus, internal and external lymph nodes, and the abomasum. The disease is virus-associated. Diagnosis includes the isolation of BLV from lymphocytes and echocardiographic evidence of a mass on the right atrium. Persistent lymphocytosis occurs in 33% of cattle infected with BLV. Bacterial endocarditis (BE) usually involves the tricuspid valve in cattle. Signs of right-sided heart failure, including dependent edema and distended jugular or mammary veins, are found in approximately one third of cases. No lymphadenopathy would be expected. A complete blood cell count (CBC) often reveals hyperfibrinogenemia, neutrophilia, and monocytosis. Similar hematologic findings may be found with traumatic reticulopericarditis. Cranial abdominal pain and poor rumen motility may also be found. *Borrelia burgdorferi* has not been definitively identified with myocarditis in cattle. In other species, other clinical findings usually occur in conjunction with cardiac signs, including lameness and fever. Cor pulmonale caused by pulmonary hypertension usually results in respiratory signs as well as cardiac signs. Neither lymphadenopathy nor lymphocytosis usually occur.

44. The answer is 2 [Chapter 17 I B 2 a (7)]. The most economic and medically sound recommendation is to cull or segregate affected animals. Lactation therapy (systemic or intramammary) is an ineffective treatment. Dry cow therapy is recommended, but it does not make economic sense to dry off all cows immediately. Stripping affected quarters is recommended for individual cows suffering from an acute or peracute episode of mastitis, but this is not appropriate with the subacute or subclinical mastitis seen on a herd basis with *Staphylococcus aureus*.

45. The answer is 5 [Chapter 7 I B 4 a]. *Mycoplasma hypopneumoniae* is the causative agent for enzootic pneumonia in growing pigs. Porcine reproductive and respiratory syndrome (PRRS) appears as respiratory distress in piglets. *Actinobacillus pleuropneumonia* can cause a chronic pneumonia but does not exhibit the same pathologic features as enzootic pneumonia. The subset of clinical and pathologic findings in the question best describes an enzootic pneumonia. Although *Pasteurella multocida* is often a secondary invader, swine influenza virus is not known as a primary initiator. Inadequate ventilation by itself does not produce enzootic pneumonia.

46. The answer is 4 [Chapter 9 I I 1]. Lactation tetany, grass tetany, grass staggers, and wheat pasture poisoning are synonyms for hypomagnesemic tetany. Milk fever is hypocalcemia. Alkali disease is selenium toxicosis. Eclampsia is hypocalcemia (e.g., in mares). "Downer" cow syndrome is recumbency without systemic signs (i.e., there is no tetany).

47. The answer is 2 [Chapter 15 II F 1]. Straining to urinate may be sufficient to prolapse the rectum, and obstructed sheep may also show tail wriggling. Signs of colic or discomfort usually abate when the bladder ruptures. A diverticulum in the penile urethra prevents the passage of a catheter. The ruptured bladder often spontaneously seals over in the steer. In sheep and goats, the blockage is usually sabulous (sandy), and the vermiform appendage may need amputation.

48. The answer is 4 [Chapter 2 III]. Squamous cell carcinoma of the stomach, malnutrition, granulomatous enteritis (lymphocytic-plasmacytic enteritis), or parasitism could all cause weight loss without other obvious clinical signs. A patient with chronic obstruction pulmonary disease (COPD) shows evidence of a compromised respiratory system (e.g., an increased respiratory rate and abnormal pattern) by the time the disease is advanced enough to cause weight loss. Liver fluke infestation (fascioliasis) is a disease of cattle, sheep, and goats. Lymphosarcoma is usually a disease of younger horses.

49. The answer is 3 [Chapter 11 I E 2–3]. These signs suggest sepsis and possible meningitis, which can be detected by a CSF sample. In a foal, these signs are not typical for neonatal maladjustment syndrome (NMS). The animal was normal up until 3 days after birth; NMS usually causes clinical signs within the first 24 hours. Signs for BVD infection are cerebellar and are noted immediately at birth. Hydrocephalus and hydranencephaly should be noted at birth, and fever and stiff neck are not part of these brain diseases.

50. The answer is 1 [Chapter 13 III A 3 e]. Sole ulcer is a circumscribed ulcer at the heel–sole junction of the foot. It is best treated by trimming to expose the ulcer or pro-truding granulation tissue and paring away excess granulation tissue followed by a pressure bandage over the site. Blocking up the unaffected claw on the lame leg will aid in ambulation and healing.

51. The answer is 2 [Chapter 14 III A 1 b]. Tumors within the spinal canal (such as lymphosarcoma) put pressure on the cord, producing signs of spinal cord disease (particularly in the hindlimbs). The bovine leukemia virus (BLV), which causes bovine leukosis, is spread via contact with blood of infected animals. There is no effective vaccine against BLV. Many cows may be infected (virus-positive), but few (possibly as low as 2%) develop solid tissue tumors (lymphosarcoma). There is no record of transmission of this disease to humans.

52. The answer is 3 [Chapter 2 I B 1, 3 f (1)–(2)]. All of the following may produce abdominal pain in foals: meconium impaction, gastric ulceration, intussusception, ascarid impaction, abdominal hernias (if a loop of bowel is entrapped within the hernial sac), and small intestinal volvulus. Cryptosporidiosis causes a nonpainful diarrhea in foals. Granulomatous enteritis causes a protein-losing and wasting enteropathy in adult horses.

53. The answer is 2 [Chapter 11 II C 1 b]. The animal most likely has polioencephalomalacia (PEM) with cortical blindness and dorsomedial strabismus. The drug of choice for this calf is thiamine (vitamin B_1). With lead toxicity, the rumen is usually static, and there should be some snapping of the eyelids. Nervous coccidiosis is not associated with cold months, and there is no sign of coccidiosis. Also, the calf is cortically blind, which suggests polioencephalomalacia or lead toxicity.

54. The answer is 3 [Chapter 17 I C 1 g]. Stripping the affected quarters as often as possible removes the endotoxin, which causes the clinical signs. Intramammary therapy is not warranted because the growth phase of the organism has passed by the time clinical signs are evident. Also, intramammary therapy does not likely diffuse well in the swollen udder. Oral fluids are not efficacious unless combined with intravenous fluids (hypertonic or isotonic). Calcium salts may be an adjunct to therapy but are not invariably necessary and can cause cardiac toxicity if administered too rapidly intravenously. Subcutaneous ad-

ministration of calcium may be considered. Dexamethasone is often indicated but only early in the course of the disease and only for one or two treatments.

55. The answer is 2 [Chapter 8 II A 1]. The calf has a ventricular septal defect (VSD). The small size of the calf suggests that the defect is large, producing a significant amount of blood that is shunted through the pulmonary circulation and a subsequent rise in venous return to the left atrium and ventricle. The murmur associated with a VSD is usually pansystolic and is heard loudest on the right side near the heart base. Cardiac catheterization reveals increased blood pressure in the right ventricle. A patent ductus arteriosus (PDA) produces a continuous heart murmur. Tricuspid valvular disease usually produces a holosystolic murmur with a point of maximal intensity (PMI) on the right side near the cardiac apex. The murmur associated with aortic insufficiency is holodiastolic, with the PMI over the aortic valve and radiating toward the left cardiac apex. Volume overload of the left ventricle may be present, resulting in impairment in left ventricular function.

56. The answer is 2 [Chapter 14 I D]. The findings of acuteness of signs, anemia, icterus, a decreased packed cell volume (PCV), plasma discoloration, and pigmenturia all support a diagnosis of acute hemolytic anemia, which can be caused by babesiosis, equine infectious anemia (EIA), red maple leaf toxicosis, and immune-mediated causes. Anaplasmosis is a hemolytic anemia of ruminants. Equine exertional rhabdomyolysis produces pigmenturia (myoglobinuria), but not anemia and icterus. Pyelonephritis is most common in sows and cows, and is associated with the discharge of pus or blood from the urinary tract.

57. The answer is 1 [Chapter 11 III A 3 a–b, d]. These signs suggest equine protozoal myeloencephalitis (EPM) because the animal is older than 3 years [the age when wobbler and equine degenerative myelopathy (EDM) have occurred] and because muscle atrophy (lower motor neuron) is present. Cervical radiographs with myelography are for vertebral malformation, which occurs earlier in life and has no muscle atrophy of unilateral nature. Green pasture and fodder with supplemental vitamin E suggests EDM, which has no muscle atrophy and usually occurs before 1 year of age. A cerebrospinal fluid (CSF) sample of high protein with the lack of inflammatory cells suggests EHV-1, which has a more sudden onset and often involves other illnesses (e.g., respiratory disease, abortion). Equine protozoal myelitis (EPM) is the likely diagnosis, but eosinophils are not a feature of the CSF cytology.

58. The answer is 1 [Chapter 13 III A 1 b]. The clinical findings best describe infectious pododermatitis or pasture foot rot. Laminitis may precede stable foot rot or underrun sole, which are conditions of the sole.

59. The answer is 4 [Chapter 9 III B 1, C]. Neonatal hypoglycemia of piglets results in hypothermia, weakness, and failure to move out of the way of sows. Lactation tetany occurs in mares, whereas vitamin E selenium deficiency, iron deficiency, or liver disease are not commonly related to piglet crushing deaths.

60. The answer is 2 [Chapter 3 II B 3 d]. *Cryptosporidium parvum* causes cryptosporidiosis in young calves. Transmission of the organism is by the fecal-oral route. Cryptosporidiosis, characterized by transient secretory diarrhea in affected calves, is usually associated with a full recovery; however, *C. parvum* can be a serious pathogen in immunocompromised individuals or those with mixed enteric infections.

61. The answer is 1 [Chapter 14 I D 1 b (1) (f)]. Neonatal isoerythrolysis in mule foals is due to the production of antibodies by the horse dam against the donkey blood antigen. Erythrocytes from any donkey would also be susceptible to lysis, and the mare's blood would contain additional antibody. Washed erythrocytes or whole blood from a horse donor would be the most effective treatment because plasma would not supply the necessary erythrocytes.

62. The answer is 3 [Chapter 2 I B 2 c (2), (3)]. Pendunculated lipoma, parasitic larval migration, and intestinal foreign body can all cause chronic, recurrent bouts of colic in horses as a result of large colon impaction. Other correct differential diagnoses include enterolith, thromboembolic infarction, sand impaction, and feed impaction. Salmonellosis may cause signs of colic, but only in the acute phases of the disease and not chronically. *Dictyocaulus arnfieldi* is a lungworm that affects donkeys and horses.

63. The answer is 1 [Chapter 11 II C 2 b]. The chronic form of lead toxicity results in recurrent choke, regurgitation of food, and aspiration pneumonia. Snapping eyelids, cortical blindness, head pressing, facial or trigeminal nerve deficits, aggressive behavior, and convulsions are signs of cranial nerve deficits and are not features of acute lead poisoning. Blindness should be accompanied by pupils that react to light (cortical blindness) in subacute lead toxicity. The differential signs between polioencephalomalacia (PEM) and lead toxicity include normal motility in PEM and an atonic rumen in lead toxicity.

64. The answer is 5 [Chapter 18 IV D 3 a (1) (b)]. An immunoglobulin G (IgG) concentration that exceeds 400 mg/dl in a healthy foal on a well-managed farm is usually considered adequate and a plasma transfusion is not required to supplement immunoglobulin. It would be futile to supplement the foal with oral immunoglobulins, because she would absorb very little at the age of 22 hours. Because the foal is not systemically ill, broad-spectrum bactericidal antibiotics are not indicated, and in fact may create resistant bacterial populations on this farm.

65. The answer is 5 [Chapter 4 II A 5 e]. Intensive deworming is not usually necessary in winter months in North America. Furthermore, repeated use of thiabendazole promotes parasite resistance to this anthelmintic. An effective intestinal parasite control program for sheep in North America would include prelambing deworming of adults with ivermectin, deworming of lambs in the spring before turning them out on pasture, raising lambs indoors and feeding hay from elevated racks, and the use of pastures grazed by cattle for rotation into sheep grazing.

66. The answer is 3 [Chapter 14 I E 1 a]. The regenerative response is most common following anemia caused by acute blood loss or hemolysis. Hemoglobin synthesis is impaired with iron deficiency anemia, and the marrow's ability to respond to anemia through increased erythrocyte production is depressed.

67. The answer is 2 [Chapter 1 II C 1 a]. Horses with dental disease often prefer grain over hay because there is less chewing involved. Symptoms of dental disease in horses include quidding; slow, painful mastication; weight loss; and choke.

68. The answer is 5 [Chapter 14 I D 2]. Hemoglobinuria is a characteristic sign of intravascular hemolysis. Major causes of intravascular hemolysis in adult cattle include postparturient hemoglobinuria, babesiosis, and leptospirosis. *Babesia* are spread by ticks, whereas leptospires can be seen on examination of urine by dark-field microscopy. Postparturient hemoglobinuria in North America is thought to be caused by phosphorus deficiency, and the severity of hemolysis with this disease can be worsened by the ingestion of oxidant-containing plants. Rickettsial parasites typically cause extravascular hemolysis.

69. The answer is 1 [Chapter 18 VI B 4 b]. A patent urachus in a foal in the absence of infection (no fever or evidence of inflammation on blood work) can be treated conservatively. Surgery is indicated if chemical cauterization has not resolved the problem within 5 days; if there is evidence of infection of the umbilical remnants on ultrasound examination (urachal abscess) or physical examination (heat, pain, purulent discharge); or if there is subcutaneous urine accumulation.

70. The answer is 1 [Chapter 14 IV B 2]. Characteristic findings in calves with leukocyte adhesion deficiency include lymphadenopathy, chronic digestive or respiratory tract infections, fever, and persistent neutrophilia.

71. The answer is 2 [Chapter 14 II B 3 a (1)]. Excessive hemorrhage after dehorning may be caused by the ingestion of moldy sweet clover. Prolonged prothrombin time or high concentrations of dicoumarol in the feed would support this diagnosis, and the administration of vitamin K_1 may decrease bleeding tendencies. Fungi can produce dicoumarol in hay or silage, and suspect feedstuffs of any type should not be fed.

Index

Note: Page numbers in *italic* indicate illustrations; page numbers followed by t indicate tables.

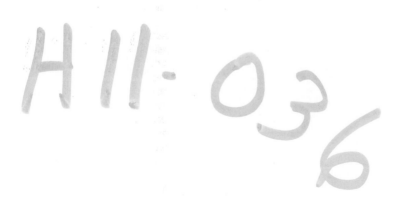